SNAKES OF MEDICAL IMPORTANCE (ASIA-PACIFIC REGION)

EDITORS
P. GOPALAKRISHNAKONE
L. M. CHOU

Published by
Venom And Toxin Research Group
National University of Singapore
and
International Society on Toxinology
(Asia-Pacific Section)

ISBN 9971-62-217-3

Typeset by International Typesetters
Printed by Vetak Services

CONTENTS

PREFACE

The Asia-Pacific region has more than it's fair share of dangerous animals and plants because of the tropical nature of the climate which supports high biodiversity. Among the dangerous creatures, the snakes both terrestial and marine are responsible for extensive morbidity and mortality as is indicated in this volume. Peasants, farmers and fisherman are among the people who suffer most from snakebite. Present medical curricula based on British and American systems place low priority on the subject of natural poisoning with very few formal lectures given to doctors or paramedical personnel. A doctor faced with a snake-bite patient in an Accident and Emergency Department usually has little knowledge of what to do with the patient and when the offending snake is produced, is unable to tell whether the snake is venomous or not.

The various chapters of this book contain much information on the identification of the dangerous venomous snakes in this region and attempts to review the various aspects of snakebite treatment as practised in the various countries. Treatment of snake still remains a controversial subject. Without identifying an ideal treatment, the various chapters deal with the "state of the art" within the different countries at the time of preparation of this book. The practises in various countries may not seem correct to some or acceptable to others; but the fact remains that these are being practised. This book therefore aims to give a true picture of the situation in these countries as described by the individual authors. An ideal method of treatment is suggested and described in the last chapter. Wherever possible, distribution maps, local names, local practises and the instruction sheets enclosed with the antivenom vials are given. The information reflects the exact situation in each country and will hopefully be of help to researchers and medical personnel in planning future strategies concerning snakebite and treatment.

P GOPALAKRISHNAKONE
L M CHOU

Dangerous Snakes Of Australia

1. P.J. Mirtschin
Venom Supplies
P.O. Box 547
Tanunda
South Australia 5352

2. G.R. Crowe
Struan House
31 Wood Tce., Whyalla
South Australia 5600

3. R. Davis
16 Andrew Avenue
Millswood
South Australia 5034

Dedication

(a) The late Eric Worrell MBE who with others, pioneered venom extraction on some of the world's deadliest snakes and on his own, wrote the first comprehensive text on snake classification in Australia.

(b) Dr S. K. Sutherland whose enthusiastic work on snake venoms in the last fifteen years, has had a major impact on the reduction in fatalities in this country. His contribution has enriched our knowledge on snake venoms and their actions. His continual review of snake bite procedures has led to a greater awareness among the medical profession and timely instruction for all to learn from.

Australia And Its Elapids

Australia is situated in the Southern hemisphere between the latitudes of 10°45' S and 43°35' S. It has an area of 7.7 million km², a maximum dimension laterally of about, 4,000 km and a maximum north-south dimension of 3,180 km. Its land mass is relatively low and the highest mountain, Mt Kosciusko, is 2,280 m high. Tasmania is separated from the mainland by Bass Strait, and lies a distance of about 230 km from Victoria.

The Eastern coast of Australia is dominated by the Eastern highlands which extend from Victoria to the northern tip of Australia. In the south, the mountain ranges experience alpine conditions in winter. Most of the inland is relatively flat with central mountain range systems in the Northern Territory and northern South Australia.

About 40% of continental Australia is situated north of tropic of Capricorn where little seasonal temperature variation is experienced. The highest

1

temperatures occur in the centre of the continent which also receives less rainfall. In summer, northern Australia experiences high temperatures and high humidity whereas the inland has a dry, hot climate. In the south, winter is a period of brief cold and windy conditions.

Generally Australia is a dry country with more than half the continent receiving less than 300 mm/year and one third receiving less than 200 mm/year. The highest rainfall of 43 cm/year is experienced near Cairns in Queensland and the lowest rainfall of 100 mm/year falls just north of Lake Eyre in South Australia.

While much is known about climatic history and geological history of Australia, fossil records of our dangerous snakes is almost non-existent. "Australian elapids may have evolved in situ or arrived early from some other Gondwanaland region. They evidently arrived in the Australian continent ahead of colubrids" (Minton 1981). Most of the fossil elapids known are from the Pleistocene and the only identifiable remains represent living forms of *Notechis*, *Pseudechis* and *Pseudonaja* (Smith 1976).

Today the ophidian populations throughout Australia are widespread. The highest densities occur in the eastern coastal areas, where combined with higher populations of people, the highest incidence of snake bite is recorded. Cogger (1987), has compiled interesting species density maps which show the number of dangerous species likely to occur in any particular area. The highest densities occur along the east coast in Central Queensland and northern New South Wales and the south west of Western Australia. Generally anywhere in Australia has a number of dangerous species of snakes inhabiting the area. Distribution maps and notes of habitat preference are supplied with each snake type within this text.

Australia has the reputation of being a snake-ridden country. It is true that Australia has a large number of snakes, however the average person in Australia may only encounter snakes very rarely, if ever, in their lifetime.

The dangerous snakes of Australia occur throughout the continent from above the winter snowline on Mt. Kosciusko to the hot central deserts. They are found in Tasmania and most large offshore islands and some of the smaller ones. The majority of the species are habitat specific, however, some, such as *Pseudonaja nuchalis*, inhabit much of the mainland continent involving a diverse range of habitats. Actual collection points for nearly all museum specimens have been published in the Atlas of Elapid Snakes of Australia (Longmore 1986).

There are over 120 species of snakes in Australia which represent about 6% of the world's snakes. About 60% of these snakes are from the Elapidae (or cobra-like) family, and being venomous these figures represent the highest ratio of venomous to non-venomous snakes in the world. Australia possesses over 40% of the world's elapid snakes and about 23% of all venomous snakes of the world.

From the many venomous snakes in Australia about twenty-nine can be considered dangerous. Twenty-seven of these species and sub-species have or are capable of causing death. Twenty-six of them can easily cause death with an average bite that is untreated. The three broad headed snakes (*Hoplocephalus* genus) have been included in this chapter because of the severe symptoms resulting from bites which in certain instances could be fatal.

In a country rich in dangerous fauna, the low mortality rate due to snake bite of 2-3 per year is largely due to the work of the Commonwealth Serum Laboratories and Dr. S. Sutherland in Victoria. Over the years they have developed highly efficient antivenoms for all of Australia's dangerous snakes. They have also produced a polyvalent antivenom which is effective against bites of all terrestrial and marine snakes. In addition, recent developments of their Venom Detection Kits enable the specific monovalent antivenom to be selected in lieu of using a greater volume of polyvalent serum. Research resulting in more efficient first aid also played a significant role in snake bite management.

Development of more efficient antivenoms using monoclonal antibodies and the possibility of prophylactic protection against snake bite could lead to even better prevention and treatment systems in the future.

Cogger (1983), discussed the implications of blurry taxonomies and the method of producing antivenoms against specific species and using them to treat snakes bites from other species. He posed the question, ".... does it really matter if the western species '(*Pseudonaja nuchalis)*' turns out not to be one but several 'species', or were likely to be, complexes of species. As a result, venom samples from many different populations were pooled to produce a composite venom which, in some cases differed significantly in its component neurotoxins from that found in any one species of population. In more practical terms, the more specific an antivenom can be made, the smaller will be the required dose of it, and the less will be the likelihood of anaphylactic and other complications."

One of the big problems with venom research is the ever changing nomenclature involved with the species and the existence of different races with varying toxicities and venom compositions. Researchers should request geographical information with venoms procured so that future reproducibility is not clouded by venom samples from different locations. Mengden (1985a) has pointed to imminent taxonomy changes with the *Pseudonaja* genus. Recent nomenclature changes to *Acanthophis* must raise serious questions to much of the earlier work on these venoms. On the other hand, some venoms show little geographical variation. Broad et al (1979) has shown the remarkable homogeneity of *Oxyuranus microlepidotus* venom in electrophoretic patterns of the crude venom. This species (formally *Parademansia microlepidotus)* underwent nomenclature changes the following year and was re-described as *O. microlepidotus* by Covacevich et al (1980). Some scientists still refer to the species by its former name, thus confusing the matter even further.

Reference to the Zoological Catalogue of Australia (Cogger et al 1983), will convey the dynamic state of flux involving nomenclature of the Australian elapids in this country's short history. With recent taxonomic work of Storr and Covacevich, genetic work of Mengden, immunological work of Schwaner and ecological studies of Shine, it is inevitable that Australian elapid nomenclature will experience a longer period of stability once the evidence is combined and the species and populations are redefined. This may lead to changes in antivenom production and provide a firmer base for future venom research.

The rate of mortality due to snake bite in Australia compared with many other countries is small. Australia experiences about 2-3 deaths per year. Figures published by Swaroop and Grab (1954) for various countries and continents are:

Africa	—	400-1,000
USA	—	10-20
Brazil	—	2,000
Venezuela	—	150
Thailand	—	200
Japan	—	100

These figures show that Australia's problem is relatively insignificant. Our small population and highly efficient antivenoms are factors that should be considered when comparisons are made. In addition, in some of the countries above, there is a great tendency to wear lighter clothes and walk around barefooted. This increases the chance of effective snake bites. White (1987) has summarized the work of Fairley (1929), Swaroop and Grab (1954), Trinca (1963), and White et al (1985) (see table 1).

TABLE 1.
Mortality figures from White (1987)

	1910 — 1926 Pre-antivenom		Antivenom Era total 1945-1949 1952-1961 and 1968-1982	
	total	Rate/yr	total	Rate/yr
Queensland	74	4.6	51	1.9
New South Wales	57	3.6	24	0.9
Victoria	43	2.7	20	0.7
Western Australia	6	0.4	16	0.6
South Australia	8	0.5	3	0.1
Tasmania	8	0.5	4	0.1
Nothern Territory	1	0.1	10	0.4
Australia Capital Territory	1	0.1	1	0.0

The mortality rates, both pre-antivenom and post-antivenom show good correlation with the dangerous snake density maps of Cogger (1985), in that more bites have occurred in areas with more snakes.

Fairley's study (1929), found that most snake bite deaths occurred later than 24 hours after the bite. These figures do not include bites from the two

Oxyuranus species or bites from *Pseudechis australis*. They were compiled in the pre-antivenom era. Today, untreated bites, die sooner than 24 hours.

One other factor often overlooked by researchers is environmental influence on snake populations. There is no doubt that snake populations are declining throughout Australia due to environmental changes and destruction. Most dangerous snakes are continually having their habitats altered, reduced and removed as a result of mans' activities. In many areas, especially around population centres, habitats have undergone gross changes. In most cases this has had detrimental effects on most reptile species. There are exceptions. For example the taipan may have increased its numbers due to introduction of the cane toad. It is thought that other large elapid snakes have preyed on cane toads thus causing a reduction in snake numbers. This has allowed taipans to expand their numbers, since they do not prey on cane toads.

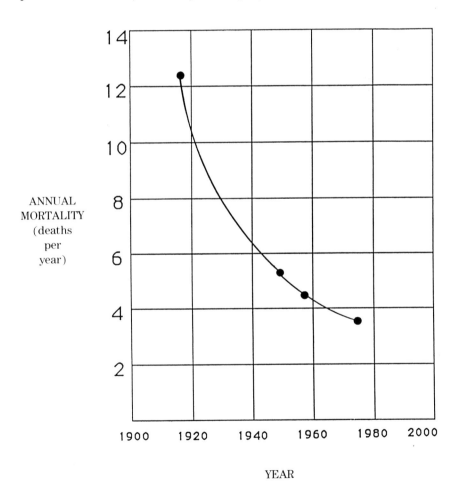

Graph 1
Decline in Mortality due to Snake Bite in Australia. (adapted from White 1987).

Given that snake populations have generally declined, snake bite frequency should also decline. This is offset as Australia's human population has increased. It is more reasonable to conclude that the reduction in snake bite has been due to:

(i)   Better first aid
(ii)   Availability of antivenoms
(iii) Venom detection kits
(iv)   Better snake bite education to the public
(v)   Reduction in snake numbers

The Problem of Snake Bite in Australia

According to Cogger (1987), some 70% of Australian snakes are venomous and apart from a few non-dangerous species from the *Colubridae* family, all our dangerous snakes are from the *Elapidae* or Cobra-like family. This group of snakes have relatively fixed front fangs which in contrast to the vipers and pit vipers, remain in the same erect position when the snake closes its mouth. A consequence of fixed fangs is the relatively short fang length when compared with vipers. Taipans, *Oxyuranus scutellatus* have the largest fangs which may exceed 12 mm in length. Brown snakes from the *Pseudonaja* genus, have the shortest fangs which are often less than 2 mm in length. From this group of elapids, 29 snake types have been described herein. All are capable of causing serious envenomation or death.

When an Australian snake bites, venom is forced under pressure through hollow fangs and out an opening near the tip. Often venom will dribble down the outside of the fang as well as through the hollow fang. This has been observed repeatedly in most Australian snakes during milking at Venom Supplies Laboratories. Thus the wearing of adequate clothing when walking, through an area inhabited by dangerous snakes, can prevent a large percentage of venom being absorbed if bitten.

There are more than 200 serious snake bites in Australia each year. All are serious enough to warrant antivenom administration. Sutherland (1983), estimates that due to failure to feedback information, a more realistic figure would be 500 cases of envenomation requiring antivenom per year. He also estimates that there may be up to 3,000 cases of bite that require no treatment because symptoms don't develop.

Identification of snakes involved in a snake bite can be difficult for the treating physician. Morrison et al (1983), demonstrated that only 19% of Australian snakes are likely to be identified correctly from typical specimens. Mirtschin and Davis (1982), and Davis and Mirtschin (1985), have displayed the colour variations that occur within the species and have discussed the confusion that arises among the partially informed.

Mengden and Fitzgerald (1987), have highlighted the potential to misidentify Brown Snakes *(Pseudonaja)*, by using colour alone. They claim there are approximately 40 species of elapid snakes in Australia that possess a degree of brown or brown markings. In addition, some species undergo seasonal colour variations. Some of these have been recorded by Banks (1981) and Mirtschin (1983). Colour alone, therefore, is an inaccurate method for snake identification.

The development of snake bite identification kits by the Commonwealth Serum Laboratories has substantially improved the probability of correctly identifying which antivenom to use. The venom detection kit (VDK) was based on the development of a micro-ELISA (enzyme linked immunosorbant assay) by Theakston et al (1977). The kit passed through a number of developmental stages, and today's version contains all equipment and reagents necessary to perform the venom detection test in about 30 minutes. The VDK can detect venom levels as low as 5-10 nanograms of venom.

The principles of today's version of the VDK is as follows:- The kit contains 6 glass tubes joined by plastic catheter tubing and connected to a 1 ml syringe. Five of the glass tubes are coated on the inside with a specific antibody for 1 of the 5 main venoms. The sixth tube is the control tube. The *venom sample* is drawn into the tubes and allowed to incubate for 10 minutes. The venom then links with its specific antibody in the appropriate tube. The sample is then washed out and the tubes filled with a solution of enzyme conjugate linked to the various antibodies. This solution is allowed to incubate for a further 10 minutes. The enzyme antibody conjugates then binds to bound venom of its type in the appropriate tube. After a further washing, the tubes are flushed with a substitute solution which reacts with any bound enzymes remaining, resulting in a colour change in the appropriate tube. Colour changes will occur after some time in the other tubes but the first one to change indicates the antivenom type to use.

The test kit is designed as a one-off type and should be discarded after use.

The kit contains a swab which can be used to soak up a sample from the bite site or from adjacent clothing on first aid bandages. The swab can be soaked in the solution in the specimen bottle of VDK and is then rubbed firmly over the bite site, adjacent clothing or bandage. A urine sample can also be used in the kit.

Although a positive result may be obtained from the kit, antivenom should be withheld if no symptoms develop in the patient. In turn, if a negative result is obtained, and symptoms develop, antivenom treatment should commence. If symptoms are present, testing the blood through the kit should yield a positive result, thus allowing selection of a monovalent antivenom.

The hospital should draw on the resources of recognised herpetologists who live in the area. Sometimes patients bring the dead (or alive) offending snakes with them to the hospital. Positive identification can then be made. However the hospital should be sure that the person identifying the snake is competent. Museums, universities, zoo's reptile parks and national parks officers are usually helpful in this regard. Failing that, the scalation records and head drawings in this book should enable anyone to at least identify the snakes' genus, which would be sufficient information to allow efficient treatment of any snake bite.

Discussion concerning the relative danger of Australian snakes has been treated in a number of publications already. The Queensland Museum has produced danger scores for Australia's most dangerous snakes by rating five aspects of snake bite. They are:

1 Venom toxicity
2 Venom yield
3 Fang length
4 Temperament
5 Frequency of bite

Each component carries a maximum of 5 points and varies from snake to snake.

A rating score for Australia's dangerous snakes can be derived using this scoring system. The following list illustrates this method.

Taipan	21
Mulga or King Brown snake	16
Death Adder	15
Common brown snake	14
Tiger Snake	14
Inland Taipan	12
Collett's Snake	10
Western brown snake	10
Copperhead	10
Bass Strait tiger snakes	9
Red bellied black snake	9
Spotted black snake	8
Rough-Scaled snake	7
Dugite	6
Small eyed snake	6

The Commonwealth Serum Laboratories in Australia, have conducted considerable research into the comparable toxicity of Australian venomous snakes. Standardised conditions for venom collection are used. Following collection of venom from the snakes, the venom is immediately freeze-dried and stored in a vacuum. This prevents break down of venom and loss of potency, which may occur if the venom is kept in a liquid form during drying. Mice are used for the tests and the venom is prepared in 0.1% bovine serum albumin in saline as diluent. These tests were carried out by Broad et al (1979) at the Commonwealth Serum Laboratories. He also conducted experiments using saline alone as diluent, but we have only used the bovine serum albumin in saline results throughout this chapter unless the saline alone figure was only available. In these cases the word saline follows the figure quoted, and the comparison is only approximate. The bovine serum results allow greater consistency and yield a more accurate assessment of toxicity. Broad used 18-21 gm mice in his experiments.

The relative danger of venomous Australian snakes can be compared by reviewing the "rating" given to each snake. This rating takes into account both the toxicity of the venom and the average venom yield. The lower the toxicity, the more venomous is the snake.

Table 2 is adapted from Broad et al (1979) and is updated using the latest venom yield figures.

TABLE 2
Relative Danger of Australian Dangerous Snakes

Common name	Scientific name	Toxicity LD_{50} mg/kg (mice)	Average yield mg	Rating (mice) total LD_{50} doses)
Inland Taipan	*Oxyuranus microlepidotus*	0.010	44.2	218 000
Taipan	*Oxyuranus scutellatus*	0.064	120.0	95 000
Reevesby Island Tiger Snake	*Notechis ater niger*	0.099	34.3	18 000
Common Tiger Snake	*Notechis scutatus*	0.118	35.0	15 000
Western Tiger Snake	*Notechis ater occidentalis*	0.124	35.0	14 500
Chappell Island Tiger Snake	*Notechis ater serventyi*	0.271	75.0	14 000
Tasmanian and King Island Tiger Snake	*Notechis ater humphreysi*	0.388 (Tas)	36.0	4 600
Kreffts Tiger Snake	*Notechis ater ater*	0.101	23.0	11 600
Common Brown Snake	*Pseudonaja textilis*	0.040	4.7	5 800
Western Brown Snake	*Pseudonaja nuchalis*	0.338	4.0	600
Peninsula Brown Snake	*Pseudonaja inframacula*		3.0	
Dugite	*Pseudonaja affinis*	0.560	5.7	520
Tanners Brown Snake	*Pseudonaja tanneri*			

TABLE 2 (cont'd)

Relative Danger of Australian Dangerous Snakes

Common name	Scientific name	Toxicity LD_{50} mg/kg (mice)	Average yield mg	Rating (mice) total LD_{50} doses)
Speckled Brown Snake	*Pseudonaja guttata*	0. 36	0.5	70
Ingrams Brown Snake	*Pseudonaja ingrami*			
Mulga Snake	*Pseudechis australis*	1.91	180.0	5 000
Red-bellied Snake	*Pseudechis porphyriacus*	2.53	35.0	700
Spotted Black Snake	*Pseudechis guttatus*	1.53	30.0	1 000
Collett's Snake	*Pseudechis colletti*	2.38 (saline)	30.0	600 approx
Butlers Snake	*Pseudechis butleri*			
Common Death Adder	*Acanthophis antarcticus*	0.338	78.0	12 000
Desert Death Adder	*Acanthophis pyrrhus*			
Northern Death Adder	*Acanthophis praelongus*		49.5	
Stephens Banded Snake	*Hoplocephalus stephensi*	1.44	4.0	140
Broad-headed Snake	*Hoplocephalus bungaroides*		12.0	
Pale-headed Snake	*Hoplocephalus bitorquatus*		1.66	
Copperhead (lowland)	*Austrelaps superbus*	0.500	24.9	2 500
Copperhead (highland)				
Copperhead (pygmy)				
Rough-scaled Snake	*Tropidechis carinatus*	1.09	6.0	300
Small-eyed Snake	*Cryptophis nigrescens*	2.67 (saline)	8.0	150 150 approx

Clearly it is necessary to take into consideration venom yield as well as venom toxicity. If only the LD_{50} was considered it would appear that the average consequences of a bite from a common brown snake would be worse than a taipan. It is well known that this is not the case, because the Taipan yield is, on average, 26-30 times higher than the common brown snake. Therefore when toxicity and yield are considered together, the overall effect is that taipan bites, on average, are 16 times more serious than Common Brown Snakes bites.

The above figures, are averages, based on mice test animals. The average yield figures were determined over many milkings of the various species. More recent work carried out by Morrison, Pearn, Coulter, Charles, Covacevich and Tanner have placed a more realistic measure of yields to be expected during the offensive hunting and defensive bites of snakes. Their work can be found in Morrison et al (1982), Morrison et al (1983a), Morrison et al (1983b), and Morrison et al (1984). They used the technique of allowing snakes to bite mice and then measuring the amount of venom injected using an enzyme-immunoassay technique. They also measured the amount of venom left on the skin of the animal. In their study with the *Tropidechis carinatus* (Morrison et al 1983b), they also used an agar gel filled vinyl glove as a bite target to simulate defense striking by the snake. They found that with *T. carinatus*, there was no difference in yield (with the first bite) between an offensive bite and a defensive bite, i.e., the amount yielded by *T. carinatus* while hunting was the same yielded when defending itself. They also found that while most snakes yielded the highest amount during the first bite, Taipans were able to maintain similar deliveries in subsequent bites. Table 3, using figures from the above information, shows the average amounts yielded by some snakes during hunting. Assuming, that all snakes are like *T. carinatus* delivering the same amount in defensive

TABLE 3

The effects of an offensive snake bite. Derived from the
work of Pearn, Coulter, Charles, Covacevich and Tanner 1983, 1984
and Broad, Coulter and Sutherland 1979.

Snake Type	LD_{50} (mg/kg) (Broad et al 1979)	Offensive bite yield (mg)	Yield LD_{50} ratio
Oxyuranus microlepidotus	0.010	17.3	1730
Pseudechis australis	1.910	62.0	32
Acanthophis antarcticus	0.338	36.0	107
Oxyuranus scutellatus	0.064	29.9	467
Notechis scutatus	0.118	5.8	49
Tropidechis carinatus	1.090	3.5	3
Pseudonaja textilis	0.041	4.0	98

11

and offensive bites; the yield/LD_{50} ratio is an indication of the deadly potential of those snake types.

The Inland Taipan, *O.microlepidotus* demonstrates a very lethal combination of yield and toxicity. To date there have been 4 human bites from the species, and no fatalities. In the first case in 1967, the victim suffered a critical illness and despite being treated with the wrong antivenom, still survived. The second and third bites have occurred with captive snakes. A bite occurred to one of the authors and the treatment and recovery were non-eventful. A third was received by a herpetologist who suffered a critical illness despite antivenom treatment. He claims that his physical condition did not return to normal for 2 years. Renal failure was experienced in the initial stages of treatment. In the 4th bite, antivenom was delayed for 8 hours. Although there was a critical illness the patient recovered.

Morrison and his co-workers found that small amounts of venom were left on the skin after bites had occurred and that there were sufficient quantities to use in the VDK tests. This venom still remained on the skin in sufficient quantities 2-3 hours after the bite.

From the work of Broad et al (1979), it is possible to compare the toxicity of some of Australia's snakes with those from other countries. The toxicity of the Indian cobra *Naja naja* can be compared with other snakes. Table 4 shows a simple comparison of Australian snakes with 3 exotic snakes using the toxicity of *Naja naja* venom as a standed equal to unity.

TABLE 4
The toxicity of 3 exotic snakes compared with Australian snakes
using the toxicity of Cobra venom as unity.

Cobra	*Naja naja*	1.00 (exotic)
King Cobra	*Ophiophagus hannah*	0.26 (exotic)
Eastern Diamond black rattle snake	*Crotalus adamanteus*	0.06 (exotic)
Red-bellied black snack	*Pseudechis porphyriacus*	0.20
King brown snake	*Pseudechis australis*	0.26
Copperhead	*Austrelaps superbus*	1.00
Dugite	*Pseudonaja affinis*	0.89
Western brown snake	*Pseudonaja nuchalis*	1.48
Death Adder	*Acanthophis antarcticus*	1.48
Chappell Is. Tiger snake	*Notechis ater serventyi*	1.85
Western Tiger snake	*Notechis ater occidentalis*	4.03
Common Tiger snake	*Notechis scutatus*	4.24
Kreffts Tiger snake	*Notechis ater ater*	9.90
Reevesby Is. Tiger snake	*Notechis ater niger*	4.76
Taipan	*Oxyuranus scutellatus*	7.81
Common Brown snake	*Pseudonaja textilis*	12.20
Inland Taipan	*Oxyuranus microlepidotus*	50.00

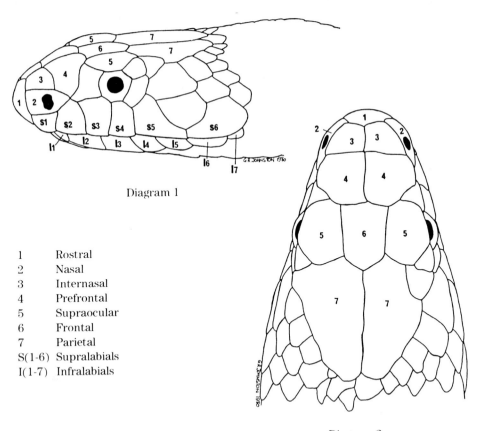

Diagram 1

1   Rostral
2   Nasal
3   Internasal
4   Prefrontal
5   Supraocular
6   Frontal
7   Parietal
S(1-6) Supralabials
I(1-7) Infralabials

Diagram 2

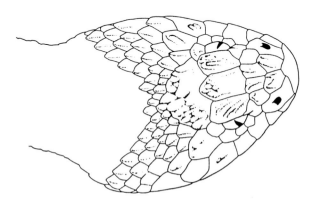

Diagram 3

NOMENCLATURE OF SCALES

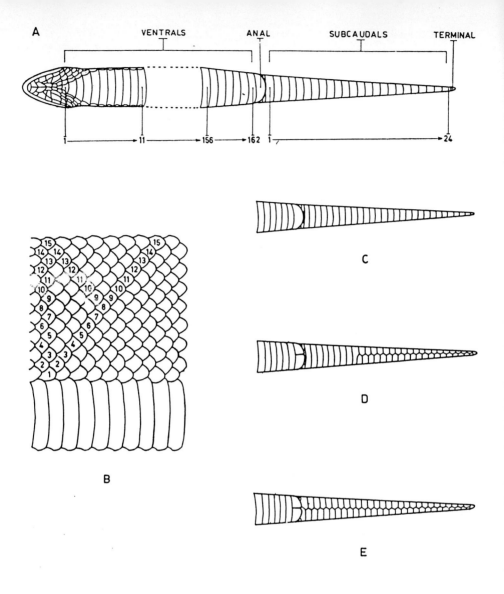

Diagram 4 *Scale counting technique* (reproduced with permission from P.A. Rawlinson and the *Victorian Naturalist*).

A   Ventral aspect of an elapid snake with scale terminology.
B   Skin removed from mid-body of a snake and spread out to show the method of making mid-body scale counts.
C   Ventral aspect of an elapid snake tail showing single anal scale and subcaudal scales.
D   Ventral aspect showing divided anal scale and subcaudals single anterior, divided posterior.
E   Ventral aspect showing divided anal scale and divided subcaudals.

The toxicity figures quoted in the form of LD$_{50}$ ratings throughout this chapter are all based on experiments with 18-21 gm mice. It should be noted that the toxicity of any snake venom varies with respect to the type of test animal used. Table 5 shows the varying toxicity with a number of different laboratory animals.

TABLE 5
Lethal lethal doses for various test animals (mg/kg).
(Mirtschin & Davis 1982).

	Guinea Pig	Rabbit	Mouse	Sheep	Rat
Notechis scutatus	0.02	0.05	0.25	0.01	0.4
Pseudechis porphyriacus	2.5	0.6		0.8	2.5
Pseudechis guttatus	0.6	0.6 — 1.0	2.5		0.7
Acanthophis antarcticus	0.15	0.15	0.7	0.025	
Austrelaps superbus	0.06	0.7	1.2	0.1	1.4
Pseudonaja textilis		0.2			

Identification of Dangerous Snakes of Australia

All snakes reviewed in this chapter are capable of inflicting a serious or lethal bite. Identification involves handling the snakes, so lay persons should not attempt to identify any snake unless it is definitely dead.

Identification entails searching through the colour photographs in the chapter until a snake of similar colour is found, then comparing the scalation count and head scales.

If no similar colour photograph is present, check the scalation with Table 6. When a match is found, check the head pattern of the snake with that on the appropriate page.

Colour variations not described in this chapter do occur. In addition, snakes may occur outside the ranges shown on the distribution maps. In either case, Australian museums will be glad to receive such information or better still, the specimen.

TABLE 6.
Scalation summary of dangerous snakes of Australia

Snake	Ventrals	Subcaudals	Anal	Mid-bodies
Common Tiger	140-190	35-65 single	single	17 or 19
Kreffts Tiger	163-173	41-50 single	single	17
Peninsula Tiger	160-184	45-54 single	single	17, 18 19 or 21
Western Tiger	140-165	36-51 single	single	17, 19
Chappel Is. Tiger	160-171	47-52 single	single	17
Tasmanian and King Is. Tiger	161-174	48-53 single	single	17, 15

TABLE 6. (cont'd)
Scalation summary of dangerous snakes of Australia

Snake	Ventrals	Subcaudals	Anal	Mid-bodies
Common Brown	185-235	45-75 divided	divided	17
Peninsula Brown	190-205	52-62 divided	divided	17
Western Brown	180-230	50-70 divided	divided	17 or 19
Speckled Brown	190-220	44-70 divided	divided	19-21
Dugite	190-230	50-70 divided	divided	19
Tanners Brown	190-230	50-70 divided	divided	19
Ingrams Brown	190-220	55-70 divided	divided	17
Taipan	220-250	45-80 divided	single	21-23
Inland Taipan	211-250	52-70 divided	single	23
Death Adder	110-130	38-55 mostly single	single	21-23
Desert Death Adder	140-160	45-60 single anterior, divided posterior	single	21
Northern Death Adder	122-134	47-57 10-39 single 14-29 paired	single	21, 23
Red-Bellied Black	180-210	40-65 first 1/3 single rest divided	divided	17
Mulga	189-220	53-70 all single or all divided or partly single and divided	divided	17
Collett's	215-235	50-70 single anterior, divided posterior	divided	19
Spotted Black	175-205	45-65 single anterior, divided posterior	divided	19
Butlers Snake	204-216	55-65 35-76%	divided undivided	17
Copperhead	140-216	35-55 single	single	15,13, 17
Stephens Banded	220-250	50-70 single	single	21
Broad-headed	200-230	40-65 single	single	21
Pale-headed	190-225	40-65 single	single	19 or 21
Rough-scaled	160-185	50-60 single	single	23
Small-eyed	165-210	30-46 single	single	15

If you are unable to identify a snake using this technique, it is possible that the specimen is either:

* A harmless snake, such as a Python, or Tree Snake.
* A venomous snake not considered dangerous.
* A legless lizard.
* An undescribed, new species of snake.
* A snake described by this chapter but having scalation outside the known range.

Tiger Snakes

Tiger Snakes are some of the better known Australian snakes since they occur in highly populated areas. They are responsible for most snake bites in Australia. Size varies from the large Chappell Island tiger snake *Notechis ater serventyi* at 1.9 m to the Pygmy tiger snake from Roxby Island, *N. ater niger* in Spencers Gulf, South Australia. They have evolved to occupy the temperate-to-cool areas of Australia. Apart from west coast of South Australia, parts of the Murray River and regions of Western Australia, they occur in localities where the average rainfall is greater than 500 mm.

Common Tiger Snakes *(N. scutatus)*, Western Tiger Snakes (*N. ater occidentalis*) (mainland), Kreffts Tiger Snake *(N. ater ater)*, and Tasmanian Tiger Snakes *(N. ater humphreysi)*, feed mainly on frogs. The presence of water from either high rainfall or from river courses supplies the necessary dampness for frogs.

Maximum average summer temperatures throughout their range vary from 18° C in parts of Tasmania and Bass Strait to 31° C in the Flinders Ranges, South Australia, the Murray River area, and parts of Western Australia.

Tiger Snakes are divided into six species and sub-species. There are, however, enough ecological immunological, and venom differences among Tiger Snakes to recognise further variations. Electrophoretic patterns of blood, venom and toxicity experiments conducted by the Commonwealth Serum Laboratories have clearly illustrated great differences with the species. Schwaner (1985) and Shine (1987), both consider Notechis to have only one taxon, explain the size differences as adaptations to food availability.

Tiger snakes *(N. ater niger)* found on the small archipelago of the Sir Joseph Banks Groups in Spencers Gulf, show ecological variations among the different island populations. The tiger snakes on Reevesby Island and Hareby Island are large and feed mainly on white-faced Storm Petrel. The tiger snakes are much smaller on nearby Roxby Island, where they feed mainly on skinks. On Hopkins Island, not far from the Sir Joseph Banks group, the Tiger Snakes are larger than those on Reevesby Island and here they feed on Mutton birds.

Common Tiger Snake *Notechis scutatus* (Peters)
Description:

Flat blunt head, slightly distinct from a robust body. Body capable of being flattened along entire length when snake is agitated or when basking.

Average length 0.9m, maximum about 1.2m but has been recorded at 2 m.

Scalation:

Scales appear like overlapping shields, especially around the neck.

VENTRALS   140-190
SABCAUDALS   35-65 all single
MID-BODIES   17 or 19 rows
ANAL   single

Colour:

Highly variable. Base colours are brown, grey, olive, green with lighter crossbands usually of a creamy yellow colour. Occasionally unbanded Tiger Snakes are found. (Figs 1-4).

Habits:

The ecology of Tiger Snakes revolves around the availability of frogs or tadpoles. Although adult Tiger Snakes have adapted well to survive on introduced mice *(Mus musculus)*, the juveniles require small frogs or tadpoles for food.

Tiger Snakes are viviparous producing about 35 young but Worrell (1963) records 80 in a single brood.

Habit and Distribution:

Tiger Snakes always occur in well-watered areas where frogs can be found; this restricts them to watercourses, swamps, lakes or wet mountain slopes.

Notes:

Although the Tiger Snake is still very common, its overall numbers have been reduced drastically. The main reason for this reduction is habitat alteration. For example, river level control along the River Murray has reduced annual flooding patterns. This has altered the water table and reduced the numbers of swamps and lagoons (Softly 1971). In south-western Victoria, the extensive stonewalls, once a haven for snakes, have been replaced by wire fences. Lakes and swamps in many areas have been drained for farming purposes. In some developed areas there are reduced but balanced Tiger Snake populations. For instance, Tiger Snakes are occasionally found in Sydney or Melbourne along watercourses or on golf courses. Tiger Snakes are still abundant in Altona, a Melbourne suburb. Fortunately Tiger Snakes are well represented in National Parks.

Food:

Predominantly frogs and tadpoles, especially in their natural state, but in man-changed environments, which applies to most of Australia today, they thrive on introduced mice *(Mus musclus)*. Other animals eaten are lizards, birds, rats, eels, and fish (Gow 1976, Worrell 1963). Tiger Snakes, because of

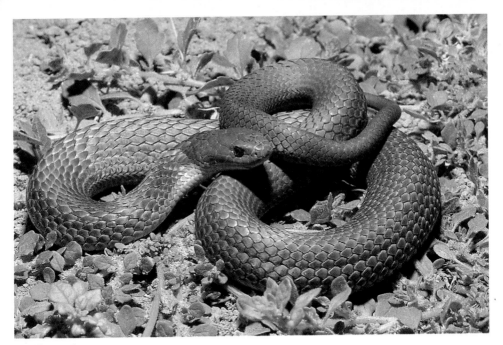

Figure 1
Notechis scutatus

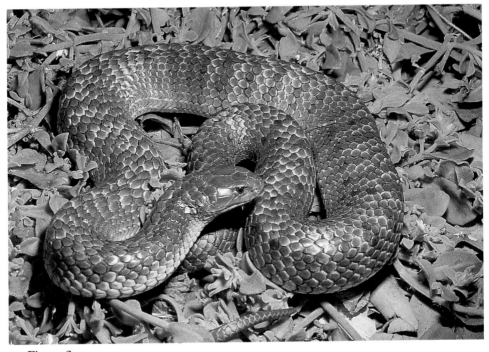

Figure 2
Notechis scutatus

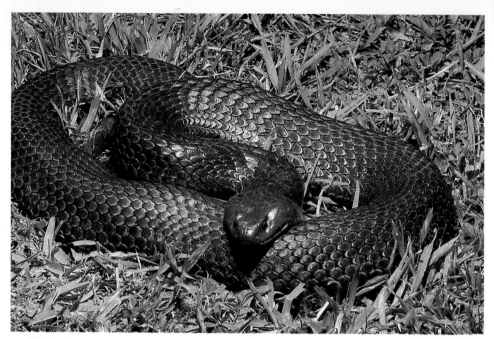

Figure 3
Notechis scutatus

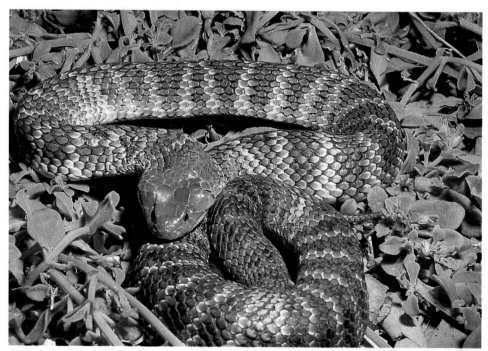

Figure 4
Notechis scutatus

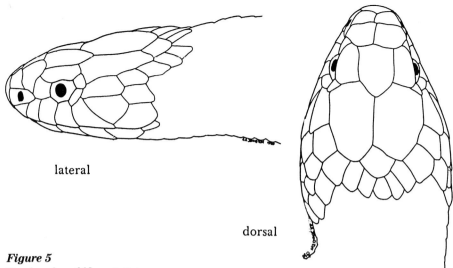

lateral

dorsal

Figure 5
Head scales of *N. scutatus,*

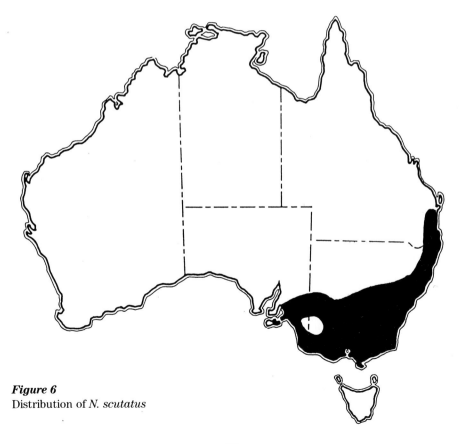

Figure 6
Distribution of *N. scutatus*

their association with water, are highly prone to trematode or fluke infestation. These flukes are transmitted by frogs and water snails and appear to be causing problems in certain areas (Giddings 1978).

Venom:

Broad (1979), determined the crude venom had a LD_{50} of 0.118 mg/kg making this venom 4.24 times more toxic than the Indian Cobra *Naja naja*.

The venom of this species has been the most actively studied Australian snake venom. Prior to the production of an effective antivenom, figures compiled by Fairley (1929), showed that 40% of all bites were fatal. It is now considered highly likely that many of the non-fatal bites were probably dry bites, as it is common for Tiger Snakes to bite without expressing venom.

Common Tiger Snakes kept at Venom Supplies Laboratories in South Australia, have shown an average yield of 27.6 mg of dried lyophilized venom. These snakes varied from 0.6 m to 1.4 m. Worrell (1963) records 35 mg as the average yield. The colour of the crude lyophilized venom is creamish.

The Neurotoxins:

Clearly, the dominant effect of Tiger Snake venom, is the effect of neurotoxins. They are divided into presynaptic and postsynaptic types. Karlsson et al (1972), described two presynaptic and two postsynaptic neurotoxins. The presynaptic neurotoxins are notexin and notechis 11-5. The postsynaptic neurotoxins are toxin 1 and toxin 2.

Karlsson (1972), found that notexin comprised 6% of the crude venom. Pluskal (1978), showed notexin had phospholipase A activity and can degranulate mast cells and release vaso-active amines. Halpert et al (1975), defined its structure as 119 amino acid residues in a single chain, crosslinked by seven disulphide bridges. Its molecular weight is 13,574.

Cull-Candy et al (1976), found that at the motor end plate, notexin appears to arrest the recycling vesicle membrane at the axolemma, resulting in omega-shaped indentations causing gross reduction of transmitter release. Notexin causes paralysis by inhibition of acetycholine release. Harris et al (1973) discovered that notexin was presynaptic at the neuromuscular junction.

Notexin is also myolytic. Harris et al (1978), found it produces a necrotizing myopathy in skeletal muscle. Harris et al (1978), showed that it is a potent Phospholipase A2, capable of hydrolysing phospholipids in micelles in fragmented bacteria membranes and in fact muscle fibre membranes. Harris et al (1978) and Harris et al (1981), established that myolytic activity was evident over a wide pH and temperature range, and was dependent on the presence of Ca++ ions. Hodd et al (1974) and Sutherland et al (1977), claimed that muscle damage was likely if administration of antivenom was delayed. It has been associated with gross elevation of serum enzymes and isoenzymes. Sutherland (1983), showed that in monkeys affected by *N. scutatus* venom, elevation of plasma creatine kinase commences two hours after S.C. injection of 120 μg/kg of venom. Daytner et al (1973), also supported their findings that the effects of notexin were difficult to reverse with antivenom if administration is delayed.

The other presynaptic neurotoxin, notechis 11-5, according to Karlsson (1972), has double the phospholipase A activity of notexin, but is only 30% as lethal in mice.

Halpert et al (1975), using amino acid sequences, demonstrated that close relation exists between notexin, notechis 11-5, porcine pancreatic Phospholipase A and phospholipase A isolated from *Naja malanoleuca.*

The two postsynaptic neurotoxins described by Karlsson (1972), toxin 1 and toxin 2 are curare-like, fast acting and have molecular weights of 6,000 and 7,000. Daytner et al (1973), found that the effects of these two neurotoxins were easily reversed by antivenom.

The Coagulant Factor:

Jobin et al (1966), confirmed that Tiger Snake venom exerted its optimal coagulant activity only in the presence of prothrombin, Factor V, a divalent metal (Ca^{++}, Ba^{++}, Sr^{++} or Mn^{++}) and a phospholipid emulsion. The venom was shown to be capable of activating prothrombin and incapable of activating Factor X. Tans et al (1985), isolated the venom activator and determined that its molecular weight was 54,000 and that it comprised 6% of the crude venom. They concluded it had a structure of light and heavy polypeptide chains, held together by one or more disulphide bridges. They found that prothrombin activation by the activator alone was very slow due to unfavourable kinetic parameters. By adding phospholipid, Ca^{++} and Factor Va, a dramatic increase in reaction rate occurred. Since the venom activity on prothrombin is greatly stimulated by the presence of phospholipid and Factor Va, this activator is useful in elucidating the mechanism of the accessory components in prothrombin activation. The prothrombin activator resembles Factor Xa in essential catalytic properties.

Sutherland (1983), reported that the pressure bandage and immobilization first aid delayed the movement of the coagulant factor. The eventual coagulation defects which occurred after the removal of restrictions were less than if the venom was unrestrained.

Haemolysins:

Sutherland (1983), suggests that haemolysis is unlikely to cause anaemia or renal damage, but the development of haemoglobinuria is an indicator of systemic envenomation.

Hyaluronidase:

Sutherland (1983), records the level of hyaluronidase at 16 IU per mg. This enzyme, or spreading factor, aids the dispersion of venom components in connective tissue.

A number of other minor components are also present. They are:

Phosphilphase A	—	Doery and Pearson (1961)
Phospholiphase B	—	Doery and Pearson (1964)

Capillary Permeability increasing factor	—	Dorey (1958)
Lymphotoxic factor	—	Campbell (1969a)
Sensory nerve ending toxin	—	Kellaway (1943b)
Smooth muscle stimulant	—	Kellaway (1929f)
Acetylcholinesterase	—	Zeller (1984)
Heat stable anticoagulant	—	Kaire (1964a)
Peptidase activity	—	Tu and Toom (1967)
Purine compounds	—	Doery (1957, 1958)

Antivenom:

Tiger Snakes antivenom — manufactured by the Commonwealth Serum Laboratories (Melbourne)

INITIAL DOSE — 3,000 units.
PHOTOGRAPH (1)

Sutherland (1983), reports that toxoided venoms have been used to stimulate antibodies to *N. scutatus* venom. The problem with this approach is that the size of the challenge from a snake bite may overwhelm the level of antibodies. Weiner (1960a), actively immunized a patient with toxoided *N. scutatus* venom and a titre of 5.2 units/ml was obtained, but it rapidly decreased after the course was completed.

Sutherland (1983), reported that Gallichio at the Commonwealth Serum Laboratories (Melbourne), has investigated the preparation of a "venoid" from *N. scutatus* venom and glutaraldehyde, with encouraging results.

Case History

Tiger Snake Notechis scutatus

(from Sutherland and Coulter, 1977)

In 1977, a 10-year-old girl was found unconscious in a paddock, in Melbourne. The differential diagnosis on admission to hospital was either head injury or drug overdose. X-rays of the skull were normal and cerebrospinal fluid was normal. Her respiration required assistance. Overnight her condition worsened and her younger brother confessed that she may have been bitten by a snake. By this time renal shutdown was established and bladder cathetization allowed collection of 300 ml of very dark urine, later attributed to myoglobin.

Drowsiness and peripheral neurological signs were compatible with snake bite. Scratches on her legs and blood on her socks suggested snake bite. Serum and urine samples and her clothing were taken to the Commonwealth Serum Laboratories (C.S.L.) and slow infusion of tiger snake and brown snake antivenom was begun.

She received 9,000 units and 1,500 units of tiger snake and brown snake antivenoms in the next few hours. Four hours after serum was taken, tiger snake venom was found by radioimmunoassay at the C.S.L. in the serum and clothing. Her muscle power increased but respiration assistance was required for a further five days. Peritoneal dialysis was necessary for six days because of the renal shutdown. Full health was regained after three weeks of extensive physiotherapy for her muscle weakness. She had no recollection of snake bite.

Laboratory findings were:

(a) 250 ng/g of venom in sock.

(b) 152 ng/g ml of venom in urine.

(c) 4.3 ng/ml of notexin in urine.

(d) serum/lactic dehydrogenase level 3,820 IU/1. (normal 70 to 140 IU/1). Elevation of isoenzymes particularly from skeletal muscle. PCK level 33,200 IU/1 (normal 0 to 80 IU/1).

(e) MM and MB bands were detected.

Note:

Today, venom type can be detected in about 30 minutes using venom detection kits. These are available for all hospitals, medical centres and laboratories.

Summary of Symptoms and Conditions Experienced from Published Notechis scutatus Bites.

— Headache
— Pain in axilla. Swollen lymph nodes.
— Nausea — vomiting. Dark material in vomit.
— Slurred speech.
— Muscle weakness.
— Desire to micturate.
— Desire to defecate.
— Dilated pupils and slow response to stimuli.
— Diplopia.
— Ptosis.
— Swollen limb.
— Haemoglobin in urine.
— Tachycardia.
— Cyanosis.
— Dysphagia.
— Short shallow respirations. Difficult respirations.
— Oozing of wounds.
— Failure of blood to clot.
— Burning sensation in mouth.
— Loss of sight.
— Paralysis of palate.
— Swollen throat.
— Sensation of lungs becoming paralysed.
— Perspiration.
— Urine — dirty brown colour (myoglobin) (some haemoglobin).
— Unconsciousness.
— Renal failure.

- Drowsiness.
- Elevated serum lactic dehyrogenase level.
- Elevation of PCK levels. MM and MB bands present.
- Diarrhoea.
- Tremors.
- Blurred vision.
- Stuporous.
- Haematuria.
- Bruising around bite site.
- Small areas of necrosis at bite site.
- Convulsions.
- Shock.
- Hypotension.
- Muscle destruction.
- Local pain.
- Numbness in mouth.
- Serum LD and AST initially elevated.
- Loss of taste (to salt).
- Restricted tongue movement.
- Reduced muscle tone.
- Local swelling.
- Small area of necrosis at bite site.

Kreffts Tiger Snake *Notechis ater ater* (Krefft)

Description:

Robust in appearance with a broad flat head which is slightly distinct from body. Average length about 83 cm.

Scalation:

Smooth scales. Appear like overlapping shields around neck.

VENTRALS	163-173
SUBCAUDALS	41-50 all single
MID—BODIES	17 rows
ANAL	single (occasionally divided)

Colours:

Seventy percent of specimens have either distinct yellow-white bands or remnant banding. The remainder are jet black. Many specimens exhibit white markings around the bottom jaw. Juveniles possess white bands. The ventral surface is dark grey to black, becoming creamish before sloughing. (Fig 7)

Habits:

These snakes can be found basking in relatively cold weather, their black colour optimising radiation absorption. In the hot weather they become aquatic and live exclusively around permanent water where they feed on

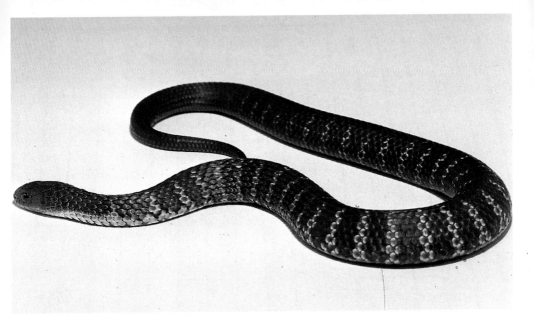

Figure 7
Notechis ater ater

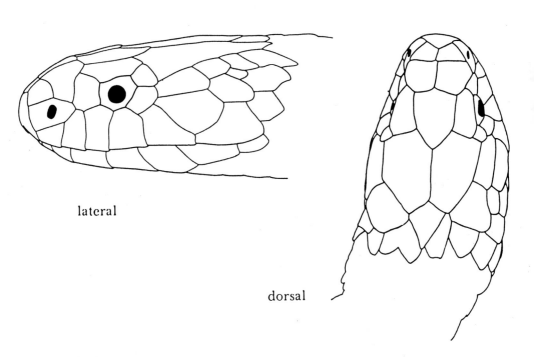

lateral

dorsal

Figure 8
Head scales of *N. a. ater*,

tadpoles and frogs. They can be seen muzzling under submerged flat rocks in search of tadpoles. Viviparous — produces 6 to 15 young.

Habitat and Distribution:

Their range is restricted to a narrow corridor of the Flinders Ranges, from Wilmington to Melrose, in the approximate confines of the 600 mm average annual isohyet. The area is typified by deep-gullied gorges, carved out by creeks dotted with River Red Gums. In summer the creeks form a series of ponds that are ideal for frogs and tadpoles. Another population occurs close to the termination of the Broughton River. The water here can be brackish. This river is the main channel capturing water from the many tributaries of the Flinders Ranges population area. There is some evidence from S. A. National Parks & Wildlife Service, that specimens still occur in some of the creek's draining from the main population area. These areas have been greatly modified by farming activities.

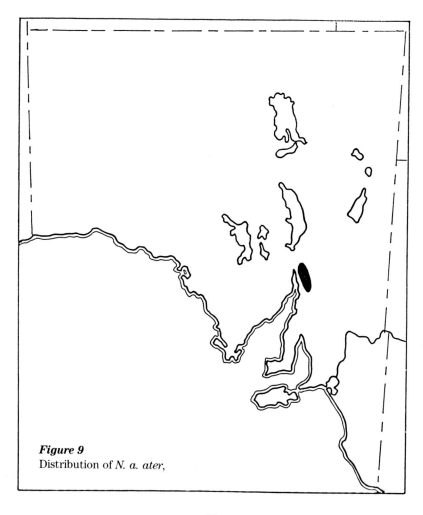

Figure 9
Distribution of *N. a. ater,*

The dependence on tadpoles and frogs by the juvenile snakes restricts the Kreffts Tiger Snake to this wet habitat, despite ability of the adult snakes to feed on mice.

Kreffts Tiger Snakes occur in Mt Remarkable National Park.

Notes:

The snake's black colour is intriguing. One theory is that radiation absorption is limited in the steep-gullied areas of its range and black helps optimise it. Moreover, the creeks containing tadpoles and frogs are relatively cool and the snakes are continually moving in and out of the water seeking to re-elevate their temperatures. In winter, snakes travel away from water and have been recorded basking on top of Mt Remarkable on warm days.

Food:

Frogs, tadpoles and lizards are the main food source. European mice *Mus musculus* are also favoured. These snakes have also been observed feeding on ducklings of *Anas supercilosa* (Black Duck).

Venom:

Kreffts Tiger Snakes kept at Venom Supplies Laboratories show an average yield of 23 mg of dried lyophilized venom.

Sutherland (1983), records a toxicity of $LD_{50} = 0.051$ mg/kg which makes this venom the most toxic (for mice), of all the Tiger Snake venoms.

The colour of the dried crude lyophilized venom is white.

Antivenom:

Tiger Snake manufactured by the Commonwealth Serum Laboratories (Melbourne).

INITIAL DOSE — 6,000 units (Sutherland 1983)

Peninsula Tiger Snake *(Notechis ater niger)* **(Kinghorn)**
Description:

Robust in appearance. Schwaner (1985) has reported the following average snout vent lengths(S.V.L.)

Franklin Is.	1.2 — 1.4 m
Goat Is.	1.1 — 1.3 m
Hopkins Is.	1.1 — 1.3 m
K.I. Islets	1.1 — 1.2 m
Hareby Is.	0.7 — 1.1 m

Surveys by Venom Supplies indicate a range from 0.4 — 1.2 m (S.V.L.) with an average of 0.8 m on Reevesby Is. and the average SVL is 0.78 m on Roxby Is. Blunt head slightly distinct from body. Adult Kangaroo Island Tiger Snake specimens have fang length of about 5 mm.

Scalation:

Smooth scales. Appear like overlapping shields around the neck.

VENTRALS	160-184
SUBCAUDALS	45-54 all single
MID-BODIES	17, 18, 19, rarely 21
ANAL	single

Colour:

Generally jet black, with adults occasionally possessing white markings around the bottom jaw. Juveniles nearly always have white cross bands. On Kangaroo Island, banding often occurs in adult specimens, and a much larger colour variation occurs ranging from brown to black with red bellies. Ventral surface dark grey to black tending to cream before sloughing. (Figs 10, 11 & 12)

Habits:

Viviparous. Surveys on Reevesby Island have shown from 3 birth records, up to 27 young are produced. The black coloration presumably allows the snake to bask more efficiently during the warmer winter days. Usually far more sluggish than the Common Tiger Snake and less vigorous when caught.

Habitat and Distribution:

Occurs on the offshore islands in Spencer Gulf, Kangaroo Island, the west coast of South Australia, and coastal sand dunes of lower Eyre Peninsula and Yorke Peninsula. Vegetation consists of coastal dunes with low shrubs, low eucalypt woodlands to eucalypt forests on Kangaroo Island. Some small islands have samphire and saltbush communities.

Notes:

Fishermen living in the Tumby Bay area have reported Peninsula Tiger Snakes swimming in the sea up to 10 km from land. This suggests they occasionally travel from island to island in the Sir Joseph Banks Group and also from the islands to the mainland. However, apparent ecological and size differences between populations suggest that these adventurers make little impact on their new found environments.

The back coloration is of interest. One explanation is that Tiger Snakes from this area are black so that optimum use of radiation can be obtained. However, good basking weather is more readily available in these habitats than, say, in Mount Gambier, where ordinary banded Common Tiger Snakes occur. Another explanation for the black colour is that it aids in more rapid digestion of food (quicker radiation absorption is required to elevate the body temperature to its optimum level for food digestion) thus allowing the snake to eat more in a shorter time span. Black would hardly be expected to provide much camouflage on white sand dunes, but at a glance a black snake could be taken as a shadow. Generally speaking the island Tiger Snakes, with the exception of Kangaroo Island are less aggressive in nature than the Common Tiger Snake,

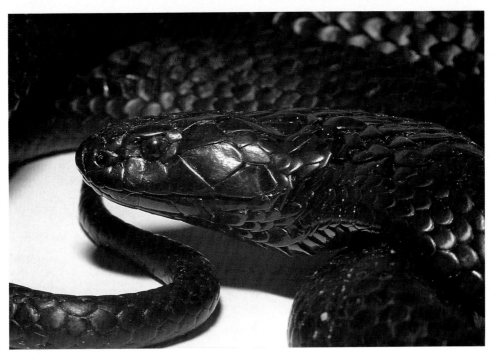

Figure 10
Notechis ater niger (Goat Is.)

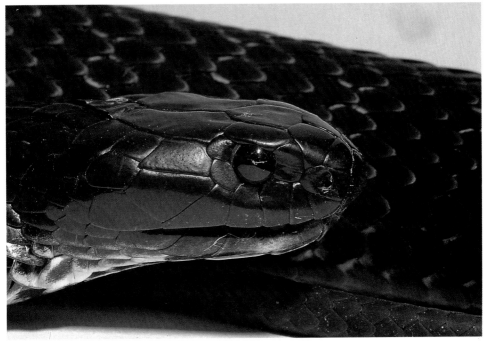

Figure 11
Notechis ater niger (Kangaroo Is)

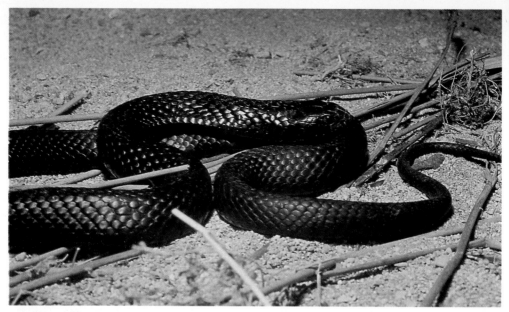

Figure 12
Notechis ater niger (Roxby Is.)

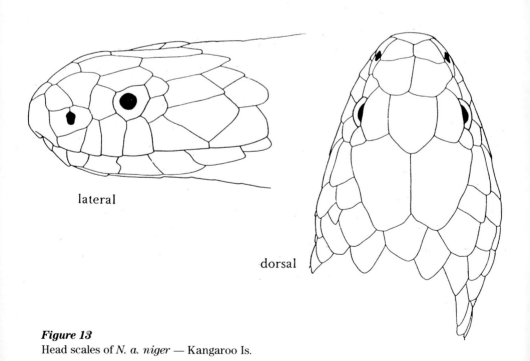

lateral

dorsal

Figure 13
Head scales of *N. a. niger* — Kangaroo Is.

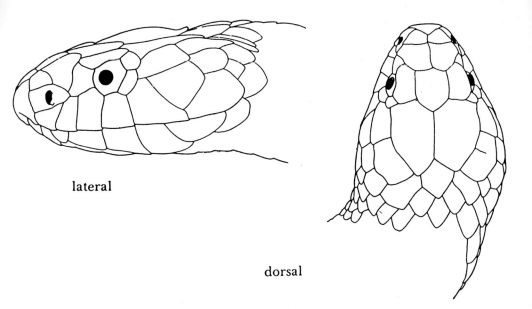

lateral

dorsal

Figure 13
Head scales of *N. a. niger* — Coffin Bay

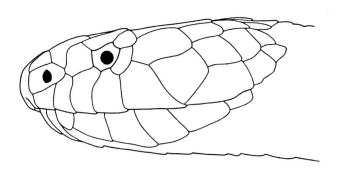

Figure 14
Head scales of *N. a. niger* — Hopkins Is.

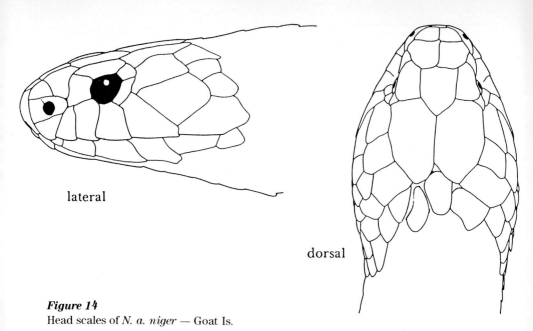

lateral

dorsal

Figure 14
Head scales of *N. a. niger* — Goat Is.

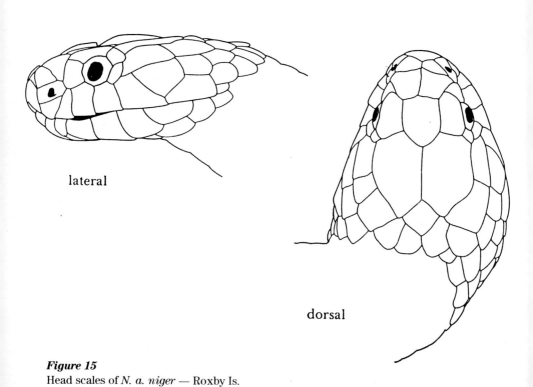

lateral

dorsal

Figure 15
Head scales of *N. a. niger* — Roxby Is.

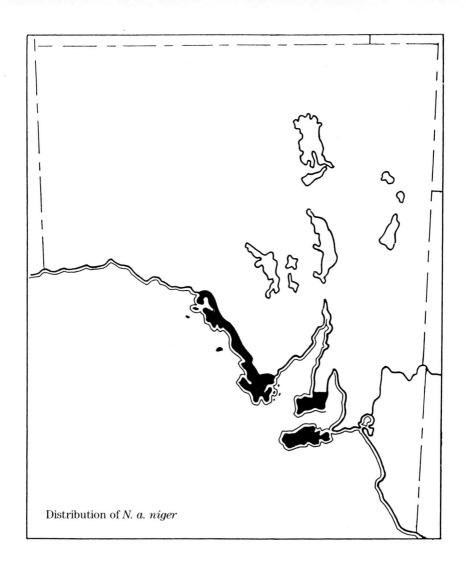

Distribution of *N. a. niger*

especially the larger ones. In the cooler weather they have been known to lie coiled up and remain motionless when approached. Freshly caught specimens appear to be less perturbed about being caught than other snakes.

Food:

Adult island snakes mainly feed on birds such as White-faced Storm-Petrels *(Pelagodroma marina)* and Muttonbirds *(Puffinus tenuirostris)*. Occasionally other birds are also eaten. Skinks are also eaten on some islands by the adult snakes. The juvenile snake feeds on small skinks. Mice have been introduced by man's inhabitation or farming activites, and these have provided another food On the mainland, birds and small mammals are eaten by these snakes.

Venom:

Morgan (1937), reports that the venom yield from Reevesby Island Tiger Snakes was 34.4 mg. The colour of the dried lyophilized venom is white. Kangaroo Island Tiger Snake's venom is creamish (same as *N. scutatus)*

Broad et al (1979), records the toxicity as LD_{50} = 0.099 mg/kg, for Reevesby Islad. Sutherland (1983) records LD_{50} = 0.105 mg/kg. for Kangaroo Island and LD_{50} = 0.164 (saline) for Hareby island.

Morgan (1937), recorded that the Reevesby Island Tiger Snakes were 2.3 times more toxic than *N. scutatus*. Sutherland (1983), could not reproduce these results.

Antivenom:

Tiger Snake — Manufactured by the Commonwealth Serum Laboratories (Melbourne).

INITIAL DOSE — 6,000 units (Sutherland 1983)

Western Tiger Snake *Notechis ater occidentalis* (Glauert)
(Storr (1982), suggests *N. scutatus occidentalis*, which is also supported by Shine (1987) and Schwaner (1985).
Description:

Broad short head slightly distinct from body. Robust body. Maximum length about 2 m.

Scalation:

Smooth scales.

VENTRALS	140-165
SUBCAUDALS	36-51
MID-BODIES	17, 19
ANAL	Single (rarely divided)

Colour:

Steel blue to black with bright yellow bands. Ventral surface yellow tending to black towards the tail. All-black specimens are common. (Fig 16).

Habits:

Viviparous can produce up to 90 young (Softly 1971). Gow records young at 15 cm from litters of 14 to 20 in November. Observations on Carnac Island suggest a mortality rate of 90 percent in the first 6 months. Lifespan has been measured at over 10 years (Softly 1971).

Habitat and Distribution:

South-western Australia and some adjacent islands including Garden and Carnac. Frogs abound in the forests and swamps in the region. Dry sclerophyll forest.

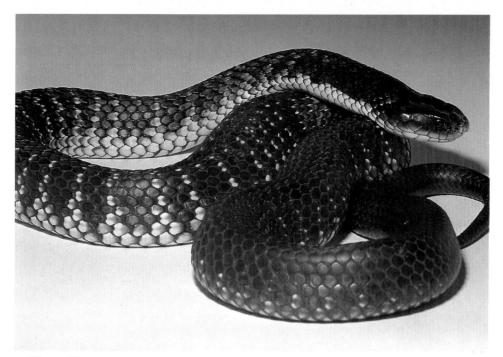

Figure 16
Notechis ater occidentalis

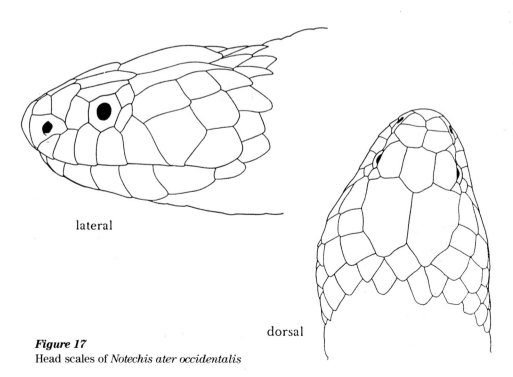

lateral

dorsal

Figure 17
Head scales of *Notechis ater occidentalis*

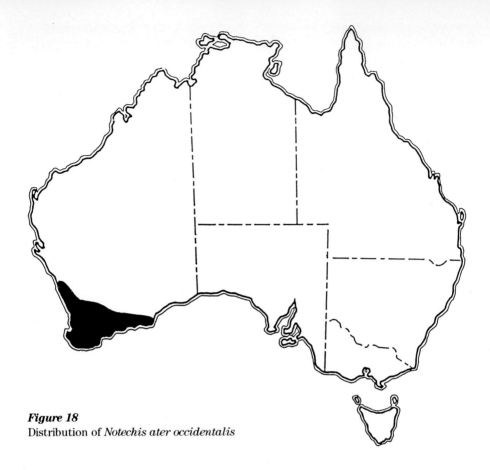

Figure 18
Distribution of *Notechis ater occidentalis*

Venom:

Broad et al (1979), records the $LD_{50} = 0.124$ mg/kg.
Softly (1971), claims the venom yield to be 35 mg.

Antivenom:

Tiger Snake — manufactured by the Commonwealth Serum Laboratories (Melbourne).

INITIAL DOSE — 6,000 units (Sutherland 1983)

Western Tiger Snake *Notechis ater occidentalis* Case History
(from Sutherland 1983)

A bite by *N. a. occidentalis* associated with epilepsy:

At 1.30 pm on the 2nd December 1978, a 12-year old girl was bitten by a snake on the ankle as she climbed through a fence in long grass at Gibson near Esperance in Western Australia.

At 2 pm she was admitted to hospital confused, vomiting and with a headache. Her blood pressure was 164/100. At 3.30 pm her pupils were dilated and not reacting to light, blood pressure was 200/120 and she was comatose. At 4.10 pm she fitted for five minutes, all limbs being involved. She became cyanosed, her pharynx was sucked out and she was given intranasal oxygen. Polyvalent antivenom (one ampoule) was given at 5.40 pm and again at 6.45 pm. Blood taken before antivenom was given would not clot over a sixty minute period. (Later analysis of this sample at the Commonwealth Serum Laboratories showed it contained 28 ng/ml of genus *Notechis* venom). She continued to fit and was paralysed, intubated and transferred to the Princess Margaret Hospital in Perth by the Royal Flying Doctor Service, whilst on intermittent positive pressure ventilation.

On admission her haemoglobin was 8.8 mmol/l, white cell count 23 x 10^9/1, (neutrophils 93%), platelet 100 x 10^9/1, partial thromboplastin time 32 seconds, and fibrin degradation products 180 mg/l.

Shortly after her arrival, her conscious state dramatically improved, she breathed spontaneously and was extubated. No further antivenom was given. Next day she still had bilateral fixed, dilated pupils, but was otherwise quite well. A day later a sluggish pupillary reflex had returned and she was discharged home and made an uneventful recovery. No serum sickness occurred.

Summary of Symptoms and Conditions Experienced with N.a. occidentalis
— Elevation of serum creatine phosphokinase.
— Vomiting.
— Coma.
— Local bruising.
— Pulmonary congestion and oedema.
— Collapsed lungs.
— Subterminal anoxic damage to myocardium.
— Congestion of organs.
— Headache.
— Dilated pupils.
— Cyanosis.

Chappell Island Tiger Snake *Notechis ater serventyi* (Worrell)
Description:

Giant race of tiger snakes averaging about 1.9 m. Head slightly distinct from neck with robust body.

Scalation:

Smooth scales.

VENTRALS	160-171
SUBCAUDALS	47-52 all single
MID-BODIES	17
ANAL	Single

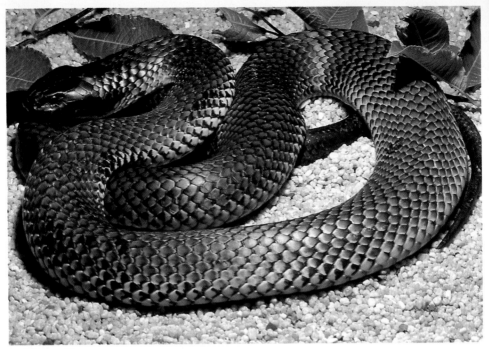

Figure 19
Notechis ater serventyi (Flinders Is.)

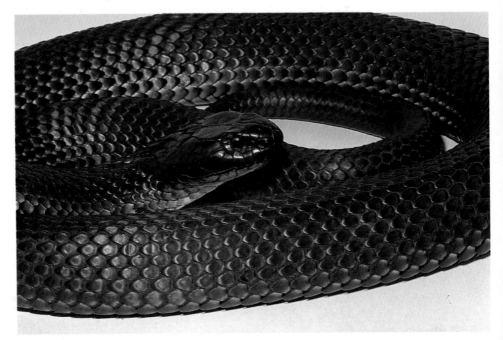

Figure 20
Notechis ater serventyi (Chapell Is.)

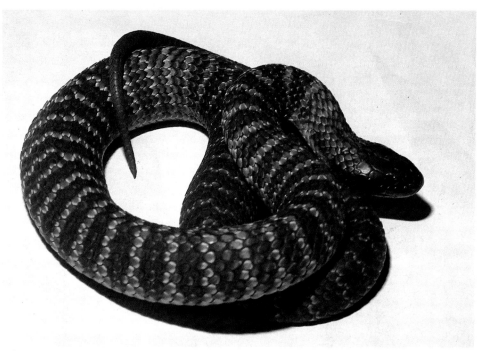

Figure 21
Notechis ater serventyi (Chapell Is. juvenile)

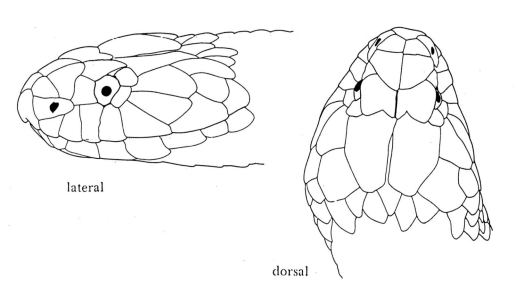

lateral

dorsal

Figure 22
Head scales of Notechis ater serventyi

Colour:

Dorsal olive brown to black. Ventral surface is usually lighter in colour. Juveniles may be banded. (Figs 19-21)

Habits:

Generally sluggish. Specimens from Chappell Island are easily kept in captivity and fed on a variety of foods such as mice, rats, strips of meat, and sausages (Worrell 1963). Viviparous. Barnett and Schwaner (1985), report a litter of 31. The young can measure 25-30 cm at birth.

Habitat and Distribution:

Occurs on Chappell Island and Badger Island of the Furneaux group. Lives in Muttonbird burrows where it finds refuge and feeds on juvenile Muttonbirds, *Puffinus tenuirostris*. Also found on Flinders Island, Cat, Babel, Florsyth and Vansittart islands.

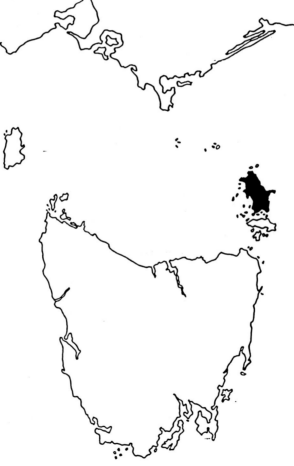

Figure 23
Distribution of *Notechis ater serventyi*

We have lumped the Furneaux group Tiger Snakes into *N. ater serventyi* purely on the basis of island proximity. Apart from the opinions of Schawaner (1985) and Shine (1987) that only one taxon of *Notechis* exists insufficient information is available to do otherwise at this stage.

Notes:

Most of work in understanding the ecology of this snake has been compiled by E. Worrell. Work on this species is currently being conducted by Schwaner. Worrell records that on Chappell Island, these Tiger Snakes feed on young Muttonbirds for several weeks and virtually starve for the rest of the year. The juveniles feed on small skinks.

Barnett and Schwaner (1985), found that the growth rate over 12 months was such that snakes kept in captivity increased from 290 mm to 1,367 mm in that period, ie., about 470% increase in length.

Venom:

Broad et al (1979), detemined the LD_{50} = 0.271 mg/kg. Sutherland (1983), determined LD_{50} = 0.542. Worrell (1963), records the average yield as 75 mg. At the Venom Supplies Laboratories 69 mg average yield has been obtained. The venom is creamish in the lyophilized form.

Antivenom:

Tiger Snake — manufactured by the Commonwealth Serum Laboratories (Melbourne).

Initial Dose — 9,000 units (Sutherland 1983)

Tasmanian and King Island Tiger Snakes
***Notechis ater humphreysi* (Worrell)**
Description:

Large adults are robust with broad blunt head. Younger snakes are slimmer to other Tiger Snakes. Maximum length about 1.5 m.

Scalation:

Smooth scales.

VENTRALS	161-174
SUBCAUDALS	48-53 all single
MID-BODIES	17 (sometimes 15). Worrell recorded that mid-body scales may count between 15 and 19 on the same snake.
ANAL	Single

Colour:

Grey with black flecks which form faint bands; black; black and yellow stripes. Ventral surface usually lighter in colour. (Figs 24, 25).

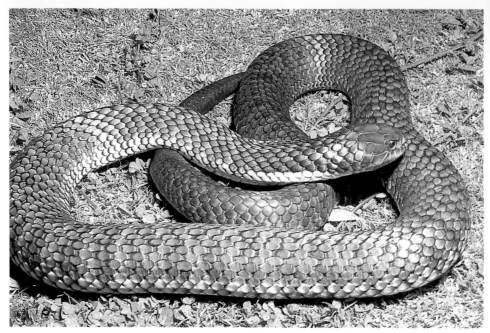

Figure 24
Notechis ater humphreysi (Tasmania.)

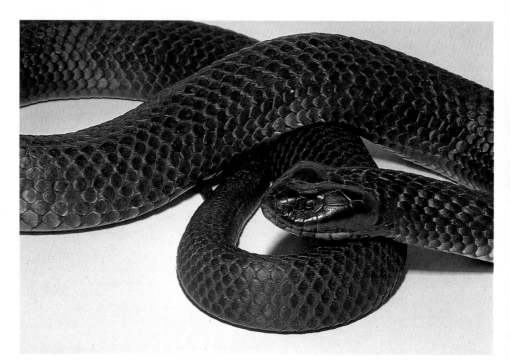

Figure 25
Notechis ater humphreysi (King Is.)

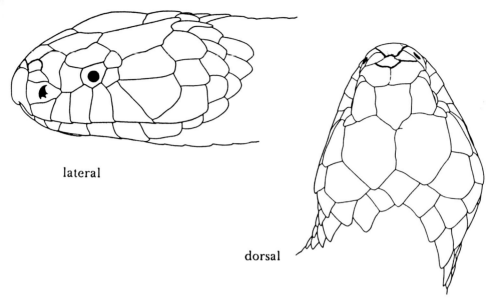

lateral

dorsal

Figure 26
Head scales of *Notechis ater humphreysi* (King Island)

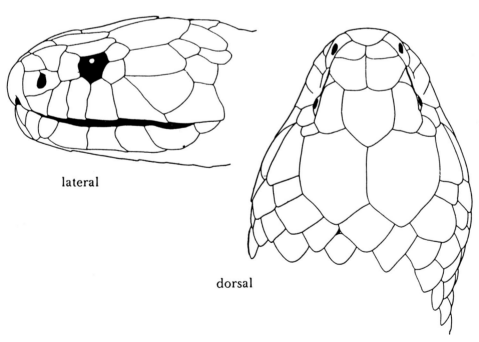

lateral

dorsal

Head scales of *Notechis ater humphreysi* (Tasmania)

45

Habits:

On Christmas and New Year Islands they feed on Muttonbird chicks. King Island Tiger Snakes have cannibalistic tendencies. Viviparous and produces large numbers of young.

Habitat and Distribution:

Sclerophyll forest, woodlands, heathland and rainforest occur on King Island, Tasmania, Seal Rocks, Christmas Island, New Year Island and Bruny Island.

Venom:

Worrell (1963), records that King Island Tiger Snakes are less toxic than other tiger snakes. Sutherland's evidence (1983), contradicts this finding. Sutherland's data show that King Island Tiger Snakes, *Notechis ater*

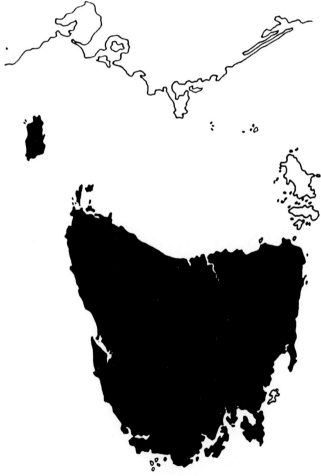

Figure 27
Distribution of *N. a. humphreysi,*

humphreysi, are more toxic than Chappell Island Tiger Snakes, *Notechis ater serventyi,* and Common Tiger Snakes, *Notechis scutatus.*

$LD_{50} = 0.111$ King Island
$LD_{50} = 0.194$ (Saline)   Tasmania
$LD_{50} = 0.147$ New Year Island

Tasmanian Tiger Snakes yield 36 mg at Venom Supplies Laboratories. The lyophilized venom is creamish.

Antivenom:

Tiger Snakes — manufactured by the Commonwealth Serum Laboratories (Melbourne).

INITIAL DOSE — 6,000 units (Sutherland 1983).

Victims bitten by Tasmanian Tiger Snakes, on average, require twice the usual dosage of antivenom for Common Tiger Snakes (Mirtschin and Davis 1982).

Case Report —
Black Tiger Snake — *N. a. humphreysi*
(from Harvey et al 1982)

At 11.45 am, 27/10/81, a 30-year-old herpetologist was bitten on the hand by a 1 m King Island Tiger Snake. He had been bitten 16 years previously by a mainland tiger snake *Notechis scutatus* and had received 3,000 units of antivenom. A slight rash followed at the time but otherwise the treatment was uneventful. On two other occasions he had been bitten by elapids but experienced no envenomation. The patient suffered from atopic eczema since childhood.

First aid was initiated immediately applied using strips of T-shirt and a few minutes later a crepe bandage was applied to the full length of the arm. He was given a 5% dextrose infusion intravenously in the ambulance and on admission to the hospital complained of pain in the bitten hand and arm, frontal headache and nasal stiffness.

He had marked truncal, facial and conjunctival erythema. He was afebrile, and vital signs were within normal limits.

At 12.40 pm, he was given promethazine (5 mg intravenously and 20 mg intramuscularly) and at 12.45 pm, a slow infusion of 3,000 units of tiger snake antivenom in 100 ml of Hartmann's solution was begun. Adrenaline and hydrocortisone were at hand for immediate use. Blood was taken for typing and crossmatch, and for biochemical and haematological studies. Thrombin time and fibrin degradation products were estimated, and then regularly over the next 3 days.

A further 3,000 units tiger snake venom diluted in 70 ml of Hartmann's solution was begun at 1.45 pm and it was noted that the cutaneous erythema had almost completely disappeared. At 2.03 pm (2¼ hours after the bite), the constructive bandage was removed and ice applied to the patient's hand, which was very painful. There were two puncture marks (one bleeding slightly) on the medial border of the hand over the front of the metacarpal head of the little finger and a surrounding area of tenderness, induration and blue discoloration 2.5 cm in diameter. The patient's upper limb was swollen and tender, but no auxiliary lymph nodes were palpable. By 3.00 pm, the patient was symptomatic, other than having severe pain in the upper limb. X-ray films of the hand, taken to exclude the presence of a fang, revealed no abnormalities.

A course of co-trimoxazole and metronidazole therapy was begun and tetanus vaccine given. The patient remained in bed under observation for 24 hours. On the second day, a transient rash was present. The patient's right hand and forearm became extremely painful, grossly swollen and oedematous, necessitating elevation and administration of pethidine. A black necrotic area, 1 cm x 2 cm, developed on the right hand over the puncture site, and there was hypoaesthesia over the distribution of the medial digited nerve of his little finger. The patient was discharged from hospital on November 2, 1981. On November 8, he presented with a mild urticarial rash and swelling of the eyelids, and was treated with antihistamines.

The results of biochemical and haematological tests remained normal throughout, with only slight elevation of the serum level of creatine phosphokinase to 466 μ/L on the second day after envenomation.

A trace of blood was present in the urine on ward testing, and microurine analysis showed from 4 to 10 red blood cells per high power field. (The patient had not been catheterised). Before release of the bandage, thrombin times were normal, and no fibrin degradation products were detected. Six hours after release, the patient's thrombin times were 8 seconds (control 7 seconds) for 10 units, and 14 seconds (control 9 seconds) for 5 units, and fibrin degradation products were 80 mg/L to 110 mg/L. By the fourth day after envenomation, these levels returned to normal.

Haemolytic and myolytic activities were not apparent in this patient, and there were no signs of renal failure. Mild haematuria, and a slight rise in thrombin time and in levels of fibrin degradation products indicated a minor coagulopathy, and frontal headache was evidence of neurotoxicity. Local necrosis of the hand with numbness in the distribution of the medial nerve of the little finger was probably due to high concentration of venom in the tissues.

Summary of Symptoms and Conditions Experienced with N.a. humphreysi Bites

— Low temperature.
— Mucous membranes blanched.
— Tachycardia.
— Headache.
— Failure of blood to clot.
— Truncal, facial, conjunctival erythma.
— Afrebile.
— Pain around bitten area.
— Local necrosis.

- Hypoaesthesia.
- Blood in urine.
- Mild haematuria.
- Slight increase in thrombin time.

The Brown Snakes

Brown snakes from the *Pseudonaja* genus are widespread throughout the mainland and occur in all type of habitats except alpine. Generally speaking they are fast moving, sun-loving (preferring higher temperature) and forage over a larger home range than most other snakes. Collectively, they are the second most common cause of snake bite in Australia.

The Brown Snakes (genus *Pseudonaja*) are a group of snakes exhibiting similar scalation, hooded threat display *(Pseudonaja* = false cobra), and methods of prey restraint. In addition to using their venom to kill their prey, Brown Snakes also constrict. The prey then either dies from the action of the venom or by suffocation. Constriction is a technique primarily used by pythons and boas for hunting, although Shine (1985), lists 16 Australian species from the elapids and colubrids that have used it. Its main effect is to stop the prey from breathing. Tight coils around the prey prevent chest expansion necessary for air intake, and so the prey dies of suffocation. Brown Snakes using this technique, either use it to supplement the action of the venom or to prevent the prey from biting while struggling to escape. *Pseudonaja modesta*, a non-dangerous but venomous Brown Snake, does not use this technique of prey restraint (Gilliam 1979).

Mirtschin and Davis (1982), claimed the taxonomy of brown snake had been questioned by taxonomists for some time. Cogger (1983), indicated that the species of *P. nuchalis* is probably a series of distinct species. Mengden (1985a), examined the chromosomes and electrophoretic patterns of blood enzymes and concluded that each of the 6 species erected by Worrell (1961) were karotypically distinct except for *P. nuchalis* which contains 7 different karomorphs, 3 of which have different diploid numbers. He concluded also that *P. nuchalis* was also distinguished by 9 different colour morphs. He found that *P. textilis* was monotypic throughout its range both chromosomally and to a lesser extent electrophoretically. He noted that *P. guttata* appeared most distinctive electrophoretically.

The Brown Snakes occur in all rainfall areas with the Dugite and the Peninsula Brown Snake occupying almost identical thermal regions with average maximum summer temperatures of 24°C-32°C.

The more southern and coastal Brown Snakes tend to be smaller and darker in colour, which may have some radiation absorption advantages.

With the exception of the top end of the Northern Territory, Western Brown Snakes tend to occupy the more arid of parts of Australia, having an average maximum temperature range of 30°C-39°C, and similar rainfalls. Mengden's work of (1985a), now suggests that the *P. nuchalis* from the Northern Territory are a different species.

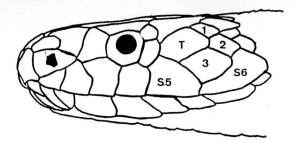

1 + 3

Head scales of *Oxyuranus scutellatus.*

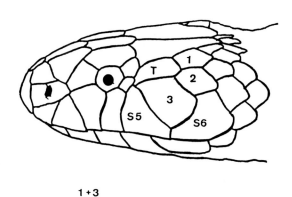

1 + 3

Head scales of *Pseudechis australis.*

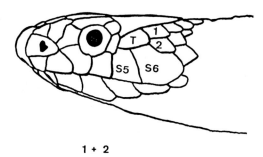

1 + 2

Head scales of *Pseudonaja nuchalis.*

Figure 28
The temporal scale formula that identifies the *Pseudonaja* genus. (Adapted from Mengden & Fitzgerald 1987)

The identification of the various species of brown snakes within the *Pseudonaja* genus is difficult. Indeed, even distinguishing a snake in the *Pseudonaja* genus presents its problems. Mengden and Fitzgerald (1987), draw attention to the many genera of Australian snakes having individuals that may be brown in colour. To assist in identification of the genus, they have devised a novel way of identifying them.

The pattern of scales in the temporal region of the head readily distinguishes the genus *Pseudonaja* from other dangerous Australian elapids. The temporal scale that borders the postoculars (T) is bordered by 2 other temporals in the *Pseudonaja* genus and 3 others in all other genera of dangerous snakes. Figure 28 shows the temporal formula for *Pseudonaja nuchalis* 1 + 2, and the temporal formulae for *Pseudonaja australis* and *Oxyuranus scutellatus* 1 + 3. The *Pseudonaja* genus does not exhibit a large temporal scale projecting down and almost separating supralabial scales S5 and S6.

Common Brown Snake *Pseudonaja textilis* (Duméril and Bibron)

Description:

Long and slender, head not distinct from body, juveniles often banded or with black heads. Can grow to more than 1.8 m. Generally southern Brown Snakes do not grow as long as northern specimens.

Gillan (1979), notes that the buccal cavity is flesh pink for Northern Territory specimens.

Scalation:

Smooth scales.

VENTRALS	185-235
SUBCAUDALS	45-75 divided
MID-BODIES	17
ANAL	Divided

Colour:

Variable in colour but usually a monotone brown. Juveniles can be banded. Light tan to dark brown. Ventral surfaces often blotched with orange, grey or brown spots. (Figs 29a, b)

Habits:

Oviparous producing about 10-30 eggs. Extremely fast-moving, alert and very difficult to catch. Of all the Brown Snakes, the common Brown Snakes *P. textilis*, probably retaliates most vigorously when threatened. This species is the most difficult to handle in captivity. Brown Snakes usually like slightly warmer weather than most other snakes and are mainly diurnal.

Habitat and Distribution:

Found in a range of habitats, from dry areas to watercourse swamps, and

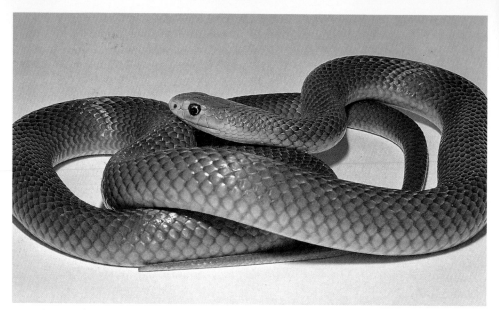

Figure 29a
Pseudonaja textilis

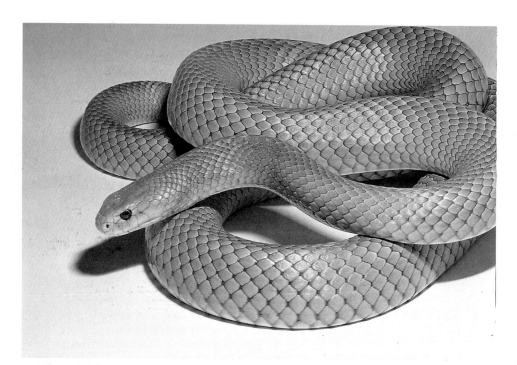

Figure 29b
Pseudonaja textilis

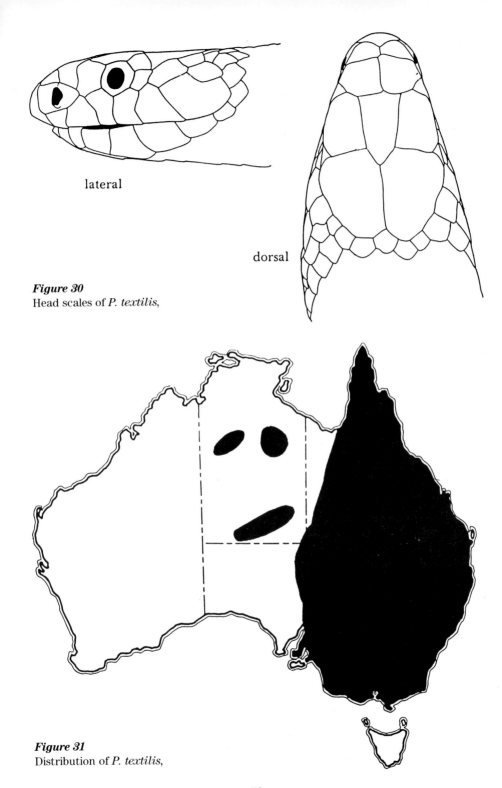

lateral

dorsal

Figure 30
Head scales of *P. textilis,*

Figure 31
Distribution of *P. textilis,*

have adapted to man-made changes to the environment. Brown Snakes are common in farmlands of the eastern States. Essentially, Brown Snakes prefer small lizards and frogs but have learnt to be extremely efficient hunters of introduced mice, *Mus musculus*.

Venom:

Common Brown Snakes kept at Venom Supplies Laboratories yield an average of 4.7 mg per milking As with most venomous snakes, the volume of venom produced, is largely dependent on the size of the snake. Worrell (1963), reports a milking of 41.4 mg from a 2.1 m specimen and Kellaway (1931), obtained 67.2 mg from a 2.1 m specimen. These records of Worrell and Kellaway are atypical. On average the Common Brown Snake yields a low volume of venom. Its generally accepted average yield is 4 mg.

Broad (1979), found the LD_{50} = 0.041 mg/kg making it more deadly than any other Australian snake except the Inland Taipan, and 12 times more toxic than the Indian Cobra *Naja naja*. Common Brown Snake venom is white in the dried lyophilized form.

Neurotoxins:

Textilotoxin, a presynaptic neurotoxin, is a very potent neurotoxin and with a molecular weight of 88,000. It represents 3% of the crude venom by weight.

Southcott and Coulter (1979), reported that textilotoxin acted on the prejunctional terminal by selectively blocking the release of acetycholine after the appearance of the action potential. This blockage had no effect on the resting membrane potential of the muscle cells, nor was the nerve conduction altered.

Sutherland (1983), reports (pers. comm. C.C.Chang 1981), "that textilotixin had direct presynaptic actions and no appreciable effect on muscle or acetylcholine receptors. The presynaptic blockade was due to the phospholipase A component of textilotoxin acting on the axolemma."

Hamilton et al (1980), showed that the crude venom produced "coated omega figures" in the axolemma of rat nerve terminals. Those figures are probably due to the action of the textilotoxin.

Barnett et al (1980), isolated a postsynaptic neurotoxin called pseudonajatoxin A. It has 117 amino acid residues and a molecular weight of 12,280. It causes irreversible blockade by firm binding to the acetylcholine receptors.

Coagulants:

Kellaway (1933), stated that *P. textilis* venom possessed a strong, highly diffusable coagulation factor. Denson (1969), concluded that the coagulation factor was a complete prothrombin activator. Masci et al (1988) found the prothrombin activator to be a major component of the venom with a high molecular weight of > 200,000. They found it was related antigenically to the prothrombin activator of *O. scutellatus* venom, able to activate citrated plasma, wartrin plasma, factor V and factor X deficient plasmas and will hydrolyse peptide p-nitroanilide substrate S-222. Ca^{++} and phospholipids have little effect on it. It was shown by Doery and Pearson (1961), that *P. textilis* venom was low in direct haemolytic properties and phospholipase A. Kaire (1964a), reported it had the least amount of heat stable anticoagulant than in any other Australian snakes.

Hyaluronidase:

Zeller (1948), found that P. textilis venom lacked hyaluronidase activity.

Myolytic Activity:

Sutherland (1983), stated there are no clinical reports of myoglobinuria resulting from *P. textilis* bites. Pearn et al (1981), reported negative findings of myolysis. Mebs and Samejima (1980), also failed to find any components in the venom that could produce myoglobinuria. These findings were also supported by Harris and Malten (1981).

Antivenom:

Brown Snake antivenom manufactured by Commonwealth Serum Laboratories (Melbourne).

INITIAL DOSE — 1,000 units

Coagulation defect, is a good guide to antivenom requirements. If near complete defibrination has occurred, use 3,000 units.

Sutherland (1983), reports that a toxoided *P. textilis* venom is available and appears satisfactory for animal use.

Common Brown Snake Bite Case History
Pseudonaja textilis (from Pearn et al 1981)

At 8.45 am on Tuesday, February 4, 1981, an experienced herpetologist, was cleaning the cage of a Common Brown Snake. This snake had laid a clutch of 33 eggs on December 8, 1980; it had last fed (two adult mice) on January 30, 1981, four days before the accident. The snake, an aggressive female 1.5 metres long, bit the herpetologist's right thumb in a single lighting strike, so quickly that there was doubt at the time that it had, in fact, struck. Two fang marks were clearly visible 30 minutes later. Immediately he was bitten, the victim applied the new first aid sequence, although the thumb itself was not covered (victim had been bitten three times in the preceding 36 months by different venomous elapids and, on each occasion, had received antivenom). The right arm was immediately ensheathed in a self applied compression bandage consisting of two rubber Esmarch's bandages, and the victim was transported to hospital by ambulance.

In hospital, the patient was given an intravenous infusion of dextrose saline. At 11 am, two hours after the bite, the patient was without any symptoms or signs of envenomation. Blood and urine samples were taken for venom assay, haematological studies, and assays, of fibrin degradation products.

The results of all investigations were within normal ranges. Immediately before the release of the compression bandage, 300 mg of hydrocortisone and 15 mg of promethazine were administered intravenously. Adrenalin was drawn up, and an experienced anaesthetist with intubation equipment was present. The compression bandage was then released. Within five minutes, the victim had developed a bursting headache, and felt nauseated. His pulse rate rose, he became very pale, and began to sweat profusely. The patient complained of an ache and tightness in his face and throat muscles, and his breathing felt subjectively "forced". (This may have been the result of postsynaptic neurotoxins). Fifteen minutes after the release of the compression bandage, the serum level of brown snake venom was 1.5 ng/ml. Thirty minutes after the release of the compression bandage, the level had risen to 4 ng/ml. After 45 minutes, venom was undetected in the serum, but urine sample obtained at this stage contained 5 ng/ml of venom.

One hour after the release of the compression bandage, one ample (50 ml) of CSL brown snake antivenom, mixed with 50 ml of dextrose saline was administered intravenously over a period of 30 minutes with no side effects (a second ampule was given one hour later as symptoms appeared to be increasing in intensity). Brown snake venom (0.5 ng/ml) was detected in the urine 5½ hours later after the bite, and two hours after the antivenom had been administered. An hour later, venom could no longer be detected in the urine. Serum creatine kinase level on the day after the accident was 45 u/L (normal range, 35u/L to 210 u/L); serum level of fibrin degradation products rose progressively from one hour after release of the tourniquet to a maximum of 1,280 ug/ml (normal range, below 10 ug/ml); thrombin clotting time rose within 50 minutes after release of the tourniquet to a maximum of greater than 60 seconds (normal range, 12 to 18 seconds); and the prothrombin time rose to 50 seconds within three hours after release of constrictive bandage (normal range, 12 to 15 seconds). Coagulation and defibrination indices were still abnormal 24 hours later.

Within six hours of administration of the first dose of antivenom, the victim was subjectively well and, apart from some feeling of weakness, especially involving the muscles of the face and throat, was without specific symptoms. He was discharged from hospital 36 hours later.

The subsequent course was uneventful, with no evidence of any rash or serum sickness. Some soreness remained in his facial muscles for several weeks thereafter. The patient had returned to work within six days.

As a result of this bite, the authors (Pearn et al) concluded that the recommended first aid for snake bite in Australia was substantiated. They also demonstrated here that "if symptoms or signs of envenomation develop, antivenom should be administered immediately in standard fashion."

Summary of Symptoms and Conditions Experienced with *Pseudonaja textilis* Bites

— Severe headache.
— Tachycardia.
— Pallor.
— Profuse sweating.
— Tightness of face and throat muscles.
— Breathing difficulties.
— Vomiting.
— Nausea.
— Abdominal pain.
— Increased respirations.
— Giddiness.
— High bowel evacuation.
— Bilateral ptosis, bulbar affection.
— Paralysis of tongue.
— Dilated pupils.
— Weakness.
— Cyanosis.
— Spasms.
— Stertorous breathing.
— Bleeding at bite site.
— Loss of consciousness.
— Haematuria.
— Haematemesis.
— Blood pigment in urine.
— Elevated FDP.
— Elevated clotting time.
— Prothrombin time elevated.

Peninsula Brown Snake *Pseudonaja inframacula* (Waite)

Description:

Similar in shape to Common Brown Snake. Slender body, head indistinct from body.

Scalation:

VENTRALS	190-205
SUBCAUDALS	52-62 divided
MID-BODIES	17 rows
ANAL	Divided

Colour:

Adult specimens range from light brown, dark brown, to almost black

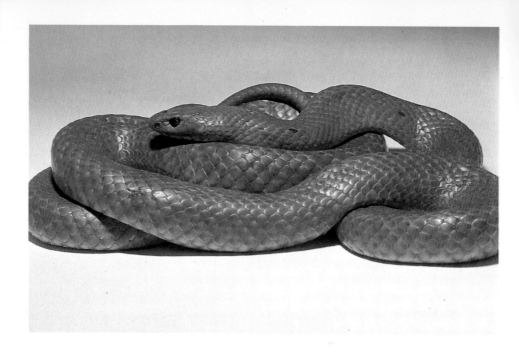

Figure 32
Pseudonaja inframacula

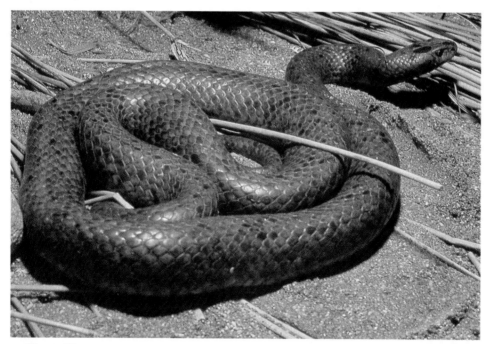

Figure 33
Pseudonaja inframacula

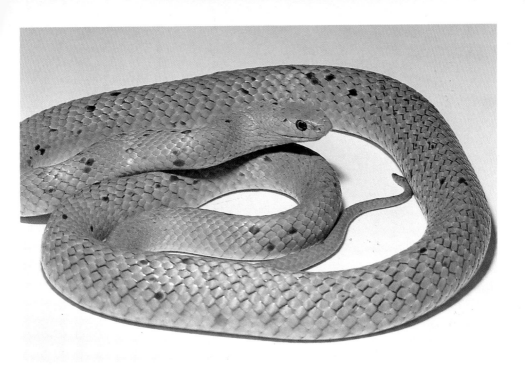

Figure 34
Pseudonaja inframacula

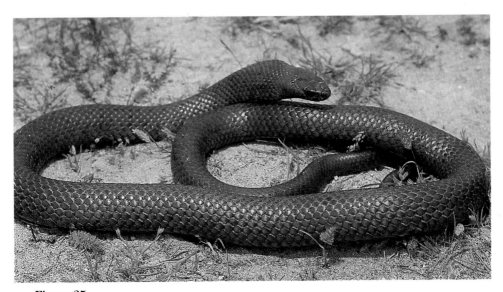

Figure 35
Pseudonaja inframacula

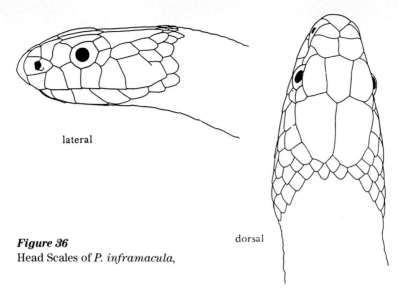

lateral

dorsal

Figure 36
Head Scales of *P. inframacula,*

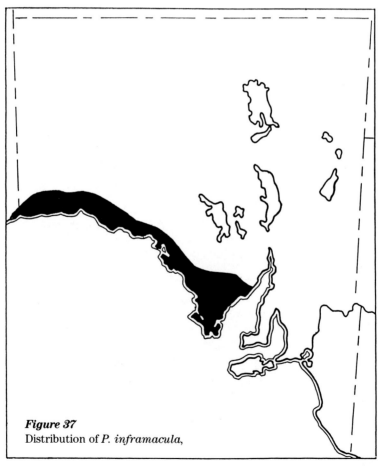

Figure 37
Distribution of *P. inframacula,*

dorsally, with grey ventral surface. Darker spots are often scattered randomly along the dorsal surface. Juveniles are usually a light tan colour. (Fig 32-35)

Habits:

Essentially a sun-loving snake, it is active in the warmer months except for days of extremely high temperature. Its dark colour enables it to be more active on cooler days than the Common Brown Snake and is probably an adaptation to the less favorable weather patterns of the more southern areas. On warm cloudy days it is not uncommon to find them basking, their dark colour optimising radiation absorption. Oviparous, producing 12-20 eggs.

Habitat and Distribution:

Generally coastal dunes and coastal farmlands of southern Eyre Peninsula. It is found on Wardang Island. Not found more than 100 km from the coastline. Very common in the Coffin Bay National Park.

Notes:

Like other Brown Snakes, it has adapted well to man's environmental changes. In fact, adult specimens, while possibly less abundant in farmed areas than virgin areas, appear to grow larger and more robust and are less affected by tick parasites. A contributory factor to their adaptation would be the abundance of pest mice, *Mus musculus* in these areas.

In temperament, the Peninsula Brown Snake in contrast to other *Pseudonaja*, is usually a very quiet snake. It is quick to retreat when approached, and if caught, its adaptation to captivity is rapid, provided an acceptable food is supplied.

The snake was elevated to species status by Mengden (1985). It was previously known as a sub-species of *Pseudonaja textilis*.

Venom:

Sutherland (1983), records that little is known about the venom. Mirtschin (1982), was bitten by a *Pseudonaja inframacula* and it caused profound sweating and breathing difficulties.

Specimens kept at Venom Supplies Laboratories yield 1.7 mg of dried venom. The dried lyophilized venom is white.

Antivenom:

Brown Snake antivenom — manufactured by the Commonwealth Serum Laboratories (Melbourne).

INITIAL DOSE — 1,000 units.

Western Brown Snake (Gwardar, Collared Brown Snake)
Pseudonaja nuchalis (Gunther)
Description:

Long slender snake, head indistinct from neck, head shorter than for

Common Brown Snake. Buccal cavity bluish-black for Northern Territory specimens (Gillam 1979). Iris red.

Mengden (1985a), found that *Pseudonaja nuchalis* contains seven different karyomorphs, three of which have different diploid numbers. He also identified nine different colour morphs.

Scalation:

Smooth scales, very shiny around head and neck. Rostral scale enlarged and strap-like; extends backwards slightly towards top of head. Head chisel-shaped when viewed from above.

VENTRALS	180-230
SUBCAUDALS	50-70 divided
MID-BODIES	17 or 19
ANAL	Divided

Colour:

Colour is highly variable. Base colour varies from yellow to pitch black. Many specimens have black markings around head or neck. Banded individuals are not uncommon. Most specimens have random spots over whole body. (Figs 38-39).

Banks (1981) and Mirtschin (1983a), have recorded seasonal colour changes in Western Brown Snakes. They tend to change to lighter colours in warmer months.

Habits:

Fast-moving, alert, mostly diurnal but occasionally nocturnal. Prefers warmer weather. Lizards form the bulk of the diet, but European mice, *Mus musculus* are now a favorite preference. Will occasionally eat small birds.

Less vigorous than the Common Brown Snake when annoyed. Oviparous, laying about 20 eggs.

Habitat and Distribution:

Lives in the drier parts of Australia and in tropical Northern Territory and part of Queensland. Due to its wide distribution and its ability to adapt to changed environments, it is one of Australia's most abundant snake.

Food:

In captivity they will feed on lizards, mice, rats and birds.

Venom:

P. nuchalis from Eyre Peninsula kept and milked at Venom Supplies Laboratories yield on average 6.5 mg of dried venom. The dried lyophilized venom is white.

Broad et al (1979) record the LD_{50} = 0.338.

Davey (1969), showed the crude venom converted prothrombin to

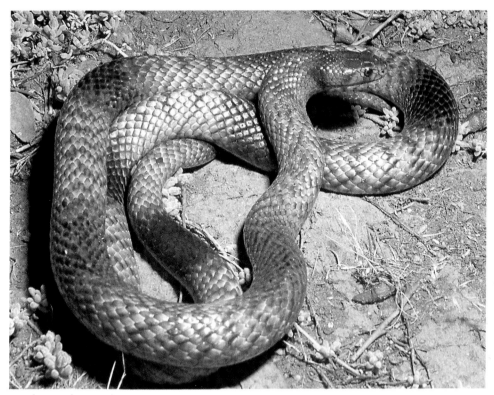

Figure 38
Pseudonaja nuchalis

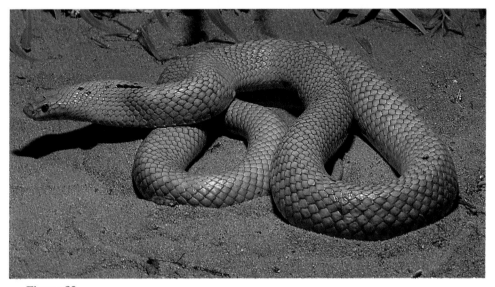

Figure 39
Pseudonaja nuchalis

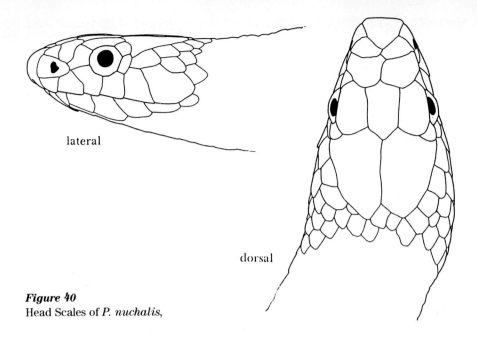

lateral

dorsal

Figure 40
Head Scales of *P. nuchalis,*

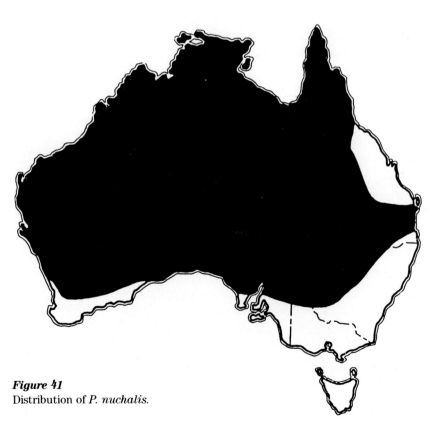

Figure 41
Distribution of *P. nuchalis.*

thrombin in the absence of co-factors. He also showed that brown snake antivenom prevented this reaction.

Sutherland et al (1981a), found that a single monkey injected with this venom developed marked ptosis and muscle weakness after 155 minutes. Full recovery after 310 minutes was evident after 460 units of brown snake antivenom. The monkey developed marked coagulopathy with a normal partial thromboplastin time of 31 seconds to 88 seconds, 150 minutes after administration of the venom. Fifty-five minutes after receiving antivenom, the coagulopathy remained the same. Sutherland (1983), suggests this is either due to the coagulation defect produced by this venom being more severe than with *P. textilis* or the venom procoagulant not being neutralised as well by brown snake antivenom.

A Venom Supplies worker also experienced this prolonged coagulopathy after being bitten by a *P. nuchalis*. He received three ampoules of antivenom before his clotting times reached normal levels. Another factor involved in this bite, was that administration of antivenom was delayed.

Cogger (1983), notes that since there are many different populations of *P. nuchalis* treatment of bites with monovalent brown snake antivenom, *P. textilis*, could require greater quantities of antivenom. It is also possible that current antivenoms are ineffective for some populations of this species.

Mengden's work (1985a), confirms the diversity within the *P. nuchalis* species. Given the evidence supporting the difficulty treating bites from this species, and the large range they inhabit, there is a suggestion that further work should be done to provide accelerated treatment of these bites.

Antivenom:

Brown snake antivenom — manufactured by the Commonwealth Serum Laboratories (Melbourne).

INITIAL DOSE — 1,000 units.

Western Brown Snake Bite Case Histories
Pseudonaja nuchalis **Case·1**
(from Chester and Crawford 1980)

This case confirms that even an immature *P. nuchalis* should be regarded as highly dangerous.

A healthy 57-year-old farmer was bitten by a snake on the side of his uncovered foot. He killed the snake and the same day attended the regional hospital. The snake was identified as a Brown snake and first aid and 1,000 units of Brown snake antivenom were given. The patient was transferred to Perth. No neurological symptoms were noted only minimal discomfort occurred at the site of the bite. Haemorrhage occurred from venepuncture sites. Afibrinogenaemia was present and, as expected, the prothrombin time and partial thromboplastin time were grossly prolonged. Factor assays performed by standard one-stage methods were as follows: XII-14%; XI-85%; IX-44%; VIII-6.5%; VII-76%; V-18.5%; II-28%.

Platelet count was normal. Fibrinogen degradation products were markedly elevated. Spherocytes were present in the blood film and intravascular haemolysis was confirmed by the presence of haemoglobinuria, reduced haptoglobin concentration and hyperbilirubinaemia without bilirubinuria. Myoglobinuria was not detected spectrophotometrically. The patient recovered uneventfully after 2,000 units of Brown snake antivenom. The dead snake was subsequently identified at the Western Australian Museum as a Gwarder. The estimated length of the snake was some 0.3 m.

Case 2
P. nuchalis Snake Bite (from a case treated at the Whyalla Hospital).

The patient was bitten in Whyalla by a large 1.4 m Western Brown snake on the back of the hand between the thumb and forefinger while attempting to milk it. There was a history of previous snake bite from *Acanthophis antarcticus* and *Pseudechis australis,* however neither of these were eventful.

Admission at the Whyalla hospital occurred about 12 minutes after the bite. Pressure/immobilisation first aid had been applied immediately after the bite. After arrival at the hospital, he was given antihistamine and a blood sample was taken for testing in a venom detection kit. The test proved negative. The compressive bandage was gradually removed after which no symptoms developed and he was allowed to go home. A couple of hours later he was readmitted in a collapsed state.

He developed respiratory paralysis and required ventilating and he had grossly abnormal coagulation studies with a prothrombin ratio of 10.5 and FDP of greater than 40. His initial APPT was also greater than 100.

He required a large dose of antivenom (4 ampoules) in order to reverse this situation but made a good recovery and fortunately did not develop any signs of renal failure. He was given tetanus toxoid before discharge.

Comments:

(i)   The patient should have been kept at the hospital for at least 24 hours after a bite from a dangerous snake.

(ii)   A negative finding using the V.D.K. does not exclude envenomation, especially if the first aid is effective.

Summary of Symptoms and Conditions Experienced with Pseudonaja nuchalis Bites.

— Haemorrhage from venepuncture.
— Afibrinogenaemia — prothrombin time elevated
                            — thromboplastin time elevated
— Hypotension.
— FDP elevated.
— Spherocytes in the blood film.
— Intravascular haemolysis.

- Reduced haptoglobin.
- Hyperbilirubinaemia without bilirubinuria.
- Headache.
- Unconsciousness.
- Heavy perspiration.
- Enlarged auxiliary lymph node.
- Weakness.
- Bite site itchy.

Speckled Brown Snake *Pseudonaja guttata* (Parker)

Description:

Grows to about 1.4 m. Buccal cavity dark bluish (Gillam 1979).

Scalation:

Smooth scales.

VENTRALS	190-220
SUBCAUDALS	44-70 divided
MID-BODIES	19-21
ANAL	Divided

Colour:

Yellow or olive to apricot with black nicks to the sides of many of the dorsal scales. Some specimens possess dark broad bands. The ventral surface is from white to yellow which is blotched with orange (Gillam 1979). (Figs 42 & 43)

Habits:

A diurnal snake about which little is known.

Habitat and Distribution:

Restricted to blacksoil plains.

Notes:

M. Gillam (1979), records that 40% of specimens examined in the Northern Territory have had parts of their tails missing. This is possibly due to their habit of leaving the tails partly exposed while seeking refuge in ground cracks. Threat attitude is a simple low arching of the nect in one bend with the section from head to the bend being flattened. J. Bredl and B. Miller (pers. com.) have recorded a juvenile *P. guttata* being regurgitated by a Curl Snake, *Suta suta* from the Goyders Lagoon on the Diamantina River.

Food:

Captive specimens prefer lizards to mammals.

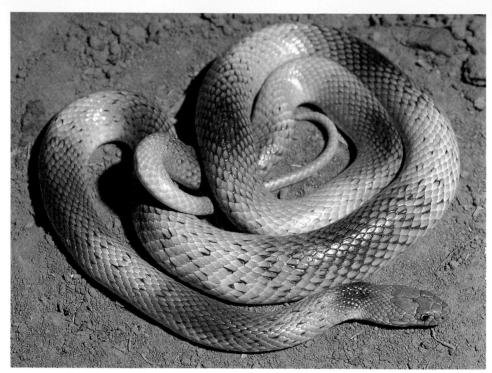

Figure 42
Pseudonaja guttata (Photo M. Gillam)

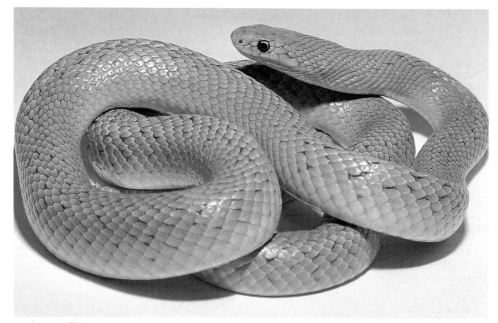

Figure 43
Pseudonaja guttata

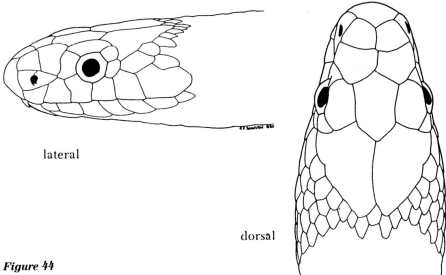

lateral

dorsal

Figure 44
Head scales of *P. guttata,*

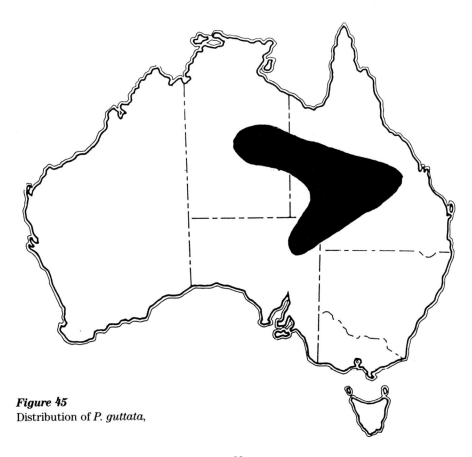

Figure 45
Distribution of *P. guttata,*

Venom:

Sutherland (1983), recorded an $LD_{50} = 0.36$.

Worrell (1963), recorded a yield of 3 mg.

Mirtschin (1982), recorded a yield of 0.5 mg from records of Howell and Naylor.

Antivenom:

Brown snake antivenom — manufactured by the Commonwealth Serum Laboratories (Melbourne).

INITIAL DOSE — 1,000 units.

Dugite *Pseudonaja affinis* (Gunther)

Description:

Similar to the Western Brown Snake but has a rounded snout rather than the chisel-shaped rostral when viewed from above. Rostral not strap-like. Grows to 2 metres.

Scalation:

Smooth scales.

VENTRALS	190-230
SUBCAUDALS	50-70 divided
MID-BODIES	19
ANAL	Divided

Colour:

Dark brown, olive, tan usually liberally marked with irregular black scales. Ventral surface is grayish white. (Fig 46, 47)

Habits:

Similar to other Brown Snakes. Oviparous with average clutch of 20 eggs.

Habitat and Distribution:

Coastal southern Western Australia and into South Australia. Occurs in metropolitan area of Perth. Dry sclerophyll and mallee.

Notes:

Feeds on lizards and mice.

Venom:

Sutherland (1983), recorded the average venom yield to be 5.7 mg with the highest record being 17 mg.

Broad et al (1979), found that the $LD_{50} = 0.56$.

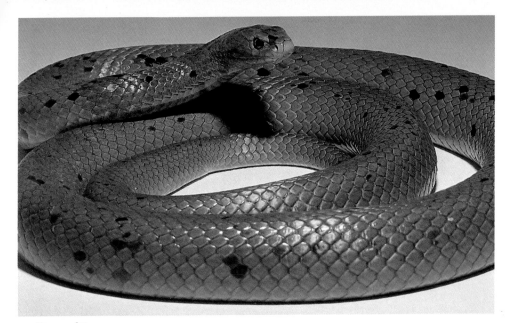

Figure 46
Pseudonaja affinis

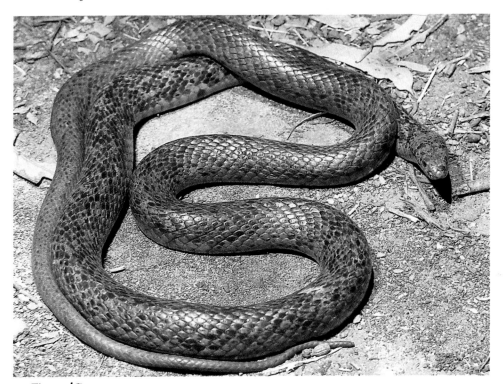

Figure 47
Pseudonaja affinis

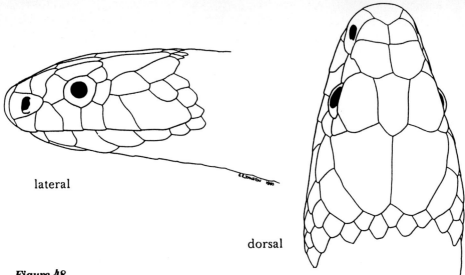

lateral

dorsal

Figure 48
Head scales of *P. affinis,*

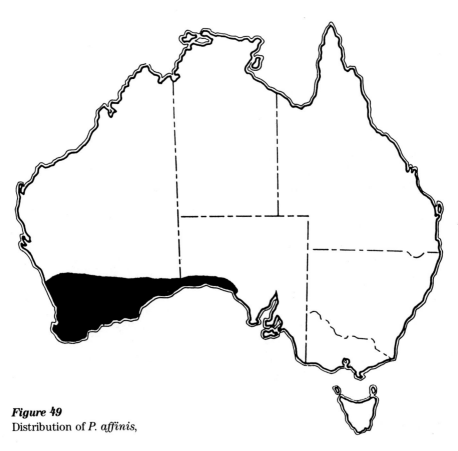

Figure 49
Distribution of *P. affinis,*

Sutherland (1983), reports that the venom is strongly neurotoxic. According to Davey (1969), an increase in blood clotting time occurs to the point where it may become incoagulable. By depletion of Factor II, V and VIII, afibrinogenaemia may be almost complete. There is no evidence of effect on erythrocytes or platelets.

Sutherland (1983), in an experiment with a single monkey, showed that the PTT extended from a normal 28 seconds to 42 seconds after 180 minutes at which time antivenom was administered. The PTT continued to rise after antivenom administration to 62 seconds at 210 minutes. Sutherland concluded that the antivenom may have difficulty in completely neutralising the procoagulant fraction in the venom. Elevation of the CK level to 2086 IU/l at 210 minutes from a normal 118 IU/l also occurred indicating some myotoxic activity.

Antivenom:

Brown Snake antivenom — manufactured by Commonwealth Serum Laboratories (Melbourne).

INITIAL DOSE — 1,000 units.

Tanners Brown Snake *Pseudonaja tanneri* (Worrell)
Description:

Grows to 1 metre.

Scalation:

Smooth scales.

VENTRALS	190-230
SUBCAUDALS	50-70 divided
MID-BODIES	19
ANAL	Divided

Colour:

Chestnut brown to black. (Fig. 50)

Habits:

Unknown.

Habitat and Distribution:

Occurs on islands of Recherche Archipelago, south-west Western Australia. Specimens from Rottnest Island are for the time being included as this sub-species.

Venom:

Unknown but considered to be dangerous because of the snake's size.

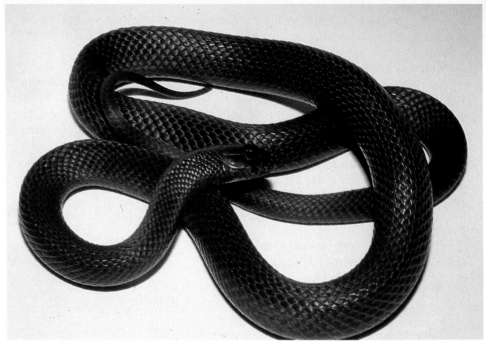

Figure 50
Pseudonaja tanneri (Photo S. Wilson)

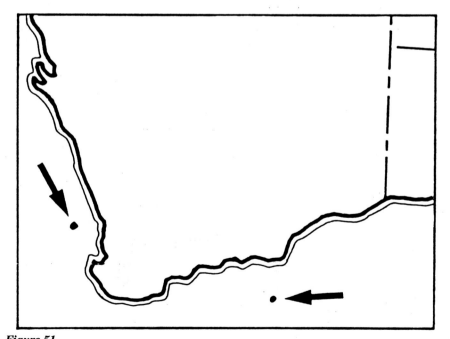

Figure 51
Distribution of *Pseudonaja affinis tanneri.*

74

Antivenom:

Brown Snake antivenom — manufactured by the Commonwealth Serum Laboratories (Melbourne).

INITIAL DOSE — 1,000 units.

Ingrams Brown Snake *Pseudonaja ingrami* (Boulenger)

Description:

Status uncertain. Buccal cavity predominantly black. Iris indistinct —entire eye appears to be black superficially. Largest specimen known 1.76 metres.

Scalation:

Smooth scales.

VENTRALS	190-220
SUBCAUDALS	55-70 divided
MID-BODIES	17
ANAL	Divided

Colour:

Gillam (1979), lists five colour forms:

1   glossy black brown
2   dark brown anteriorly, golden brown posteriorly
3   uniform golden brown
4   head and nape grey brown to dark brown body light to rich yellow brown
5   pale olive brown

Scales in all forms are darker at tips. (Fig 52)

Habits:

Diurnal. Preys predominantly on small mammals, mainly rats and mice, especially the long-haired rat, *Rattus villosissimus* and European mouse, *Mus musculus*.

Habitat and Distribution:

Seeks refuge in deep earth cracks. Black soil plains subject to seasonal flooding. Barkly Tableland.

Notes:

Activity mostly in early morning from 8 am to 10.30 am. Gillam (1979), justifies species as distinct from *P. textilis* by iris colour, buccal cavity colour, and number of infralabials. Forty-five percent of specimens examined by Gillam had damaged tails or up to 10% missing. This could be due to their habit of leaving their tails partially exposed when they seek refuge in ground cracks.

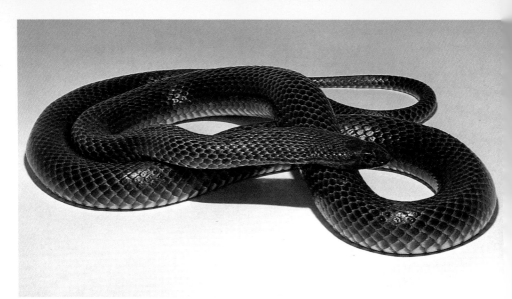

Figure 52
Pseudonaja ingrami

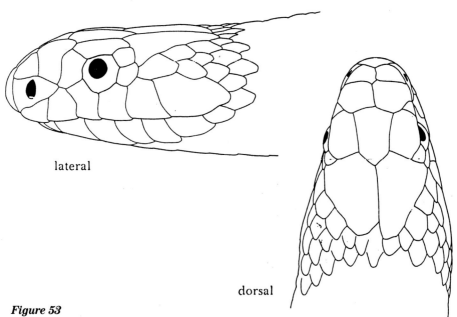

lateral

dorsal

Figure 53
Head scales of *P. ingrami,*

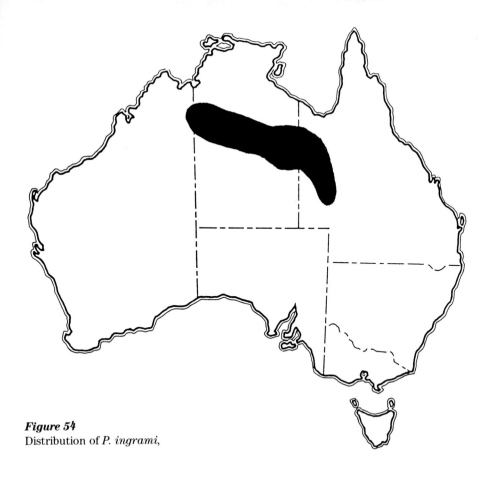

Figure 54
Distribution of *P. ingrami,*

Gillam suggests this is due to predation as snakes leave their tails partially exposed after entering cracks in the ground.

Venom:
Nothing known at this stage but assumed to be dangerous because of the snake's size.

Antivenom:
Brown Snake antivenom — manufactured by the Commonwealth Serum Laboratories (Melbourne).

INITIAL DOSE — 1,000 units.

The Taipans
The Taipans (genus *Oxyuranus)* are the largest Australian dangerous snakes with long heads, distinct from the slender neck, and distinguished from other snakes by scalation, dentition, hemipenis structure and venom.

Two species occur in Australia. They have some similar physical and ecological features, but their habitat preferences are quite different.

Taipan *Oxyuranus scutellatus* (Peters)
Description:

Large rectangular shaped head, narrow neck, cylindrical body and red eyes. Taipans have been recorded up to 2.8 metres in length. Fangs range from 7.9 mm — 12.1 mm in length. Taipan fangs are long in comparison to the other elapid fangs and the lower jaw has small sockets for the fangs to project through the jaw when the mouth is closed.

Scalation:

Dorsal scales feebly keeled (especially on the neck and the vertebral region) to smooth and small on the neck.

VENTRALS	220-250
SUBCAUDALS	45-80 divided
MID-BODIES	21-23
ANAL	Single

Colour:

Taipans always exhibit a pale creamish colour around the head. The heads of juveniles are predominantly pale, but the head darkens so that only the front remains pale in mature Taipans. Dorsally, Taipans have been recorded in colours of light brown, dark brown to black, coppery red, and olive. They have been recorded to undergo seasonal colour variation (Banks, 1981; Mirtschin, 1983) changing to lighter colours during summer. (Fig 55, 56, 57)

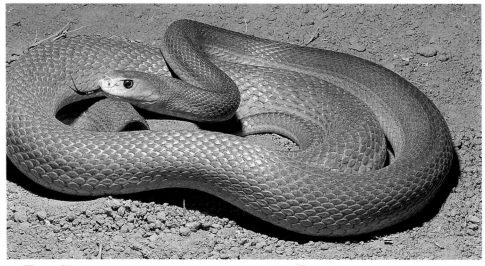

Figure 55
Oxyuranus scutellatus

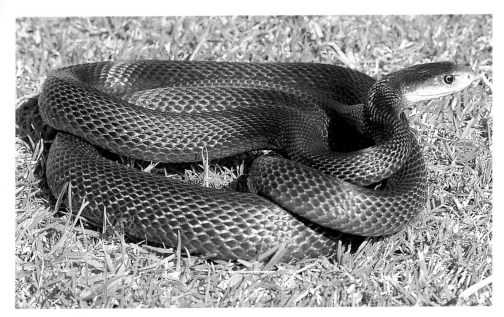

Figure 56
Oxyuranus scutellatus

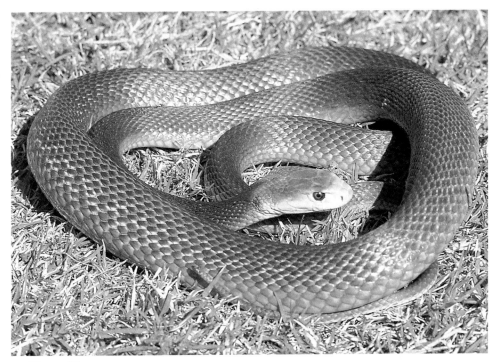

Figure 57
Oxyuranus scutellatus

Habits:

From observations in captivity, the Taipan is an efficient hunter, with a lightning strike, an acute sense of smell and extremely acute eyesight. It moves rapidly in on its prey, strikes, retracts slightly and waits for the venom to immobilise its victim, thus increasing its chance of success without injury to itself from the prey animal. In a defensive situation, the Taipan will often bite more than once. Taipans are oviparous, producing 7-20 eggs. They occasionally lay 2 clutches of eggs in quick succession Mirtschin (1986) with less than 2 months between clutches. Male combat has been observed with specimens kept in captivity. Of all the Australian Snakes, the Taipan is the most intelligent, nervous and alert.

Habitat and Distribution:

The wetter coastal areas of Queensland, the Northern Territory and Western Australia, with 800 - 1600 mm rainfall. Does not occur where average maximum winter temperature falls below 18°C. The Taipan prefers undulating country, but on Cape York Peninsula inhabits open woodland areas. Introduced lantana is also a favoured habitat. The sugar cane fields in Queensland abound with rats, *Rattus rattus* and *Melomys*, which provide an excellent food source.

Notes:

Because of the Taipan's keen senses, they will generally retreat if they have the chance, and consequently they are rarely encountered by humans. In the unfortunate cases where people have been bitten by Taipans, usually the snake has been approached suddenly or was cornered and felt threatened. In these circumstances, Taipans viciously defend themselves, often inflicting multiple bites.

Food:

Rats, especially *Melomys (spp)* are the preferred food of Taipans. However, small birds, mice, bandicoots and lizards are all recorded as food items. Covacevich and Shine (1983), have suggested that the introduction of the cane toad, *Bufo marinus* in the range of the Taipan, has allowed it to increase in population. This happened as a result of other elapid species being displaced as they preyed on and succombed to the poisonous cane toad. Taipans have no preference for amphibians.

The destruction of rat population by poisoning in the sugar cane areas potentially could affect Taipan numbers. Also, the habitat destruction due to erosion and soil degradation by the sugar industry may also have a long term effect.

Venom:

Taipans kept at Venom Supplies Laboratories yield about 120 mg of dried

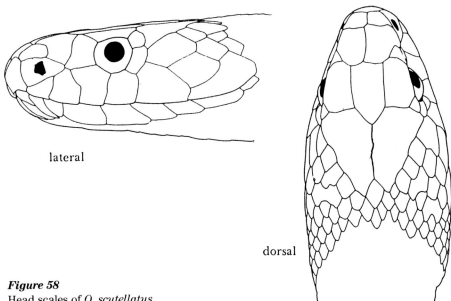

lateral

dorsal

Figure 58
Head scales of *O. scutellatus,*

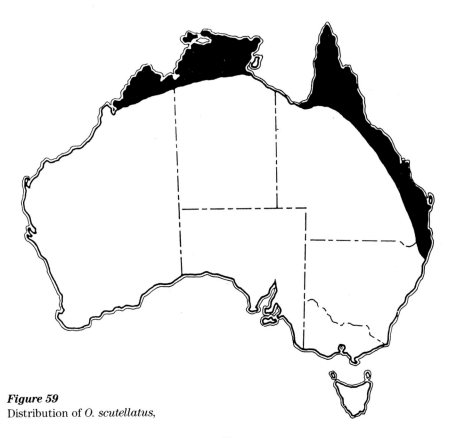

Figure 59
Distribution of *O. scutellatus,*

81

venom. The dried lyophilized venom has a slight pink coloration. Trinca (1969), records the maximum yield for a single Taipan to be 400 mg of dried venom.

Broad (1979), found that the crude venom had a $LD_{50} = 0.064$ mg/kg.

Neurotoxins:

Fohlman et al (1979), isolated a potent presynaptic neurotoxin called taipoxin with a molecular weight of 45,600. It was shown to have three sub-units, and with only the sub-unit producing neurotoxic activity.

Cull-Candy et al (1976), showed that taipoxin caused omega-shaped indentations in the axolemma at the motor nerve end plates and suggested the toxin interferes with the recycling of synaptic vesicles resulting in the neuromuscular block. A postsynaptic neurotoxin was found by Mebs et al (1979).

Myotoxin:

Harris et al (1977), showed that taipoxin was also myotoxic. Sutherland (1979b), demonstrated a marked elevation of plasma creatine kinase after 120 minutes in monkeys injected with the crude venom. Brigden and Sutherland (1981), confirmed experimental results, when myoglobinuria was detected in a snake bite victim.

Coagulants:

Denson (1969) and (1971) showed that unlike Tiger Snake venom, Taipan venom was a complete prothrombin activator and could be used as a one-staged prothrombin assay.

Pirkle et al (1972), confirmed the results of Denson, but in contrast, found the yield of thrombin to be independent of venom concentration. They also found that within wide limits of sample dilution and incubation time, the method was consistent.

Aronson et al (1984), found that a crude Taipan venom prothrombin assay, could measure prothrombin 2 if a small amount of serum was present.

Denson (1976), showed that Taipan venom was about a 1,000 times stronger prothrombin activator than that of *Echis carinatus* venom in the presence of Ca^{++}. Walker et al (1980), demonstrated that the venom contained a specific hydrolase which can hydrolyze the factor Xa substrate S2222 while not hydrolyzing the thrombin (S2160) or plasmin (S2251) substrates. They also, proposed that a protease was directly involved in the prothrombin activities.

Other Components:

Kaire (1964), found a heat stable anticoagulant in Taipan venom. Phospholipase A was found by Doery and Pearson (1961), but little haemolytic activity was recorded. Tu et al (1965), noted peptidase activity in Taipan venom.

Hyaluronidase activity is recorded for this venom and averages 7.5 units/mg. (Broad et al 1979).

Antivenom:

Taipan antivenom — manufactured by the Commonwealth Serum Laboratories (Melbourne).

INITIAL DOSE — 12,000 units.

Coastal Taipan Case Histories
Oxyuranus scutellatus
Case 1 (from Sutherland 1980b)

At 9 am on October 4, 1979, a 4-year-old boy was playing under trees near his home at Kindura Beach, some 30 miles north Townsville. Shortly after 9 am, the child walked up to his aunt complaining that he was tired. He vomited the water she gave him to drink and then collapsed. Help was summoned and mouth-to-mouth resuscitation was commenced with no response. The child was declared dead at the Townsville General Hospital at 10.15 am.

At post-mortem examination, 12 puncture marks were noted, eight on the anteromedial aspect of the right upper thigh and four on the right buttock. No specific findings were made other than acute venom congestion of most organs. Samples of skin and subcutaneous fat from the bitten area and whole blood were sent to Melbourne for venom analysis.

The tissues were found to be saturated with Taipan *(Oxyuranus scutellatus)* venom. When the radioimmunoassay method was used, approximately 2 mg of venom/g of tissue was detected. The rapid enzyme immunoassay (EIA) was positive of both Taipan venom and Eastern Brown snake *(Pseudonaja textilis)* venom when undiluted extracts were tested. This false positive result for Brown snake venom was eliminated by appropriate dilution of the sample.

As a result of this finding, it was recommended that in areas of Queensland and the Northern Territory where these two species coexist, samples tested by EIA should be examined both in the concentrated and well-diluted state. Although this cross-reaction is found when high concentrations of venom are present, there is no cross-protection between the two antivenoms. Hence clinically it is important to distinguish between the two venoms and this can be achieved by an appropriate dilution step.

Since it has been estimated that 120 mg of Taipan venom could kill 12,000 adult guinea pigs, it is not surprising that a small child receiving the multiple bites (and hence more venom) in a highly vascular area should succumb so rapidly.

Unfortunately, circumstances did not allow the use on this child of the recommended first-aid measures, but the case clearly indicates the necessity for prompt safe first-aid measures in snakebite. Such recommended measures should be maintained until the patient has come under adequate medical care.

This case demonstrates the extreme urgency involved in first-aid application and subsequent antivenom treatment involved in bites from this species.

Case 2

Oxyuranus scutellatus Snake Bite (from Brigden and Sutherland 1981)

On 10 April 1980, a 39-year-old tobacco farmer presented to Mareeba Hospital, Queensland, with a history of nausea and vomiting for 1 hour. Some 48 hours earlier he had eaten the contents of a tin of savoury mince.

The morning before admission, he had been out on his farm, working barefoot. Six hours after admission he developed fixed dilated pupils and bilateral ptosis. Progressive muscle paralysis developed rapidly, involving the respiratory muscles, and necessitated intubation and artificial ventilation. He was transferred to Cairns Base Hospital with a provisional diagnosis of acute botulism.

On arrival at Cairns Base Hospital he was totally paralysed. Pupils were fixed and dilated, tone was flaccid and tendon reflexes were absent. He was afebrile, his pulse was 90 beats per minute, and his blood pressure 22.7 kPa/15.3 kPa (170 mmHg/115 mmhg). Examination of his chest and abdomen showed nothing abnormal. There was no ecchymoses or petechiae. There were no obvious puncture marks, although his feet were covered with cuts, grazes and minor trauma. Investigations on admission demonstrated a marked leucocytosis, and laboratory investigations showed a severe coagulopathy. On this evidence it was felt that snake bite was the most likely diagnosis, occurring between 6 am and 9 am that day, unnoticed by the patient.

He was given 4 units of polyvalent antivenom, after blood and urine samples had been taken for specific venom assay. Over the next twelve hours he became hypotensive and oliguric. Further investigations the next day showed a markedly elevated creatine phosphokinase (19,600 IU/l) and reversal of his coagulopathy. He was maintained for 19 days on mechanical ventilatory support, hyper-alimentation and peritoneal dialysis, being discharged with no residual problems 27 days after admission.

The results of venom assay on serum performed in Cairns were negative. Assays performed at the Commonwealth Serum Laboratories in Melbourne on the serum samples also gave negative results, but a urine sample was strongly positive for Taipan *(Oxyuranus scutellatus)* venom. Myoglobin was also present in this urine sample. Investigations by the Commonwealth Pathology Laboratory in Cairns of the savoury mince from the suspected can, and of unopened cans of savoury mince from the same batch code, proved negative for botulinus toxin and *Clostridium botulinum*. This finding was confirmed by the Commonwealth Institute of Health, Sydney.

This case demonstrates the difficulties sometimes experienced in diagnosing snake bite on accounts given by the patient. The victim emphatically denied having been bitten by a snake.

Summary of Symptoms and Conditions Experienced with Oxyuranus scutellatus Bites

— Vomiting.
— Collapse.
— Venous congestion of organs.

84

— Nausea.
— Fixed dilated pupils.
— Bilateral ptosis.
— Muscle paralysis
  respiratory muscles paralysis.
— Flaccid tone.
— Absence of tendon reflexes.
— Weakness of masseter muscles.
— Weakness of sterno-mastoid muscles.
— Afebrile.
— Coagulopathy.
— Hypotension.
— Oliguria.
— Elevated creatine phosphokinase.
— Presence of myoglobin in urine.
— Blurred vision.
— Severe headache.
— Tachycardia.
— Swollen bite site.
— Salivation.
— Cyanosis.
— Rigor.
— Local necrosis.
— Pallor.
— Drowsiness.
— Abdominal pain.
— Oozing of blood at bite site.
— Diplopia.
— Albumin in urine.

Inland Taipan *Oxyuranus microlepidotus* (McCoy)

Description:

Large snake up to 2.5 metres, averaging about 2 metres. Narrow neck similar to the Taipan but more robust. Head shape long and rectangular like a Taipan, but slightly shorter with a greater slope from the frontal scale to the rostral. The black eyes of the Inland Taipan are smaller in proportion to those of the Taipan. Fang length is 3.5 — 6 mm whereas in the Taipan (*O. scutellatus*), it is 7.9 — 12.1 mm.

Scalation:

Smooth scales. Small dorsal neck scales.

VENTRALS	211-250
SUBCAUDALS	52-70 divided
MID-BODIES	23
ANAL	Single

Colour:

Nearly all specimens have a dark brown to black head. Some have lighter coloured heads. Dorsal coloration pale to dark brown with dark flecks that often form distinct bands posteriorly. Ventrals surface yellow. Seasonal colour changes have been recorded. (Mirtschin 1983) (Figs 60, 61)

Habits:

Very little is known about this snake since it occurs in a remote part of Australia and is rarely observed. Its ecology is thought to be closely associated with the occurrence of the Plague Rat, *Rattus villosissimus*, on which it feeds (Mirtschin 1981). It has a similar prey catching technique to the Taipan, *O. scutellatus*, in that it strikes, then holds back until the prey succumbs to the venom. Compared with other venomous snakes, it is fairly placid in nature.

Habitat and Distribution:

Occurs in dry area of less than 300 mm average annual rainfall and average maximum winter temperature of about 18°C. Occurs in the Channel country of south-west Queensland and the north-east of South Australia. It has been collected from blacksoil plains and flood plains where it lives in solution holes (Mirtschin 1982), gibbers, and sand dunes. It appears that areas of greatest population occur on or near the flood plains and channels of the Diamantina River and Copper Creek. Major vegetation in the area is low saltbush, giant saltbush *(Altriplex nummularia)*, and lignum bush.

Notes:

The Inland Taipan has also been known as the Western Taipan, Fierce Snake, Small-scaled Snake and Lignum Snake. Similarly, the generic history of the snake has been just as unstable. Originally it was referred to as *Diemenia microlepidota* by McCoy in 1879. Since then it has been called one of the Brown Snakes *(Pseudonaja)* and more recently in 1976 it was described by Covacevich et al as *Parademansia microlepidotus* (Covacevich and Wombey 1976). Covacevich et al (1980), defined the Taipan and the Inland Taipan as congeneric on the basis of the external and cranial morphology, venom, head musculature, hemipenis structure, behaviour and karyotyping.

The original specimens were collected at the junction of the Murray and Darling Rivers before 1879. All other known specimens are from the Channel country of the Diamantina River and Cooper Creek area. The collection point of the original specimens is so far from the present known habitats that it is now in doubt.

Rediscovery of the snake followed a serious snake bite in 1967 in the Channel country of south-western Queensland. The snake was thought to be a

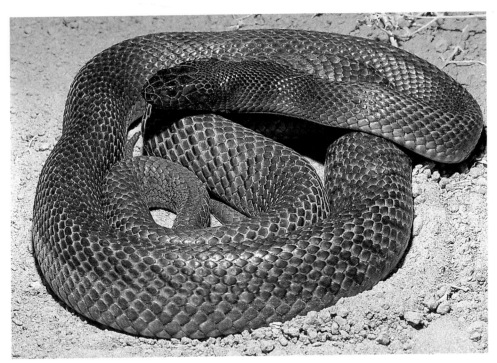

Figure 60
Oxyuranus microlepidotus (winter colour)

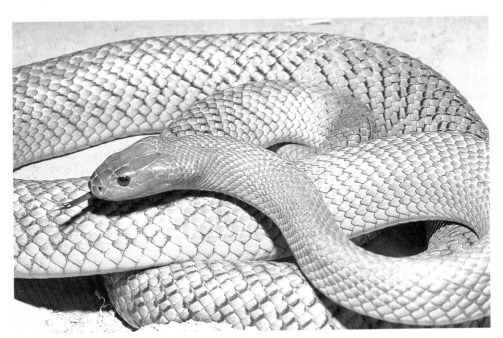

Figure 61
Oxyuranus microlepidotus (summer colour)

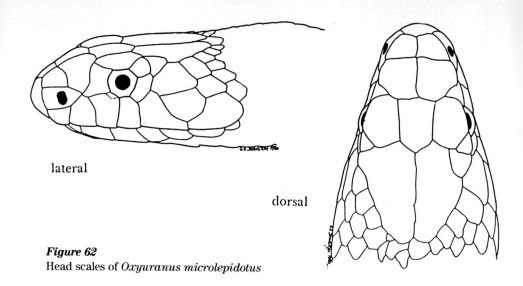

lateral

dorsal

Figure 62
Head scales of *Oxyuranus microlepidotus*

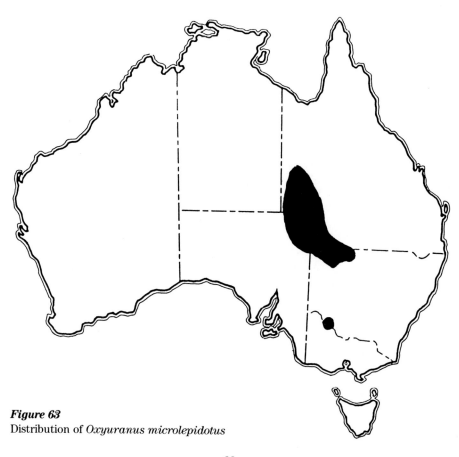

Figure 63
Distribution of *Oxyuranus microlepidotus*

Common Brown Snake and the patient received Brown Snake antivenom, but responded poorly and suffered a critical illness. The snake was later identified as *Oxyuranus scutellatus*. This greatly extended the range of the Taipan. Covacevich in 1976 described specimens from this area as *Parademansia microlepidotus*, and later in 1980 as *Oxyuranus microlepidotus*.

Small-scaled Snake is sometimes used as a common name, but Inland Taipan is a more appropriate name because (1) it is less confusing from a medical standpoint; and (2) small scales occur on both *Oxyuranus scutellatus* and *Oxyuranus microlepidotus*.

Venom:

Fohlman (1979), suggested the venoms of *Oxyuranus scutellatus* and *Oxyuranus microlepidotus* were similar and suggested the two snake types were congeneric. Work in the same year by Broad et al (1979), concluded that due to differences in electrophoretic patterns in venoms of the two snake types, they were from different genera, namely *Oxyuranus* and *Parademansia*. A re-assessment of available venom data and examination of other taxonomic characters, allowed Covacevich et al (1980) to conclude that the two snake types were congeneric and redefined the *Oxyuranus* genus to include this species.

The average yield of most of the *O. microlepidotus* kept at Venom Supplies Laboratories is 64 mg. We do have one specimen that repeatedly registers a nil yield. When fed rats, this particular snake requires the rats to be killed first since it rarely ever injects venom into its prey animals. Other specimens in other collections are known to be the same. One other specimen regularly produces 90 — 100 mg per milking. The dried lyophilized venom is white.

LD_{50} = 0.01 mg/kg (Broad et al 1979). Toxicity work carried out by the Commonwealth Serum Laboratories has shown that the Inland Taipan is far more toxic than any other snake venom known. Compared with the Indian Cobra, *Naja naja*, *Oxyuranus microlepidotus* venom is 50 times more toxic. It is also 770 times more toxic than the Eastern Diamondback Rattlesnake, *Crotalus adamanteus*.

Hamilton et al (1980), showed that the venom was strongly neurotoxic being presynaptic in mode of action.

Paradoxin, a presynaptic neurotoxin, was isolated by Fohlman (1979) and found it very similar to taipoxin from *O. scutellatus*. It is composed of $\propto$, β and δ components like taipoxin. Fohlmann also found that, like Taipan venom, *O. microlepidotus* had a prothrombin activator.

Broad et al (1979), found that *O. microlepidotus* venom had a higher hyaluronidase activity (11.8 units/mg) than *O. scutellatus* venom.

Sutherland's work with monkeys (1979), indicated that no marked prolongation of the partial thromboplastin time over three hours of observation occurred with this venom. (In contrast to *O. scutellatus* venom). It should be noted however, that in a well documented snake bite from this species in 1967, the patient, 17 hours after the bite, did experience a failure of his blood to clot after one hour. Twenty-four hours after the bite, his clotting time was twenty minutes. Also White et al (1988), records coagulupathy in a bite from this species.

No myolytic activity has yet been found due to this venom.

Antivenom:

Taipan — manufactured by the Commonwealth Serum Laboratories (Melbourne). — Photo

INITIAL DOSE — 12,000 units.

Inland Taipan Case History *Oxyuranus microlepidotus*

There have been four bites recorded from this highly dangerous species. Three of the bites have been published. Sketchy details exist regarding the other bite.

Case 1 (from Trinca 1969)

In 1967, a naturalist attempted to capture a snake he thought was *P. textilis*. He was bitten twice on the right thumb, a tourniquet was applied above the elbow, the bitten area was incised and sucked and the snake killed.

The unfortunate man suffered a critical illness from which he took some four weeks to recover. There were a number of factors which influenced his clinical course. He was mistaken in his identification of the snake. Some months later, the snake was identified initially as *O. scutellatus* and later as *P. microlepidota* (Covacevich and Wombey, 1976). Thus, when eventually he received antivenom, it was Brown Snake antivenom which was quite inappropriate.

The bite occurred in a very remote area in south-west Queensland. It took forty minutes to reach the nearest homestead and it was five hours from the time of the bite before the Flying Doctor reached him from the Base at Broken Hill, some 724 km to the south. By this time, the patient was unconscious and incontinent. He regained consciousness again and complained of the pain caused by the tourniquet which was briefly released from time to time.

The third factor, which contributed to a near fatal outcome, was the decision to withhold antivenom until he reached the Flying Doctor Base, because of his known history of severe allergy to horse serum. During the flight back he became more confused and disorientated and suffered a cardiac arrest when being taken off the plane, some nine hours after the bite. He was resuscitated and was given 500 units of Brown Snake antivenom when he reached hospital. He was moderately paralysed and was given intermittent positive pressure respiration. Seventeen hours after the bite, he developed haematuria and bloody diarrhoea. His blood failed to clot after one hour. Platelet count was within normal limits and he was transfused with whole blood.

Twenty-four hours after the bite, his clotting time was twenty minutes. He remained dependent upon the respirator and was transferred to large

Adelaide hospital. He slowly improved and was discharged a month after the bite had occurred.

This case highlighted the mistakes which can be made, even by someone experienced with snakes. The naturalist's survival, considering the circumstances and the lack of specific antivenom, is quite remarkable.

Case 2
Oxyuranus microlepidotus Snake Bite (from Mirtschin et al 1984)

After the successful breeding of *Oxyuranus microlepidotus* at Venom Supplies Laboratories, one of the authors was bitten by a juvenile *O. m.* while trying to feed it.

On March 23, 1984, when the snakes were about three weeks old, they were forcibly fed by a 37-year-old man. After he had finished feeding three of the juvenile snakes, he attempted to feed the fourth, a male. Two attempts to restrain it failed, and the snake became agitated, whipped its body towards the handler's restraining hand, and bit the back of the middle finger of his left hand between the first and the second joint. It was a severe bite by an excited snake. After an attempt to suck the venom from the wound was made, the finger was bandaged and the local hospital was informed about the emergency. The patient went to the hospital on his own, and arrived there about 12 minutes after he was bitten.

About 20 minutes after the bite, he developed a severe headache, and complained of a sensation of pressure behind his ears and feeling flushed; he also had difficulty in speaking and had an uncomfortable feeling in his chest.

On examination, the patient was fully alert, and had no muscle weakness. Some periorbital swelling was noted, especially on the left side. He had tachycardia (80 —120 beats/min), his respiratory rate was 22/min, and his axillary temperature was 36.4°C. His blood pressure was 130/70 mmHg.

Despite the risk of an anaphylactic reaction (he had a childhood history of a reaction to anti-tetanus serum and was bitten by a tiger snake in 1977, for which he had not received antivenom), 12,000 units of taipan antivenom (B548, 47-031-1) in Hartmann's solution were administered immediately by way of an intravenous infusion. At the same time, he received an intramuscular injection of promethazine (50 mg) and a subcutaneous injection of adrenaline (1:1000, 1 ml).

The patient's recovery was uneventful, and he had no significant signs of proteinuria. He was discharged from hospital well, two days after admission. After discharge from hospital, he received prednisolone (15 mg three days a week) for two weeks for the prevention of serum sickness.

Notes:

Sucking the venom from the site of the bite is unnecessary and generally, is not advisable, because the surface venom can be used for identification in venom detection kits.

It would have been better to seek assistance in getting to hospital rather than the victim driving himself.

Summary of Symptoms and Conditions Experienced from *Oxyuranus microlepidotus* Bites

— Unconciousness.
— Incontinence.
— Cardiac arrest.
— Paralysis.
— Haematuria.
— Bloody diarrhoea.
— Blood failure to clot.
— Breathing difficulty.
— Severe headache.
— Pressure behind ears.
— Difficulty in speaking.
— Uncomfortable feeling in chest.
— Periorbital swelling.
— Tachycardia.
— Increased respiratory rate.

The Death Adders

There are three species of Death Adders (genus *Acanthophis)* in Australia; the Common Death Adder, Desert Death Adder, and Northern Death Adder. They are very similar in appearance and between the three they occupy nearly all of the Australian mainland.

The Common Death Adder occurs closer to the coast, preferring areas with greater than 250 mm rainfall and slightly cooler areas to those inhabited by the Desert Death Adder. The Northern Death Adder occurs in Northern Australia.

Habitat destruction or alteration has greatly reduced populations of the Common Death Adder in some areas. Mirtschin (1983b), observed the decline of Death Adders in South Australia and related it to land clearing activities. This is further supported by Mirtschin (1985), where habitat destruction throughout Australia is listed as a cause for population decline. The Cane Toad *Bufo marinus* in north Queensland is believed to be responsible for the decline of *A. praelongus* and *A. antarcticus*.

Common Death Adder *Acanthophis antarcticus* (Shaw)
Description:

Broad triangular head distinct from neck. Short stubby body with a small thin rat-like tail terminating in a sharp curved spine. Pupils elliptical. Specimens over 0.915 metres have been recorded, but average length is about 0.5 — 0.6 metres.

Scalation:

Scales on head are almost rugose.

VENTRALS	110-130
SUBCAUDALS	38-55 mostly single.
MID-BODIES	21-23 rows
ANAL	Single

Colour:

General colour highly variable throughout Australia — colour variations exist within localities. Base colour varies from earthy grey to red. Darker transverse bands occur on all Death Adders. Tip of tail is either black or white and is banded in juveniles. Tip of tail usually black in southern Australia and white in the northern extent of their range. (Figs 64-67)

Habits:

Seeks refuge in leaf litter or loose sand and is nocturnal, being mainly active on hot nights. Captures prey by wriggling grub-like tail as a lure to attract insectivorous creatures. Will not usually retreat if approached by humans. Death Adders are viviparous producing 10 — 33 young. Shine (1980), concludes that Death Adders only reproduce in alternative years. However, in captivity, one specimen in Whaylla reproduced for four successive years (Mirtschin 1985). Other specimens in captivity, mated at nineteen months gave birth to young at twenty-one months.

Shine (1980), found that sexual maturity was twenty-four months for males, and forty-two months for females based on examination of museum specimens.

Habitat and Distribution:

Death Adders occur in coastal sand dunes, mallee country, and tropical forests. Virgin habitats appear to be necessary in southern populations and hence no evidence exists of long term adaptations to drastically modified areas. Their reliance on leaf mulch for refuge and native reptile, mammal and bird fauna for food, makes it difficult for Death Adders to tolerate any major changes to their environment.

Notes:

It is possible that sometimes Death Adders lose their tails to their prospective prey, since two specimens found on Eyre Peninsula, South Australia, had only partial tails. This, however, could be a result of incomplete sloughing of skin on the tail causing it to wither and drop off. This has happened to one specimen kept in captivity in Whyalla.

The Death Adder is unique in Australia in both its appearance and habits. Although having a resemblance to a true adder, Death Adders are really elapids, with relatively fixed venom fangs that are not capable of being rotated to the same degree as Viper fangs. Compared with other Australian snakes, Death Adders have long fangs for snakes of their size, averaging about 6 mm.

Food:

In the wild, Death Adders feed on native insectivorous prey such as birds,

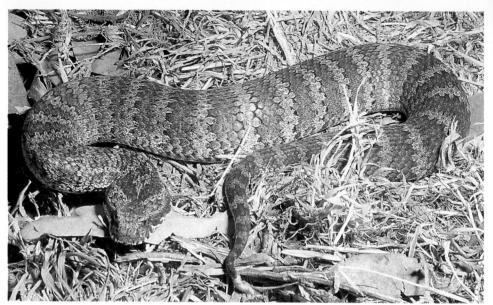

Figure 64
Acanthophis antarcticus (QLD)

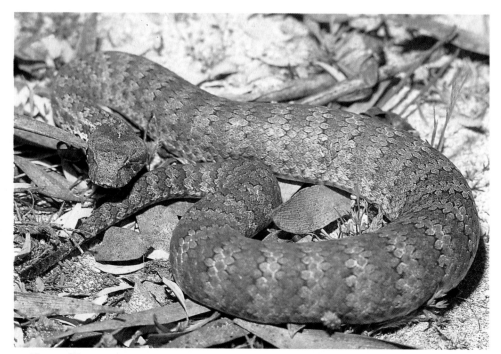

Figure 65
Acanthophis antarcticus (South Australia)

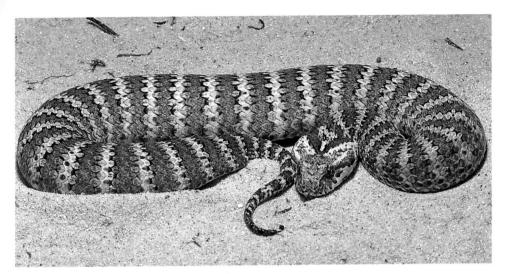

Figure 66
Acanthophis antarcticus (South Australia)

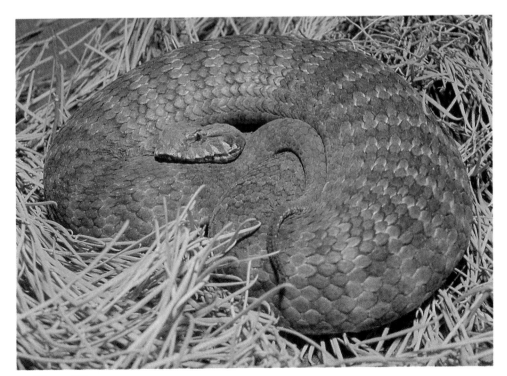

Figure 67
Acanthophis antarcticus (South Australia)

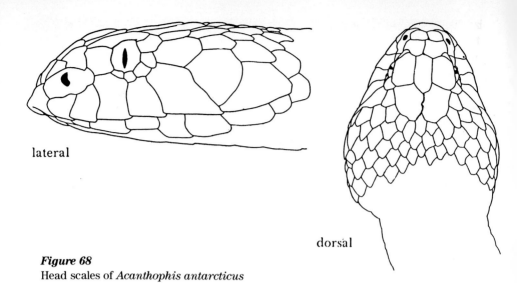

lateral

dorsal

Figure 68
Head scales of *Acanthophis antarcticus*

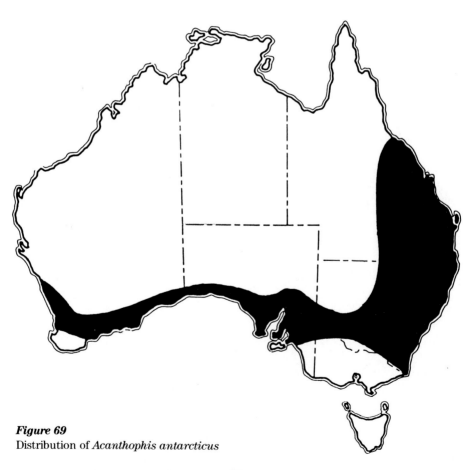

Figure 69
Distribution of *Acanthophis antarcticus*

lizards, and hopping mice. In captivity, they thrive on the introduced mouse, *Mus musculus*, but it is doubtful that they prey on them in the wild since these mice are not insectivorous and are therefore not attracted by the wriggling tail.

The Death Adder population on Reevesby Island in Spencers Gulf, South Australia is smaller in size than its nearby mainland relations. It also shows less colour variation than is displayed by mainland specimens and its disposition is less aggressive when disturbed. Tindale (1924), noted a massacre of Death Adders on Reevesby Island in 1923, when 89 were killed in a small area in that year. Since the population is still thriving today, this activity had no long term effect.

Venom:

Venom milked from Common Death Adders from South Australia kept at Venom Supplies Laboratories yield 80.5 mg on average. A group from the northern New South Wales/southern Queensland population, yield on average 65 mg. The maximum yield is reported to be 236 mg (Fairley and Splatt 1929). The South Australian Death Adder dried lyophilized venom is cream coloured, whereas the other group has venom of a much paler cream colour.

Broad et al (1979), found the LD_{50} = 0.338 mg/kg.

Kellaway (1929), noted the venom as being highly neurotoxic and also had weak haemolytic and anticoagulant activity. Sutherland (1983), suggested that the neurotoxin is entirely postsynaptic.

Sheumack et al (1979), isolated a lethal peptide neurotoxin 'acanthopin a' consisting of 63 amino acid residues cross linked by four disuphide bridges. They concluded that 'acanthopin a' accounted for the symptoms seen in the crude venom envenomation.

Sutherland (1979), could find no evidence of myotoxic poisoning in monkeys inoculated with this venom. This was supported by Mebs and Samejima (1980) in their work with mice.

Denson (1969), found the venom to be an incomplete prothrombin activator and Sutherland's work in (1979b) showed that prothrombin time in monkeys increased due to *A. antarcticus* envenomation.

Local pain around the bite site, is associated with Death Adder bites during recovery stages. One of the authors received a bite from a large 900 mm specimen in 1986 and experienced intense pain at the bite site after all other symptoms had subsided following antivenom treatment. This pain remained for four days. Mertens (pers. com.), also experienced similar local pain after *A. antarcticus* bites. In Mertens' case, which was his second bite from the species, he experienced muscular loss and numbness in the bitten finger. This condition was still evident twelve months after the bite.

Antivenom:

Death Adder antivenom — Commonwealth Serum Laboratories (Melbourne).

INITIAL DOSE — 6,000 units.

Common Death Adder Case History
Acanthophis antarcticus

Case 1 (The following case history details were supplied by Ted Mertens from the Bowmans Park Trust near Clare S.A.)

On 15/6/86, a 39-year-old Caucasian male of 60 kg weight and 1.82 m height, was bitten by an adult Death Adder during venom extraction. He was bitten on the right index finger by 1 fang of the snake.

1430 hrs Bitten by Death Adder.

1431 hrs Compression bandage applied as recommended

1432 hrs Sharp pain in finger experienced.

1435 hrs Dizziness and onset of nausea.

1440 hrs Incontinent/loss of bowel control. Speech slurred. Sight impaired. Loss of limb co-ordination.

1450 hrs Admitted to Port Pirie Hospital. Constrictive bandage left in place. Oxygen given — Pulse 116.

1455 hrs 6,000 units of Death Adder antivenom in saline commenced intravenously over 30 minutes.

1510 hrs Constrictive bandage removed.

1512 hrs Pulse 100.

1520 hrs Pulse 88, respirations 16. 15 minutes observations. Admitted to ICU.

1600 hrs Pulse 98, respiration 14. Blood pressure 85/55.

1645 hrs Pulse 88, respiration 18. Blood pressure 110/85, temperature 35.8°C.

1800 hrs Pulse 84, respirations 16. Blood pressure 120/65, temperature 38°C.

1900 hrs Pulse 88, respirations 20. Blood pressure 110/60, temperature 37.9°C.

2000 hrs Pulse 88, respirations 16. Blood pressure 115/65, temperature 38°C.

2100 hrs Observations reduced to 30 minute intervals. Pulse 72, respirations 18, blood pressure 115/65.

2200 hrs Pulse 72, respirations 18. Blood pressure 110/65, temperature 37.3°C.

2300 hrs Severe pain in bitten finger and area, 15 mg morphine and 10 mg Maxolon (metoclopamide) given intravenously.

16/6/87 Patient allowed to eat and drink. I.V. therapy continued.

17/6/87 I.V. discontinued. Venflow left in situ.
Transferred to ward.

18/6/87 Pain in finger and hand still acute. Limb elevated. Severe discoloration of bite site.

19/6/87 Patient discharged.

After discharge, the bitten finger was numb, and in the upper section, badly necrotised. Antibiotics were taken for a period of three weeks after which the necrosis ceased and a section of dead tissue and skin 3 cm x 1.5 cm approx. fell from the digit. During this period there was pain and numbness in the finger after which only the numbness was experienced in the top joint, as well as continued muscle pain in the entire right arm.

The numbness and pain was particularly bad on cold days. On the worst of these, the arm only had half normal strength. Normal functioning of the hand

and finger was achieved through practice although some disability remains. Lack of strength and stiffness of the arm were still present in August 1987.

Case 2
Acanthophis antarcticus Snake Bite

A 39-year-old male from Venom Supplies was bitten twice in quick succession on the left middle finger by a 0.91 m specimen of *A. antarcticus* while trying to assist it with a skin slough. The accident occurred in September 1986.

Compression and immobilisation first aid was applied, an ambulance summoned by an assistant, and arrival at the hospital was achieved in about 15 minutes. He felt hot and flushed, was sweating and a tachycardia developed. The following drugs were administered:

(a) Phenergan (promethanzine HCl) 25 mg I.V.
(b) Hydrocortisone 100 mg I.V.
(c) Adrenaline 1/1000 0.5 ml S.C.

6,000 units of Death Adder antivenom were administered I.V. undiluted.

Tachycardia increased after administration of the adrenaline, but subsided upon receiving the antivenom. Tetanus toxoid vaccine 0.5 ml was given S.C.

Recovery was uneventful, the painful finger improving over a week.

Since it is expected that venom from *Acanthophis pyrrhus*, *Acanthophis praelongus* and *Acanthophis laevis* (New Guinea) are similar, the following list of symptoms and experiences covers bites from the whole genus. In many bites, the species concerned was not identified precisely.

Summary of Symptoms and Conditions Experienced with Acanthophis Bites.

— Pain in bitten area which can persist for weeks.
— Headache.
— Severe pain in regional lymph nodes.
— Blurred vision.
— Ptosis.
— Paralysis.
— Depressed ventilation.
— Vomiting
— Excessive salivation.
— Dizziness.
— Nausea.
— Incontinence.
— Tachycardia.
— Hypotension.

Desert Death Adder *Acanthophis pyrrhus* (Boulenger)

Description:

Similar in appearance to the Common Death Adder but with a flatter head and the body is more elongate. Grows to 0.75 metres.

Scalation:

Body scale keeled, head scales rugose and keeled.

VENTRALS	140-160
SUBCAUDALS	45-60 single anterior, divided posterior
MIDBODIES	21
ANAL	Single

Colour:

The specific name refers to the brick-red colour of the snake and means fire. Dark indistinct cross bands. Ventrally whitish. Tail can be black or white. (Fig 70).

Habits:

Assumed to be similar to Common Death Adder. However, little is known about this snake because it occurs in such remote areas.

Habitat and Distribution:

Occurs in dry areas, rocky slopes, and porcupine grass *(Triodia)* areas of inland Australia.

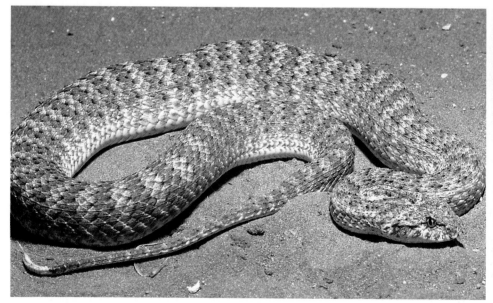

Figure 70
Ancanthophis pyrrhus

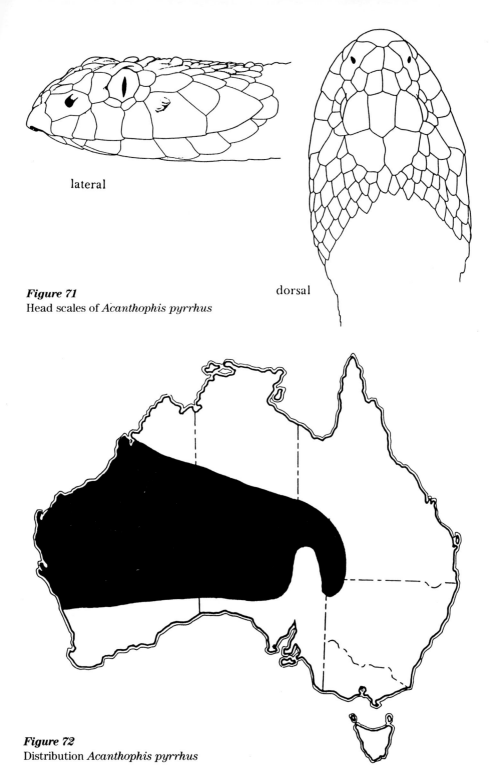

lateral

dorsal

Figure 71
Head scales of *Acanthophis pyrrhus*

Figure 72
Distribution *Acanthophis pyrrhus*

Notes:

The Aborigines have great fear of the snake and call it 'Mythunda' (Waite 1928). Its nature is less predictable than that of the Common Death Adder.

Venom:

Nothing is known about the venom except that its effect on laboratory animals appears to be rapid.

Antivenom:

Death Adder — Commonwealth Serum Laboratories (Melbourne).

INITIAL DOSE — 6,000 units.

Northern Death Adder *Acanthophis praelongus* **(Ramsey)**

Description:

Moderately stout, intermediate between the Common Death Adder and Desert Death Adder in rugosity of head shields, keeling of dorsals, and number of ventrals and subcaudals (Storr 1981). Average length is 0.4m. Grows up to 0.7m.

Scalation:

VENTRALS	122-140
SUBCAUDALS	39-57 (19-39 single)
MID-BODIES	Usually 23 (rarely 19, 21)
ANAL	Single

Colour:

Darker than the Common Death Adder and Desert Death Adder, stronger colour pattern. Ventral surface, whitish with dark spots (Storr 1981, Gow 1982). (Fig 73, 74)

Habits:

Assumed to be similar to the Common Death Adder.

Habitat and Distribution:

Sub-humid and semi-arid zones of Kimberley Ranges. North of Northern Territory and Queensland and in southern New Guinea (Storr 1981).

Notes:

It is viviparous.

Venom:

While there is nothing documented on the effects and properties of this venom, it is assumed that since the elevation of these populations to species

102

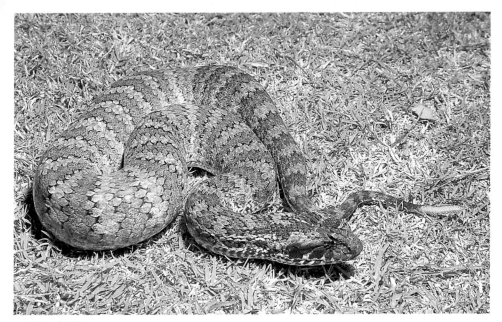

Figure 73
Acanthophis praelongus

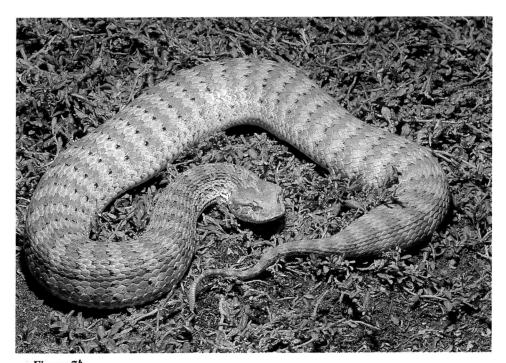

Figure 74
Acanthophis sp undescribed from the Barkley Tableland.

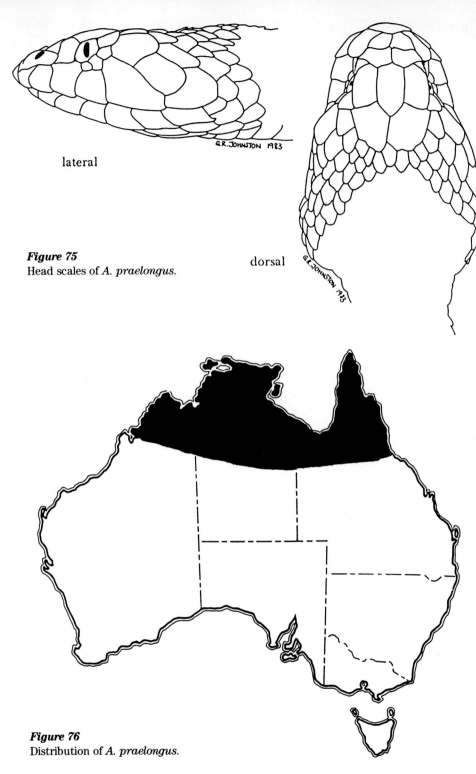

lateral

Figure 75
Head scales of *A. praelongus*.

dorsal

G.R. JOHNSTON 1983

Figure 76
Distribution of *A. praelongus*.

status is only recent, it is inevitable that some of its venom would have been supplied to the researchers investigating *A. antarcticus* venom. Therefore, it is reasonable to conclude that the findings for *A. antarcticus* venom would be similar to *A. praelongus* venom.

Bredl (pers. com.), experienced pain in the arm after being bitten on the finger.

Antivenom:

Death Adder — Commonwealth Serum Laboratories (Melbourne).

INITIAL DOSE — 6,000 units.

The Black Snakes

The genus *Pseudechis* has two black-coloured snakes, the Red-Bellied Black Snake, *P. porphyriacus* and the Spotted Black Snake, *P. guttatus*. The Mulga or King Brown Snake, *P. australis* is normally brown to coppery red but does have a black phase in some southern areas. The Collet's Snake, *P. colletti* has varied colour patterns on its dorsal surface. *P. butleri* is similar to *P. porphyriacus*, being very dark in colour. The common group name for the genus is therefore somewhat misleading.

Despite marked colour differences, all the *Pseudechis* genus have relatively small frontal scales. This genus occupies nearly all habitat types in Australia with Mulga Snake *Pseudechis australis* being the most widespread and diverse species with possible sub-species differences. The Red-Bellied Black Snake, *P. porphriacus* and the Spotted Black Snake, *P. guttatus* both occur in areas with rainfall greater than 500 mm per year except in some dry areas along the Murray River where *P. porphyriacus* is resident. This suggests that both of these species are frog-dependent for their food. Mengden et al (1986), suggests *P. porhyriacus* is the most divergent from the rest based on cytogenetics, scalation, general morphology and electrophoretic patterns of blood proteins . It is also viviparous whilst the others are ovoviviparous.

Red-Bellied Black Snakeporphyriacus (Shaw)
Description:

Average length about 1.25 m, maximum length 2.5 m. Head slightly distinct from body.

Scalation:

Smooth scales.

VENTRALS	180-210
SUBCAUDALS	40-65 first one-third single, remainder divided.
MID-BODIES	17
ANAL	Divided

Colour:

Fairly uniform in coloration in separate areas throughout its range. Purplish black dorsally with a red to orange ventral surface tending to white in the north. The red is more intense on the outer edges of the belly fading to a lighter colour towards the centre. Underside of tail is black. (fig 77)

Habits:

This is the only essentially diurnal snake of the genus. It is usually shy by nature, flattening out its neck when alarmed; it may even attempt mock strikes. Viviparous producing 8 — 40 young (Cogger 1975). Shine et al (1981), records male combat for this species.

Food:

In the wild, the food consists mainly of frogs, but small mammals, other snakes, lizards, fishes, eels and birds are taken. The species is recorded to be cannibalistic. It has a distinct body odour.

Very easy to maintain in captivity and a voracious feeder.

Habitat and Distribution:

Prefers wet areas: swamps, lagoons, streams, and wet forests of eastern Australia and south to south-eastern S.A.

Venom:

Red-Bellied Black Snakes kept at Venom Supplies Laboratories yield on average 32 mg of dried lyophilized venom. Martin and Smith (1892), recorded a maximum yield of 94 mg from this species. The dried lyophilized venom is a rich golden colour.

Broad et al (1979), determined LD_{50} = 2.53 mg/kg which makes it only moderately toxic (only about one twentieth the toxicity of the Cobra *Naja naja*).

Fong and Tirrel (1979), demonstrated that the crude venom enhanced the formation of fibrin in plasma, while other components had varying degrees of coagulation activity.

Vaughan et al (1981), isolated a toxin called Pseudexin which accounted for 25% of the venom. This toxin showed phospholipase A activity and caused indirect haemolysis of washed erythrocytes. Pseudexin directly haemolysed erythrocytes under conditions in which phospholipases were normally non-haemolytic. This toxin caused paralysis and evidence suggested it may be a presynaptic neurotoxin.

Sutherland et al (1981), reported that this venom was powerfully myolytic. Mebs and Samejima (1980), isolated a phospholipase component that was myolytic to mice.

Mild coagulating defects have also been reported by Sutherland (1979c) and Davey et al (1967). It contains phospholipase A and a direct haemolysin. (Doery and Pearson 1961). Sutherland (1981), suggested that since monkeys

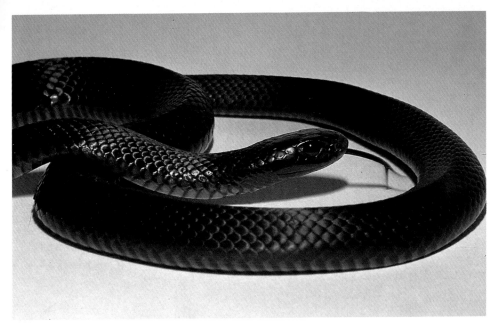

Figure 77
Pseudechis porphyriacus

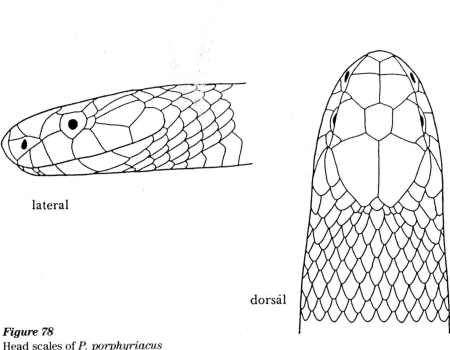

lateral

dorsal

Figure 78
Head scales of *P. porphyriacus*
(Drawing courtesy of P. Rawlinson)

which had received 1,200 µg of *P. porphyriacus* venom only showed slight changes in the PTT and none in the PT significant coagulation defects should not result from a bite of this species.

At least one death has occurred due to a bite from this species (Fairley 1929). With administration of antivenom, death from this snake is an unlikely event. The young and elderly, as with all snake bites, are at greater risk with this species.

Antivenom:

Tiger Snake or Black Snake — manufactured by the Commonwealth Serum Laboratories (Melbourne).

INITIAL DOSE — Tiger Snake — 3,000 units.
OR Black Snake — 6,000 units

Sutherland (1983), advises the use of Tiger Snake antivenom in preference to the larger volume Black Snake antivenom vial which should be reserved for treating other *Pseudechis* species.

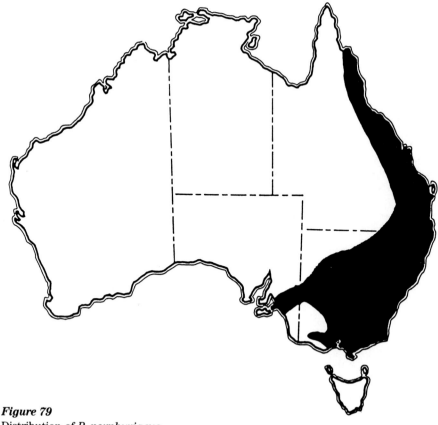

Figure 79
Distribution of *P. porphyriacus*.

Red-Bellied Black Snake — Case Histories

Pseudechis porphyriacus (The following case histories are taken from Sutherland (1983)

(a) On 12 March 1978, a 15-year-old male was bitten on the left index finger when trying to catch *P. porphyriacus*. He developed local swelling of the finger associated with tenderness in the axilla. He vomited once. Headache and pain persisted, and eight hours later he was given 6,000 units of Black snake antivenom and made an uneventful recovery. This bite occurred near Kirra in Queenland.

(b) A 23-year-old male welder was bitten on the left foot by a 0.8 m *P. porphyriacus* at 11.45 am near Bundaberg, Queensland, on 21 March 1978. He accidentally stood upon the snake. He developed local pain at the bite site and moderate pain in the axillary lymph nodes. No general symptoms developed, but he was given 9,000 units of Black snake antivenom shortly after arrival in hospital.

(c) At 5 pm on 16 January 1979, a 7-year-old child lifted a sheet of iron at his home near Dungong, New South Wales. He was bitten on his left second toe. He suffered local pain and swelling, vomiting and severe abdominal pain. Local pressure was applied to the foot and he received 6,000 units of Black Snake antivenom. The response was described as excellent. He was discharged from hospital the next day with some local swelling still present.

(d) A 23-year-old man was bitten by *P. porphyriacus* at 5 pm on 27 December 1980 whilst fishing on a river bank at Yetman, Queensland. Shortly after the bite he became nauseated and vomitted repeatedly. Traces of blood were seen in the bile stained vomitus. He applied a tourniquet to his upper arm, but did not occlude the circulation. One hour after the bite, pain extended up his arm and he complained of a painful lump in his armpit. By this time he had abdominal pain and blood stained diarrhoea. Three hours after the bite, twitching of the extremities was observed. He was conscious with a slight headache but no respiratory distress. He had haematuria and was incontinent of faeces. He responded well to an infusion of 6,000 units of Black snake antivenom which was given at the Texas Hospital.

Summary of Symptoms and Conditions Experienced with Pseudechis porphyriacus Bites

— Short of breath.
— Local swelling.
— Tenderness in axilla (lymph nodes).
— Vomiting (sometimes traces of blood and bite in vomit).
— Headache.
— Local pain and in bitten limb.
— Severe abdominal pain.
— Unconsciousness (brief).
— Nausea.
— Tachycardia.
— Blurred vision.

— Microscopic haematuria.

— Dizziness.

Mulga or King Brown Snake *Pseudechis australis* (Gray)

Description:

Average maximum length varies from area to area. Maximum length recorded has been in excess of 2.7 m. Average length is about 1.5 m. A robust snake, relatively slow-moving. Very broad head especially with larger specimens. Head slightly distinct from body, sometimes with bulbous cheeks.

Scalation:

Large scales.

VENTRALS	189-220
SUBCAUDALS	53-70 all single or all divided, or partly single and divided
MID-BODIES	17
ANAL	Divided

Colour:

Variable depending on locality. Ranges from light to dark brown, coppery red to nearly yellow. Southern specimens tend to be darker to almost black. Scales are either lighter or darker tipped. Ventral surface usually yellow or yellow-green. Sometimes with orange blotches. (Fig 80, 81).

Habits:

Temperament appears to vary with locality. In southern areas of Eyre Peninsula and west coast of South Australia, it is a shy, quiet snake. Northern specimens are be quite excitable when disturbed. They are diurnal in warm weather and become nocturnal in the hotter weather. Worrell (1963) and McPhee (1979), records that they are viviparous, however, Fitzgerald and Pollitt (1981) and Mirtschin (1986) record oviparity. This is probably due to undescribed speciation from different geographical regions. Mirtschin (1986) records maximum of 15 eggs in specimens from Eyre Peninsula S.A. Southern specimens (dark coloured) have been observed basking in the winter.

Habitat and Distribution:

Found over most habitat ranges. Woodlands, mallee, and grass lands, mulga, tropical forests. Rare in Victoria and absent in Tasmania. Does not occur in swamps or alpine regions. Makes its home under large rocks, logs, in rabbit warrens and other animal holes.

Notes:

Mulga Snake venom has a devastating effect on other Australian venomous snakes, but from our experience at Venom Supplies, the venom of other Australian snakes has no apparent effect on Mulga Snakes. This is probably an

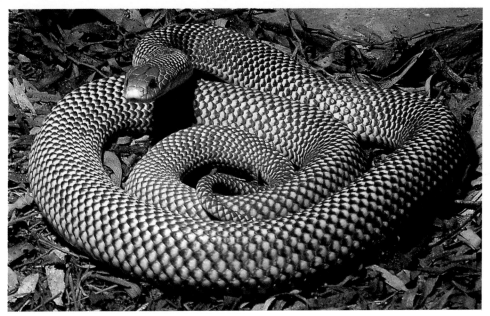

Figure 80
Pseudechis australis (South Australia)

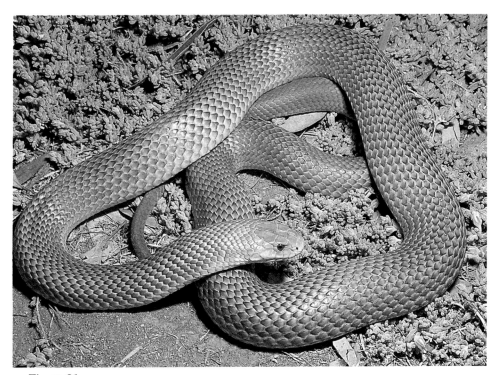

Figure 81
Pseudechis australis (Northern Territory)

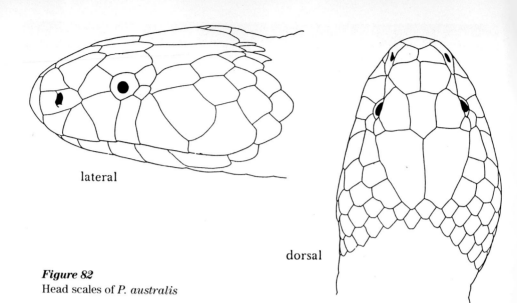

lateral

dorsal

Figure 82
Head scales of *P. australis*

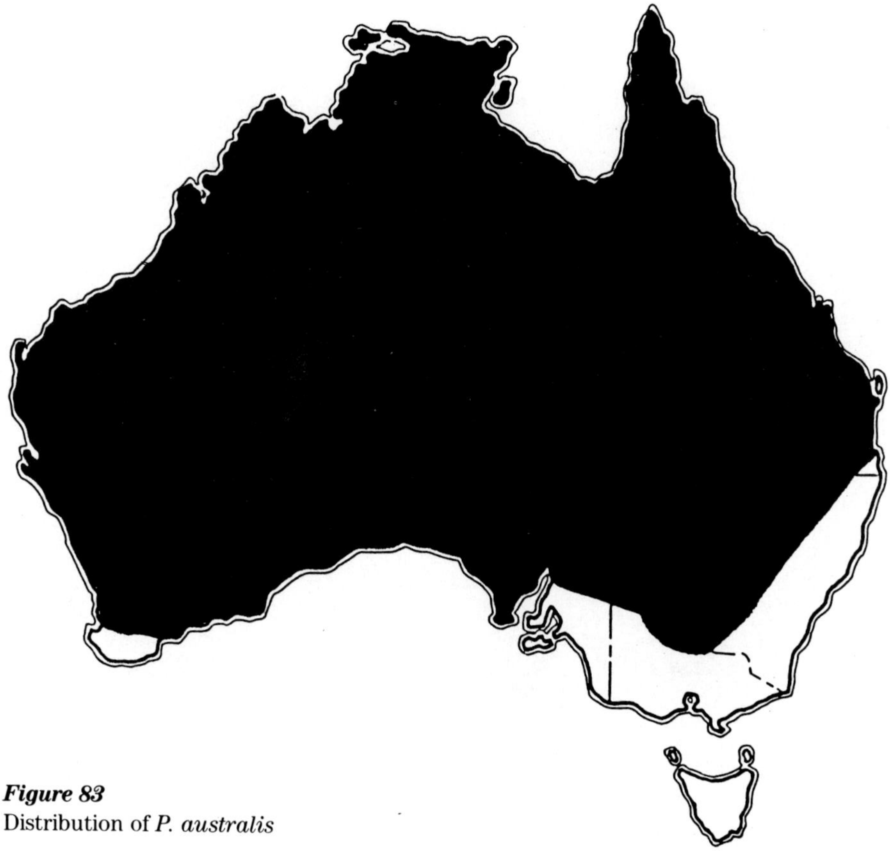

Figure 83
Distribution of *P. australis*

adaptation resulting from the habit of eating other snakes. When biting, the Mulga Snake has the characteristic of hanging on and chewing into its prey. Mulga Snakes from some areas can emit unpleasant odours when frightened.

Food:

Rats, mice, lizards and snakes. In captivity *P. australis* has been found to eat other species of snakes.

Venom:

Mulga Snakes kept at Venom Supplies Laboratories have yielded the following amounts.

South Australian Mulga Snakes   —   average 190 mg
Northern Territory Mulga Snakes (less than 2 m in length)   —   average 190 mg

The venom is bright yellow in the dried lyophilized form. The Northern Territory Mulga Snakes can be expected to yield additional venom when they grow to maximum size.

Worrell (1963), notes a maximum yield of 600 mg for this species.

Broad et al (1979), determined the $LD_{50} = 1.91$ mg/kg.

Kellaway and Thompson (1930), carried out extensive testing on a number of different laboratory animals and found the *P. australis* venom caused a marked delay in coagulation time. The absence of any evidence of neurotoxins contrasted this venom with most other Australian dangerous snake venoms. They also demonstrated haemolytic activity.

Masci et al (1989), isolated and characterised the coagulation inhibitors. They found two different inhibitors called P_A-serpin™ — 1 and P_A—serpin™— 2 of molecular weights 18,000 and 27,000 each being a single chain polypeptide. Both blocked the generation of factor Xa and the action of factor Xa on prothrombin. Both inhibitors are able to block platelet aggregation completely in response to collagen, adrenalin, arachidonic acid, ristocetin, A23187 and U44069, but only secondary aggregation in response to ADP.

They found that platelet release inhibition was variable. ADP induced release of serotonin was completely inhibited whereas there was only a minimal effect upon A23187 induced platelet release. Both fractions inhibited thromboxane production. The inhibitors varied only in the speed of inhibition, were non-competitive, heat stable and had no haemolytic or neurotoxic activity. Their action was enhanced but not dependent on the presence of lipids. Masci et al (1989), suggested they could be useful in elucidating a role for factor Xa in platelet function. The results suggest the 2 anticoagulants are in serine protease inhibitors and have been shown to be toxic with bleeding at the injection site in 20gm mice at a loading dose of 20 μg. Death is prevented in pre-heparinized animals. Both P_A-serpin™ products are produced by Venom Supplies Laboratories.

After a fatal snake bite in 1969 in Western Australia indicating gross rhabdomyolysis (Rowlands et al 1969), alternative recommendations were made regarding antivenom selection for bites involving this species (Sutherland 1983).

Doery and Pearson (1961), found the venom to be rich in phospholipase and direct haemolysin. Nashida et al (1985), isolated two phospholipases A_2 from *P. australis* venom. One group, Pa-11 was lethal to mice, whereas the other, Pa-13 showed no lethal activity. Leonardi et al (1979), isolated a strong myotoxin called mulgotoxin from *P. australis* venom. It is a basic toxin with a single polypeptide chain of 122 amino acid residues cross linked by seven disulphide bridges.

Mebs and Samejima (1980) and Sutherland and Campbell (1980), both confirmed the presence of myolytic toxicity with *P. australis* envenomation. An interesting finding of Sutherland et al (1981), was that when a monkey was injected with 1,200 μg of *P. australis* venom, it developed significant coagulopathy which later resolved. The fluctuating absorption of the venom unexplained by Sutherland was probably due to the different kinetics associated with the two coagulation inhibitors isolated by Masci et al (1989).

Sutherland et al (1981), also noted that a serosanguineous discharge occurred at the venom injection sites of his test animals. This phenomenon has not been recorded for other Australian snake venoms studied. Sutherland et al (1981) mentions that painful swelling can be associated with the bite and Vines (1978), indicates that the swelling may cause the skin to burst. Observations at Venom Supplies Laboratories on juvenile rats envenomated by juvenile *P. australis* and not eaten, had swollen to 2 to 3 times their initial size in 12 hours.

Antivenom:

Black Snake antivenom — manufactured by the Commonwealth Serum Laboratories (Melbourne).

NB   This antivenom is manufactured by immunizing horses with *P. australis* venom (Sutherland 1983).

INITIAL DOSE — 18,000 units.

Mulga or King Brown Snake Case History
***Pseudechis australis* (from Rowlands et al 1969)**

A 20-year-old farm labourer was bitten on the hand by a 1.82 m *P. australis*. The bite occurred at night on a veranda in a township in the wheatbelt some 320 km from Perth. The unfortunate man had been reaching underneath his bed for a packet of cigarettes.

Two hours after the bite, when he was nauseated and vomiting, he sought medical aid. He twice received intravenous injections of Brown (500 units), Death Adder (6,000 units) and Tiger Snake (3,000 units) antivenoms. His condition steadily worsened, and at thirty-seven hours after the bite he was admitted to the Royal Perth Hospital, where he died three hours later. At post mortem gross rhabdomyolysis was present. Cardiac muscle showed

114

widespread myolysis, confirming the experimental studies of Kellaway and Thompson (1930).

The investigations carried out on this patient at thirty-seven hours post bite showed renal failure due to myoglobinaemia, although its existence was not positively proved. At thirty-seven hours the haemoglobin was 9.4 mmol/l, white cell count 40 x 10^9/l, platelet count 19 x 10^9/l and the coagulation time five minutes.

Summary of Symptoms and Conditions Experienced with Pseudechis australis Bites.

— Nausea.
— Vomiting.
— Rhabdomyolysis.
— Renal failure.
— Myoglobinuria.
— Extended coagulation.
— Paleness.
— Tachycardia.
— Enlargement of lymph nodes.
— Ptosis.
— Reduced consciousness.
— Cyanosis.
— Blood in urine.
— Swelling of bitten limb.
— Pink maculopapular rash.
— Severe local reaction, gangrene.

Colletts Snake Pseudechis colletti (Boulenger)

Description:

Robust body with broad blunt head slightly distinct from body. Average maximum length 2 m.

Scalation:

Smooth scales.

VENTRALS	215-235
SUBCAUDALS	50-70 anterior single, posterior divided.
MID-BODIES	19
ANAL	Divided

Colour:

Is probably the most colourful of our venomous snakes. Light brown, dark brown to black with salmon to red scales forming irregular bands. Cream to orange ventrally. (Figs 84, 85).

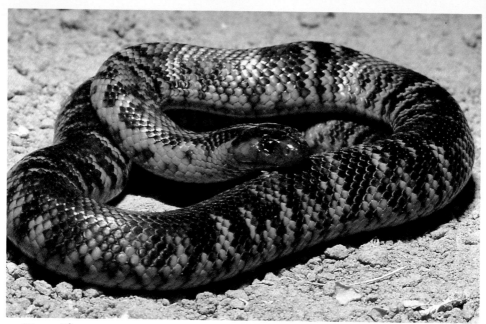

Figure 84
Pseudechis colletti

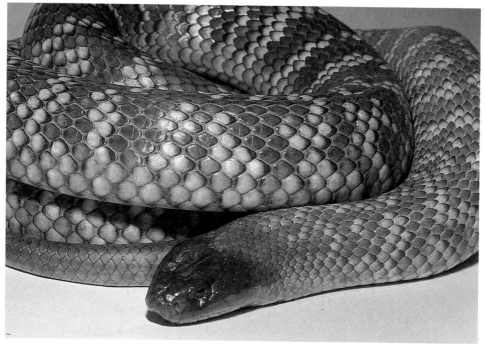

Figure 85
Pseudechis colletti

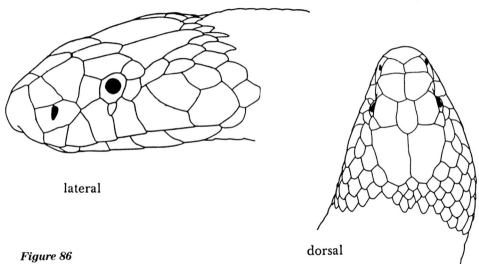

lateral

dorsal

Figure 86
Head scales of *P. colletti*

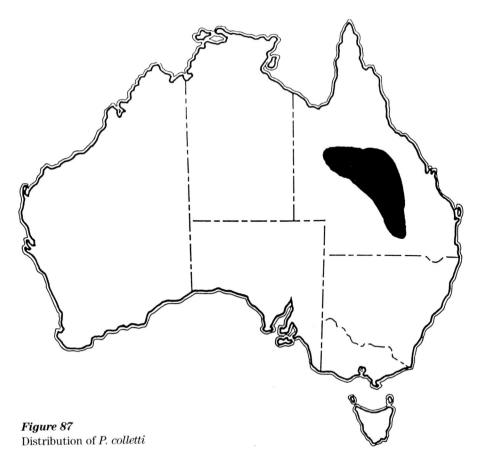

Figure 87
Distribution of *P. colletti*

Habits:

Very little is known about this snake, probably because it occurs in remote areas. Like other members of this genus, it has an offensive odour when handled. Oviparous producing 12 or more young. Specimens kept at Venom Supplies Laboratories exhibited have male combat. Known to be cannibalistic. Feeds on lizards and small mammals.

Habitat and Distribution:

Central Queensland, non-swampy drier inland areas.

Venom:

Collett's snakes, *P. colletti*, maintained at Venom Supplies Laboratories yield on average 48 mg. The venom is a rich yellow colour in the lyophilized dried form.

Broad et al (1979), recorded LD_{50} = 2.36 mg/kg (saline) for this species.

Mebs (1969), found a number of low molecular weight toxins and Mebs and Samejima (1980), isolated 2 separate myolytic phospholipase A groups from it.

Bernheimer et al (1986), found that *P. colletti* venom had high direct haemolytic activity and proposed that Phospholipase B may be responsible for direct lysis of erythrocytes.

Antivenom:

Tiger Snake antivenom
Black Snake antivenom

Both manufactured by the Commonwealth Serum Laboratories (Melbourne).

Sutherland (1983), suggests that Tiger Snake antivenom be used in preference to a larger quantity of Black Snake antivenom.

INITIAL DOSE — Tiger Snake — 3,000 units
OR Black Snake — 18,000 units.

Spotted Black Snake *Pseudechis guttatus* (De Vis)
Descritpion:1

Head indistinct from body. Grows to about 2 m. Fang length about 3.5 mm.

Scalation:

Smooth scales.

VENTRALS	175-205
SUBCAUDALS	45-65 anterior single, posterior divided.
MID-BODIES	19
ANAL	Divided

Colour:

Dorsally, this snake is usually glossy black, sometimes exhibiting a few cream coloured scales. Some specimens are cream with black tipped scales. Ventral surface blue grey. (Fig 88)

Habits:

Oviparity has been reported by Charles et al (1979) and Gow (1976) and Venom Supplies Laboratories. Up to 16 eggs have been recorded in one oviposition.

The species like many other Australian elapids is capable of flattening the whole body when annoyed. The species, when annoyed will expel air from its lung with a hissing sound and will often mimic a strike with closed mouth.

Venom:

The average yield from *P. guttatus* maintained at Venom Supplies Laboratories is 32 mg. The colour of the dried lyophilized venom is a rich yellow.

Broad et al (1979), found LD_{50} = 1.53 mg/kg.

Kellaway (1929), carried out extensive laboratory tests on a number of different laboratory animals and found that the venom contained a coagulant, haemolysin, haemorrhagin and neurotoxin. He found the coagulant to be weaker for *N. scutatus* and *P. porphyriacus*. The venom was greater in haemolytic activity than for *N. scutatus*.

Despite the 4 general toxic activities described by Kellaway, no other recent work has been carried out with this venom to characterise and quantify the specific active fractions.

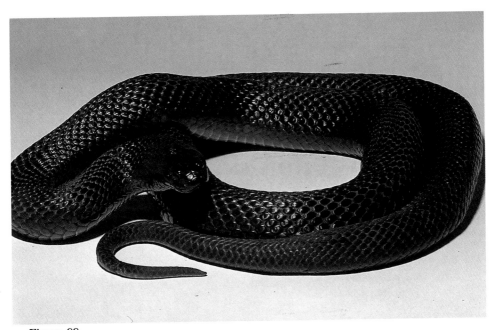

Figure 88
Pseudechis guttatus

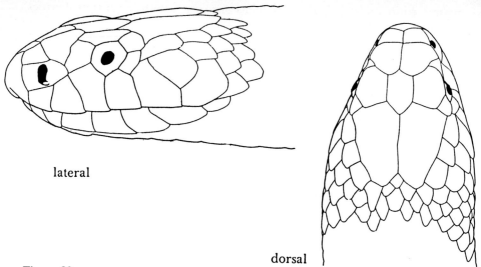

lateral

dorsal

Figure 89
Head scales of *P. guttatus*

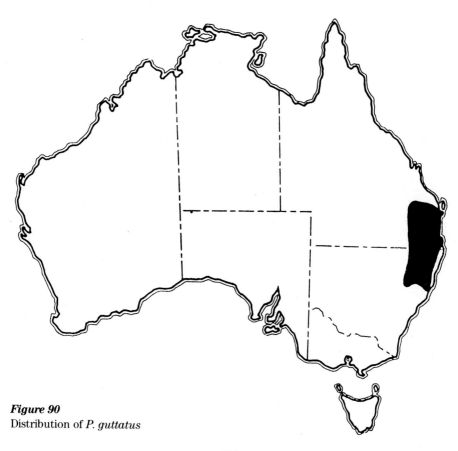

Figure 90
Distribution of *P. guttatus*

Antivenom:

Tiger Snake antivenom
Black Snake antivenom

Both antivenoms are manufactured by the Commonwealth Serum Laboratories (Melbourne).

Sutherland (1983), recommends the use of the Tiger Snake antivenom in preference to Black Snake antivenom based on the quantities involved for neutralization of the venom.

INITIAL DOSE — Tiger Snake — 3,000 units
OR Black Snake — 6,000 units

Butlers Snake *Pseudechis butleri* (Smith)

Description:

A large snake growing to a maximum of 1.6 m in length. Head moderately distinct from body.

Scalation:

VENTRALS	204-216
SUBCAUDALS	55-65 (35%-76% undivided)
MID-BODIES	17
ANAL	Divided

Colour:

Reddish-brown on the rostral, nasals, preoculars, labials (except for a short black subocular streak bordering orbit), chin shields, and gulars. Black on the remainder of head and nape with reddish-brown tinge. Reddish-brown on head and neck more prominent in juveniles. Remainder of dorsal scales black with yellow centres. Ventrals surface bright yellow with black flecks and an uneven black edge at base (Smith 1982). (Fig 91)

Habits:

Unknown.

Habitat and Distribution:

Arid mid-west of Western Australia (Smith 1982).

Venom:

Nothing is known about the venom, at this stage. However since it is closely related to *P. australis* (Smith 1982), their venom may be similar.

Antivenom:

Tiger Snake antivenom
Black Snake antivenom

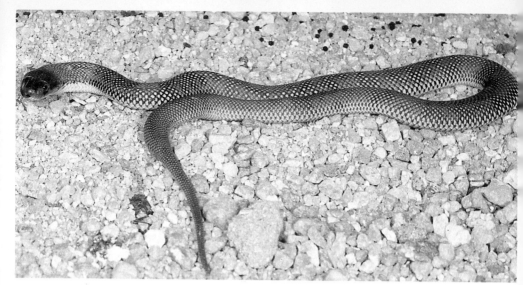

Figure 91
Pseudechis butleri (Photo M. Cermak)

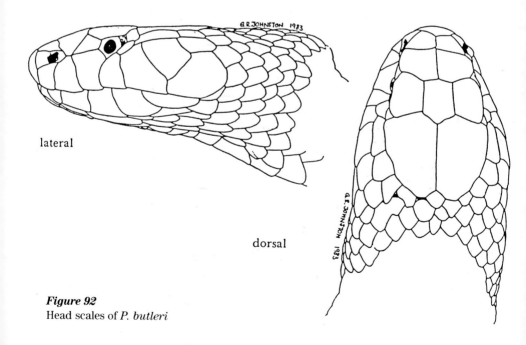

lateral

dorsal

Figure 92
Head scales of *P. butleri*

122

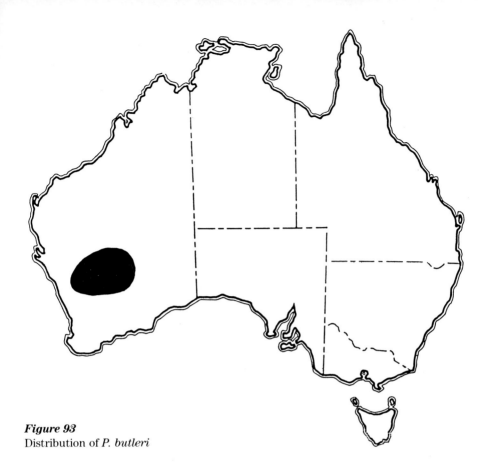

Figure 93
Distribution of *P. butleri*

Both are manufactured by the Commonwealth Serum Laboratories (Melbourne).

INITIAL DOSE   Tiger Snake — 3,000 units.
                      Black Snake — 18,000 units.

The Copperheads

Storr (1982), included Copperheads *Austrelaps* in his concept of *Notechis*.

Mengden (1985a), noted that *Notechis, Austrelaps* and *Tropidechis* have the same karymorph.

The comparative work carried out by Coulter and his co-workers, cited below, add further weight to the close relationship between *Notechis* and *Austrelaps*. This was supported by Minton and da Costa (1975) with their immunology comparison.

Rawlinson (pers comm), suggests there could be three separate forms of *Austrelaps* which are probably justify separate species. They are:

1   Highland form

2   Lowland form
3   Pygmy form (Adelaide Hills and Kangaroo Island)

The lowland and highland forms occur in areas of greater than 450 mm rainfall annually with average summer maximum temperatures ranging from 18°C —21°C in Tasmania Bass Strait Islands, to 24°C — 33°C on the mainland of Australia.

The pygmy species occurs in areas with 600 — 800 mm rainfall per year and a mild summer maximum of 23°C — 25°C average.

Copperhead *Austrelaps superbus* (Gunther)

Description:

Head small and slightly distinct from body. Attains 1.7 metres, but averages about 0.9 metres. Pygmy Copperheads are much smaller. They eye is large, and has a round pupil.

Scalation:

Smooth scales.

VENTRALS	140-165
SUBCAUDALS	35-55 single
MID-BODIES	15 (rarely 13 or 17)
ANAL	Single

Colour:

Dorsal colour variations are: black, brown, tan, coppery and light grey. Some specimens possess a dark vertebral stripe and dark band across the nape. Belly is cream to gray. The labial scales are often strikingly barred. (Figs 94, 95, 96).

Habits:

One of the features of the Copperhead is its low temperature tolerance (or preference). Copperheads are active earlier in spring and later in autumn than other snakes. Nocturnal during warm weather. Usually inoffensive, quick to retreat. Occur in large colonies. Viviparous; up to 20 young have been recorded. Shine (1980), recorded male combat in this species in the mating season.

Habitat and Distribution:

Occurs in the south-eastern highlands and surrounding swamplands. Has been recorded from mainland Tasmania, Kangaroo Island, Adelaide Hills, Flinders Island, King Island, Hunter Island, Preservation Island and Great Dog Island.

Notes:

The main diet, comprises either frogs or tadpoles. On occasions they will eat snakes, mice and lizards.

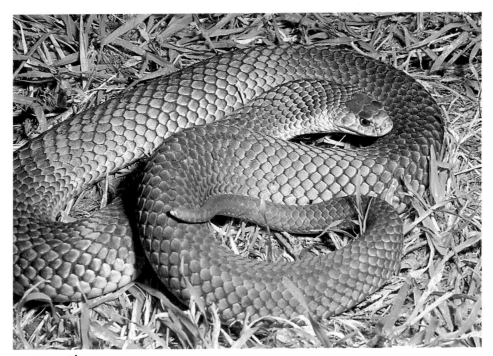

Figure 94
Austrelaps superbus (Lowland)

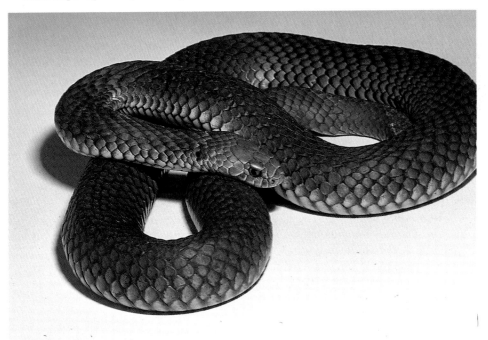

Figure 95
Austrelaps superbus (Lowland)

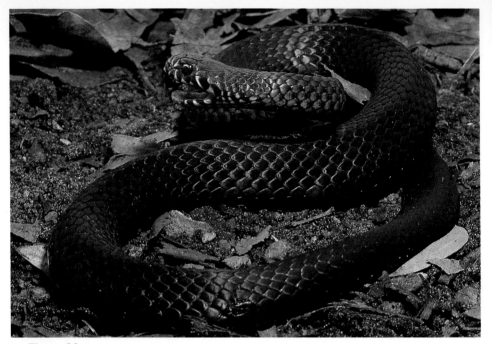

Figure 96
Austrelaps superbus (Pygmy)

Venom:

Austrelaps superbus maintained at Venom Supplies Laboratories yield on average 32 mg of dried venom. The maximum yield for the species was 84.6 mg (Fairley and Splatt 1929).

The dried lyophilized venom was cream in colour similar to *Notechis scutatus* venom.

Broad et al (1979), found that the LD_{50} = 0.5 mg/kg.

Considerate variations in toxicity have been reported in venom taken from *A. superbus* from different geographical locations (Sutherland 1983 and Mebs et al 1978). This is probably due to undescribed speciation which Sutherland (1983), has foreshadowed in his treatment of *A. ramsayi*. (Formal publication of this proposed new species by Rawlinson has not been forthcoming).

Kellaway (1929a) and Kellaway (1929e), demonstrated the venom had neurotoxic, anticoagulant, haemorrhagic and haemolytic properties. No coagulants were found.

Sutherland (1979b), showed that pronounced extension of PPT occurred in monkeys inoculated with this venom.

Doery and Pearson (1961), confirmed the presence of a direct haemolysin and phospholipase A.

Kaire (1964a), detected a heat stable anticoagulant.

Mebs et al (1978), found five toxic fractions in *A. superbus* venom, four of which were postsynaptic neurotoxins which were not cardiotoxins.

Figure 97
Head scales of *Austrelaps superhus*

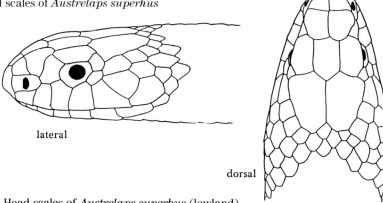

lateral

dorsal

Head scales of *Austrelaps superbus* (lowland)

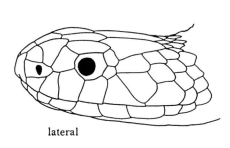

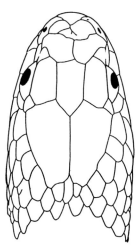

lateral

dorsal

Head scales of *Austrelaps superbus* (pygmy)

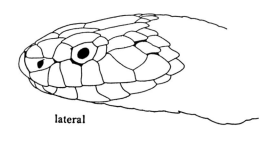

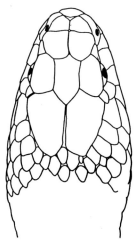

lateral

dorsal

Head scales of *Austrelaps superbus* (highland)

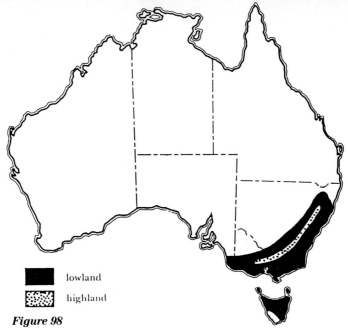

Figure 98
Distribution of *Austrelaps superhus*

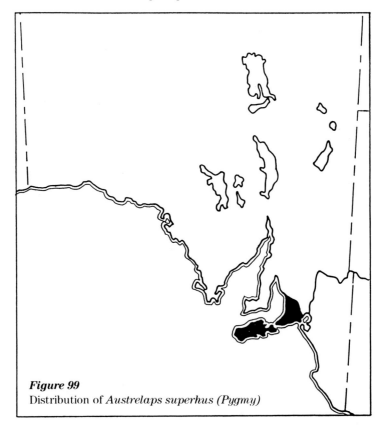

Figure 99
Distribution of *Austrelaps superhus (Pygmy)*

128

Coulter et al (1981), found that antibodies prepared against the presynaptic notexin from *N. scutatus* venom, reacted against one of the fractions in *A. superbus* venom. This provided further evidence for the proposal for Storr (1982), that *Austrelaps* genus could be absorbed into the *Notechis* genus. Mebs and Samejima (1980), isolated tow myolytic components. Sutherland et al (1981), also showed strong myolytic activity of the venom.

Bernheimer (1986), proposed that the haemolytic activity in *A. superbus* venom was due to phospholipase B.

Antivenom:

Tiger Snake Antivenom — manufactured by the Commonwealth Serum Laboratories (Melbourne).

INITIAL DOSE — 3,000 units

Copperhead *Austrelaps superbus* Case History (from Sutherland 1983)

This case demonstrates the development of a near fatal paralysis within five hours of the bite.

At 9 am on 26 November 1978 near Omeo in Victoria, a heavily built 22-year-old man jumped off a plough and trod on an *Austrelaps*. It bit him on the ankle and he killed it by jumping up and down upon it, thus increasing the rate of venom absorption. By the time he reached the Bairnsdale Hospital some five hours later, he was semiconscious and with marked cyanosis. He was intubated and given one ampoule of polyvalent antivenom, and then two ampoules of both Brown snake antivenom and Tiger snake antivenom. He was transferred to a Melbourne hospital where a further dose of both Tiger and Brown snake antivenom was given. The next day he was extubated and he made a good recovery.

Summary of Symptoms and Conditions Experienced with Austrelaps superbus Bites.

— Loss of consciousness.
— Cyanosis.
— Respiratory distress.
— Fluid on lungs.
— Paralysis.

The Broad-headed Snakes

The Board-headed snakes (genus *Hoplocephalus*) all occur along the eastern coast and are characterized by their broad heads, keeled ventral scales, and smooth dorsal scales.

Throughout their range the average rainfall exceeds 800mm and the summer average maximum is about 30°C.

Pale-headed Snake *Hoplocephalus bitorquatus* (Jan)

Description:

Broad flat head distinct from body. Varies in length from 0.5 — 0.9 m.

Scalation:

Smooth scales.

VENTRALS	190-225 keeled
SUBCAUDALS	40-65 single
MID-BODIES	19 or 21
ANAL	Single

Colour:

The dorsal colour is light brown to grey with a white or cream band on the nape. There is lighter grey colouring on the head interspersed with dark grey scales. The ventral surface is creamy grey, occasionally with darker flecks. (Fig 100).

Habits:

Mostly arboreal and lives under tree bark where it feeds on geckoes and

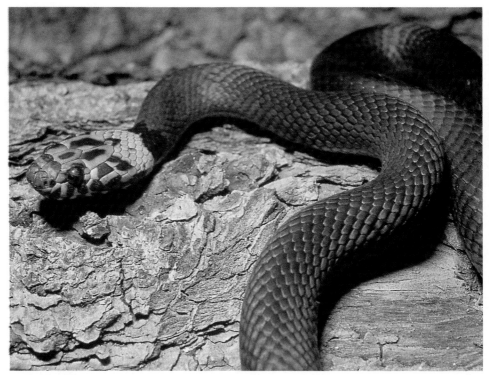

Figure 100
Hoplocehalus bitorquatus

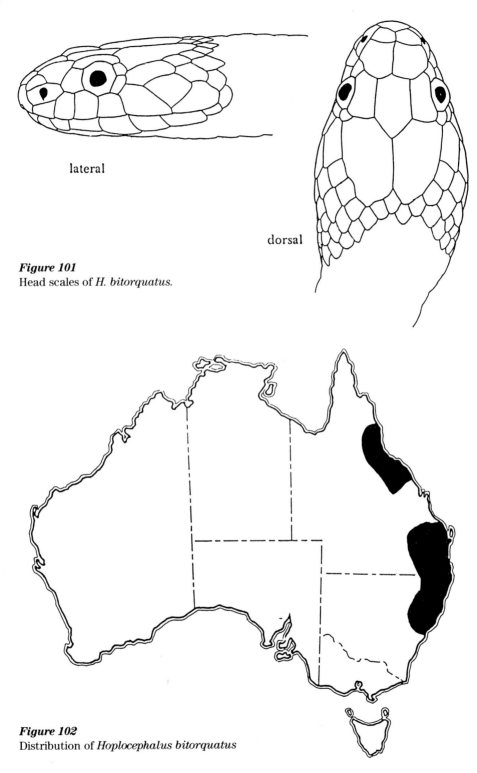

lateral

dorsal

Figure 101
Head scales of *H. bitorquatus.*

Figure 102
Distribution of *Hoplocephalus bitorquatus*

lizards. Easily aroused assuming a threat posture at the slightest disturbance. Viviparous.

Habitat and Distribution:

Rain forest, wet sclerophyll forest to dry sclerophyll forest and woodlands.

Venom:

Yield 1.66 mg (Single milking record). Very little known at this stage.

Joe Bredl (pers. com.) suffered blurred and double vision, sweating, breathing difficulty, and headache within 10 minutes of bite from a specimen 0.76 m long.

Antivenom:

Tiger Snake Venom — manufactured by the Commonwealth Serum Laboratories (Melbourne).

Sutherland (1983), reports that it is unlikely that antivenom would ever be necessary.

INITIAL DOSE — Tiger Snake antivenom — 3,000 units.

Stephens Banded Snake *Hoplocephalus stephensi* (Krefft)
Description:

Broad flat head, distinct from body. Varies from 0.5 m to 1 m length.

Scalation:

Smooth scales.

VENTRALS	220-250 keeled
SUBCAUDALS	50-70 single
MID-BODIES	21
ANAL	Single

Colour:

Dorsally black with narrow cream crossbands. Unbanded specimens occur on occasions. On the ventral surface they are cream with black spots tending to uniform black at the tip of tail. (Fig 103).

Habits:

Ill-tempered snake, usually difficult to keep in captivity. An arboreal snake that takes refuge behind loose bark or in tree hollows. Nocturnal.

Habitat and Distribution:

Wet sclerophyll or rainforests of the east coast.

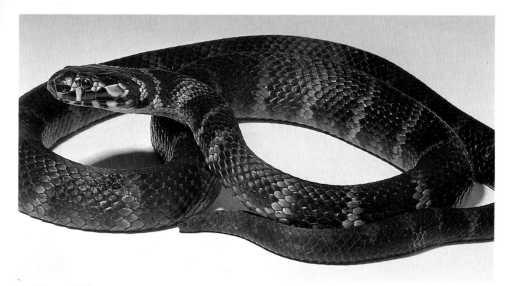

Figure 103
Hoplocephalus stephensi

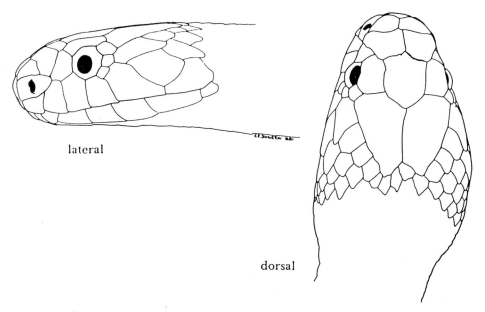

lateral

dorsal

Figure 104
Head scales of *Hoplocephalus stephensi*

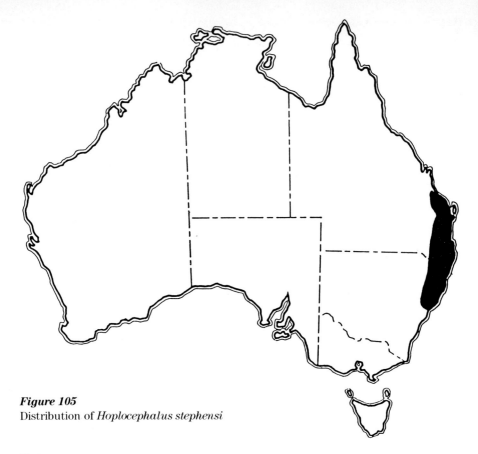

Figure 105
Distribution of *Hoplocephalus stephensi*

Notes:

Viviparous — 5 young have been observed. The main threat to its survival lies in the future of the rainforests in its range.

Feeds on geckoes and skinks, sometimes large specimens in captivity accept mice.

Venom:

Kellaway (1934b), indicated yields, of a single 0.7 m specimen from 2 —6 mg.

Broad et al (1979), found the venom to have LD_{50} = 1.44 mg/kg.

Kellaway (1934b), described the venom as powerfully coagulant, mildly neurotoxic and feebly haemolytic.

Antivenom:

Tiger Snake antivenom — manufactured by the Commonwealth Serum Laboratories (Melbourne).

Sutherland (1983), is of the opinion antivenom would rarely be necessary for bites from this species.

INITIAL DOSE — 3,000 units.

Broad-headed Snake *Hoplocephalus bungaroides* (Schlegel)

Description:

Head distinct from body. Broad head. Maximum length is about 0.6 m.

Scalation:

Smooth scales.

VENTRALS	200-230 keeled
SUBCAUDALS	40-65 single
MID-BODIES	21
ANAL	Single

Colour:

Jet black dorsally with narrow yellow cross bands. Labial scales barred with black and yellow. Head black with yellow spots (Fig 106).

Habits:

Feeds on lizards and frogs. Nocturnal. Herpetologists find this one of the more difficult snakes to handle.

Habitat and Distribution:

Lives in a restricted area of about 250 km radius of Sydney, mainly living under sandstone rocks. Its main population occurs in the Hawkesbury sandstone formation. Worrell (1963) noted that it also lives in hollow trees during summer.

Notes:

Viviparous giving birth to 8 - 20 young. Because of restricted range, much of which is situated in a highly populated area, it is the opinion of the authors that this snake is an endangered species and its legal protection must be fully supported.

Venom:

Kellaway (1934b), studied the effects of this venom with a venom sample 23 years ago. He noted a yield of 12 mg and that the venom contained a strong coagulant activity which altered with heat application, and neurotoxic activity. It was also feebly haemolytic. He found the venom was effectively neutralised by antivenom made against *N. scutatus* and to a lesser extent by *A. superbus* antivenom.

Worrell (1963), reported that a bite caused a violent headache, vomiting, partial blindness, perspiration and general weakness.

Antivenom:

Tiger Snake antivenom — manufactured by the Commonwealth Serum Laboratories (Melbourne).

INITIAL DOSE — 3,000 units.

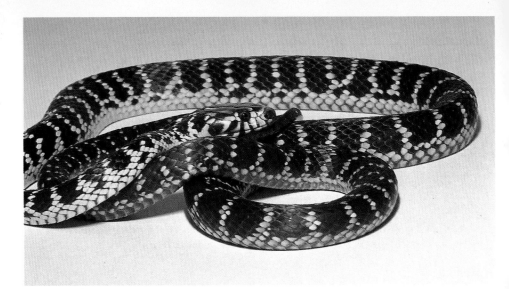

Figure 106
Hoplocephalus bungaroides

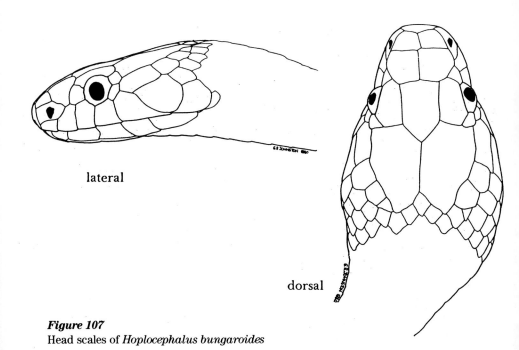

lateral

dorsal

Figure 107
Head scales of *Hoplocephalus bungaroides*

136

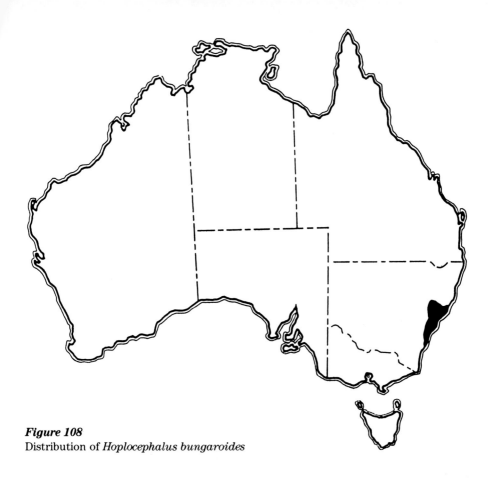

Figure 108
Distribution of *Hoplocephalus bungaroides*

Broad-headed Snake Case History
Hoplocephalus bungaroides (from Worrell 1958)

Worrell received a bite from a 0.7 m long specimen. His account is as follows:

"At the time I was living in Sydney and weighed a healthy eleven stone. I didn't bother to treat the bite as it was a quick snap, and seemed inconsequential. I was running late for a city appointment so immediately ran five hundred yards to a tram stop and jumped on a moving tram. Five minutes after the bite I developed a violent headache, my vision blurred, and everything seemed dark. I vomited, and lost my powers of speech. My hands were icy cold, yet my clothes were soaked with perspiration. Even breathing was difficult. Ten minutes after the bite I decided I needed medical attention, but could not convey my wishes to the sole fellow passenger."

"I was aware of the guard asking for fares. "Probably back from New Guinea with a wog". I heard the passenger explain. "He'll be all right. I'll keep an eye on him.""

"Gradually within the next twenty minutes the condition subsided, and within thirty minutes had disappeared, leaving me weakened and shivering."

Summary of Symptoms and Conditions Experienced with *Hoplocephalus bungaroides* Bites

— Drowsiness.
— Violent headache.
— Blurred vision.
— Vomiting.
— Lost powers of speech.
— Cold hands.
— Perspiring.
— Difficulty breathing.
— Local swelling and pain.
— Flushing.
— Pyrexia.
— Sore joints.
— Difficulty opening mouth.
— Dysphagia.
— Nausea.

Other Snakes
Rough-scaled Snake *Tropidechis carinatus* (Krefft)

Mengden (1985b), noted that *Notechis Austrelaps* and *Tropidechis* have the same karymorph. Storr (1985), presented an argument to include *Tropidechis* in the *Notechis* lineage. The comparative venom studies listed below carried out by Sutherland, Trinca, Morrison and their co-workers, add further weight to the close relationship between *Notechis* and *Tropidechis*. This is further supported on ecological grounds by Shine (1985).

Description:

Broad head, distinct from body. Grows to almost 1 m but averages about 0.7 m. Large eyes. Superficially resembles the harmless fresh water snake *(Styporhynchus mairii)* and is sympatric with it in part of its range. Possesses large fangs up to 5 mm (Reilly 1963).

Scalation:

Dorsal scales strongly keeled.

VENTRALS	160-185
SUBCAUDALS	50-60 single
MID-BODIES	23
ANAL	Single

Colour:

Dorsally, it is olive green to dark brown with dark blotches forming cross bands. Ventral surface is creamish with darker blotches (Fig 109).

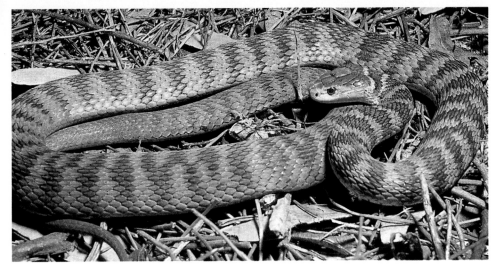

Figure 109
Tropidechis carinatus

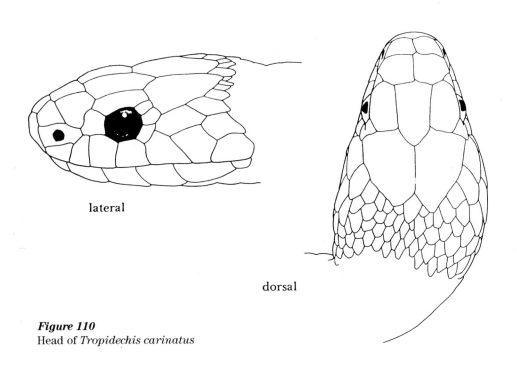

lateral

dorsal

Figure 110
Head of *Tropidechis carinatus*

Habits:

Feeds mainly on frog but also takes lizards and mice in captivity. Very alert and nervous. Herpetologists find it very difficult to handle safely. Both diurnal and nocturnal.

Habitat and Distribution:

Prefers areas near water. Found in wet sclerophyll forests or rainforests. Most common in the Clarence River district of New South Wales. Limited to areas with rainfall exceeding 800 mm/year. Often referred to as the Clarence River snake. Will defend itself vigorously if molested or threatened. Very nervous snake when kept in captivity.

Venom:

T. carinatus maintained by Venom Supplies Laboratories yield on average 11 mg of dried lyophilized venom (3 snakes). The colour of the venom was similar to that of *N. scutatus*.

Broad et al (1979), found that LD_{50} = 1.09 mg/kg.

Sutherland (1983), reported that the venom of *T. carinatus* cross reacts strongly with *N. scutatus* crude venom, notexin from *N. scutatus* venom, and crude venoms of *P. porphyriacus* and *A. superbus*.

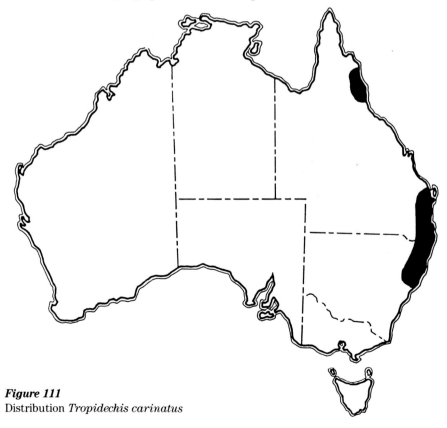

Figure 111
Distribution *Tropidechis carinatus*

Millar (1963), studied the effects of *T. carinatus* venom in a number of animals and concluded it was neurotoxic and affected coagulation.

Trinca et al (1971), reported a powerful coagulant (slightly weaker than in *N. scutatus* venom). and the presence of a potent phospholipase.

Sutherland (1981) and Pearn (1987) both reported myotoxicity. Sutherland (1981), recorded the CK levels of 3,044 IU/1 between 150 and 180 minutes after inoculation in monkeys. Sutherland (1983), also observed the CK levels at 5,000 IU/1 after 6 hours.

Morrison et al (1984), studied the venom of *T. carinatus* and found 5 fractions of which only 2 were significant to envenomation. They discovered the major toxic effect arose from one of the fractions and it proved to possess both potent presynaptic and postsynaptic activity. They proposed that this neurotoxin was similar to notexin from *N. scutatus* venom based on its similar LD_{50} rating, and molecular weight. They also found that there was a marked difference in toxicity in the other potent fraction with the age of the mice test animals, and that it was postsynaptic in action.

Morrison et al (1984), also found that *T. carinatus* venom was fairly robust when challenged by a variety of "physical insults" such as heat, sonication, and freeze-thaw cycles.

Antivenom:

Tiger Snake — manufactured by the Commonwealth Serum Laboratories (Melbourne).

INITIAL DOSE Tiger Snake antivenom — 3,000 units.

Rough Scaled Snake — *Tropidechis carinatus* (from Patten et al 1985)

On July 28, 1978, a 9-year-old boy was playing in long grass near his home at Kin Kin, 10 miles west of the Cooloola coast, in south-east Queensland. He felt a sharp prick on his hand and within minutes felt weak, vomited and lost consciousness. When the ambulance attendants arrived, they noted that faecal incontinence had occurred, and that he was very pale and limb; he soon regained consciousness and was able to move all his limbs.

At the local hospital, the boy complained, during the subsequent 24 hours, of intermittent abdominal, chest and limb pains, and of progressive weakness. He was noted to be in a disturbed conscious state, with dilated pupils, muscular incoordination and weak pulse, and suffered an episode of acute bronchospasm, which responded to treatment with bronchodilator agents. Twenty-four hours after the bite he began to pass dark red urine. Over the next twelve hours his clinical state deteriorated until cardiopulmonary arrest occurred, 38 hours after the bite. This was successfully managed with intermittent positive pressure ventilation (IPPV), external cardiac massage and the administration of inotropic agents. IPPV had to be maintained for about 10 weeks before it was gradually withdrawn. Thirty-nine hours after the bite, decerebrate spasms occurred for two hours.

Fifty to sixty hours later, some further historical details of the circumstances relating to his initial collapse had become available, and at 10 am, 60 hours after the bite, he received an intravenous infusion of less than half a 50 ml ampoule of Australian Polyvalent Snake Antiserum (containing 3,000 units of tiger snake antivenom), diluted (1 in 10) in 500 cm^3 saline. No noticeable improvement occurred, and when hypotension developed, the administration of antivenom was stopped. By 72 hours, the patient had developed oliguric renal failure, and hyperkalaemia and hypertension were noted. Several hours later, an unknown quantity of polyvalent antivenom was administered by intravenous infusion, again with no apparent clinical improvement. On day 4, the boy was transferred to the Royal Children's Hospital, Brisbane. On his admission, at 8 am, 88 hours after the bite, he was suffering from gross oedema, anuria, hypothermia and flaccid paralysis. IPPV was maintained. The boy's blood pressure was 120/100 mmHg. Abnormal oozing from previous venepuncture sites was noted. There was no muscle fasciculation or fibrillation. A small puncture with associated scratch marks was seen near the base of the right finger, which was consistent with a snake bite.

The results of initial laboratory investigations were as follows; haemoglobin concentration, 146 g/L (several hours post-transfusion); white cell count, 42.8 x 10^9/L (neutrophils, 86%); platelet count, 290 x 10^{9}L; coagulation screening test results were normal, except for thrombin time, 15 s (normal, 9-11 s); plasma fibrinogen, 2.3 g/L (normal, 1.5 — 4.0 g/L), fibrin degradation products, 20 mg/L (normal, less than 20 mg/L). Tests for intravascular haemolysis produced negative results, and there was no haemoglobinuria. The urine contained gross amounts of myoglobin. The serum sodium level was 131 mmol/L; serum potassium level, 5.4 mmol/L; serum calcium level, 1.30 mmol/L; serum phosphate level, 1.56 mmol/L; serum urea level, 19.5 mmol/L; serum creatine level, 0.21 mmol/L; serum lactic dehyrogenase, 11,500 μ/L (normal, 1.25 — 3.25 μ/L); creatine phosphokinase, 380,000 μ/L, (normal, 0.35 — 2.10 μ/L). A chest x-ray showed collapse of the right upper lobe of the lung. An ECG showed an abnormal sinus rhythm.

Within one hour after the boy's admission to the Royal Children's Hospital, the content of one ampoule of polyvalent antivenom was administered, undiluted, intravenously over 30 minutes. Within 15 minutes there was a dramatic improvement in muscle power, particularly in the lower limbs, but this was no longer sustained one hour later. Three further ampoule doses of polyvalent antivenom were given at 92, 94 and 98 hours after the bite.

The improvement observed after the first administration of antivenom in Brisbane was seen again with the second, but did not occur after the third and fourth doses.

On the day following the child's admission to the hospital in Brisbane, the result of an ELISA assay for snake venom in samples in blood and urine collected on July 31, 1978 (59 hours) became available. No venom was detected in the blood. Venom was detected in the boy's urine, and reacted with Tiger snake antivenom at concentrations of 3 ng/ml in the urine. At the time, it was known that this result could have been due to either Tiger snake or Rough-scaled snake envenomation. Tiger snake antivenom (or polyvalent antivenom, which contains tiger snake antivenom) is the appropriate antivenom for the management of envenomation by both these species.

Renal failure occurred within 48 hours after the bite. Peritoneal dialysis was instituted on day 4 to correct the hyperkalaemia and fluid retention. With the aid of the instillation of intragastric ion-exchange resin, the hyperkalaemia settled on day 5. Despite the intravenous administration of calcium gluconate, and an increase in the calcium content of the dialysate to 4 mmol/L with calcium chloride, the serum calcium level on day 5 was only 1.67 mmol/L.

From day 6 to day 8, gross palpable myokymia occurred. An ECG on day 8 showed grossly abnormal profuse slow activity. Total paralysis remained, and gross generalized muscle wasting was present from the third week. An EMG showed a total loss of many motor units, with residual units showing myopathic (low voltage, polyphastic) potentials. Other complications early in the clinical course included gastrointestinal haemorrhage and stasis, diarrhoea, hypoproteinaemia, chest infections, possible septicaemia, and hypertension from day 15 to day 18, which necessitated the intravenous administration of hydralazine. The serum calcium level remained below 2 mmol/L until day 16. Complete anuria persisted until day 21, controlled by peritoneal dialysis. Myoglobinuria had cleared by day 35.

The return of voluntary power occurred in a striking centripetal direction. Very weak but definite movement in the legs returned during the second week. In the subsequent nine weeks, movement gradually returned in the arms, in the hands, then in the face (four weeks,) the external ocular muscles (five weeks), the palate (nine weeks) and the pharynx and respiratory muscles (eleven weeks).

Respiratory function showed the slowest improvement, and palatal movement and swallowing were also very slow to recover. Artifical ventilation was gradually diminished from week 7, and was no longer necessary at the beginning of week 11.

An intravenous pyelogram at week 13 showed changes consistent with earlier medullary necrosis. The glomerular filtration rate remained at 43 ml/min at week 13, and the creatinine clearance was 26 ml/min at week 16, indicating significantly reduced renal function (both serum urea and creatinine levels were normal at this time).

Serial EMG studies showed delayed terminal latency consistent with a peripheral neuropathy, and some myopathic changes were still evident at week 16. Late complications included two episodes of aspiration pneumonia, one during week 14, which necessitated bronchial aspiration. Eighteen weeks after the bite, the patient was well enough to be discharged from hospital. Generalized muscle wasting was still present, and muscle power (particularly swallowing) was still well below normal. His blood pressure was normal.

Six months after his discharge from hospital, the boy was back at school and leading a relatively normal life. The only long-term complication was an oesophageal stricture necessitating dilation to allow the normal passage of solid food.

Three years later, full psychological assessment revealed an IQ in the normal range (WISC-R Full Scale IQ 95; Verbal sub-scale, 96; Performance sub-scale, 95). He has remained clinically well since.

Summary of Symptoms and Conditions Experienced with Tropidechis carinatus Bites

— Vomiting.
— Loss of consciousness (rapid).
— Incontinence.
— Paleness.
— Abdominal, chest and limb pains.
— Weakness.
— Dilated pupils.
— Muscular inco-ordination.
— Weak pulse.
— Acute bronchospasm.
— Dark red urine.
— Cardiopulmonary arrest.
— Decerebrate spasms.
— Hypotension.
— Oliguric renal failure.
— Hyperkalaemia.
— Hypertension.
— Gross oedema.
— Anuria.
— Hypothermia.
— Flaccid paralysis.
— Oozing from venepunctures.
— Myoglobinurea.
— Abnormal sinus rythmn.
— Staggering gait.
— Breathing difficulty.
— Nausea.
— Micturition.
— Dysphonia.
— Coughing spasm.
— Blindness.
— Tachycardia.
— Dark brown urine.
— Dizziness.
— Blurry vision.
— Sweating.
— Bleeding of gums.
— Diarrhoea.
— Prolonged coagulation.
— Amnesia.

Small-Eyed Snake *Cryptophis nigrescens* **(Gunther)**

Description:

Grows to 1.2 m. Head distinct from body.

Colour:

Shiny blue-black dorsally. Ventrally white, cream, or pink, sometimes with darker blotches. (Fig 112)

Scalation:

Smooth scales.

VENTRALS	165-210
SUBCAUDALS	30-46 single
MID-BODIES	15
ANAL	Single

Habits:

Nocturnal. Feeds mainly on geckoes and small skinks, occasionally frogs. Viviparous, producing up to 5 young. The young measure 10 — 20 cm.

Habits and Distribution:

Sandstone areas, well timbered country, rocky areas. Found under rocks, in

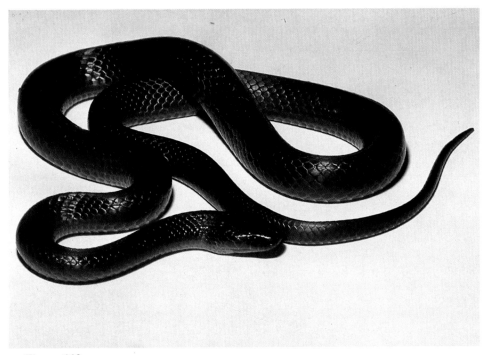

Figure 112
Cryptophis nigrescens

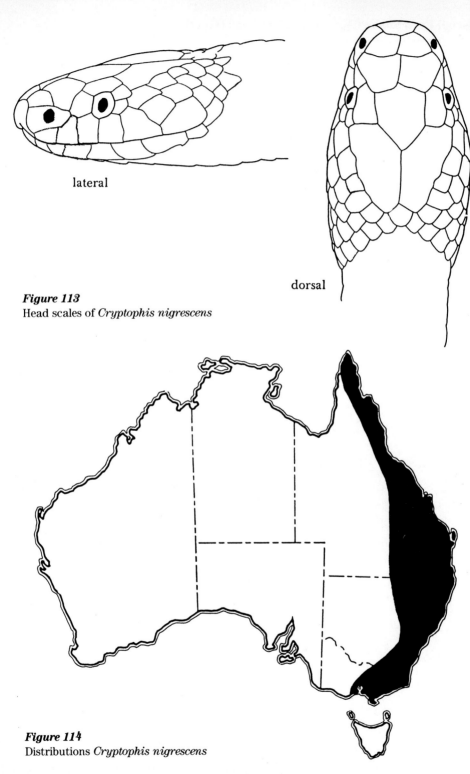

lateral

dorsal

Figure 113
Head scales of *Cryptophis nigrescens*

Figure 114
Distributions *Cryptophis nigrescens*

crevices, earth cracks, or under the bark of fallen trees. They have been found hibernating together in large numbers.

Venom:

Sutherland (1983), reported the average yield on this snake to be about 5 mg. Pollitt (1980), reported a higher yield of 8 mg using a plastic capillary tube for venom extraction.

Broad et al (1979), recorded a LD_{50} = 2.67 mg/kg (saline).

Sutherland (1983), noted that *C. nigrescens* venom contained a notexin-like component. Pollitt (1980) suggested that this fraction, called cryptoxin, might be similar to notexin but has no neurotoxic effect but instead, only myotoxic. In a monkey experiment described by Sutherland (1979b), very little toxic effect was experienced by inoculation of 1,200 μg of *C. nigrescens* venom. Myolytic activity was registered when the CK increased to 16 times its normal level in 170 minutes after inoculation. This could be rated as moderate myotoxic effect in comparison to myotoxic envenomation from other snakes. Pollitt (1980), concluded that destruction of muscle tissue continues for days after envenomation. Death may result due to renal failure, dehydration or inhalational pneumonia.

Antivenom:

Tiger snake — manufactured by the Commonwealth Serum Laboratories (Melbourne).

INITIAL DOSE — 3,000 units

Small Eyed Snake Case History
Cryptophis nigrescens (from Furtado and Lester 1968)

On the 9th of May 1965, a 20-year-old male, whose hobby was collecting reptiles, was bitten on the left index finger by a *C. nigrescens*. He ignored the bite because he believed the snake to be harmless, an opinion supported by the fact that he had received bites previously with no apparent effects. Three days later he was admitted to the local hospital complaining of a stiff neck and inability to open his mouth. These complaints could not be demonstrated objectively and he was discharged after an injection of tetanus toxoid.

He was readmitted to hospital five days after the bite with severe muscle pain and weakness of his lower limbs. He was transferred to Cairns Base Hospital where a diagnosis of leptospirosis was made on the basis of pyrexia, dark urine and muscle pain. He was commenced on crystalline penicillin. Over the next few days the muscle power and weakness increased and his output of dark brown urine fell.

He died on 19 May 1965 of renal failure secondary to myoglobinaemia. Although a muscle biopsy of the left deltoid performed on 18 May showed areas of muscle necrosis, no changes were detected in post mortem samples from either quadriceps.

Summary of Symptoms and Conditions Experienced with *Cryptophis nigrescens* Bites

— Stiff neck.
— Inability to open mouth.
— Severe muscle pain.
— Weakness of lower limbs.
— Pyrexia.
— Dark urine.
— Renal failure.
— Myoglobinaemia.
— Widespread hyaline degeneration of muscles.

EDITOR'S NOTE:- The following section on the treatment of snake bite is given without any comments from the editor. It is true not only to Australia but also to the other countries. This will allow the reader to understand the actual practise and method of treatment in that particular country. Even though the editor not necessarily agree with some of the steps they are allowed to show the present status.

First Aid Treatment of Snake Bite

"In practical terms, venom movement can be effectively delayed for long periods by the applications of a firm crepe bandage to the length of the bitten limb combined with immobilisation by a splint. Pressure alone or immobilisation did not delay venom movement." (Sutherland et al 1979).

Optimal first aid treatment of snake bite is the immediate application of a firm broad pressure bandage to the limb. The limb should also be kept still and immobilised by a splint. Clothing or towels can be used as makeshift bandages and rolled up newspaper used for a splint.

Compression Bandage

For research, Sutherland et al (1979), used an experimental model of an adult monkey restricted in a well-padded frame. He showed that following the injection of Tiger Snake *(Notechis scutatus)* venom into a limb, which was immobilised and compressed, only low levels of circulating venom resulted. The reason for the low plasma levels of venom appeared to be due to immobilising the venom by compressing lymphatics at the bite site and thus reducing lymph flow. Compression of superficial veins may also help in restricting venom movement. The pressure used during the experiment was 55 mm mercury and this is equivalent to applying a firm bandage to a sprained ankle. Both crude venom and neurotoxin levels were measured. Snake venom is usually injected subcutaneously and the lymphatics are largely responsible for the venom's absorption. First aid measures aim to decrease and slow down central lymphatic movement.

This has been clearly demonstrated in a number of real snake bite emergencies (Pearn et al 1979, Harvey et al 1982 and Mirtschin et al 1984).

The victim should rest, not walk around, and should be transferred to hospital with minimal delay. If possible, bring transport to the patient rather than vice versa. In remote areas, aerial transport and medical retrieval teams should always be considered (Davis et al 1979). Snake identification and early hospital notification are valuable adjuncts to therapy.

Following snake bite, hypotension (low blood pressure) and collapse may occur. For this reason it is best to position the patient lying down during transport. Also, if the patient does collapse, his blood pressure and circulation can be improved by raising his legs. It is essential that the victim's airway be maintained and safeguarded. If paralysis is rapid and breathing ceases, mouth to mouth ventilation, applied by untrained personnel in a car, will probably be ineffective. In this case, the car should stop and ventilation maintained with the patient lying on the ground. Help should be summoned and an ambulance with trained first aiders, if possible including a medical team with antivenom supplies, be brought to the patient.

Incising and excising snake bite is absolutely contraindicated (Sutherland 1979a). There is no evidence to show that incising snake bite is of any use and clearly it runs the risk of damaging tissues.

Cryotherapy and placing the bitten limb in ice are also contraindicated. Alcohol, food, and drugs which depress respiration should not be given.

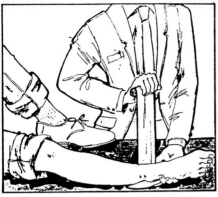

1. Apply a broad pressure bandage over bite site.

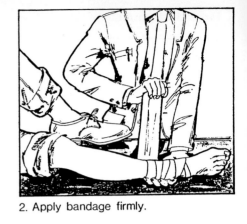

2. Apply bandage firmly.

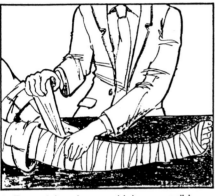

3. Extend bandage as high as possible.

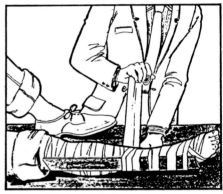

4. Immobilise the limb.

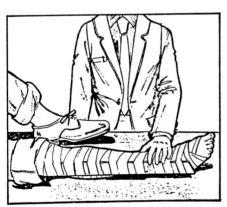

5. Limb immobilised with pressure bandage in place.

Sutherland has shown that the use of arterial tourniquets is impractical because even short usage causes intense distress (Sutherland 1979b). In addition, he points out that when the tourniquet is released, there is a surge of blood into the limb causing reflex hyperaemia which results in rapid central movement of the venom. Tourniquets reduce the central movement of the lympatics; arterial tourniquets very effectively but venous tourniquets in an uncertain manner. Venous tourniquets will limit venous and lymphatic return, but venous congestion, discomfort in the limb and increased lymphatic production will result. The inevitable result is that the victim releases the tourniquet, potentially causing an emergency.

Many snake bites would not occur if adequate prophylactic measures and greater caution were taken. Where possible, always wear protective clothing including long trousers and boots. Avoid long grass and at night time use a torch when walking about in the bush. Cut grass around houses and playgrounds and clear away rubbish. Most important, children should be taught to leave snakes alone. When travelling in remote areas a radio transmitter is valuable for many reasons, including medical communication (Sutherland 1979c).

The question is often asked, "We are going for a holiday in the country; should we take antivenom with us?" It is a calculated risk but usually antivenom should not be taken for a number of reasons. It is expensive, needs to be kept in a refrigerator, and if used should be given intravenously with resuscitation equipment and drugs available to treat anaphylaxis if it occurs.

Antivenoms

Antivenom is the only specific treatment of snake bite and today virtually all snake-bite deaths are due to lack of adequate correct antivenom. Antivenoms should never be withheld when there are clear indications for their use. On occasions, antivenoms may not be available, but usually where tragedies occur, too little antivenom has been given, often too late.

Unfortunately, some doctors still believe that antivenoms 'are more dangerous than the disease itself', but this is not correct. Sutherland (1977), reviewed all serious reactions to antivenoms over a fifteen year period and found no deaths related to anaphylaxis. More recently, Sutherland et al (1979), followed up 181 out of 203 (89%) cases where antivenom was used to treat snake-bite victims during the twelve-month period from July 1978 to June 1979 and again, there were no deaths from antivenom anaphylaxis.

Nevertheless, reactions to antivenom are reasonably common and this is why patients should be premedicated with an antihistamine and adrenaline. The antivenom should be given as a slow dilute infusion. In early days when antivenoms were very crude preparations and many people had been sensitised to equine proteins following the use of antisera (eg. for tetanus and diphtheria immunisation), severe reactions were more worrying. Trinca (1963), noted that a decade earlier, three deaths had occurred from anaphylactic reactions. Since this report, there has been no death due to anaphylactic reactions to snake antivenom in Australia. Today, because reactions are less severe and less common, it is a mistake only to use antivenom in desperate situations.

To make the antivenom, a constant supply of snake venom is required, and this is acquired from suppliers such as Venom Supplies Laboratories in South Australia. Here, many snakes used for venom extraction are kept, bred and regularly milked for their venom. The liquid venom is lyophilized, stored refrigerated under vacuum and dispatched to the Commonwealth Serum Laboratories in Victoria as required. Venom produced at Venom supplies is also used for medical research all over the world.

The initial step in antivenom production is the immunisation of horses with the venom. The Commonwealth Serum Laboratories own a 616 — hectare farm where some 250 French-bred Percheron horses are regularly injected with venoms from snakes. The snake venom is injected at increasing dosages until the horse has developed sufficient antibodies. The serum is then collected and fractionated. The horse immunoglobulins are purified, concentrated, and standardised to contain a minimal number of units. A unit of antivenom will neutralise 0.01 mg of dried snake venom.

Antivenom should be stored away from the light in a refrigerator between 0°C and 10°C. It should not be frozen and its shelf life is three years. Antivenom is available for sale to the hospitals and anyone authorised to write a prescription.

In Australia, all snake-bite antivenoms are of equine origin and contain large volumes of protein. One ampoule of Australian polyvalent antivenom contains more than 40 ml of 17% equine protein. This is greater than any other overseas polyvalent antivenom and also has the highest protein concentration. Such an enormous quantity of antivenom is required because of the potency and yield of Australia's dangerous snakes.

Antivenom possess considerable anti-complementary activity and it is believed that anaphylactic reactions are due, at least in part, to this activity (Sutherland 1977b). The more protein infused, the greater the chance of an immediate or a delayed reaction.

Campbell (1969), reviewed 61 cases of snake bite treated at the Moresby General Hospital and 28 patients (46%) developed some side effect, including five (8%) who suffered a serious anaphylactic-type reaction. Delayed reactions were more common following large doses of antivenom. Sutherland et al (1979), has reported that 79% of unexpected reactions to antivenom occur following usage of the large volume polyvalent antivenom. In these same series Sutherland noted 13% of patients suffered some untoward effects when giving antivenom. Patients receiving polyvalent have a 10% or greater chance of developing a significant delayed reaction. Clearly, where the snake has been accurately identified, it is preferable to use the small volume monovalent antivenom. Severe, acute and delayed reactions are more common in older snake-bite victims suggesting that prior exposure to equine protein may be a factor.

Antivenom should be given when there are definite signs or symptoms of systemic envenomation. It is likely that all patients who have been effectively bitten by a mature, dangerous, snake will need antivenom. Children become critically ill faster than adults because of their small body weight and because they more frequently have suffered multiple bites. The dose of antivenom for a child is the same as for an adult and that is enough to neutralise the venom.

Details on how to give antivenom are listed on the package by the Commonwealth Serum Laboratories. The antivenom should be diluted 1 in 10 in saline solution and then slowly infused over twenty minutes. Prior to starting the infusion the patient should receive an antihistamine, eg. Phenergan 25 — 50 mg (promethazine HCI) and subcutaneous adrenaline. Anaesthetists frequently give adrenaline as a slow careful intravenous infusion under E.C.G. Control. Adrenaline is the drug par excellence in reducing anaphylactic shock and the dose in adults is about 0.3 mg. Steroids are recommended for patients likely to develop serum sickness, which includes those persons with a relevant allergic history, asthma sufferers, and those who have received equine protein previously. Wherever possible, it is recommended that antivenom be given by medical personnel in hospital where there are satisfactory facilities for resuscitation. When these precautions are taken, serious reactions to antivenom are unlikely. Preliminary sensitivity tests are not accurate and skin testing with antivenom is not recommended.

When determining the dose of antivenom required, the following facts should be kept in mind. The quantity of antivenom in an ampoule is the amount required to neutralise the venom from an 'average yield' milking, in vitro. The quantity of venom injected into a snake-bite victim is unknown but may be more than an 'average yield' milking. If five times the quantity of venom has been injected, five ampoules of antivenom would be required. Where delays in using antivenom have occurred, more antivenom may be required. No patient is too ill to receive antivenom.

In 1929 the first national distribution of antivenom took place in Australia. It was an antivenom for the treatment of Tiger Snake bite. Following this, other specific monovalent antivenoms were produced and this culminated in 1962 with the release of polyvalent antivenom for use in Australia and Papua New Guinea. Since the introduction and distribution of polyvalent antivenom it has no longer been essential to identify the snake involved.

Reactions to antivenoms may be immediate or delayed and can be mild to severe. Immediate mild symptoms and signs include pyrexia, rash, sweating, headache, mild bronchospasm, cough and vomiting. Severe immediate problems are usually cardiovascular, such as hypotension and collapse, or respiratory, causing bronchospasm and wheezing. Patients with delayed mild illness complain of urticaria, mild arthralgia and polylymphadenopathy. However, some patients develop serum sickness and are very ill with pyrexia, joint and muscle pains and gross urticaria.

Using monovalent snake antivenoms is preferable to polyvalent antivenom if the identity of the snake is definitely known or the venom is identified using a venom detection kit. This is because serum reactions are more likely when using polyvalent antivenom. Polyvalent antivenom should not, however, be withheld if systemic envenomation is evident and the venom identity unknown.

TABLE 7.
Amount of monovalent antivenom where snake identity is known.

Snake	Appropriate monovalent antivenom	Initial Dose
Common Tiger Snake *Notechis scutatus*	Tiger Snake	3,000 units
Western Tiger Snake *N. ater occidentalis*	Tiger Snake	6,000 units
Kreffts Tiger Snake *N. ater ater*	Tiger Snake	6,000 units
Peninsular Tiger Snake *N. ater niger*	Tiger Snake	6,000 units
Tasmanian Tiger Snake King Island Tiger Snake *N. ater humphreysi*	Tiger Snake	6,000 units
Chappell Island Tiger Snake *N. ater serventyi*	Tiger Snake	9,000 units
Taipan *Oxyuranus scutellatus*	Taipan	12,000 units
Inland Taipan *Oxyuranus microlepidotus*	Taipan	12,000 units
Copperhead *Austrelaps superbus*	Tiger Snake	3,000 units 6,000 units (in Tasmania)
Common Brown Snake *Pseudonaja textilis*	Brown Snake	1,000 units
Dugite *Pseudonaja affinis*	Brown Snake	1,000 units
Western Brown Snake *Pseudonaja nuchalis*	Brown Snake	1,000 units
Peninsula Brown Snake *Pseudonaja inframacula*	Brown Snake	1,000 units
Ingrams Brown Snake *Pseudonaja ingrami*	Brown Snake	1,000 units
Speckled Brown Snake *Pseudonaja guttata*	Brown Snake	1,000 units
Death Adder *Acanthophis antarcticus*	Death Adder	6,000 units
Desert Death Adder *Acanthophis pyrrhus*	Death Adder	6,000 units
Northern Death Adder *Acanthophis praelongus*	Death Adder	6,000 units

TABLE 7. (cont'd)
Amount of monovalent antivenom where snake identity is known.

Snake	Appropriate monovalent antivenom	Initial Dose
Mulga Snake		
Pseudechis australis	Black Snake	18,000 units
Red-Bellied Black Snake	Tiger Snake or	3,000 units
Pseudechis porphyriacus	Black Snake	6,000 units
Spotted Black Snake	Tiger Snake or	3,000 units
Pseudechis guttatus	Black Snake	6,000 units
Collett's Snake	Black Snake or	18,000 units
Pseudechis colletti	Tiger Snake	3,000 units
Butlers Snake	Black Snake or	18,000 units
Pseudechis butleri	Tiger Snake	3,000 units
Rough Scaled Snake		
Tropidechis carinatus	Tiger Snake	3,000 units
Broad-headed Snakes		
Hoplocephalus (sp)	Tiger Snake	3,000 units
Small-eyed Snakes		
Cryptophis nigrescens	Tiger Snake	3,000 units

Note:

Contents of one ampoule of polyvalent antivenom should be used initially if monovalent antivenoms are not available.

TABLE 8

Antivenom dosage and combination where identity of snake is unknown.

Snake	Antivenom	Initial Dose
Tasmania	Tiger Snake	6,000 units
Victoria	Tiger Snake	3,000 units
	Brown Snake	1,000 units
New South Wales Queensland South Australia Western Australia Northern Territory	Polyvalent	Contents of one ampoule

Notes:

Contents of one ampoule of polyvalent antivenom should be used initially if monovalent antivenoms are not available.

Snake Bite Management
Diagnosis

Patient Assessment

In most cases, patients are unable to accurately identify snakes. Colour alone should be avoided as a guide for identification. Any area of Australia usually has a variety of dangerous snakes. Cogger (1987), has made a relevant assessment of the numbers of snakes in the various sub-divisions of Australia. He has also presented a map predicting the number of dangerous species in any area. Most areas have at least 2 dangerous species and some areas have up to 6 species. A trained herpetologist, competent zoo staff, museum curators, reputable reptile keepers or National Parks and Wildlife Service staff, are often available for accurate snake identification. All hospital casualty departments would do well to make arrangements so that they can readily contact experts in an emergency. Venom detection kits are a major breakthrough in assisting with identification of the correct monovalent antivenom type. Their real advantage is the decreased need to use the large volume polyvalent antivenoms when the identity of the snake involved is unknown.

Generally, the identity of the offending snake is unknown, however herpetologists and snake keepers are exceptions to this rule. They often give informative histories of snake bite, and are usually more efficient with their first aid and present to hospital in a calmer manner.

Many victims are children, who for varied reasons may wish to hide the fact that they have received a snake bite. Parents and doctors should always be wary of the snake bite possibility with a child, especially if symptoms develop. There is a common association between heavy alcohol intake and snake bite and this often masks the real problem of snake bite. The patient may be seriously ill, even unconscious and only the alert physician will consider snake bite as a possible diagnosis.

Without treatment with antivenom, there is a distinct chance the patient will die if envenomation has occurred. Fairley in 1929, in quoting work of Tidswell and Ferguson, claimed the overall expected mortality rate from all snake bites would be about 12% from all effective bites. Higher mortality rates would be expected if bites from certain species are considered in isolation. For instance, survival from an untreated *O. scutellatus* or *O. microlepidotus* bite is unlikely.

The Amount of Antivenom Required

The contents of one ampoule of antivenom produced by the Commonwealth Serum Laboratories is sufficient to neutralise in vitro the average amount of venom obtained during milking for the species concerned. Table 7 shows initial amounts required for the various snake species where positive identification has been made.

Local Reactions

Compared with many non-Australian snakes, Australia's dangerous snakes produce insignificant proteolytic enzymes so their bites produce minimal local reaction. In most bites the patient does not experience local pain, bruising or swelling, however, in a number of cases small local reactions adjacent to the bitten area have occurred. Classic fang and teeth marks rarely ever occur. Usually, the snake bites, through clothing and the victim may pull away when the sharp pain of the needle-like teeth are felt. This produces a series of scratches or even a single scratch which only to the very skilled eye may resemble a snake-bite. Although snake bite should be suspected, identification of the offending snake from these marks is impossible.

Fairley in 1929 reviewed 281 snake bites and found that 57% were on the lower limbs, 42% on upper extremities and the remainder on the body and face.

Bites on the fingers and ankles are more painful than elsewhere (Sutherland 1983). The anticoagulant fractions in *P. australis* bites may cause continued bleeding especially if swelling occurs. Swelling to the bite site can occur, accompained by pain with *A. antarcticus* bites. Local reactions can be complicated by prolonged use of pressure immobilisation first aid measure (Sutherland 1983).

Systemic Signs

Systemic signs of envenomation may be acute or delayed. Effective bites usually produce obvious problems within twenty minutes and certainly two hours. However, delayed onset of serious illness may occur, particularly when first aid treatment has been effective in slowing lymphatic movement. Some patients have been discharged from hospital only to be readmitted several hours later, very ill. In any suspected case of snake bite, the patient should be admitted to hospital for 24 hours.

Lymph Nodes Enlarged

Tender, enlarged or painful regional lymph nodes are a definite indication of envenomation, however, these symptoms alone do not indicate the use of antivenom. For example, one of the authors was bitten by a *Suta suta* (not considered dangerous). The bite resulted in a swollen lymph gland in the arm pit and a stiff finger. No other symptoms developed. If this snake had been unidentified, the symptoms alone would not justify administration of antivenom.

Headache, Nausea & Sweating

Common early signs and symptoms following an effective dangerous snake bite are nausea, vomiting, sweating and headaches. Often headache is severe. One of the authors experienced severe headaches in bites from *Oxyuranus microlepidotus* and *Acanthophis antarcticus*. Bites from *Notechis scutatus* are also noted for causing severe headaches (Sutherland 1983). Also bites from P. textilis cause headaches. Epilepsy has also been recorded after snake bite (Sutherland 1983).

Hypotension

Low blood pressure may occur. In extreme cases it can be profound, occurs within minutes of the bite and may result in partial or complete loss in consciousness. This condition will be accentuated by strenuous exercise of the bitten limb (Sutherland 1983; Mirtschin and Davis 1982). The condition is usually transient, but may require rapid infusion of antivenom in children (Sutherland 1983).

Allergic Reaction

An anaphylactic reaction or allergic reaction to the actual venom has been reported and this can be lethal. Allergic reactions are more likely to occur in people who have been bitten previously by the same species. Herpetologists and snake handlers are prone to such reactions (Mirtschin and Davis 1982), and would certainly benefit from the commercial development of snake bite vaccines.

Cardiovascular Changes

Cardiotoxins are found in the venom of some elapids, for example, *Naja nigricollis*. However there has been no formal assessment of cardiotoxins in Australian elapids to date. Sutherland (1983), reports that snake bite usually involves a sinus tachycardia and that cardiovascular changes are only mild. Both hypotensive and hypertensive changes could be due to minor cardiotoxins in the venoms.

Paralysis

Motor nerve blockade, resulting in muscular weakness, is the major action of Australian elapid venom. The neurotoxins work at the neuromuscular junction by two distinct methods, one presynaptically and the other postsynaptically. Progressive, ptosis, diplopia, dysphagia and then the insidious onset of diaphragmatic paralysis occurs which lead to respiratory failure. Paralysis of the tongue and palate may precipitate death from respiratory obstruction (Mirtschin and Davis 1982). Generally significant neurological signs take at least an hour to develop (Sutherland 1983). Sutherland (1983), proposes that the postsynaptic neurotoxins produce paralysis faster than the slower acting presynaptic neurotoxins, however, the presynaptic neurotoxins are harder to treat and reverse.

Abdominal Pain

Sutherland (1983), suggests that the frequent experience of abdominal pain associated with snake bite could be due to involvement of the lymph nodes as the venom moves centrally, or the direct effect of the smooth muscle of the gut. Kidney pain due to myoglobinaemia may be another reason for abdominal pain.

Haematological Changes

The most important coagulation problem is defibrination of the blood.

Many of the venoms convert prothrombin to thrombin and in turn fibrinogen to fibrin. The fibrin is then destroyed resulting in fibrin degradation products (FDP) and low levels of fibrinogen. In this condition, clotting times are lengthened and the blood becomes unclottable in vitro. Snake venoms with anticoagulant activity such as with *Pseudechis australis*, possess coagulation inhibitors which in themselves slow down clotting (Masci 1989). The action of the Copperhead, *Austrelaps superbus*, anticoagulant activity is yet to be described.

Classic evidence of coagulopathy is continuous bleeding from the bite site and venepuncture sites. Multiple bruising or large blood collections under the skin can occur. Blood in vomit, faeces, coughed up or in urine all indicate coagulopathy (Knyvett and Molphy 1959, Schapel et al 1971, Crawford 1980, Trinca 1969, Frost 1980).

White (1987), expressed a concern at the potential for brain haemorrhages associated with a coagulopathy, and recommended aggressive antivenom treatment to prevent this condition. Sutherland (1983), suggests that usually serious haemorrhage is restricted to elderly patients with a pre-existing condition such as a peptic ulcer or hypertension.

Unlike many exotic snake venoms, Australian snake venoms cause little damage to the blood vessels themselves and the platelet level remains adequate (Sutherland 1983).

Myotoxins

The effect of Australian snake venoms on the skeletal muscle is now well established (Rowlands et al 1969, Hood and Johnston 1975, Furtado and Lester 1968, Brigden and Sutherland 1981 and Pattern et al 1985). Myoglobinuria can lead to oliguria and acute renal failure if treatment is delayed (Sutherland 1983). Sutherland et al (1981), studied the effects of various Australian snake venoms on monkeys and found the plasma CK levels for all venoms studied showed myolytic activity. Myolysis is caused by the release of the muscle protein myoglobin, which is excreted in the urine causing it to darken to a mahogany colour. The damaged muscle loses the enzyme creatine kinase which can be measured in the plasma (CK levels). This can be used as an index for muscle damage (Sutherland 1983). Acute tubular necrosis can arise because of myoglobin deposition in the renal tubules.

Sutherland's studies with monkeys (1983), suggest that not until two hours after envenomation, does biochemical evidence of myolysis occur. Antivenom arrests myolytic activity. Sutherland (1983), concluded in retrospect that myoglobinaemia resulting in renal failure has been the cause of a number of snake bite deaths.

Hospital Treatment

"The essence of proper treatment of snake envenomation is simple — give the appropriate antivenom in adequate amounts by the correct route without unnecessary delay."

Editorial, Med. J. Aust. February 1978

On admission to hospital, patients may be severely ill, moderately unwell, or show no signs or symptoms at all. Particularly where first aid treatment has been effective; initially it may be difficult to tell how seriously the patient is envenomated. It is important that hospitals have well defined policies on the management of snake bites.

(A) Severely Ill Patients

Established intravenous line—	Keep resuscitation drugs at hand.
Premedication	— Adrenaline, steroids, Phenothiazines (promethazine HCI).
Administer antivenom	— See table 7 and table 8.
Intensive card	— transfer to major hospital.

Antivenom should be diluted 1 in 10. Normal saline or 5% dextrose are used to dilute the antivenom. If the snake type is not known, use polyvalent antivenom. Do not wait for the results from the venom detection kit. These results will be useful if further antivenom is required. The antivenom should be given intravenously over about 20 minutes. Absorption via the subcutaneous and intramuscular routes is too slow and these routes should not be used.

Prior to giving the antivenom, patients should be premedicated with adrenalin and 5 ml of blood should be taken for snake identification purposes. Adrenaline is the drug of choice to protect against, and for the treatment of severe anaphylactic reactions (Munro Ford 1977, Morrow and Luther 1976, and Fisher 1980). Adrenaline can be given subcutaneously or intramuscularly in a dose of 0.3 ml of 1,000 solution (less for a child 0.01 mg/kg). Warn the patient of a mild headache and tachycardia. If possible monitor the patients electrocardiogram when giving adrenaline.

If serum sickness or anaphylaxis is likely, steroids (eg. hydrocortisone 100 mg) should be given intravenously. Serious reactions are common where there has been prior sensitisation to horse protein. A antihistamine is recommended (eg promethazine HC1 25 — 50 mg) given intravenously or intramuscularly.

Avoid hypoxia — Give oxygen therapy. Be prepared to perform endotracheal intubation and prolonged ventilation. Tracheostomy is contra indicated since bleeding may occur. Monitor blood gases if possible. Remove airway obstructions.

Maintain pressure to bitten area — For severely ill patients, this can delay absorption of the venom until the antivenom has neutralised all the circulating venom and is at sufficient levels to deal with a further venom onslaught.

More Antivenom — If signs or symptoms of envenomation recur or persist another ampoule of antivenom is indicated as soon as possible. Sutherland (1983), claims that venom has been detected in untreated patients as late as 56 hours after snake bite has occurred. Therefore it is important to remember:-

"It is never too late to administer antivenom, except when the patient is dead" (Sutherland 1977).

The number of ampoules of antivenom required to effectively neutralise the venom will be determined by the persistence of symptoms. Australian antivenoms may be effective even when given to moribund patients and a number of case reports vividly illustrate this (Gaynor 1977 and Sutherland 1977).

Patients requiring prolonged ventilation, suffering from bleeding diathesis or renal failure should be considered for transfer to a major hospital with full intensive care facilities.

(B) Moderately Unwell Patient or No Symptoms

Leave pressure bandage in place — If the correct first aid has been used, leave it in place for the time being.

Establish I.V. line — Assemble premedication drugs — adrenaline hydrocortisone, and promethazine. (see above for dilutions).

Establish the facts — If dead snake is available, have it identified by proper experts but do not delay any subsequent treatment while awaiting this information. Identification can proceed simultaneously with all the other necessary hospital priorities.

Admit to intensive care   — Confine patient to bed.
                             — Observations as for head injury.
                             — Awaken hourly and check vital signs.

Determine exact symptoms, eg   — headache
                                   — ptosis
                                   — vomiting etc.

Establish time of bite.

Arrange antivenom — If possible identity is known, arrange for initial antivenom and back up ampoules.

Arrange venom detection — Bite — site swab, (if not covered by first aid), urine or blood sample if systemic envenomation is obvious. Sample should be tested in a Commonwealth Serum Laboratories Venom Detection Kit.

Blood is also required for clotting and enzymes studies. If systemic envenomation is not obvious, wait until first aid bandages are removed so that a site swab can be taken.

Assemble resuscitation drugs and apparatus.

If envenomation significant —

(i)   Premedicate with adrenalins and hydrocortisone as above. Five to ten minutes later commence antivenom infusion diluted in saline or 5% dextrose with appropriate precautions. Infuse antivenom over 15 — 20 minutes.

(ii)   Remove compression bandages so that there are no restrictions on the venom movement. If the patient's condition rapidly deteriorates, replace bandages and allow the antivenom to take effect, before removing it again.

Patient with no symptoms — Remove the compression bandage and

splints and monitor closely. If symptoms develop, reinstate the first aid and commence antivenom treatment as above. Remove bandages and splints later and repeat above if symptoms recur.

When no changes occur and after removal of first aid bandages, then they may be left off permanently.

When the bandage is off, take a bite swab for venom detection in the VDK.

After the first aid bandages have been removed for a while and no symptoms develop, monitor the patient as for a "head injury" for at least twenty four hours. The patient must be carefully monitored for signs of anaphylaxis or muscle paralysis. When the patient is in a state of peripheral shock, absorption of the venom may also slow down or cease only to recommence when the condition is rectified (Sutherland 1983).

The dose of antivenom depends on the amount of venom injected and not on the patients age or size. Children require the same dose as adults. Sometimes children or the elderly may even require more as the consequences of snake bite in these groups are more severe.

In extreme emergencies, antivenom has to be given more rapidly.

Initial doses of antivenom are shown in table 7 and 8. The use of venom detection kits is now superseding the use of table 8, however, if a kit isn't available or the result is inconclusive, table 8 should be used. The large volume of polyvalent antivenom diluted at 1:10 necessitates a faster flow rate. It should be used administered over thirty minutes if time permits. In critical situations near neat antivenom should be used (Sutherland 1983).

As stated previously, antivenom quantities have been based on volumes of venom obtained from average milkings of snakes. Morrison and his co-workers (1982- 1984) have shown that in a bite situation, less venom on average is involved than is obtained when snakes are milked, therefore, in most cases, the contents of one ampoule of antivenom should be more than adequate to neutralise circulating venom from a snake bite. Exceptions occur, and the treating physician should always be alert to the occasional need for further antivenom. In addition, if treatment is delayed , the patient will probably require more antivenom, as much as four times the normal amount.

Sutherland (1982), considers slight coagulation defects caused by immature dangerous snakes, in many cases does not warrant antivenom treatment if other evidence of poisoning is absent. Using this evidence to determine the treatment is a sound approach, however, there is a tendency among herpetologists and snake handlers to treat bites from juvenile snakes fairly indifferently. Evidence presented on some overseas species shows that young snakes possess more toxic venoms than do older snakes (Meier 1986). This feature could well be true for some Australian species, but has not been tested yet. In the meantime, all bites from dangerous snakes, even juvenile snakes should be regarded with the same degree of emergency.

Concern about acute anaphylaxis and serum sickness are the two main reasons why doctors hesitate in giving antivenom. However, as will be discussed later in the section on antivenoms, if the patients are premedicated with adrenalin and promethazine HC1 and the antivenom diluted, serious reactions are unlikely. Fears about antivenom are largely unfounded and are a hangover of the past when they were far less pure. The real danger today is that antivenom occasionally is not given at all, or that it is given too late and in inadequate amounts (Mirtschin and Davis 1982).

Victims should always be observed for twenty four hours because there are reports of patients being seen and discharged from hospital, only to be re-admitted some hours later in a moribund state. The patient should be nursed like a head injury and examined hourly. The patient's tetanus immunisation status should be checked and if the wound is dirty, antibiotics are recommended. Pain relief is normally not required but if pain is very severe and opiates used, respiratory depression must be carefully watched for (Mirtschin and Davis 1982).

The most common cause of death following snake bite is respiratory failure. Death from renal failure or bleeding diathesis is uncommon. For seriously ill patients, supportive measures in addition to the giving of antivenom may be needed. Peritoneal dialysis and haemodialysis may be life saving in cases of renal failure (Hood and Johnson 1975 and Harris et al 1976).

When coagulopathy persists, it should be treated with more antivenom. Plasma should not be administered before adequate antivenom has been used, since massive clotting and thrombosis may follow.

Avoidable deaths and unnecessary suffering due to snake bite continue to occur and the reasons remain the same as listed by Sutherland (1975). They are:-

1. Antivenom withheld despite clear evidence of envenomation.
2. The wrong antivenom is administered; occasionally when the snake has been mis-identified.
3. The appropriate antivenom given but in insufficient quantity.
4. The dose of antivenom is not repeated when the signs and symptoms of envenomation persist or recur.
5. The victim is not under medical surveillance for an adequate period.

Laboratory Investigations

Laboratory tests are important in the management of suspected or definite snake bite. Often such tests will demonstrate changes due to envenomation very soon after the bite has occurred. Deterioration in the patient's clinical condition may even be preceded by abnormal laboratory results.

Identification samples must be collected prior to giving antivenom. Specimens should include 5 ml of blood, 5 ml of urine, a saline (or distilled water) swab of the bite site, and of any venom stained clothing.

TABLE 9
Summary of samples and testing

Blood and Serum
1. 5 ml of blood.
2. Bleeding time, clotting time, partial thromboplastin time (P.T.T.K.), prothrombin time.

3. Fibrinogen levels.
4. Presence of F.D.P.
5. C.K. levels.
   M.M. and M.B. isoenzymes if facilities available.
6. Estimation of blood gases.
7. Blood urea estimation.
8. White cell count.
9. Electrolytes

Urine

1. 5 ml urine.
2. Hourly output.
3. Haemoglobin.
4. Myoglobinuria.
5. Erythrocytes.

Bite Site

1. Saline (or distilled water) swab of bite site and/or adjacent clothing or bandages.

Bleeding and clotting studies are a sensitive guide to the patient's condition, and if altered, should be repeated frequently. If inadequate antivenom has been given in the presence of severe envenomation, the activated partial thromboplastin time (P.T.T.K.) is prolonged, the fibrinogen level drops, the fibrin degradation products increase, and the platelet count remains normal. The correct treatment of altered bleeding and clotting studies is more antivenom not administration of fibrinogen, fresh blood, heparin or epsilon amino caproic acid (Mirtschin and Davis 1982).

Haemoglobin in the urine indicates haemolysis of erythrocytes and should be differentiated from myoglobin. Erythrocytes in the urine is a pointer towards a bleeding and clotting problem developing. Myoglobin in the urine indicates lysis of muscle cells (Mirtschin and Davis 1982).

C.K. in serum associated with snake bite is common. Sutherland (1981), demonstrated that all snake venoms tested showed myolytic activity. Sutherland (1983), suggests the C.K. will rise within two hours. Severe cases will rise to 5,000 IU/1 or more.

Sutherland (1983), states that it is very rare for snake bite victims to require infusions of whole blood. Coagulopathy status should be checked. Bleeding time, clotting time, partial thromboplastin time, prothrombin time, and lowered fibrinogen levels of FDP indicates coagulopathy. Only when the venom has been neutralised by antivenom should an infusion of fresh frozen plasma or cryoprecipitate be considered. Whole blood is only necessary, if there has been a significant haemorrhage. Sutherland (1983), reports that there is a risk of gangrene and death because of infusion of fresh blood before the procoagulants have been neutralised by the antivenom.

Electrocardiograms should be taken for older patients. Snake bite usually involves a sinus tachycardia (Sutherland 1983).

Follow Up Management

In the two serious snake bites experienced by one of the authors, a period of general weakness and feeling of being run down followed. This is typical for most bites. Sometimes irritability and short temperedness will follow. Most of these effects take about a month to resolve themselves.

Serum Sickness — Can occur from a few days after treatment to fourteen days or later. The range of presentations include:-

— Minor rash.
— Multi-systemic disease involving kidneys, swollen lymph nodes, stiff joints.
Urticaria.

Serum sickness is an immune complex disease and the discomfort can be minimised by the use of steroids (eg. prednisolone). Reactions are more likely when the patient has received a large volume of antivenom (monovalent or polyvalent).

Allergy to venom — Sutherland (1983) and White (1987), both agree that allergic reactions to snake venoms can occur. They both point out that people who have previously been bitten by snakes, especially from juvenile snakes where only minor quantities of venom are involved, face the risk of becoming sensitised, not only to the venom of the particular species involved in the bite, but a range of other venoms. In these cases, there is an even greater need to premedicate with adrenaline antihistamines and steroids.

The dead snake — If a snake, no matter in what condition, is brought in to hospital for identification, it should never be thrown out. Preserve the animal in spirit and try to have it identified quickly by an experienced herpetologist. These experienced people should be known to the hospital before any emergency. The snake should be lodged in the States Museum if not required for any medico-legal reasons or coronal enquiry.

References Cited

Aronson, D.L., Franza, B.R. and Bagley, J. (1984). 'The use of Prothrombin Activating Snake Venoms to Measure Human Prothrombin 2: Absence of Prothrombin 2 in Serum.' Thrombosis Research, 34, 419-429.

Banks, C. (1981). 'Notes on seasonal colour change in a Western Brown Snake.' Herpetofauna, 13(1), pp 29-30.

Barnett, D., Howden, M.E.H. and Spence, I. (1980). 'A neurotoxin of novel structural type from the venom of the Australian common brown snake.' Naturwissenschaften, 67, 405.

Barnett, B. and Schwaner, T.D. (1985). 'Growth in captive born Tiger Snakes *(Notechis ater serventyi)* from Chappell Island: Implications for field and Laboratory studies.' Trans. R. Soc. Sth. Aust., 109(2), 3-36.

Bernheimer, A.W., Weinstein, S.A. and Linder, R. (1986). 'Isoelectric analysis of some

Australian Elapid Snake venoms with special reference to Phospholipase B and Haemolysis.' Toxicon, 24(8), 841-849.

Brigden, M.C. and Sutherland, S.K. (1981). 'Taipan bite with myoglobinuria.' Med. J. Aust., 2, 42-44.

Broad, A.J., Sutherland, S.K. and Coulter, A.R. (1979). 'The lethality in mice of dangerous Australian and other snake venoms.' Toxicon, 17, 661-667.

Broad, A.J., Sutherland, S.K., Tanner, C. and Covacevich, J. (1979). 'Electrophoretic, enzyme and preliminary toxicity studies of the venom of the Small-Scaled snake, *Parademansia microlepidotus* (Serpentes: Elapidae), with additional data on its distribution.' Mem. Queens, Mus., 19(3): 319-329.

Campbell, C.H. (1969a). 'Clinical aspects of snake bite in the Pacific area.' Toxicon, Vol. 7, 25-28.

Campbell, C.H. (1969b). 'A clinical study of venomous snake bite in Papau.' M.D. Thesis, Univ. of Sydney.

Charles, N., Whitaker, P. and Shine, R. (1979). 'Oviparity and captive breeding in the Spotted Blacksnake, *Pseudechis guttatus* (Serpentes: Elapidae).' Aust. Zool. 20, 361-364.

Chester, A and Crawford, G.P.M. (1980). 'Envenomation by a juvenile gwardar.' Med. J. Aust., 2, 462.

Cogger, H.G. (1975). 'Reptiles of Australia.' A.H. & A.W. Reed, Sydney.

Cogger, H.G. (1983). 'A Case of Mistaken Identity.' Med. J. Aust., (2), 2, 51-53.

Cogger, H. (1987). 'The Venomous Land Snakes' in Toxic Plants and Animals. A guide for Australia. Eds. J. Covacevich, P. Davie and J. Pearn. Qld. Museum 340-355.

Cogger, H.G., Cameron, E.E. and Cogger, H.M. (1983). Zoological Catalogue of Australia Vol. 1. 'Amphibia and Reptilia.' Aust. Govt. Publishing Service.

Coulter, A.R., Harris, R.D., and Sutherland, S.K. (1981). 'Enzyme immunoassay and radioimmunoassay: Their use in the study of Australian and exotic snake venoms.' In: Proceedings of the Melbourne Herpetological Symposium, 19-21 May 1980 (ed. C.B. Banks and A.A. Martin). Zoological Board of Victoria, Melbourne.

Covacevich (1981). 'Australia's Most Dangerous Snakes.' Queensland Museum Colour Transparencies, No. 2.

Covacevich, J., McDowell, S. and Tanners, C. (1980). 'Relationship of the Taipan, *Oxyuranus scutellatus* and the Small-Scaled snake *Oxyuranus microlepidotus*.' Proc. Herp. Symposium, Melbourne, Zoo. Fds. Banks & Martin, 160-168.

Covacevich, J. and Wombey, J. (1976). 'Recognition of *Parademansia microlepidotus* (McCoy).' Proc. Royal Soc. Qld., 87: 29-32, Pls 1-2.

Crawford, G.P.M. (1980). 'Envenomation by a juvenile Gwardar.' Med. J. Aust., 2, 158.

Cull-Candy, S.G., Fohlman, J., Gustavsson, D., Lullman-Rauch, R. and Thesleff, S. (1976). 'The effects of taipoxin and notexin on the function and fine structure of the murine neuro-muscular junction.' Neuroscience, 1, 175-80.

Davey, M.G. (1969). 'Activation of human prothrombin by Australian snake venoms.' Minutes Annual Meeting. Haematology Society of Australia, Adelaide.

Davey, M.G. and Luscher, E.G. (1967). 'Effects of some coagulant snake venoms upon human platelets.' Proc. 10th Cong. Europ. Soc, Haemat. Strasborg. 1965. Karger. Basel/New York Part II. 1118-1123.

Davis, R., Fennell, P. and Mirtschin, P.J. (1979). 'Poisonous Snakes of South Australia's Eyre Region — Identification and Treatment. A Co-ordinated Approach.' Whyalla Press, Whyalla, S.A.

Davis, R. and Mirtschin, P.J. (1985). 'Snake Bites.' A Guide to Treatment. Emergency Medicine. Patient Management, 91-99.

Daytner, M.E. and Gage, P.W. (1973). 'Australian Tiger snake venom — an inhibitor of transmitter release.' Nature (New Biology and Nature), 241, 246-247.

Denson, K.W.E. (1969). 'Coagulant and anticoagulant action of snake venoms.' Toxicon, 7, 5-11.

Denson (1976). 'Clot-inducing substances present in snake venoms with particular reference to *Echis carinatus.*' Thrombosis Research, Vol. 8, 351-360.

Denson, K.W.E., Borrett, R. and Biggs, R. (1971). 'The specific assay of Prothrombin using taipan snake venom.' British J. Haematology, 21, 219-226.

Doery, H.M. (1957). 'Additional purine compounds in the venom of the tiger snake *(Notechis scutatus).*' Nature (London), 180, 799-800.

Doery, H.M. (1958). 'The separation and properties of the neurotoxins from the venom of the tiger snake, *Notechis scutatus scutatus.*' Biochem. J., 70, 535-543.

Doery, H.M. and Pearson, J.E. (1961). 'Haemolysins in venoms of Australian snakes. Observations on the venoms of some Australian snakes and the separation of phospholipase A from the venom of *Pseudechis porphyriacus.*' Biochem. J., 78, 820-827.

Doery, H.M. and Pearson, J.E. (1964). 'Phospholipase B in snake venom and bee venom.' Biochem. J., 92, 599-602.

Fairley, N.H. (1929). 'The present position of snake bite and the snake bitten in Australia.' Med. J. Aust., 1, 296-313.

Fairley, N.H. and Splatt, B. (1929). 'Venom yields in Australia's poisonous snakes.' Med. J. Aust., 1, 336-348.

Fisher, M.M. (1977). 'The Management of Anaphylaxis.' Med. J. Aust., Vol. 1, 793.

Fitzgerald, M. and Pollitt, C. (1981). 'Oviparity and Breeding in the Mulga or King Brown snake *Pseudechis australis (Serpentes: Elapidae).*' Aust. J. Herp., 1(2), 57-61.

Fohlman, J. (1979). 'Comparison of two highly toxic Australian snake venoms: The Taipan *(Oxyuranus s. scutellatus)* and the Fierce snake *(Paeademansia microlepidotus).*' Toxicon, 17, 170-172.

Fohlman, J., Eaker, D., Karlsson, E. and Thesleff, S. (1976). 'Taipoxin, an extremely potent presynaptic neurotoxin from the venom of the Australian snake taipan *(Oxyuranus s. scutellatus).* Isolation, characterization, quarternary structure and pharmacological properties.' Eur. J. Biochem., 68(2), 457-469.

Frost, J. (1980). 'Tiger snake envenomation.' Med. J. Aust., 1, 440.

Futardo, M.A., and Lester, I.A. (1968). 'Myoglobinuria following snake bite.' Med. J. Aust., 1, 674-676.

Gaynor, B. (1977). 'An unusual snake bite story.' Med. J. Aust., Vol. 2, 191-192.

Giddings, S.(1978). "Some notes on Trematode infestation in tiger snakes in South Australia." Herpetofauna, 10(1), 7-8.

Gillam, M.W. (1979). 'The genus, *Pseudonaja* (Serpentes: Elapidae) in the Northern Territory,' Territory Parks and Wildlife Commission Research Bulletin, No. 1.

Gow G.F. (1976). 'Snakes of Australia.' Angus and Robertson, Sydney.

Gow G.F. (1982). 'Australia's Dangerous Snakes.' Angus and Robertson, Sydney.

Guido Tans, Govers-riemslag, J.W.P., van Rijin, J.L.M.L. and Rosing, J. (1985). 'Purification and Properties of a Prothrombin activator from the venom of *Notechis scutatus scutatus.*' The Journal of Biological Chemistry, 260, 16, 9366-9372.

Halpert, J. and Eaker, D. (1975). 'Amino acid sequence of a presynaptic neurotoxin from the venom of *Notechis scutatus scutatus* (Australian Tiger Snake).' J. Biol. Chem., 250, 6990-6997.

Hamilton, R.C., Broad, A.J. and Sutherland, S.K. (1980). 'Ultrastructural effects of the venom of the small scaled snake *(Parademansia microlepidotus)* on the nerve terminals of the rat diaphragm.' Aust. J. Exp. Biol. Med. Sci., 48, 377-380.

Harris, J.B. and Johnson, E. (1975). 'Pathological responses of a rat skeletal muscle to a single subcutaneous injection of a toxin isolated from the venom of the Australian tiger snake, *Notechis scutatus scutatus.*' Clin. Exp. Pharmacol. Physiol., 2, 383-404.

Harris, J.B. and Johnson, M.A. (1978). Further observations on the pathological response of rat skeletal muscle to toxins isolated from the venom of the Australian tiger snake, *Notechis scutatus scutatus.*' Clin. Exp. Pharmacol. Physiol., 5, 587-600.

Harris, J.B., Johnson, M.A. and MacDonell, C.A. (1977). 'Taipoxin, a presynaptically active neurotoxin destroys mammalian skeletal muscle.' Br. J. Pharmacol., 61, 133.

Harris, J.B., Karlsson, E. and Thesleff, S. (1973). 'Effects of an isolated toxin from the Australian tiger snake *(Notechis scutatus scutatus)* venom at the mammalian neuro-muscular junction.' Br. J. Pharmacol., 47, 141-146.

Harris, J.B. and MacDonell, C.A. (1981). 'Phospholipase A_2 activity of notexin and its role in muscle damage.' Toxicon, 19, 419-430.

Harris, J.B. and Maltin, C.A. (1981). 'The effects of the subcutaneous injection of the crude venom of the Australian common brown snake *Pseudonaja textilis* on the skeletal neuro-muscular system.' Br. J. Pharmacol., 73, 157-163.

Harris, R.C., Hurst, P.E. and Saker, B.M. (1976). 'Renal failure after snake bite.' Med. J. Aust., 2, 409-411.

Hood, V.L. and Johnson, J.R. (1974). 'Acute renal failure with myoglobinuria following tiger snake bite.' Aust. N.Z. J. Med., 4, 415-437.

Hood, V.L. and Johnson, J.R. (1975). 'Acute renal failure with myoglobinuria after tiger snake bite.' Med. J. Aust., Vol.2, 638-641.

Jobin, F. and Esnouf, M.P. (1966). 'Coagulant activity of tiger snake *(Notechis scutatus scutatus)* venom.' Nature, 211, 873-875.

Kaire, G.H. (1964). 'A Heat-stable anticoagulant in snake venoms.' Med. J. Aust., 2, 972.

Karlsson, E., Eaker, D. and Ryden, L. (1972). Purification of a presynaptic neurotoxin from the venom of the Australian Tiger Snake, *Notechis scutatus scutatus.* Toxicon, 10, 405-413.

Kellaway, C.H. (1929a). 'A preliminary note on the venom of the Australian copper-head *(Denisonia superba)*: Its toxic effects in the common laboratory animals.' Med. J. Aust., 1, 358-365.

Kellaway, C.H. (1929b). 'A preliminary note on the venoms of *Pseudechis guttatus.*' Med. J. Aust., 1, 372-377.

Kellaway, C.H. (1929c). 'The action of the venoms of the Copperhead *(Denisonia superba)* and the death adder *(Acanthophis antarcticus)* on the coagulation of the blood.' Med. J. Aust., 1, 772-781.

Kellaway, C.H. (1929d). 'Observations on the certainly lethal dose of the venom of the death adder *(Acanthophis antarcticus)* for the common laboratory animals.' Med. J. Aust., 1, 764-772.

Kellaway, C.H. (1929e). 'The action of Australian snake venoms on plain muscle.' Br. J. Exp. Pathol., 10, 281-303.

Kellaway, C.H. (1931). 'Observations on the certainly lethal dose of the venom of the common brown snake *(Demansia textilis)* for the common laboratory animals.' Med. J. Aust., 2, 747-751.

Kellaway, C.H. (1933). 'Some peculiarities of Australian snake venoms.' Trans. R. Soc. Trop. Med. Hyg., 27, 9-21.

Kelllaway, C.H. (1934a). 'The peripheral action of Australian snake venoms. 4. Action on sensory nerve endings in frogs.' Aust. J. Exp. Biol. Med Sci., 12, 177-186.

Kellaway, C.H. (1934b). 'The venoms of the broad-headed snake *(Hoplocephalus bungaroides)* and the yellow-banded snake *(Hoplocephalus stephensi).*' Med. J. Aust., 2, 249-255.

Kellaway, C.H. and Thomson, D.F. (1930).'Observations on the venom of a large Australian snake, *Pseudechis australis* (Gray). 2. Venom yield and venom.' Aust. J. Exp. Biol. Med. Sci., 7, 134-150.

Knyvett, A.F. and Molphy, R. (1959). 'Respiratory paralysis due to snake bite; Report of two cases,' Med. J. Aust., 2, 481-484.

Leonardi, T.M., Howden, M.E.H. and Spence, I. (1979). 'A lethal myotoxin isolated from the venom of the Australian King Brown snake *(Pseudechis australis).*' Toxicon, 17, 549-555.

Longmore, R. (1986). 'Atlas of elapid snakes of Australia.' Aust. Govt. Pub. Service. Canberra.

Martin, C.J. and Smith, J.McG. (1892). 'The venom of the Australian black snake *(Pseudechis porphyriacus).* ' J. Proc. R. Soc. N.S.W., 26, 240-264.

Marshall, L.R. and Herrmann, R.P. (1983). 'Coagulant and anticoagulant actions of Australian snake venoms.' Throm. Haemostas. (Stuttgart), 50(3), 707-711.

Masci. P.P., Whitaker, A.N. and de Jersey, J. (1988). 'Purification and Characterisation of a prothrombin activator from the venom of the Australian Brown Snake, Pseudonaja textilis textilis. Biochem. International 17(5). 825-835.

Masci, P.P., Whitaker, A.N., Madaras, F., Mirtschin, P.J. and de Jersey, J. (1989). 'Characterisation and purification of two anticoagulant components in the venom of the Australian King Brown Snake. Pseudechis australis. X11th Cong. of the I.S.O.T.A.H. Tokyo. Japan.

McPhee, D.R. (1979). 'The observers' book of snakes and lizards of Australia.' Jacaranda press.

Mebs, D. (1969). 'Preliminary studies on small molecular toxic components of elapid venoms.' Toxicon, 6, 247-253.

Mebs, D., Chen, V.M. and Lee, C.Y. (1978). 'Biochemistry and pharmacology of toxins from Australia snake venoms.' Toxicon Suppl., (1), 365-373.

Mebs, D., Chen, V.M. and Lee, C.Y. (1979). 'Biochemical and pharmacological studies on Australian snake venom toxins.' In: Neurotoxins, Fundamental and Clinical Advances (ed. I.W. Chubb and L.B. Geffen). Adel. Univ. Union Press, Adelaide.

Mebs, D. and Samejima, Y. (1980). 'Purification, from Australian elapid venoms, and properties of phospholipases A which cause myoglobinuria in mice.' Toxicon, 18, 443-454.

Meier, J. (1986). 'Individual and Age-dependent. Variations in the venom of the Fer-De-Lance *(Bothrops atrox).*' Toxicon, 24(1), 41-46.

Mengden, G.A. (1985a). 'A chromosomal and electrophoretic analysis of the genus, *Pseudonaja.* ' In Biology of Australian frogs and reptiles.' Eds. G. Grigg, R. Shine and H. Ehmann, Roy. Zoo. Soc. of N.S.W., 193-208.

Mengden, G.A. (1985b). 'Australian elapid phylogeny: A summary of the chromosomal and electrophoretic data.' In 'Biology of Australian frogs and reptiles.' Eds. G. Grigg, R. Shine and H. Ehmann. Roy. Zoo. Soc. of N.S.W., 185-192.

Mengden, G.A., Shine, R. and Moritz, C. (1986). 'Phylogenetic Relationships within the Venomous Snakes of the Genus Pseudechis. Herpetologica, 42(2): 215-229.

Mengden, G.A. and Fitzgerald, M. (1987). 'The Paradoxical Brown Snakes.' In 'Plants and Animals. A guide for Australia.' Eds. J Covacevich, P. Davie and John Pearn. 458-469.

Millar, D.B. (1963). 'A preliminary study of the habits and venom of *Tropidechis carinatus* (Serpentes: Elapidae).' Herpetofauna, 1, 3-7.

Minton, S.A. and Da Costa, M. (1975). 'Serological relationships of sea snakes and their evolutionary implications.' In 'Biology of Sea Snakes'. Ed. by W.A. Dunson. Univ. Park Press: Baltimore. 35-55.

169

Minton, S.A. (1981). 'Evolution and distribution of venomous snakes.' 55-59 in Banks, C.B. and Martin, A.A. (eds). Proc. Melb. Herp. Symp. 1980. Melb. Zoo. Board of Victoria.

Mirtschin, P.J. (1981). 'South Australian records of the inland taipan *(Oxyuranus microlepidotus)* McCoy, 1879.' Herpetofauna, 13(1), 20-23.

Mirtschin, P.J. and Davis, R. (1982). 'Dangerous snakes of Australia.' Rigby, Adelaide.

Mirtschin, P.J. (1982). 'Occurrence and distribution of the Inland Taipan, *Oxyuranus microlepidotus* (Reptilia: Elapidae) in South Australia.' Trans, Roy. Soc. of S.A., Vol. 106, pt. 4, 213-214.

Mirtschin, P.J. (1983a). 'Seasonal colour changes in the Inland Taipan *Oxyuranus microlepidotus* McCoy 1879.' Herpetofauna, 14(2). 97-99.

Mirtschin, P.J. (1983b) 'The common death adder, *Acanthophis antarcticus* in South Australia. Its Status and Conservation.' Sth. Aust. Nat., Vol., 58, No. 2.

Mirtschin, P.J., Crowe, G.R. Thomas, M.W. (1984). 'Envenomation by the Inland Taipan, *Oxyuranus microlepidotus.*' Med. J. Aust., 141, 850-851.

Mirtschin, P.J. (1985). 'An overview of captive breeding of common death adders, *Acanthophis antarcticus* (Show), and its role in conservation.' In 'Biology of Australian frogs and reptiles.' Eds. Gordon Grigg, Richard Shine and Harry Ehmann. Royal Zoological Society of N.S.W., 505-509.

Mirtschin, P.J. (1986). 'Captive breeding and oviparity in the King Brown snake *Pseudechis australis* (Serpentes: Elapidae) from Eyre Peninsula South Australia.' 10th International Herp. Symposia on Captive Propagation and Husbandry. San Antonio, Texas, 141-148.

Mirtschin, P.J. (1986). 'Double egg laying of *Oxyuranus scutellatus scutellatus.*' 10th International Herpetological Symposia on captive propagation and husbandry. San Antonio, Texas. 149-157.

Morgan, F.G. (1937). Director of the Commonwealth Serum Laboratories. "The venom of *Notechis scutatus* variety *niger* (Reevesby Island)." Proc. Roy. Soc. Vic. 50(2). 303-413.

Morrison, J.J., Pearn, J.H., Charles N.T. and Coulter, A.R. (1983). Further Studies on the mass of venom injected by elapid snakes. Toxicon, 21(2). 279-284.

Morrison, J.J., Pearn, J.H. and Coulter, A.R. (1982). 'The mass of venom injected by two elapidae: The Taipan *(Oxyuranus scutellatus)* and the Australian Tiger snake *(Notechis scutatus).*' Toxicon, Vol. 20, No. 4, 739-745.

Morrison, J.J., Pearn, J.H., Covacevich, J., Tanner, C. and Coulter, A.R. (1984). Studies on the venom *(Oxyuranus microlepidotus)* Clin. Toxicology, 21(3), 373-385.

Morrison, J.J., Charles, N.T. and Pearn, J.H. (1983). 'The use of experimental models to study the biting habits of the Australian snakes on both "Defensive" and "Hunting" bites.' Toxicon, Suppl., 3, 305-308.

Morrison, J.J., Pearn, J.H., Covacevich, J. and Nixon, J. (1983). 'Can Australians Identify Snakes?' Med. J. Aust., 2(2), 66-70.

Morrison, J.J., Tesseraux, I., Pearn, J. and Masci, P.P. (1984). 'Venom of the Australian rough-scaled snake, *Tropidechis carinatus:* Lethal potency and electrophysical actions.' Toxicon, 22(5). 759-765.

Morrow, D.H. and Luther, R.R. (1976). 'Anaphylaxis-Aetiology and guidelines for management.' Anesthesia and Analgesia: Current Researches, Vol. 11, 494-499.

Munro Ford, R. (1977). 'The management of acute allergic disease including anaphylaxis.' Med. J. Aust., Vol. 1, 222-223.

Nishida, S., Terashima, M., Shimazu, T., Takasaki, C. and Tamiya, N. (1985). 'Isolation and properties of two phospholipase A_2 from the venom on an Australian Elapid snake *(Pseudechis australis).*' Toxicon, Vol. 23, No.1, 73-85.

Pattern, B.R., Pearn, J.H., De Buse, P., Burke, J. and Covacevich, J. (1985). 'Prolonged intensive therapy after snake bite. A probable case of envenomation by the rough-scaled snake.' Med. J. Aust., 142-467-469.

Pearn, J., Morrison, J., Charles, N. and Muir, V. (1981). 'First aid for snake bite. Efficacy of a constrictive bandage with limb immobilization in the management of human envenomation.' Med. J. Aust., 2, 293-295.

Pearn, J. (1987). 'The rough-scaled snake *(Tropidechis carinatus)*, in Toxic Plants & Animals. A guide for Australia.' Eds. J. Covacevich, P. Davie and J. Pearn. Qld. Museum, 174-479.

Pirkle, H., McIntosh, M. Theodor, I. and Vernon, S. (1972). 'Activation of prothrombin with taipan snake venom.' Thrombosis Research, Vol. 1, 559-568.

Pluskal, M.G., Harris, J.B., Pennington, R.J. and Eaker, D. (1978). 'Some biochemical responses of rat skeletal muscle to a single subcutaneous injection of a toxin (Notexin) isolated from the venom of the Australian tiger snake. Notechis sculatus sculatus Clin. Exp. Pharmacol. Physiol., 5, 131-141.

Pollitt, C.C. (1980). 'Studies on the venom and the blood of the Eastern Small-eyed Snake *Cryptophis nigreceus* (Gunther). In Proc. of Melb. Herp. Syup. 19-21 May 1980 (ed. C.B. Banks and A.A. Martin). Zoo. Board of Vic. Melb.

Reilly, V.M. (1963). 'The rough scaled snake (*Tropidechis carinatus*).' North. Qld. Nat., 34,4.

Rowlands, J.B., Mastaglia, F.L., Kakulas, B.A. and Hainsworth, D. (1969). 'Clinical and pathological aspects of a fatal case of mulga *(Pseudechis australis)* snake bite.' Med. J. Aust., 1, 226-230.

Schwaner, (1985). 'Population structure of black tiger snakes, *Notechis ater niger*, on offshore islands of South Australia.' In 'Biology of Australian frogs and reptiles.' Eds. G. Grigg, R. Shine and H. Ehmann. Roy. Zoo. Soc. of N.S.W., 177-184.

Sheumack, D.D., Howden, M.E.H. and Spence, I. (1979). 'Isolation and partial characterisation of a lethal neurotoxin from the venom of the Australian death adder *(Acanthophis antarcticus)*'. Toxicon, 17, 609-616.

Shine, R. (1980). 'Ecology of the Australian Death Adder, *Acanthophis antarcticus* (Elapidae): Evidence for convergence with the Viperidae.' Herpetologica, 36, 281-289.

Shine, R. and Allen, S. (1980). 'Ritual combat in the Australian Copperhead, *Austrelaps superbus* (Serpentes: Elapidae).' Victorian Nat. 97, 188-190.

Shine, R., Grigg, G.C., Shine, T.G. and Harlow, P. (1981). 'Mating and male combat in Australian Black snakes, *Pseudechis porphyriacus.* ' Journal of Herpetology, 15(1), 101-107.

Shine, R. and Covacevich, J. (1983). 'Ecology of highly venomous snakes: The Australian genus *Oxyuranus* (Elapidae). Journal of Herpetology, Vol. 17, No. 1, 60-69.

Shine, R. (1985a). 'Ecological evidence on the Phylogeny of Australian Elapid snakes.' In 'Biology of Australian frogs and reptiles.' Eds. G. Grigg, R. Shine and H. Ehmann. Roy. Zoo. Soc. of N.S.W., 255-260.

Shine, R. (1985b). Prey Constriction by venomous snakes. A review and data on Australian species. Copeia (4) 1067-1071.

Shine, R. (1987). Ecological comparisons of island and mainland populations of Australian Tiger Snakes. (Notechis. Elapidae). Herpetologica 43(2), 233-240.

Smith, L.A. (1982). 'Variations in *Pseudechis australis* (Serpentes: Elapidae) in Western Australia and description of a new species of *Pseudechis.* ' Rec. West. Aust. Mus., 10(1), 35-45.

Smith, M.J. (1976). 'Small fossil vertebrates from Victoria Cave, Naracoorte, South Australia,' IV. Reptiles. Trans. R. Soc. Sth. Aust., 100(1), 39-51.

Softly, A. (1971). 'Necessity for Perpetration of a Venomous Snake.' Biological Conservation, Vol. 4, No. 1, Applied Science Publishers, Great Britain, 40-42.

Southcott, R.N. and Coulter, A.R. (1979). 'The action of textilon on neuoromuscular transmission in the murine diaphragm.' In: Neurotoxins, Fundamental and Clinical Advances (ed. I.W. Chubb and L.B. Geffen). Adelaide Univ. Union Press, Adelaide.

Storr, G.M. (1981). 'The genus *Acanthophis* (Serpentes: Elapidae) in Western Australia.' Rec. West. Aust. Mus., 9(2), 203-210.

Storr, G.M. (1985). 'Phylogenetic relationships of Australian Elapid snakes: External morphology with emphasis on species in Western Australia.' In 'Biology of Australian frogs and reptiles.' Eds. G. Grigg, R. Shine and H. Ehmann. Roy. Zoo. Soc. of N.S.W., 221-222.

Sutherland, S.K. (1975). 'Treatment of snake-bite in Australia. Some observations and recommendations.' Med. J. Aust., Vol. 1, 30-32.

Sutherland, S.K. (1977a). 'Antivenoms: Better late than never.' Med. J. Aust., Vol. 2, 813.

Sutherland, S.K. (1977b). 'Acute untoward reactions to antivenoms.' Med. J. Aust., 2(17), 841-842.

Sutherland, S.K. (1977c). 'Serum reactions: An analysis of commercial antivenoms and the possible rate of anti-complementary activity in de-novo reactions to antivenoms and antitoxins.' Med. J. Aust., Vol. 1, 613-615.

Sutherland, S.K. and Coulter, A.R. (1977). 'Three instructive cases of tiger snake *(Notechis scutatus)* envenomation — And how a Radioimmunoassay proved the diagnosis.' Med . J. Aust., (2), 177-180.

Sutherland, S.K., Harris, R.D. and Coulter, A.R. (1979). 'Rationalisation of first aid measures for Elapid snake-bite.' Lancet, 183-186.

Sutherland, S.K. (1979a). 'First aid for snake bite in Australia.' Commonwealth Serum Laboratories publication, Melbourne.

Sutherland, S.K. (1979b). 'First aid for snake bite in Australia.' Editorial, Med. J. Aust., Vol.1 (19), 437-438.

Sutherland, S.K. (1979c). 'Australian venoms and care of the envenomed patient.' MD thesis, Univ. of Melbourne.

Sutherland, S.K. and Lovering, K.F. (1979). 'Antivenoms. Use and adverse reactions over a 12 month period in Australia and Papua New Guinea.' Med. J. Aust., Vol. 2, 671-674

Sutherland, S.K. (1980). 'First aid for snake bite in Australia with notes on first aid for bites and stings by other animals.' 2nd Revision. October 1980. Commonwealth Serum Laboratories Publications, Melbourne.

Sutherland, S.K. and Campbell, D.G. (1980). 'Myolytic effects of Australian snake venoms in monkeys, *Macaca fascicularis.* 'Proceedings of the Australian Society for Clinical Experimental Pharmac., 19-21 May, Dept. Pharmacology, Univ. of Melb.

Sutherland, S.K., Campbell, D.G. and Stubbs, A.E. (1981). 'A study of the major Australian snake venoms in the monkey, *(Macaca fascicularis).*' 2. 'Myolytic and haematological effects of venoms.' Pathology, 13, 705-715.

Sutherland, S.K., Coulter, A.R., Harris, R.D., Lovering, K.E. and Roberts, I.D. (1981). 'A study of the major Australian snake venoms in the monkey *(Macaca fascicularis).*' 1. 'The movement of injected venom, methods, which retard this movement, and the response to antivenoms.' Pathology, 13, 13-27.

Sutherland, S.K. (1983). 'Australian Animal Toxins. The creatures, their toxins and care of the poisoned patient.' Oxford University Press.

Swaroop, S. and Grab, B. (1954). 'Snake bite mortality in the world.' Bulletin of the World Health Organisation, 10, 35-76.

'The management of snake bite.' (1978). Editorial, Med. J. Aust., Vol. 6, 11 Feburary, 137-138.

Theakston, R.D.G., Lloyd-James, M.J. and Reid, H.A. (1977). 'Micro-ELISA for detecting and assaying snake venom and venom antibody.' Lancet 2, 639-641.

Tindale, N.B. (1924). 'Visit to the islands of the Sir Joseph Banks Group.' Sth. Aust. Nat., 5(3), 130-133.

Trinca, G.F. (1963). 'The treatment of snakebite.' Med. J. Aust., 1, 275-280.

Trinca, J.C. (1969). 'Report of recovery from a taipan bite.' Med. J. Aust., 514-516.

Trinca, J.C., Graydon, J.J., Covacevich, J. and Limpus, C. (1971). 'The rough-scaled snake *(Tropidechis carinatus)* a dangerously venomous Australian snake.' Med. J. Aust., 2, 801-809.

Tu, A.T., James, G.P. and Chua, A. (1965). 'Some biochemical evidence in support of the classification of venomous snakes.' Toxicon, 3, 5-8.

Tu, A.T. and Toom, P.M. (1967). 'Hydrolysis of peptides by snake venoms of Australia and New Guinea.' Aust. J. Exp. Biol. Med. Sci., 45, 561-567.

Venomous bites and stings. (1979). Use of antivenom. C.S.L. Medical handbook. Ch. 11.

Vines, A. (1978). 'Severe local reaction to bite of king brown snake.' Med. J. Aust., 1, 657.

Waite, E.R. (1928). Reptiles and Amphibians of South Australia. Govt. Printer Adelaide.

Walker, F.J., Owen, W.G. and Esmon, C.T. (1980). 'Characterisation of the prothrombin activator from the venom of *Oxyuranus scutellatus scutellatus* (taipan venom).' Biochemistry. 19, 1020-1023.

Weiner, S. (1960a). 'Active immunization of man against the venom of the Australian tiger snake *(Notechis scutatus).* ' Am. J. Trop. Med. Hyg., 9(3), 384-392.

Weiner, S. (1960b). 'Venom yields and toxicity of the venoms of male and female tiger snakes.' Med. J. Aust., 2, 740-741.

Wells, R.W. and Wellington, R.C. (1983). 'A synopsis of the class Reptilia in Australia.' Australian Journal of Herpetology, Vol. 1, (3-4), 73-129.

White, J., Pounder, D., Pearn, J.H. and Morrison, J.J. (1985). 'A perspective on the problems of snake bite in Australia.' In 'Biology of Australian frogs and reptiles.' Eds. G. Grigg, R. Shine and H. Ehmann. Roy. Zoo. Soc. of N.S.W., Sydney, 351-514.

White, J. (1987). 'Elapid snakes: Aspects of envenomation in Toxic Plants and Animals. A guide for Australia.' Qld. Museum, 391-429.

White, J. Intensive Care Staff of the Royal Adelaide Hospital. (1988). The Western Taipan: Human Case Report in The World's Most Venomous Snake. eds Jeanette. Covacevich, John Pearn and Julian White.

Worrell, E. (1958). 'Song of the Snake' Angus and Robertson, Sydney.

Worrell, E. (1961). 'Herpetological name changes.' West. Aust. Nat., 8(1), 18-27.

Worrell, E. (1963). 'Reptiles of Australia.' Angus and Robertson, Sydney.

Zeller, E.A. (1948). 'Enzymes of snake venoms and their biological significance.' In: Advances in Enzymology, Vol. 8, (ed. F.F. Nord). Interscience Publishers Inc., New York.

Acknowledgements

J. Pearn, N. Charles, P. Windsor, S. Sutherland, R. Davis, G. Clothier, F. Madaras, A. Gallus, P. Masci, H. Zola, Rex Jordan, J. Rumpf, G. Johnston who holds the copyright on head scale drawings, Pamela Yates, Jacqui Littlewood, Elizabeth Sowry, Marion Norman and Lisa Mettjes.

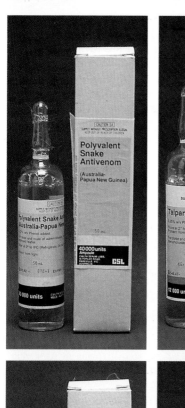
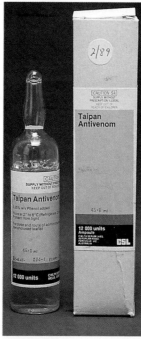
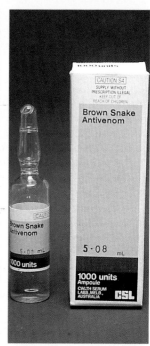
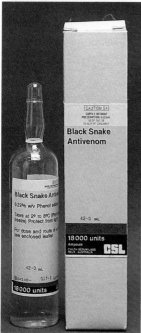
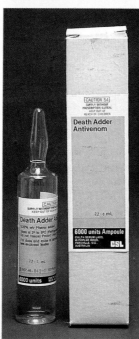
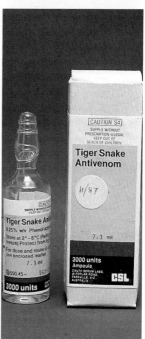

Types of Antivenin produced by Commonwealth Serum Laboratories

Venomous Snakes of Medical Importance in Australia: Clinical Toxinology

by Julian White

Introduction

Australia has the most diverse elapid snake fauna of any continent on Earth, and all of these snakes are technically venomous. While most are not dangerous to man, there are many common species which have proved capable of killing humans, and their venoms rank amongst the most toxic snake venoms known to man. Snake bite has been a perennial topic of interest, both in the lay press and the medical journals produced within Australia. The impression is given that snake bite is an ever-present and frequently encountered hazard in Australia. The true facts suggest otherwise. A full discussion on snake bite and its management in Australia is available in several recent books or monographs. The most important of these are "Toxic Plants and Animals; A Guide for Australia", edited by J. Covacevich, P. Davie and J. Pearn, Queensland Museum 1987; "Australian Animal Toxins", by S.K. Sutherland, Oxford University Press 1983; "Ophidian Envenomation; a South Australian Perspective", by J. White, Records of The Adelaide Children's Hospital 1981.

Epidemiology

The epidemiology of snake bite in most regions of the world is usually a 'guesstimate' based on available information, acknowledging the fact that complete and accurate statistics are not available. Australia is no exception. Snake bite is not a notifiable disease in Australia, and many country hospitals have not in the past kept statistics on types of presentation. Details of all deaths are recorded, but the notified cause of death may be only a supposition, and undoubtedly some deaths ascribed to snake bite are in fact due to other causes, and vice versa. Estimates of cases requiring treatment have been generated from information returned to the antivenom manufacturer in Australia. While these data are probably amongst the best available, they will nevertheless miss many cases where the correct information is not received. In 1929 Fairley reported an annual death rate from snake bite in all of Australia of 12.4 cases per year. By 1949 the World Health Organisation (Swaroop and Grab 1954) estimated the death rate had dropped to 5.6 cases per year. The most recent figures (White *et al* 1985) suggest 3.7 fatalities per year. The WHO study published in 1954 estimated a fatality rate from snake bite in Australia of 0.07 per 100,000 population, a similar rate to that in France (0.05 per 100,000 population). Thus it may be seen that snake bite is not a significant cause of death in Australia and it is probable that the vast majority of Australians will never see a poisonous snake other than in a zoo or reptile park.

Australian Elapid Snakes

In considering snake bite in Australia it is important to understand certain characteristics of Australian dangerously venomous snakes. Firstly, all are elapid snakes, having fangs at the front of the mouth on a modified maxilla capable of only a small degree of rotation (Figure 1). This limits the length of the fang, and for many dangerous species in Australia fangs are less than 5 mm, and sometimes less than 3 mm even in adult snakes. Table 1 documents adult fang length for some of the important species. The mobile maxilla nevertheless allows sufficient rotation for fang movement during the act of biting (Figure 2). This may result in the fang leaving a track of venom under the skin, or a scratch mark through the skin surface. This, plus the variety of other teeth in both the upper and lower jaw, frequently results in a complex bite pattern often associated with scratch marks rather than two distinct fang entry points (Figure 3). The determination of the type of snake which has bitten a snake bite victim from the appearance of the fang marks alone is therefore not a practical proposition. Furthermore the small size of the fangs in some species, combined with the glancing nature of most snake bites, may result in a local skin injury which is either difficult or impossible to identify with the naked eye. Thus the absence of visible fang marks does not preclude a diagnosis of snake bite.

For practical purposes the dangerously venomous snakes of Australia may be divided into five major groups which correspond with some characteristics of their venom, and the five monovalent antivenoms available for treatment. This grouping does not imply taxonomic relationships, but in reality does reflect our current knowledge of the phylogeny of these snakes. The five groups are listed in Table 2.

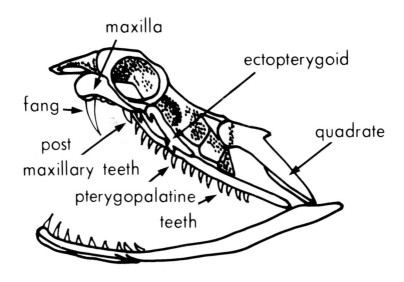

Figure 1
Lateral view of the skull of a death adder, *Acanthophis antarcticus* (after White 1981).

TABLE 1
Length of fangs of various snakes
(after Fairley 1929, Covacevich et al 1981, Kellaway and Thompson 1930)

Snake	Average length of fang (mm)	Range of length of fang (mm)
Taipan (*Oxyuranus scutellatus*)		7.9 – 12.1
Inland Taipan (*Oxyuranus microlepidotus*)		3.5 – 6.2
Mulga Snake (*Pseudechis australis*)	6.5	
Death Adder (*Acanthophis antarcticus*)	6.2	5.0 – 8.3
Red-bellied Black Snake (*Pseudechis porphyriacus*)	4.0	3.5 – 5.0
Tiger Snake (*Notechis scutatus*)	3.5	2.0 – 5.5
Copperhead (*Austrelaps superbus*)	3.3	3.0 – 4.5
Brown Snake (*Pseudonaja textilis*)	2.8	2.0 – 4.0

Snake Venom

The most important purpose of snake venom appears to be the subduing and digestion of prey. The venom is produced in a gland in the upper head situated posterior to the eye, and surrounded by a variety of muscles which can contract and compress the gland (Figure 4). Venom is thus forced from the gland through a venom duct to the base of the fang where it usually enters a closed groove in the fang, exiting near the tip of the fang. There is extensive clinical experience that snakes may bite without injecting a significant quantity of venom, and recent experimental research (Morrison *et al* 1982, 1983, 1983/84) confirms that snakes do inject significantly variable amounts of venom, and may be able to control the quantity injected. The average and maximum quantities of venom produced for each species are shown in Table 3.

The problem of determining how toxic a given snake venom is has vexed toxinologists for many years. Researchers working on the same venom, and using the same assay, may produce significant differences in apparent venom toxicity. Recently attempts have been made to define standard assay procedures for the toxicity and characterisation of snake venoms (Theakston and Reid 1983). The standard method remains the LD50, that is, the minimum dose of venom which will cause death in 50% of the test animals (usually mice) administered by the technique listed for the assay (e.g. IV, IM, SC, IP). This

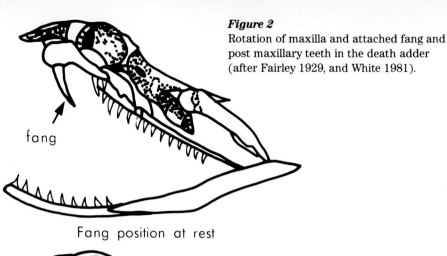

Figure 2

Rotation of maxilla and attached fang and post maxillary teeth in the death adder (after Fairley 1929, and White 1981).

fang

Fang position at rest

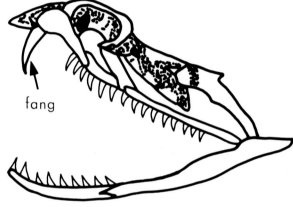

fang

Fang position at maximum elevation

situation is made more complex due to several characteristics of snake venom. Firstly snake venom is not a single component, but is a mixture of a variety of components with varying actions, which working together may have a different toxicity to the same components working in an isolated assay. There is also a variability in the relative quantities of components, and sometimes even in the type of components within the venom of a single species depending on where each individual specimen of that species was found. Thus research work done on the toxicity and actions of the venom from a particular species of snake using specimens from one part of Australia may not fully represent the action of the venom of the same species, but from a geographically distant part of Australia. Bearing these problems in mind, there is information on the relative toxicity of important dangerous snakes in Australia, based on the work of Broad *et al* 1979, shown in Tables 4 and 5, and mortality rates based on data collected before specific (antivenom) therapy was available, shown in Table 6 (after Fairley 1929, White 1987).

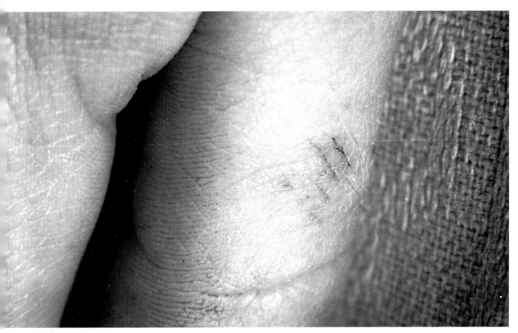

Figure 3
Result of a single snake bite on the thumb of a seven year old boy, bitten by a brown snake, *Pseudonaja* sps. The bite resulted in significant systemic envenomation. Note the series of scratch marks.

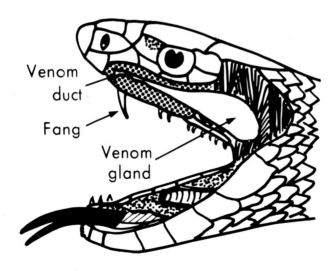

Venom duct

Fang

Venom gland

Figure 4
The relative position of the venom gland, venom duct and fang in an Australian elapid snake (after White 1981).

TABLE 2

The five major groups of Australian snake venoms, based on neutralisation by monovalent antivenoms.

Snake Group	Major Species in Group
Brown Snake Group	Brown Snake (*Pseudonaja textilis*)
	Western Brown Snake (or Gwardar) (*Pseudonaja nuchalis*)
	Dugite (*Pseudonaja affinis*)
Tiger Snake Group	Tiger Snake (*Notechis scutatus*)
	Black Tiger Snake (*Notechis ater*)
	Copperhead (*Austrelaps* sps)
	Rough-scaled Snake (*Tropidechis carinatus*)
Death Adder Group	Death Adder (*Acanthophis antarcticus*)
	Desert Death Adder (*Acanthophis pyrrhus*)
	Northern Death Adder (*Acanthophis praelongus*)
Taipan Group	Taipan (*Oxyuranus scutellatus*)
	Inland Taipan (Small-scaled or Fierce Snake)
	(*Oxyuranus microlepidotus*)
Black Snake Group	Red-bellied Black Snake (*Pseudechis porphyriacus*)
	Mulga Snake (*Pseudechis australis*)
	Collett's Snake (*Pseudechis colletti*)
	Blue-bellied Black Snake (*Pseudechis guttatus*)

Australian snake venoms may have numerous components with varied actions, but the important clinical consequences of snake bite can be related to just a few principal venom actions. Some of these disparate actions may in fact be caused by a single venom component, though this is not so in all cases. The most important actions of Australian snake venoms in man are:

1. Neurotoxicity

In the past paralysis was thought to be the major cause of death from snake bite in Australia, although more recent evidence (White *et al* 1985, White 1987) casts some doubt on this. Not all Australian snakes have neurotoxins, but where they are present they may cause severe paralysis even of the respiratory muscles, and without respiratory support a patient in this situation will die. There are two important classes of neurotoxins causing this paralysis, namely the more common, rapidly acting, but less toxic post-synaptic neurotoxins, and the more potent pre-synaptic neurotoxins. The pre-synaptic neurotoxins in Australian snake venoms all appear to have a phospholipase A2 as a principal component, and are either single chain, such as notexin from *Notechis scutatus*, the Tiger Snake, or multi-chain, such as taipoxin, from *Oxyuranus scutellatus*, the Taipan.

2 Myotoxins

Several Australian snake venoms have potent myolytic or muscle destroying

TABLE 3
Venom production in various snakes based on milking of venom
(after Broad *et al* 1979, Fairley and Splatt 1929)

Snake	Average Yield (mg)	Maximum Yield (mg)
Mulga Snake (*Pseudechis australis*)	180	
Taipan (*Oxyuranus scutellatus*)	120	400
Death Adder (*Acanthophis antarcticus*)	78	236
Chappell Island Black Tiger Snake (*Notechis ater serventyi*)	75	388
Inland Taipan (*Oxyuranus microlepidotus*)	44	110
Red-bellied Black Snake (*Pseudechis porphyriacus*)	40	75
Tiger Snake (*Notechis scutatus*)	35	189
Copperhead (*Austrelaps superbus*)	20	85
Rough-Scaled Snake (*Tropidechis carinatus*)	6	
Common Brown Snake (*Pseudonaja textilis*)	2	67
Indian Cobra (*Naja naja*)	169	610
Eastern Diamond Back Rattlesnake (*Crotalus adamanteus*)	410	848

TABLE 4
Relative toxicity of snake venoms in mice (after Broad *et al* 1979)

(S = sea-snake; E = elapid snake;
EA = Australian elapid snake; V = viperid snake)

Snake		LD_{50} (Saline) in mg/kg	LD_{50} (bovine serum albumin)
Inland Taipan			
(*Oxyuranus microlepidotus*)	EA	0.025	0.010
Common Brown Snake			
(*Pseudonaja textilis*)	EA	0.053	0.041
Taipan			
(*Oxyuranus scutellatus*)	EA	0.099	0.064
Tiger Snake			
(*Notechis scutatus*)	EA	0.118	0.118
Reevesby Island Tiger Snake			
(*Notechis ater niger*)	EA	0.131	0.099
Beaked Sea Snake			
(*Enhydrina schistosa*)	S	0.164	0.173
W.A. Tiger Snake			
(*Notechis ater occidentalis*)	EA	0.194	0.124
Chappell Island Tiger Snake			
(*Notechis ater serventyi*)	EA	0.338	0.271
Death Adder			
(*Acanthophis antarcticus*)	EA	0.400	0.338
Western Brown Snake			
(*Pseudonaja nuchalis*)	EA	0.473	0.338
Copperhead			
(*Austrelaps superbus*)	EA	0.560	0.500
Indian Cobra			
(*Naja naja*)	E	0.565	0.500
Dugite			
(*Pseudonaja affinis*)	EA	0.660	0.560
Papuan Black Snake			
(*Pseudechis papuanus*)	E	1.09	1.36
Stephens Banded Snake			
(*Hoplocephalus stephensii*)	EA	1.36	1.44
Rough-scaled Snake			
(*Tropidechis carinatus*)	EA	1.36	1.09
King Cobra			
(*Ophiaphagus hannah*)	E	1.80	1.91
Blue-bellied Black Snake			
(*Pseudechis guttatus*)	EA	2.13	1.53
Collett's Snake			
(*Pseudechis colletti*)	EA	2.38	—
Mulga Snake			
(*Pseudechis australis*)	EA	2.38	1.91
Red-bellied Black Snake			
(*Pseudechis porphyriacus*)	EA	2.52	2.53
Small-eyed Snake			
(*Cryptophis nigrescens*)	EA	2.67	—
Eastern Diamond Back Rattlesnake			
(*Crotalus adamanteus*)	V	11.4	7.70

TABLE 5
Average venom yields and various species of snake (LD_{50} for mice)
(after Broad *et al* 1979)

Snake	Average Venom Yield		Maximum Venom Yield	
	mg	LD_{50} doses	mg	LD_{50} doses
Inland Taipan (*Oxyuranus microlepidotus*)	44	217,821	110	544,554
Taipan (*Oxyuranus scutellatus*)	120	94,488	400	314,961
Brown Snake (*Pseudonaja textilis*)	2	2,469	67	80,426
Chappell Island Tiger Snake (*Notechis ater serventyi*)	75	13,838	388	71,587
Indian Cobra (*Naja naja*)	169	16,900	610	61,000
Death Adder (*Acanthophis antarcticus*)	78	11,538	236	34,911
King Cobra (*Ophiaphagus hannah*)	421	11,050	(500?)	13,123
Eastern Diamond Back Rattlesnake (*Crotalus adamanteus*)	410	2,662	848	5,505

TABLE 6
Mortality rate for various snakes, if no antivenom used
(after Fairley 1929)

Snake	Number of Patients	Deaths	% Mortality
*Taipan (*Oxyuranus scutellatus*)	8	6	75%
Death Adder (*Acanthophis antarcticus*)	10	5	50%
Tiger Snake (*Notechis scutatus*)	45	18	40%
Brown Snake (*Pseudonaja textilis*)	70	6	8.6%
Red-bellied Black Snake (*Pseudechis porphyriacus*)	125	1	0.8%

* Based on review of published cases, prior to availability of antivenom.

properties and with these species rhabdomyolysis may be an important clinical problem, particularly if it causes secondary renal failure. It appears that some of the potent pre-synaptic neurotoxins also have potent myotoxic activity.

3   Haemotoxins

This is a rather broad term covering venom components acting in some way on the normal processes of haemostasis and blood clotting. This therefore includes actions on blood platelets as well as the clotting pathway, and fibrinolytic pathway. While some Australian venoms do have components with potent action on platelets (White and Williams, in preparation) clinically it is the action of some venoms on blood clotting which is the most important. In particular several venoms cause activation of the common pathway in the blood coagulation cascade, particularly by the activation of prothrombin to thrombin, and the subsequent formation of fibrin and its rapid degradation to fibrin degradation products. This apparent powerful coagulant action *in vitro* causes a severe hypo-coagulability *in vivo*, and the patient's fibrinogen is rapidly destroyed, thus severely impairing clot formation in the body. This process is basically a defibrination, and the platelet count is rarely significantly affected. Probably because of this lack of effect on platelets, major haemorrhage as a result of defibrination is rarely seen, but a review of fatal cases of snake bite in Australia (White *et al* 1985, White 1987) suggests that, left untreated, this coagulopathy has the potential for major and even fatal haemorrhages, particularly in the central nervous system.

In addition to these powerful coagulant actions of Australian snake venoms, some venoms may also contain components which specifically inhibit sections of the coagulation pathway. Relatively little work has been done to isolate these, a reflection of their relative unimportance clinically.

A number of these venoms may also be directly toxic to blood cells, particularly red cells, causing intravascular haemolysis. Snakes of the genus *Pseudechis* have the most powerful haemolytic action amongst Australian snakes, but haemolysis is rarely described clinically, and is not a major problem with Australian snake bite.

4   Local Actions

While many non-Australian dangerous venomous snakes cause significant local tissue injury at the site of the bite, such injuries are rarely seen following snake bite in Australia, and local tissue destruction is not a significant problem in Australian snake bite.

5   CNS Actions

It is a common finding in major snake bite in Australia, particularly in children, for the patient to have had a brief period of unconsciousness, and a more prolonged period of impaired conscious state, usually defined as irritability. Because the period of brief unconsciousness often occurs prior to admission to hospital, and in a situation of a severe snake bite there are more important things to do with the patient than research the cause of their consciousness problems, detailed information on the cause of these CNS changes is not available. It may be that an early and brief hypotension may cause the brief period of loss of consciousness, and hypoxia may be responsible for some cases of continued irritability, but this author doubts that this is the complete explanation, and suspects that other venom components with direct or indirect actions on the CNS are at work. In addition, convulsions following snake bite, particularly in children have been recorded numerous times in Australia and the cause of these convulsions is not understood.

Venom research in Australia has been scattered in both time and place, and is sporadic in nature. In recent years three groups have consistently contributed to the literature on snake venom and snake bite in Australia. Firstly there has been a group at the Commonwealth Serum Laboratories in Melbourne, producers of Australia's antivenoms. Much eminent research has come from this institution, stimulated and led by Dr S.K. Sutherland who for a number of years was head of immunology research at these laboratories. Within Australia Dr Sutherland is the best known medical expert on snake bite. The second group is based in Brisbane, headed by Dr J Pearn of the University of Queensland. The third group is in Adelaide, headed by Dr J. White at the Adelaide Children's Hospital. The important contribution of Australian museums in each of the capital cities to our understanding of Australian venomous snake taxonomy cannot be underestimated. Furthermore in recent years some museums have contributed directly to venom research, in particular Dr J. Covacevich of the Queensland Museum working with Dr Pearn in Brisbane, and Dr T. Schwaner of the South Australian Museum working with Dr White in Adelaide. There are a number of other researchers who have contributed in recent times to the literature on Australian snake venoms or snake bite, but a full discussion of this field is beyond the scope of this chapter.

First Aid for Snakebite

Recommended first aid for snake bite in Australia underwent major changes from 1979 onwards as a result of extensive animal experimentation by Dr S. Sutherland and colleagues, and subsequent development of field usage Venom Detection Kits by the same team. Using a sensitive radioimmunoassay to follow venom appearance in the blood stream, they showed that the combination of local pressure bandage plus immobilisation, the "pressure-immobilisation technique", was as effective as all other methods, but also safer, easier to apply, and more practical for the Australian situation (Sutherland *et al* 1979, Sutherland *et al* 1981). The current recommended first aid for snake bite in Australia is therefore:

1. Immediately apply a broad firm bandage to cover the bitten area. In the case of a limb, as much of the limb as possible should be bound. The bandage should be bound as tightly as for a sprained ankle. (Figure 5)
2. Immobilise the affected limb with some form of splint. Leave the bandage and splint on until medical care is reached.

3. Bring transport to the victim if possible; do not permit the victim to move around more than is necessary.
4. If the snake can be killed safely, then bring it along with the victim.
5. Do *not* wash the bite site.

Figure 5
The application of pressure immobilisation first aid in the treatment of snake bite.

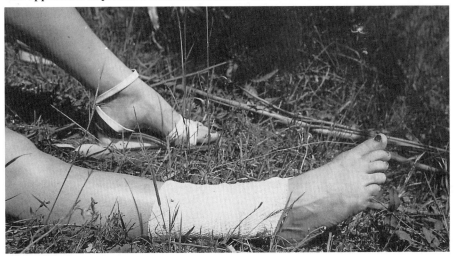

Figure 5(a)
The patient is laid down if possible and a broad elastic bandage or similar (pantyhose, torn strips of clothing) is firmly applied over the bite site at the same pressure as used for a sprained ankle.

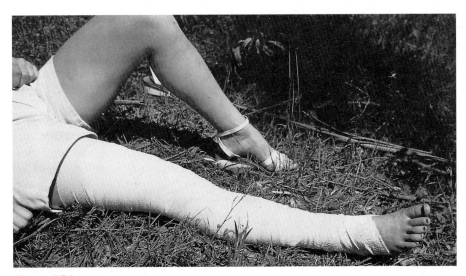

Figure 5(b)
The bandage is then applied to involve as much of the bitten limb as possible, being applied firmly, but not so tightly that blood circulation to the whole limb is impaired.

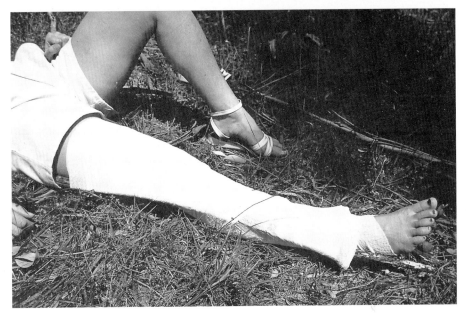

Figure 5(c)
The limb is positively immobilised using further bandage and any available implement as a splint.

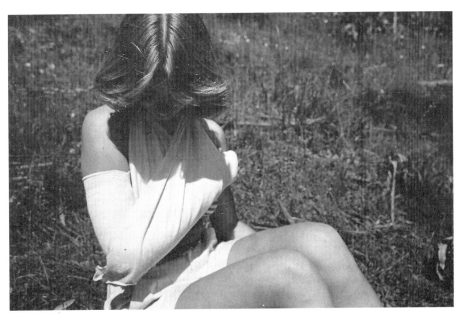

Figure 5(d)
In the case of a bite to the hand or arm the same form of bandage is applied, and the arm immobilised with a splint and sling.

The use of arterial tourniquets, cutting open the bite area, and use of local applications such as Condy's crystals, are not appropriate treatment for snake bite.

The first aid bandage, once applied, should not be removed until the patient is in a medical facility fully equipped to treat snake bite.

Envenomation and Medical Management of Snake Bite

Envenomation is the spectrum of problems which occurs in the victim of a bite or sting by a venomous animal, and ascribable to the effects of the venom. Envenomation will only occur when enough venom has been injected into the victim to cause a detectable problem. In this context it is important to remember that in a significant number of snake bites in Australia insufficient venom is injected by the snake into its human victim to cause problems, therefore envenomation does not occur, and in these cases there is no need for antivenom treatment. Indeed the use of antivenom in such cases is contra indicated and would constitute medical malpractice. It therefore becomes quite important to determine whether a patient is envenomed or not as this determines the whole treatment strategy. Clearly this subject is of great importance, and a full discussion of the topic and the related subject of medical management may be found in the three major reviews quoted at the beginning of this chapter. However, in terms of medical decision making, when managing a case of suspected snake bite the important elements of diagnosis on which subsequent management will be based remain history, examination and laboratory investigation.

History

It is important to note the circumstances of the bite. In particular it should be noted when the patient was bitten, or thought they may have been bitten, and the events surrounding the bite, which may give a clue about the probability of the bite actually having occurred. If possible a description of the snake may be useful, and it is important to know the region of Australia that the bite occurred in as this will in many cases define the potential species, involved. A single glancing bite may be trivial, though not necessarily so, but multiple bites are nearly always associated with major envenomation. Thus a history of whether the snake struck once, twice or more is important. A strike through clothing may minimise the effect of the bite.

Details of first aid should be noted, and the patient or companions questioned about development of general and specific symptoms of envenomation. Of particular importance as general symptoms are headache, nausea, vomiting, abdominal pain, loss of consciousness, difficulty with vision, and convulsions. The presence of any of these symptoms suggests that envenomation has probably occurred. Specific problems relate to specific actions of snake venom. Thus snakes with neurotoxins in their venom may cause paralysis and the patient may relate this initially as blurred vision, drooping or sleepy eyelids, distortion of speech, general weakness, and difficulty with breathing. The myotoxins causing muscle destruction will result in muscle pain, muscle weakness, and the passing of dark urine. The coagulant components in the venom may result in a coagulopathy, but this rarely causes obvious symptoms and signs, at least in the first few hours following the bite. Nevertheless persistent bleeding from the bite site is suggestive of a coagulopathy, and a history of haemoptysis, haematemesis, haematuria, or melaena, is an indication of severe coagulopathy.

In addition to the history relating to the snake bite, it is important to further determine if the patient has any other important medical problems, especially heart problems, kidney problems, or history of allergic reactions or asthma, the latter two suggesting a potential problem with antivenom treatment.

Examination

In examining a patient with possible snake bite it is important both to note the local wound, and evidence of systemic spread of the venom. Thus the local wound should be inspected, looking for bruising, tenderness, swelling and signs of a multiple snake bite. Note that the local wound may be very hard to identify, with no obvious fang puncture marks or other marks, and no local pain, tenderness, swelling, or erythema. The absence of notable local symptoms and signs does not necessarily exclude the diagnosis of snake bite. In particular bites by Brown Snakes (genus *Pseudonaja*) are often associated with no or minimal local pain and local reaction despite major envenomation.

Spread of the venom initially is largely via the lymphatic system, and enlarged or tender draining lymph nodes may be an early sign of venom spread. Specific signs of envenomation include evidence of paralysis such as diplopia, paralysis of medial gaze, ptosis, lack of facial muscle expression, dysarthria, generalised muscle weakness, and evidence of respiratory muscle paralysis. Muscle weakness may also be caused by myolysis however, associated with pain on muscle movement. Impairment of CNS function has already been mentioned, the most common finding being irritability, with or without some degree of drowsiness. As previously mentioned signs of coagulopathy are rarely evident even though a major coagulopathy may be present.

The examination should also include assessment of respiratory function, including auscultation, as pulmonary oedema may occur following snake bite. Where the patient is unconscious a thorough neurological examination may be warranted to elicit the focal signs.

Investigations

The Commonweatlth Serum Laboratories in Melbourne have introduced a snake venom detection kit based on the ELISA technique (Theakston *et al* 1977, Coulter *et al* 1980, Chandler and Hurrell 1982). This kit is designed to detect nanogram quantities of snake venom, and determine which of the five major groups of snakes is involved, corresponding to the five monovalent antivenoms available (Figure 6). The best test results are from samples taken at the site of bite, and the kits are completely self contained, with all required components, and no need of laboratory facilities (Figure 7). If the patient has systemic envenomation then some venom may be excreted in the urine and in this situation the test kit may also be used to test urine. The test kit has proved unreliable for testing either plasma or serum for the presence of venom.

The value of the snake venom detection kit lies in its ability to identify the type of snake involved in the snake bite, corresponding to the appropriate monovalent antivenom which will neutralise the snake venom (Table 7). This allows treatment with monovalent antivenom rather than using the more costly and more hazardous polyvalent antivenom. This is an important advance in treatment as it has been shown that the incidence of untoward side effects following antivenom therapy is significantly greater following polyvalent antivenom therapy than for therapy with most monovalent antivenoms in Australia. The most reliable detection of venom will be a swab from the region

TABLE 7

Specificities of C.S.L. ELISA snake venom detection kits (V.D.K.)

Tube (specific antibody)	Species giving positive reaction
1) Yellow	Tiger Snake (*Notechis sps*) Red-bellied Black Snake (*Pseudechis porphyriacus*) Copperhead (*Austrelaps sps*) Rough-scaled Snake (*Tropidechis carinatus*)
2) Red	Brown Snake Western Brown Snake (or Gwardar) Dugite (*Pseudonaja sps*)
3) Blue	Mulga Snake (*Pseudechis australis*) Papuan Black Snake (*Pseudechis papuanus*) Red-bellied Black Snake (*Pseudechis porphyriacus*) Copperhead (*Austrelaps sps*)
4) Green	Death Adder (*Acanthophis sps*)
5) White	Taipan (*Oxyuranus scutellatus*) Inland Taipan (*Oxyuranus microlepidotus*) Rough-scaled Snake (*Tropidechis carinatus*)

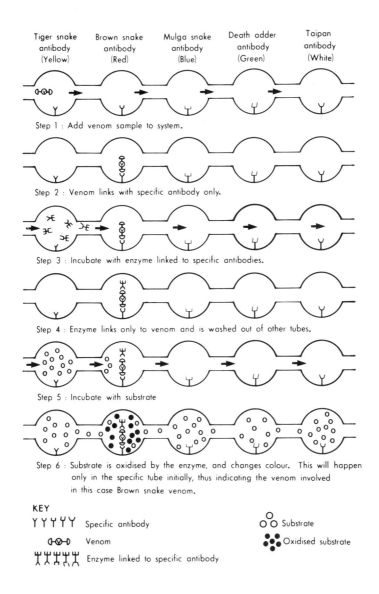

| Tiger snake antibody (Yellow) | Brown snake antibody (Red) | Mulga snake antibody (Blue) | Death adder antibody (Green) | Taipan antibody (White) |

Step 1 : Add venom sample to system.

Step 2 : Venom links with specific antibody only.

Step 3 : Incubate with enzyme linked to specific antibodies.

Step 4 : Enzyme links only to venom and is washed out of other tubes.

Step 5 : Incubate with substrate

Step 6 : Substrate is oxidised by the enzyme, and changes colour. This will happen only in the specific tube initially, thus indicating the venom involved in this case Brown snake venom.

KEY

ΥΥΥΥΥ Specific antibody

О-⊗-О Venom

ΥΥΥΥΥ Enzyme linked to specific antibody

O O Substrate

Oxidised substrate

Figure 6

Diagrammatic representation of the mechanism of action of the ELISA venom detection kit (after White 1981).

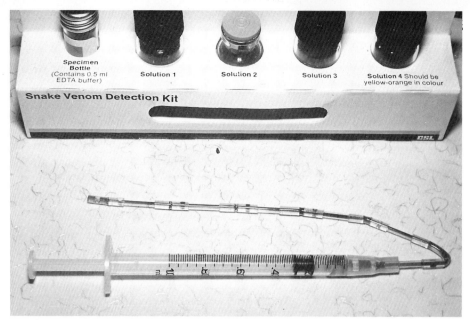

Figure 7
The Commonwealth Serum Laboratories (Melbourne) ELISA venom detection kit. All
reagents required are supplied in the kit.

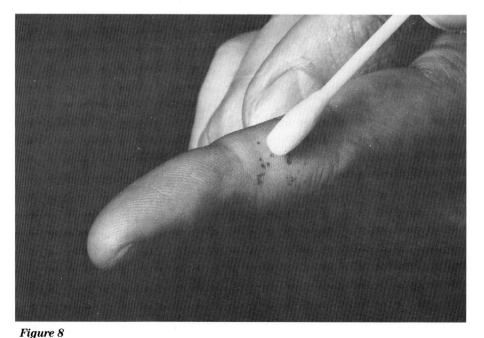

Figure 8
The best sample for venom detection is a swab of the skin over the bite site. Swab stick
and moistening solution are supplied in the venom detection kit. Rub the moistened
swab firmly over the skin directly over and adjacent to visible fang marks.

of the bite site detecting venom remaining on the skin surface (Figure 8). It is possible for an Australian venomous snake to bite a victim without injecting significant amounts of venom, and in this situation it is possible for venom to be deposited on the skin in sufficient amounts to give a positive reaction with the snake venom detection kit. Thus a positive venom detection result from a skin swab does not imply systemic envenomation and is not an indication for antivenom therapy. It is merely an indication of which antivenom is most appropriate to use should the patient have or develop evidence of systemic envenomation. The criteria for systemic or significant envenomation remain as discussed earlier.

Apart from venom detection the other useful tests are either common laboratory tests or tests of blood clotting function. While there are a wide range of coagulation laboratory tests which may be applied in a case of snake bite, the key tests to determine the presence or absence of a significant coagulopathy are the prothrombin time (prothrombin ratio), activated partial thromboplastin time (APTT, PTTK etc), fibrinogen level, and fibrin degradation products. In addition a complete blood picture including platelet count should be performed particularly looking for thrombocytopenia and evidence of a microangiopathic haemolytic anaemia. These latter two problems are usually only encountered in severe envenomation associated with renal failure. A standard blood electrolyte and enzyme screen (LDH etc, and including creatine phosphokinase if possible) and renal function screen should be performed. Blood transfusion is very rarely required as treatment for snake bite, but in cases of major envenomation a group or group and screen should be considered. Urine output should be measured, and urine checked for proteinuria and haemoglobinuria, and if there is systemic envenomation also tested for myoglobinuria.

Antivenom Therapy

Antivenom therapy is the treatment of choice in patients with significant systemic envenomation and in such cases should be given without delay. The aim of such treatment is to neutralise all circulating venom and venom yet to reach the circulation. Patients who do not have evidence of significant systemic envenomation do not require antivenom therapy. While in most cases a patient will show definite evidence of systemic envenomation within one to two hours of the snake bite, there are cases where the patient will appear initially well, and will not develop evidence of systemic envenomation for several hours. In this situation the patient will initially not receive antivenom during the symptom free period, but on later development of symptoms antivenom therapy should be commenced. Obviously in some cases this will mean delaying antivenom therapy in cases who ultimately require it, but providing adequate therapy is given as soon as evidence of systemic envenomation occurs, this will not cause the patient harm, and is much preferable to the less selective administration of antivenom to all patients presenting with snake bite, irrespective of whether they require it or not, a policy unofficially practised by some medical practitioners in Australia in the past. Figure 9 illustrates the time between snake bite and death in cases not treated with antivenom (statistics from pre-antivenom era) illustrating that few patients die in the first hours, nearly half taking 24 hours or more to die.

Snake antivenoms in Australia are manufactured by the Commonwealth Serum Laboratories in Melbourne using the standard technique of hyper-immunising horses. The resultant antivenom is therefore a horse serum product with all the attendant antigenic implications, and thus all patients receiving such antivenom should do so in a carefully controlled environment with every precaution taken to treat allergic reactions including anaphylactic shock, should this develop.

There are currently antivenoms covering all known dangerous species of Australian snake divided into five subgroups, and with a polyvalent antivenom available covering all five groups. The details for each antivenom are listed in Table 8. The quantity of antivenom per vial is based on the average amount of venom milked from the relevant species of snake, and is a guide only in determining dose. A severe snake bite will require multiple vials of antivenom, while a minor systemic envenomation may be controlled with a single vial of antivenom. As there is relatively little cross-reactivity between the five

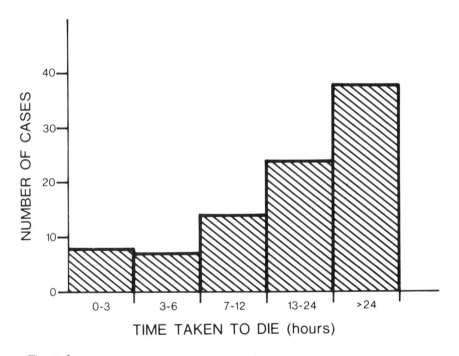

Figure 9
Graph illustrating statistics on time between bite and death in 81 cases of snake bite treated (without antivenom) in the pre-antivenom era (after Fairley 1929).

TABLE 8
Antivenoms available to Australian elapid venoms, produced by C.S.L.

Antivenom (AV)	Species effective for	Units per vial	Average volume per vial (mls)
Brown Snake AV	Brown Snake *Pseudonaja textilis* Western Brown Snake (or Gwardar) *Pseudonaja nuchalis* Dugite *Pseudonaja affinis*	1000 μ	4
Tiger Snake AV	Tiger Snake *Notechis scutatus* Black Tiger Snake *Notechis ater* Copperhead *Austrelaps sps* Rough-scaled Snake *Tropidechis carinatus* Red-bellied Black Snake *Pseudechis porphyriacus* Collets Snake *Pseudechis colletti* Blue-bellied Black Snake *Pseudechis guttatus*	3000 μ	6.8
Death Adder AV	Death Adder *Acanthophis antarcticus* Desert Death Adder *Acanthophis pyrrhus* Northern Death Adder *Acanthophis praelongus*	6000 μ	20
Taipan AV	Taipan *Oxyuranus scutellatus* Inland Taipan (Small-scaled or Fierce Snake) *Oxyuranus microlepidotus*	12000 μ	40
Black Snake AV	Red-bellied Black Snake *Pseudechis porphyriacus* Mulga Snake *Pseudechis australis* Collets Snake *Pseudechis colletti* Blue-bellied Black Snake *Pseudechis guttatus*	18000 μ	35
Polyvalent AV	Equivalent to: Brown Snake AV Tiger Snake AV Death Adder AV Taipan AV Black Snake AV	1000 μ 3000 μ 6000 μ 12000 μ 18000 μ	48

195

monovalent antivenoms, it is essential that the correct antivenom is used for the species of snake involved (Table 9). The major exception to this are bites by the Red-bellied Black Snake (*Pseudechis porphyriacus*) which are equally well controlled by Tiger Snake antivenom as by the more specific Black Snake antivenom, the latter being much higher volume and more expensive, and therefore Tiger Snake antivenom is preferable in such cases. Multiple bites will virtually always require multiple vials of antivenom. Children require the same dose of antivenom as adults.

Antivenom should always be administered intravenously, preferably diluted in a standard intravenous solution such as Hartmann's solution or normal saline solution. The extent of dilution will depend on the volume involved, but is usually in the range of 1:5 to 1:10. It should then be given over a twenty to thirty minute period through an established intravenous line, and not through a temporarily placed needle in a vein. Adrenalin should be drawn up in a syringe ready for subcutaneous administration should an anaphylactic reaction occur. Some authors suggest the use of a small dose of subcutaneous adrenalin, and of intravenous antihistamine prior to giving any antivenom, to further reduce the chance of allergic reaction (Sutherland 1983). This policy is controversial, and is not adopted by some experts. Intravenous antihistamines usually have a sedative effect on the patient, which may mask important symptoms and signs of envenomation, and adrenalin is probably best reserved to treat a severe reaction should it occur. If there is a history of previous exposure to antivenom, or allergy to horse serum, or history of severe allergic reactions or asthma, extra care must be taken with antivenom administration. In this situation consideration should be given to prior treatment with subcutaneous adrenalin and intravenous antihistamine as previously discussed, and possibly intravenous hydrocortisone as well. However, for most patients the combination of dilution of antivenom, and slow administration through the intravenous line will not result in significant side effects.

Not all venom will reach the circulation at the same time, and it is possible for a trickle of venom to reach the circulation over several hours. Therefore an initial dose of antivenom may neutralise the first quantity of venom to reach the circulation, but further antivenom therapy may be required in an hour or so to neutralise further venom which has reached the circulation. If the venom has caused a coagulopathy, serial coagulation tests to follow the progress and resolution of the coagulopathy may assist in determining if further antivenom is required. Failure to show resolution of coagulopathy, or worsening coagulopathy, two hours after administration of antivenom is evidence of continuing circulating venom, and an indication for further antivenom therapy.

Where the venom concerned contains neurotoxins, antivenom may not reverse paralysis already established at the time of antivenom therapy, but may prevent further progression of that paralysis. In this situation the early signs of paralysis such as ptosis and double vision may remain unaltered by antivenom therapy, but the patient will not go on to develop more severe and life threatening paralysis.

If antivenom therapy fails to give the expected response in the patient this

TABLE 9
Recommended minimum doses of antivenom (intravenous).
Note that many times this dose may be needed.
Child's dose the same as for adults.
(after White 1981, Sutherland 1983)

Snake		Appropriate Antivenom	Minimum Dose
Brown Snake	)	Brown Snake	1000μ
Western Brown Snake (Gwardar)	)	AV	
Dugite	)		
Tiger Snake	)	Tiger Snake	
Copperhead	)	AV	3000μ
Rough-scaled Snake	)		
Black Tiger Snake	)	Tiger Snake AV	6000μ
Chappell Island Black Tiger Snake		Tiger Snake AV	12000μ
Red-bellied Black Snake	)	Tiger Snake AV	3000μ
Blue-bellied Black Snake	)	OR	
Collett's Snake	)	Black Snake AV	6000μ
Mulga Snake		Black Snake AV	18000μ
Death Adder	)	Death Adder	
Desert Death Adder	)	AV	6000μ
Northern Death Adder	)		
Taipan	)	Taipan	12000μ
Inland Taipan (Small-scaled or Fierce Snake)	)		

may indicate one of several problems. First of all if a monovalent antivenom has been used, it may indicate that the wrong monovalent antivenom has been chosen. This is most likely to occur when the patient presents with the snake which has bitten them, and someone inexperienced in snake identification incorrectly identifies the serpent. While further attempts should be made to correctly identify the snake, the immediate needs of the patient in this situation are best met by the use of polyvalent antivenom. A second common problem is that insufficient antivenom is given. Occasionally inactive antivenom is used, but if the expiry date is checked before use this problem should not occur. Antivenom given by the wrong route, typically intramuscularly, will fail to reach therapeutic doses quickly, and this has been a cause of problems in the past. It is uncertain if it is ever too late to give antivenom, but the greater the delay between envenomation and treatment, the greater the chance of an unfavourable outcome for the patient. Nevertheless favourable effects of antivenom therapy have been observed for up to sixty hours after envenomation.

The decision on which variety of antivenom to use, once a decision to use antivenom has been taken, is a most important one. As mentioned earlier polyvalent antivenom covers all snake species, and therefore does not suffer

197

from the problem of incorrect antivenom type. However the cost is considerable, both in monetary terms, and more importantly side effects for the patient. The polyvalent antivenom inevitably is of larger volume, and thus is associated with a much higher incidence of unwanted side effects. In one series the average volume of polyvalent antivenom used was 70 mls, with a 22% rate of untoward reaction (Sutherland and Lovering 1979). This compared with an average of 4.2 mls of Brown Snake antivenom with a 5% untoward reaction rate. However if polyvalent antivenom is not to be used, then one must know with confidence the type of snake involved in the snake bite incident. This may be achieved by detection of venom using the previously mentioned venom detection kit. A snake brought in with the patient may also provide information, but it must be identified by an expert herpetologist, and not by a keen amateur. In most hospital settings such an expert may not be readily available. In any case a dead snake is rarely presented with the victim. A further possibility involves combining expert herpetological knowledge including accurate knowledge of the distribution of snakes, together with an understanding of symptoms and signs of envenomation specific for each

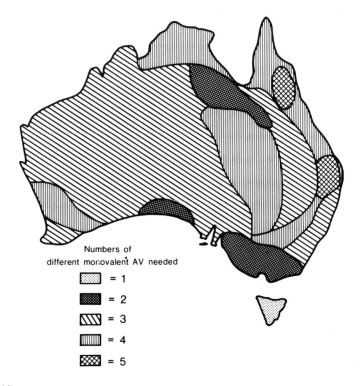

Numbers of
different monovalent AV needed

▦ = 1

▩ = 2

◩ = 3

▥ = 4

▨ = 5

Figure 10.
Map of Australia illustrating the relative diversity of snake venom types in different regions of Australia, reflected in the number of monovalent antivenom types required to fully cover all possibilities. This map is a rough guide only. Expert clinical toxinologists should generate more detailed maps for their own hinterland, showing which monovalent antivenoms are appropriate for each area.

species group (Figure 10). This level of knowledge and expertise should be available through clinical toxinologists, who may be able to determine the type of snake involved using this information, or narrow the possibilities down to just two different venom groups requiring only the mixture of two monovalent antivenoms, which is certainly preferable to the use of polyvalent antivenom. Unfortunately such expert clinical toxinologists are not readily available in Australia at present, but their advice is available in some centres, and should be sought early in the management of any case of suspected or definite envenomation. The availability of such an expert may be determined through contact with the local State Poisons Information Centre.

Untoward reactions to antivenom are numerous in type, but fortunately serious reactions are rarely seen. Of these anaphylaxis remains the most important, and may occur even in a patient who has never previously been exposed to horse serum. Sensitivity to antivenom is not accurately predicted by prior skin testing, and skin testing prior to use of antivenom is not a recommended procedure in Australia. Other reactions noted following antivenom therapy include urticaria, itching, oedema, rigors, shivering, fever, colicky abdominal pain, headache, sweating, and bronchospasm. There may also be delayed reactions including arthralgia and polylymphadenopathy. In one series (Campbell 1969) 46% of cases receiving antivenom therapy developed some form of untoward reaction, fortunately most being minor, but with a 3% rate of anaphylaxis. A more recent study by the Commonwealth Serum Laboratories (Sutherland and Lovering 1979) showed a much lower incidence of side effects. It is important that the patient who has received antivenom therapy be made aware of the possibility of delayed reactions to antivenom, and in particular the possibility of serum sickness. This is most likely to occur if a large volume of antivenom has been infused, such as occurs with polyvalent antivenom therapy, and onset may be delayed from four to ten days. The symptoms may mimic 'flu, and if the patient is not aware of this, may lead to inappropriate diagnosis and treatment by another medical practitioner not involved in the treatment of the snake bite. Detailed discussion of serum sickness and its management may be found in general textbooks of medicine.

General Management of Snake Bite

In addition to the specific management of systemic envenomation, using antivenom therapy, several other points should be noted. Local pain at the bite site is usually not a major problem, but colicky abdominal pain may be a problem in some cases, and this may not be completely relieved by antivenom. Pain relief with morphine is contra-indicated in such cases, but less potent analgesics may be used. Pulmonary oedema may occasionally occur in severe snake bite, and requires appropriate therapy including diuretics in some cases. As vomiting is a frequent accompaniment of systemic envenomation, the patient should be nursed on their side if there is significant impairment of conscious state, to avoid the possibility of aspiration pneumonia. For similar reasons, oral fluids should either be withheld or limited to clear fluids, and food should be withheld until the situation is stabilised. Fluid requirements can be maintained via intravenous therapy. Infection following snake bite is rarely a problem, but should be treated with appropriate antibiotic therapy if it occurs. Tetanus immunisation status should be determined on admission, and managed appropriately. All staff including junior medical staff and nursing staff should be made aware of the potential problems of snake bite, on admission of the patient, and alerted to watch for specific signs of developing systemic envenomation, particularly the early signs of developing paralysis. It should be impressed on these staff that as soon as such signs are observed they should be reported to the medical officer in charge. Resuscitation facilities should be readily available. In all cases of systemic envenomation it is best to manage the patient in a high intensity nursing area such as an Intensive Care Unit.

Management of Neuromuscular Paralysis

Most cases of snake bite in Australia today should receive appropriate antivenom therapy before significant paralysis has occurred. However some cases will not reach appropriate medical care until major paralysis has developed, and this may necessitate a period of assisted ventilation. Appropriate antivenom therapy should still be given in such cases, to neutralise other effects of the snake venom, despite the fact that the paralysis may not be reversed by such therapy. As a general rule the last muscles to be paralysed by snake venom in man are those involved in respiration, and their period of paralysis may be short, lasting only a few hours. It therefore may be necessary to maintain the patient on assisted ventilation for less than 24 hours. There are of course exceptions to this, where the patient will require assisted ventilation for many days. The first muscles paralysed, such as the fine muscles around the eye, are usually the last muscles to recover from such paralysis, and indeed recovery may take many weeks. Such impairment of eye function should be documented prior to discharge of the patient, and may be of relevance in determining when the patient may recommence normal activities, in particular driving.

Management of Coagulopathy

As mentioned previously coagulopathy following snake bite in Australia is usually a defibrination syndrome, and primary treatment of this is by neutralisation of all circulating venom with appropriate antivenom. Indeed the response of the coagulopathy to antivenom therapy may be used to titrate the quantity of antivenom required by the patient. If a coagulopathy has been documented, it is advisable to re-test coagulopathy parameters approximately two hours following the dose of antivenom, to determine if there has been any change. If these parameters have showed improvement over this time, with substantial movement towards normality, then further antivenom therapy for the coagulopathy may be withheld, pending re-testing a further two hours later. If however there has been insignificant resolution, or worsening of the coagulopathy, then further antivenom therapy should be given, again with re-testing two hours later. The use of blood product replacement therapy has been suggested as ancillary treatment in cases of severe coagulopathy following snake bite in Australia, but this will rarely if ever be indicated, as use of the correct antivenom in sufficient quantity will almost invariably allow correction of the coagulopathy. Rarely a true disseminated intravascular coagulation with platelet consumption will occur, usually in association with a microangiopathic haemolytic anaemia as seen in cases of renal failure following snake bite. The best treatment plan for such cases has not been established, and the role of heparin in this situation remains uncertain. Where renal failure occurs it may be necessary to institute haemodialysis (White and Fassett 1983).

Reptile Keepers and Snake Bite

Throughout Australia there are a number of amateur reptile keepers who maintain private collections of venomous snakes. Most of these collectors are very careful with their pets, and are rarely if ever bitten. A few individuals engage in inappropriate bravado, resulting in repeated bites. These individuals may present two major problems. The first, and fortunately rarest, is the development of true allergy to snake venom akin to that seen with severe allergic reaction to bee venom. In this situation the reptile keeper may collapse within minutes of a further snake bite due to an anaphylactic reaction to the venom rather than primary venom toxicity. Such a situation may be rapidly fatal. Less severe allergic reactions including bronchospasm may be seen, and alert the medical practitioner to the potential for tragedy in the future. Such individuals should be strongly advised to cease keeping or handling venomous snakes. A more common problem, though nevertheless infrequently encountered, is developing allergy to horse serum following multiple treatments of snake bite with antivenom. This may provide major problems in managing a severe snake bite, where the only available therapy is antivenom, to which the patient is allergic. Such patients should be premedicated with hydrocortisone and subcutaneous adrenalin, before antivenom therapy. Sutherland (1983) has suggested that in this situation the antivenom should be infused as rapidly as possible as it may play the role of a blocking antibody as well as reducing any toxic effects of the venom.

Effects of the bites of each major snake group in Australia

In this section brief information on local and systemic effects observed for each snake group will be discussed, although it must be stressed that snake bite is unpredictable, and occasionally patients will present with symptoms and signs atypical of those usually seen for a given species. The salient points for each group are summarised in Table 10.

Brown Snakes (*Pseudonaja species*)

The major species in this group are the Common or Eastern Brown Snake (*Pseudonaja textilis*); the Western Brown Snake or Gwardar (*P. nuchalis*); and the Dugite (*P. affinis*). Brown Snakes are probably responsible for the majority of snake bites in Australia, but due to the small size of their fangs, and the small quantity of venom they produce, despite its high toxicity, the majority

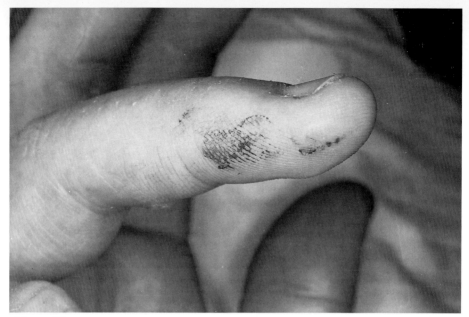

Figure 11
A brown snake (*Pseudonaja textilis*) bite to the tip of the ring finger of a 24 year old herpetologist. Note the lack of local reaction such as swelling or bruising.

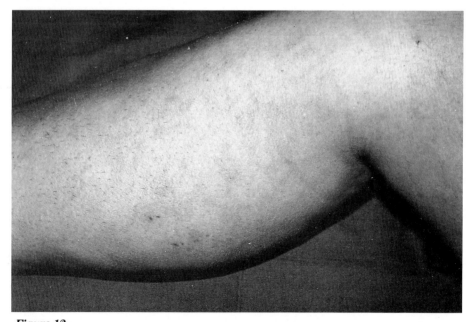

Figure 12
A brown snake (*Pseudonaja* sps) bite to the calf of a 42 year old woman. No local swelling or bruising. Systemic envenomation with defibrination syndrome developed in this patient.

of Brown Snake bites will not result in major envenomation. Nevertheless severe and potentially fatal envenomation following Brown Snake bite can occur, and indeed serious envenomation including collapse of the patient may be seen within fifteen minutes of the bite in some cases, particularly in children. The site of bite may be hard to locate due to the small size of the fangs and other teeth, and usually there is minimal or no local pain, no local swelling, and no local bruising around the area of the bite (Figures 11, 12, 13). Collapse or unconsciousness is common in significant systemic envenomation, as is coagulopathy, usually a defibrination. In cases with delayed treatment, paralysis may develop, but in most cases paralysis is not a significant feature. Muscle destruction is unlikely to occur following Brown Snake bite, but several cases of renal failure have been reported.

Tiger Snake Group

This group includes the Mainland Tiger Snake (*Notechis scutatus*), and the Black Tiger Snake (*N. ater*). In addition the Australian Copperheads (*Austrelaps* species), and the Rough-scaled Snake (*Tropidechis carinatus*) appear to cause similar problems to the Tiger Snake, and their venom is neutralised by the same antivenom. Tiger Snakes have moderate sized fangs and a moderate to large quantity of potent venom, and major envenomation is a frequent accompaniment of Tiger Snake bite. This is usually associated with a

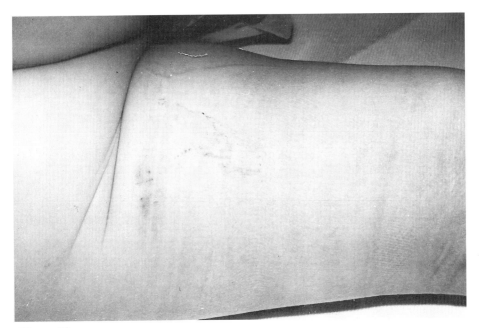

Figure 13
A brown snake (*Pseudonaja* sps) bite to the upper posterior thigh of a 2 year old boy. The snake bit the child twice, and major life threatening systemic envenomation ensued. Despite this, there is no significant local swelling or bruising, and the bite marks are indistinct.

TABLE 10

Summary of clinical effects of envenomation by Australian elapid snakes
(after WHITE, 1981, 1986: WHITE and POUNDER, 1984)

Snake/Venom Group	Local Problems at the bite site			Systemic Problems			
	Pain	Swelling	Bruising (³ mild necrosis)	Unconsciousness	Paralysis	Coagulopathy	Muscle destruction (Muscle movement pain/myoglobinuria)
Brown Snakes (*Pseudonaja sps*)	Absent or minimal	Nil	Nil	Usual (³convulsions)	Uncommon	Usual, severe	Nil
Tiger Snakes (*Notechis sps*)	Frequent	Frequent but mild	Often present	Usual (³convulsions)	Usual and sometimes severe	Usual, severe	Frequently present
Mulga Snake (*Pseudechis australis*)	Often minor	Usually severe	Usually absent or minimal but necrosis may occur	Usual	True paralysis not seen	Frequent, but often mild	Usual and sometimes severe
Red-bellied Black Snake (*Pseudechis porphyriacus*)	Often minor	Usual	Variable	Occasionally	Not seen	Unlikely	Frequently present, though often minor
Death Adders (*Acanthophis sps*)	Frequent	Minimal or absent	Absent	Unusual	Usual and sometimes severe	Unlikely	Not seen
Taipans (*Oxyuranus sps*)	Variable, sometimes absent	Often minimal	Unusual	Usual (³ convulsions)	Usual and sometimes severe	Usual, severe	Probably frequently present

mild to moderate local reaction with local pain frequently seen, together with a mild degree of local swelling, and frequent association of local bruising, and on occasion a minor degree of superficial necrosis around the fang entry points (Figure 14). Collapse or unconsciousness is frequently seen in cases with major envenomation, especially in children, where it may occur within thirty minutes of the bite. Coagulopathy is usually seen if there is systemic envenomation, and is usually a defibrination. Paralysis is seen in most cases with systemic envenomation, and may be severe (Figures 15, 16). A mild degree of muscle destruction is frequently present, and cases with major destruction of skeletal muscle due to myotoxins have been reported.

Black Snake Group (Genus *Pseudechis*)

The most important member of this group is in fact the King Brown or Mulga Snake (*Pseudechis australis*), the other members being the Red-bellied Black Snake (*P. porphyriacus*), Collett's Snake (*P. colletti*), and the Spotted Black Snake (*P. guttatus*). The Mulga Snake venom is best neutralised by specific Black Snake antivenom, but venom of the other three species is adequately neutralised by Tiger Snake antivenom. Bites by the Mulga Snake are usually associated with moderate to severe local swelling, this being the most obvious local feature of Mulga Snake bite, and distinctive for this species group (Figure 17, 18). Although one case of local necrosis following Mulga Snake bite has been reported (White 1981), there is usually no significant necrosis or even bruising in the region of the bite, and indeed the fang marks may be hard to

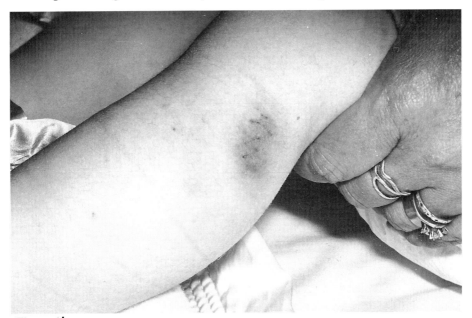

Figure 14
A tiger snake (*Notechis scutatus*) bite on the upper calf of a 2 year old girl. The snake bit twice, and there is local swelling and bruising. This child developed severe life threatening envenomation.

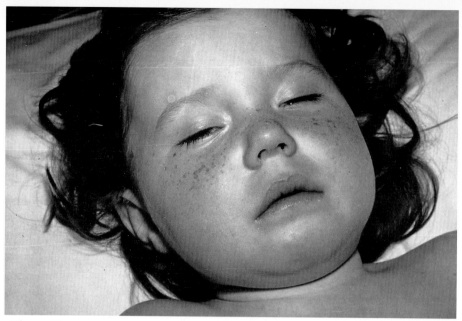

Figure 15
The same child as in Figure 14. Bilateral ptosis and lack of facial muscle expression can be seen, evidence of early neuromuscular paralysis.

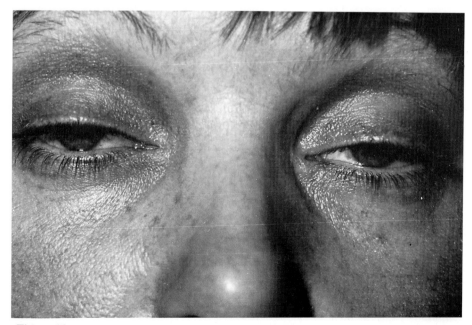

Figure 16
A tiger snake (*Notechis scutatus*) bite to a 27 year old woman, showing bilateral ptosis, a sign of early neuromuscular paralysis.

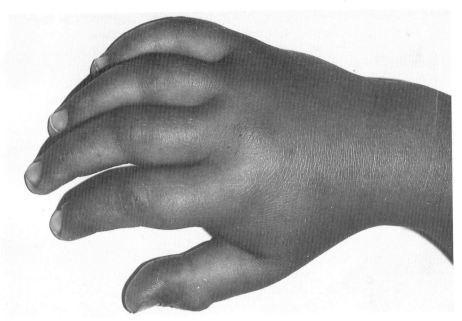

Figure 17
A mulga snake (*Pseudechis australis*) bite to the thumb of an 11 year old boy. There is extensive swelling of the whole hand, but no local bruising.

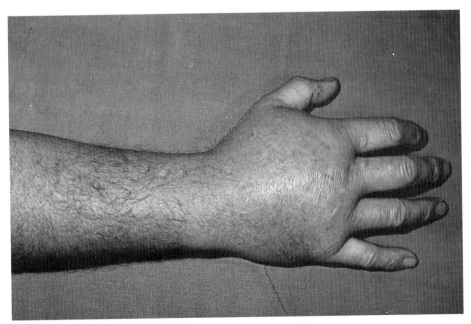

Figure 18
A mulga snake (*Pseudechis australis*) bite to the hand of a 48 year old man, showing extensive local swelling.

locate despite the severe swelling. Pain may be severe, but in most cases there is little local pain associated with the swelling, and no impairment of vascular function. The swelling will resolve over several days. If systemic envenomation develops then collapse is a frequent accompaniment, and there is usually some muscle destruction, which may be quite severe. This in itself may mimic paralysis, but there is no current evidence that true paralysis can occur following Mulga Snake bites. Coagulopathy may occur, and indeed may be a frequent accompaniment, but data presently available suggest that it would be limited to a mild defibrination. Bites by the Red-bellied Black Snake show a similar though less severe local effect, and major systemic problems are rarely encountered (Figure 19). Usually the systemic problems may be minor only, such as headache and abdominal pain, which will frequently resolve over an hour or so without the need of antivenom therapy.

Death Adder Group

This group includes the three species of Death Adder (*Acanthophis antarcticus*, *A. pyrrhus* and *A. praelongus*). All Death Adders have moderate to large fangs and are capable of producing large amounts of venom. Thus Death Adder bites will frequently be associated with systemic envenomation. Pain at the bite site is frequently encountered, but swelling is minimal if present, and local bruising is not usually seen. The main systemic problems are those associated with paralysis, as muscle destruction and coagulopathy are not encountered with Death Adder bites. The paralysis may develop rapidly and can be severe.

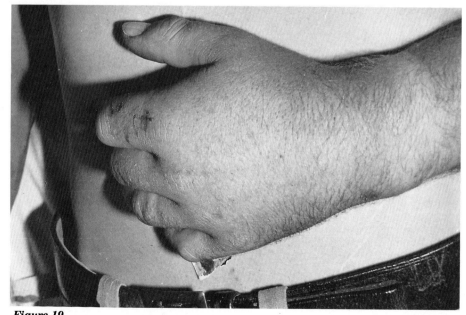

Figure 19
A red-bellied black snake (*Pseudechis porphyriacus*) bite to the index finger of a 28 year old amateur herpetologist. There is extensive local swelling of the whole hand.

Taipans

This group contains the Queensland or Common Taipan (*Oxyuranus scutellatus*), and the Inland Taipan or Small-scaled or Fierce Snake (*O. microlepidotus*). The Taipans are potentially the most dangerous snakes in Australia, having large fangs and capable of injecting large amounts of very potent venom. The effects of Taipan bite appear quite variable, but it is likely that the vast majority of Taipan bites result in significant and potentially fatal envenomation. Early and adequate antivenom therapy is particularly important for bites by Taipans. The local effects of Taipan bite have not been well documented, and vary from trivial local effects as seen with Brown Snake bite through to more significant local pain and reaction as seen with Tiger Snake bite. The systemic problems are legion, including rapid collapse, convulsions, severe and rapidly developing paralysis, severe coagulopathy, and major muscle destruction.

Acknowledgements

The author acknowledges with gratitude the help and support of the Adelaide Children's Hospital in production of this manuscript, particularly the Department of Haematology, especially Mrs O. Lammas for her expert typing, and the Department of Photography for preparing reproductions of the author's original photographs and artwork. The illustrations in this manuscript have been previously published in either Records of the Adelaide Children's Hospital or Queensland Museum book (Toxic Plants and Animals: A Guide for Australia), and their respective editors are thanked for their co-operation in re-publishing these illustrations.

References

1. Broad A. J., Sutherland S.K., Coulter A. R. (1979). The lethality in mice of dangerous Australian and other snake venoms. Toxicon, 17, 661-664.
2. Campbell C. H. (1969). Clinical aspects of snake bite in the Pacific area. Toxicon, 7, 25-28
3. Chandler H. M. and Hurrell J.G.R. (1982). A new enzyme immunoassay system suitable for field use and its application in a snake venom detection kit. Clinica Chimica Acta, 121, 225-230
4. Coulter A.R., Harris R.D., Sutherland S.K. (1980). Enzyme immunoassay for the rapid clinical identification of snake venom. Medical Journal of Australia, 1, 433-435.
5. Fairley N.H. (1929). The present position of snake bite and the snake bitten in Australia. Medical Journal of Australia, 1, 296-313.
6. Morrison J.J. Pearn J.H., Coulter A.R. (1982). The mass of venom injected by two elapidae: the Taipan (*Oxyuranus scutellatus*) and the Australian Tiger Snake (*Notechis scutatus*) Toxicon, 20, 739-745.
7. Morrison J.J., Pearn J.H., Charles N.T., Coulter A.R. (1983). Further studies on the mass of venom injected by elapid snakes. Toxicon, 21, 279-284.

8. Morrison J., Pearn J., Covacevich J., Tanner C., Coulter A. (1983-84). Studies on the venom of *Oxyuranus microlepidotus*. Clinical Toxicology, 21(3), 373-385.
9. Theakston R.D.G., Lyoyd-James M.J., Reid H.A. (1977). Micro-ELISA for detecting and assaying snake venom and venom antibody. Lancet, 2, 639-641.
10. Theakston R.D.G., Reid H.A. (1983). Development of simple standard assay procedures for the characterisation of snake venom. Bulletin of the World Health Organisation, 61, 949-956.
11. Sutherland S.K., Coulter A.R., Harris R.D. (1979). Rationalisation of first-aid measures for elapid snake bite. Lancet, 183-186.
12. Sutherland S.K. and Lovering K.E. (1979). Antivenoms; use and adverse reactions over a 12 month period in Australia and Papua New Guinea. Medical Journal of Australia, 2, 671-674.
13. Sutherland S.K., Coulter A.R., Harris R.D., Lovering K.E., Roberts I.D. (1981). A study of the major Australian snake venoms in the monkey (*Macaca fascicularis*); in the movement of injected venom; methods which retard this movement, and the response to antivenoms. Pathology, 13, 13-27.
14. Sutherland S.K. (1983). Australian Animal Toxins. Oxford University Press, Melbourne.
15. Swaroop S. and Grab B. (1954). Snake bite mortality in the world. Bulletin of the World Health Organisation, 10, 35-76.
16. White J. (1981). Ophidian envenomation; a South Australian perspective. Records of The Adelaide Children's Hospital, 2(3), 311-421.
17. White J. and Fassett R. (1983). Acute renal failure and coagulopathy after snake bite. Medical Journal of Australia, 2, 142-143.
18. White J., Pounder D., Pearn J.H., Morrison J.J. (1985). A perspective on the problems of snake bite in Australia. In Biology of Australasian Frogs and Reptiles, pages 551-614, editors Grigg G., Shine R., Ehmann H., Royal Zoological Society of New South Wales.
19. White J. (1987). Elapid snakes; venom production and bite mechanism. In Toxic Plants and Animals; a guide for Australia, pages 357-367, editors Covacevich J., Davie P., Pearn J., Queensland Museum.
20. White J. (1987). Elapid snakes; venom toxicity and actions. In Toxic Plants and Animals; a guide for Australia, pages 369-389, editors Covacevich J., Davie P., Pearn J., Queensland Museum.
21. White J. (1987). Elapid snakes; aspects of envenomation. In Toxic Plants and Animals; a guide for Australia, pages 391-429, editors Covacevich J., Davie P., Pearn J., Queensland Museum.
22. White J. (1987). Elapid snakes; management of bites. In Toxic Plants and Animals; a guide for Australia, pages 431-457, editors Covacevich J., Davie P., Pearn J., Queensland Museum.

Note: A more complete list of references may be found in White 1987, Sutherland 1983, and White 1981.

Venomous Snakes of Medical importance in Burma

Dr Maung Maung Aye

Introduction

Burma is a tropical country in South East Asia inhabited by about 144 species of snakes, of which only a few are venomous. Two species in particular, Russell's viper and the common cobra, are deadly. Every species that is medically important, is described in detail for reference. Each year a large number of snake bite occurs and about ten percent of the cases are fatal. Farmers are the usual victims. The snake bite problem is of national importance as Burma is an agricultural country. The epidemiology of snake bite is presented to illustrate the severity and magnitude of the problem. The clinical aspects of the snake bite is discussed in great detail especially on Russell's viper bite. The clinical features and management of snake bite patients by different species are also described. A brief review of research activities on snake bite is also given.

The prophylactic measures against snake bite are outlined in detail. The prevention of snake bite, reduction of serpent population and prophylaxis by active immunisation are discussed. When prevention fails and snake bite occurs, prompt effective treatment for the victim must be made available. Immediate adequate treatment of the patient is the next best option to prevention.

Snakes of Burma

Burma, situated between latitude 28° 29' N to 9° 58' N and longitude 101° E to 92° 11' E, is part of Southeast Asia with a tropical climate (Fig. 1). The country has three seasons — summer, rainy monsoon and winter but nevertheless the weather is generally hot and humid all year round except for the northern and eastern hilly regions of the country. It has a long coast line bordering the Bay of Bengal and the Andaman Sea. The country is made up of central plains where rivers Irrawaddy and Chindwin traverse and lead to a southern low lying delta region where a number of rivulets and estuaries intermingle. The area is hot, humid, wet and marshy, particularly in lower delta region. The soil is especially fertile and the climate suitable for paddy growing. Middle and upper Burma have a hot and dry climate, and fertile land suitable for paddy growing with the aid of irrigation systems, and other agricultural farming such as wheat, cotton, maize and beans. Varieties of birds and small mammals including rodents and other animals make the region their homeland.

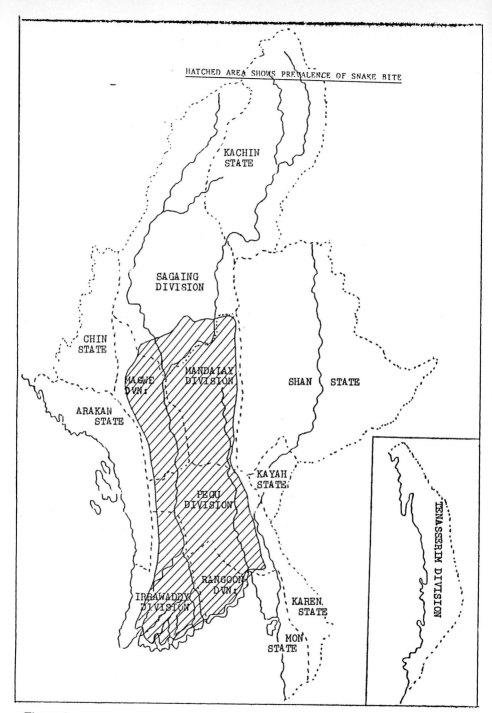

Figure 1
Map of Burma

In Burma, 144 species of snakes belonging to 52 genera and 9 families are found (table 1).

TABLE 1

List of snakes of Burma (based on Smith, 1943)

	Family	Sub family	Genus	Species
1	Typhlopidae	0	*Typhlops*	4
2	Leptotyphlopidae	0	0	0
3	Uropeltidae	0	0	0
4	Anilidae	0	*Cylindrophis*	*rufus burmanus*
5	Xenopeltidae	0	*Xenopeltis*	*unicolor*
6	Boidae	0	*Python*	2
7	Colubridae	5	32	89
8	Dasypeltidae	0	*Elachistodon*	*westermanni*
9	Elapidae	0	3	11
10	Hydrophiidae	2	8	22
11	Viperidae	2	4	13
	Total Family 9	9	52	144

Snakes of medical importance

Family Elapidae Boie 1827

Bungarus fasciatus (Schneider) 1801
(Banded Krait) NGAN-DAW-GYAR MWE

A venomous protoglyphous snake whose body is triangular in cross-section, and covered with black and yellow (or buff) rings (Fig. 2). Head is not distinct and the tail blunt, thick and slightly bulbous at the tip. Even though it is a venomous snake, the behaviour is mild and inoffensive. It is a cannibalistic snake often found in great numbers and when caught, does not make any attempt to escape. When disturbed they coil loosely and hide the head beneath the body. This snake does not bite except on extreme provocation. The venom is 10 to 15 times less potent than the cobra venom but nonetheless is neurotoxic and could be deadly.

Callophis macclellandi Form 1 (Reinhardt) 1844
(Coral Snakes) THANDAR MWE

This is a colorful and beautiful snake. It has a small cylindrical body and the head is not distinct. Head is black except for a broad white transverse bar behind the tiny eyes with round pupil. There are narrow black regularly placed bars on the dorsum; the belly is studded with irregular patches of black quadrangles or narrow bars throughout the whole length. There are five forms based on colour pattern. They are mostly found in Maymyo region, 1000 m above sea level. They are timid in disposition, nocturnal in habit and partially burrow into the soft earth beneath the logs. Their main food appears to be

213

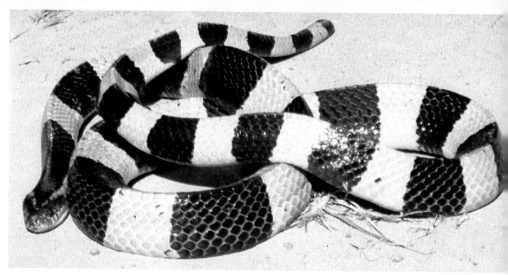

Figure 2
Banded Krait (*Bungarus fasciatus*)

worm-snakes and possibly insects. They are poisonous and the venom is neurotoxic, but practically harmless.

Naja naja kaouthia Lesson 1831
(Common Cobra) MWE HAUT

This is a very common Elapid found all over Burma. It has a monocellate diamond shape or rather broad-based pyramid-like marking on the hood (Fig. 3). On the ventral aspect, there is a small black spot on either side nearer towards the edge. A broad black band runs across the belly of the neck, otherwise the ventrals, are pale throughout the entire length. The snake is generally black or dark coloured, and always ready to slither away if given a chance. When cornered, it rears up and hisses which is a threat display and often strikes with a closed mouth. The effective striking distance is short and man can easily keep out of the range. It is nocturnal in habit and its actions and strikes are more precise and fast during the night. The cobra is usually more than a metre long and feeds chiefly on rats, mice, toads and frogs. It tends to stay in tree holes and rodent habitats, hence most people get bitten when they push their hands carelessly into these holes. It is not necessary for the cobra to rear and strike to produce a fatal bite, and a number of cases bitten that way while hunting for rodents have been reported. Cobra bites on human are effective only in about 30% of cases and it is responsible for 5% of deaths due to venomous snake bite in Burma. It is found in most habitats particularly in the vicinity of human habitations and heavily populated areas.

Mating takes place in January and February, 10 to 20 eggs are usually laid in May, and incubation period takes two to three months.

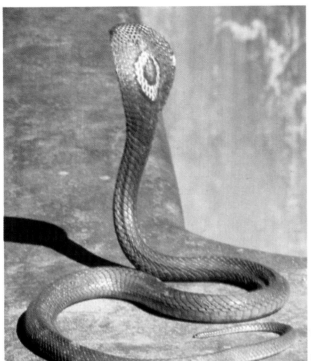

Figure 3
Monocellate Cobra
(*Naja naja kaouthia*)

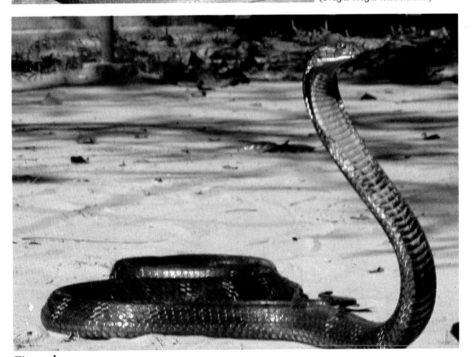

Figure 4
King Cobra (*Ophiophagus hanna*)

Ophiophagus hanna (Cantor) 1836
(King Cobra, Jungle Cobra)
TAW-GYI MWE HAUT

The King Cobra (Fig. 4) is a giant serpent exceeding 4 or 5 m easily and usually found only in thick jungles and tropical forest. It is a dangerous, deadly and aggressive snake particularly so when brooding. It shows strong parental instinct and is keen to protect its eggs and offsprings. There are many accounts of people having been chased and attacked, however it usually makes an escape without delay when encountered. There are records of pythons having been attacked and eaten.

It is cannibalistic and diurnal in habit. It preys entirely on snakes both venomous and nonvenomous. The colour is dark grey or black, crossed by speckled narrow white bars; the belly is rather pale. It probably mates in January — February, 20 — 40 eggs are laid in April and takes 2 — 3 months to hatch. Man has been rarely bitten and people who are exposed to this danger are those working in thick jungles, as reptile attendants in zoos and those who earn their living by giving snake shows. I have witnessed an isolated instance (though it happens time and again) where a snake charmer was bitten by a king cobra during the snake show. He died almost instantaneously. If a man is bitten by a king cobra, he probably has no chance to survive. There are records that even elephants succumb to king cobra bite. The venom is neurotoxic and produces respiratory paralysis.

Family Hydrophiidae Boie 1903
Sub Family Hydrophiinae Smith 1926

Enhydrina schistosa (Daudin) 1803
Hydrophis spiralis (Shaw) 1803
Hydrophis microcinctus Daudin 1803
Hydrophis stricticollis Gunther 1864
PIN-LE GYAT MWE

All sea snakes are venomous, with oar like tails and about 1 m long. Head is relatively small, eyes minute with round pupils and the nostrils placed on the upper surface of the snout. Sea snakes may be divided into two sub families, the Laticaudinae which is semiaquatic and the Hydrophiinae which is entirely aquatic. They are graceful swimmers.

Members of the Hydrophiinae are rather slow and awkward in movements on land as the ventral shields are small (about one quarter of the breadth of the body) or absent completely. Occasionally they are found many miles away from the shore though their preference is the vicinity of the coast where waters are comparatively sheltered. Estuaries and river mouths are their favourite places. The Hydrophiinae are viviparous. Members of the Laticaudinae are not found far from the shore and some of them move about and spend a good deal of time on land as their ventrals are large, a third to half of the breadth of the body. They are oviparous.

Sea snakes feed on fish, are diurnal in habit and some species with small head and slender forebody live exclusively on eels. Although all sea snakes are poisonous, Hydrophiinae venom is said to be much more potent and lethal than that of the Laticaudinae. Fishermen are the occasional victims and death is due mostly to myonecrosis and acute renal failure. Identification of the species of a snake is particularly difficult as the scales are so small that precise numbers cannot be counted. The colour is often grey and black with rather faint patterns of cross bars.

Family Hydrophiidae Boie 1803
Sub Family Laticaudinae Smith 1926

Laticauda colubrina Smith 1926
PIN-LE GYAT-LONE

This sea snake is semiaquatic, swims in the sea and crawls on the land with ease. The body is sub-cylindrical, only slightly compressed, The colour is light or dark bluish grey above, yellowish below with uniform black bands slightly narrowing over the belly. The head is not distinct; the snout is yellow in colour which extends backwards on each side of the head leaving a dark bar in between the two. These black bars fuse with the black band behind the eye. It is about a metre long and usually found near the shore. They feed on fish and are oviparous.

Family Viperidae Bonaparte 1840
Sub Family Viperinae

Vipera russelli siamensis Smith 1917
(Russell's Viper, Daboia, Tic-Polonga)
MWE PWE

This is a true viper of deadly repute and perhaps the most venomous. It is about a metre long and the body is fat; head enlarged, stumpy and broadly triangular, covered with small and strongly keeled scales similar to the ones on the body. The tail is short.

There are five colour forms:

(1). *Vipera russelli russelli*, (2). *Vipera russelli siamensis*, (3) *Vipera russelli formosensis*, (4). *Vipera russelli limitis* and (5). *Vipera russelli pulchella*.

Vipera russelli siamensis is abundant and poses a severe health problem to Burma than any other country. The distinction of *V. r. siamensis* is that there are triangular or oval spots present between the dorsal and lateral chains. Generally, they are yellow or light brown above matching the colour of the soil of that particular region (Fig. 5). On the head are large symmetrical dark brown triangular markings intervened by light broad lines, two of which unite at the snout (Fig. 6). On the body are three longitudinal series of large

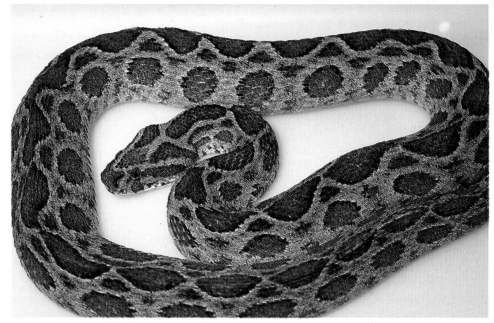

Figure 5
Russell's Viper (*Vipera russelli siamensis*)

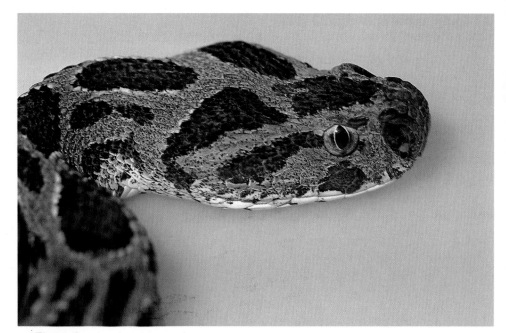

Figure 6
Russell's Viper's head region
(Figure 5 & 6 Copyright @ D.A. Warrell)

oval dark brown patches with black margins which are separated by yellow white lines from the general background. The vertebral row or chain is largest and sometimes confluent with one another forming an open chain. When this happens, it is believed locally that the serpent is so deadly that once bitten, no treatment will avail. The lateral row of patches are more oval in shape, smaller and less uniform in size. In addition, in *V. r. siamensis*, triangular dark spots occur in between the chains. Ventrally, it is yellowish white sprinkled with semilunar black spots all throughout the entire length. It is solenoglyphous i.e. with forward mobile canalized fangs about 1.5 to 2 cm long and they usually possess replacement fangs. The fangs are folded backwards when the mouth is closed and when it opens to strike, the fangs spring up by the action of muscles. The snakes strike very forcefully and buries the fangs deep into the body of the victim, while the jaw muscles contract, squeezing the venom sac and injecting large amounts of venom instantaneously. It then draws back its fangs without holding onto the prey unlike in other snakes and waits for the victim to succumb to envenomation, before trailing it by scent and devouring it. The food consists mainly of rodents, lizards and frogs. In captivity, they often refuse to eat on their own even when hungry. They rarely breed in captivity.

The snake is nocturnal in habit and hunts most actively during the early evening. Its movements are slow and it often waits quietly for the prey to pass nearby. Even when it is disturbed it usually maintains its ground. When it is angry it hisses loudly and assumes a striking posture with a lateral S-shaped loop of the neck. When it strikes, it does so with great force and determination, sometimes literally hurling itself at its victim. The bite is tenacious, powerful and certain to inflict damage by the injecting a large amount of venom deep into the tissues of the victim.

Its distribution is variable, being abundant in some districts and much less frequent or rare in the adjoining areas. They prefer the plains where paddy and other agricultural cultivation take place. It is a prolific, ovoviviparous snake, producing 20 — 40 young at a time. Mating occurs in January-February and the young are mostly born in June-July. The gestation period is about six months.

The venom of Russell's viper is very potent, a very powerful coagulant and contains a number of enzymes. Detoxification, toxoid production and active immunization are in progress in Burma. Although immunization may be effective there is one reservation which is that snake bite is a massive assault of venom injection unlike that of bacterial or viral infection where toxins are slowly released from the infected area. Hopefully, envenomation will be less severe in the immunised person and can buy him more time if he is bitten, so that treatment may still be effective even after a lapse of time. The average venom yield on extraction is about 140 mg and the subcutaneous LD_{50} for a 70kg man extrapolated from mouse-value is 516.6 mg. In man, viper bites usually produce subcutaneous injection; intravenous injection invariably causes a fatal outcome.

In Burma, Russell's viper is responsible for 85% of poisonous snake-bites and produces significant envenomation in 70% of the bites. When fatal cases are analysed, Russell's viper is the cause of death in 95% of the cases.

Family Viperidae Bonaparte 1840
Sub Family Crotalinae

Trimeresurus erythrurus (Cantor) 1839
(Dry Tail Green Snake)
MWE SEIN MEE CHAUT

This is a pit viper, solenoglyphous and venomous but not fatal. Envenomation by *Trimeresurus* species cause consumption coagulopathy and non-clotting of blood for a few days.

The head is large and irregular with a local pit, and it is covered by subequal tuberculate scales though those in the temporal region are strongly keeled. Supraocular and internasals are distinctly large, usually a small scale separating the two large internasals, subocular is elongated. On the average, it is about 60 cm long with slender body covered by strongly keeled scales; the colour is leaf-green on the dorsal aspect whereas the ventrals are uniformly fresh pale green with a yellow tinge (Fig. 7 & 8). There is a white line adjacent to the ventrals on each side. The prehensile tail is usually spotted with brown and looks dry compared to the leafy-green body, hence it is called locally, the 'dry-tailed green snake'.

Its habit is mostly arboreal though it frequently comes down to the ground in search of food. Although the species is fairly common, the bite is uncommon, constituting a little more than 3% of poisonous snake bites in Burma. There has been no fatality.

Among the species of *Trimeresurus*, identification and assignment of a particular snake is difficult as many species are alike with unstable morphological characters. Therefore, one has to be contented sometimes with assigning the snake only to the genus *Trimeresurus*.

SNAKE BITE PROBLEM IN BURMA

It is known from the literature that by the size of its population, Burma is the country with the highest incidence and death rates due to snake bite in the world.

Morbidity and Mortality Rates

The magnitude of the snake bite problem can be ascertained by looking at the annual incidence of snake bite and case fatality rates over a period of a few years. Table 2 shows morbidity and mortality rates due to snake bites for the 5-year period from 1969 — 1973.

Age Incidence

The incidence of snake bite can be expected to be highest among the age groups that are most exposed to venomous snakes. Table 3 shows the age groups among the victims of snake bite for the period of 5 years. The table reveals that persons belonging to the age group (15-45) who are most active and exposed to the risk, are the most commonly bitten. Death rate is proportional to the incidence.

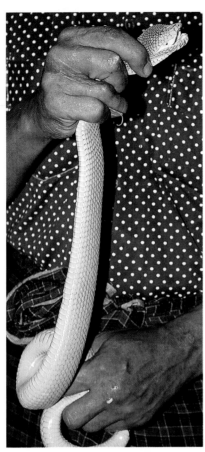

Figure 7
Trimeresurus erythrurus
(Copyright @ D.A. Warrell)

Figure 8
Dry Tail Greensnake
(*Trimeresurus erythrurus*)

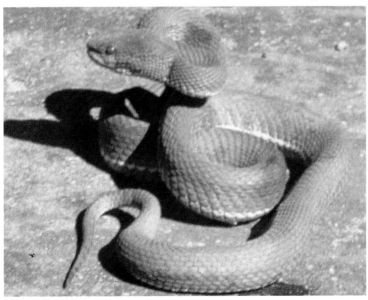

TABLE 2
Snake bite Morbidity and Mortality Rate in Burma (1969-1973)
(Note the high incidence of snake bite and considerable number of victims that succumbed)

Year	Incidence	Mortality Rate No.	Mortality Rate Percentage
1969	6823	543	7.96%
1970	7860	637	8.10%
1971	8511	732	8.60%
1972	9978	679	6.80%
1973	9097	845	9.29%

TABLE 3
Age incidence of snake bite in Burma (1969 — 73)

Age Group	Incidence No.	%	Mortality Rate No.	%
0 — 4	526	1.3	6	0.2
5 — 14	5,176	12.5	490	15.2
15 — 24	13,949	33.8	1,299	40.3
25 — 34	9,007	21.8	678	21.0
35 — 44	6,515	15.8	292	9.1
45 — 54	3,551	8.6	286	8.9
55 — 64	1,799	4.4	141	4.4
65 — 74	725	1.8	30	0.9
+	41,248	100.0%	3,222	100.0%

Sex Incidence

Since snake bite is commonest among the age of 15 to 45 who are most active at work and also since it is a hazard to a certain group of people, it is logical to expect that males will dominate females in sex distribution. In fact, snake bite among males is 2 to 3 times higher than among females (Table 4).

TABLE 4
Sex incidence in snake bite cases in Burma (1969 — 73)

Year	1969	1970	1971	1972	1973
Sex	M : F	M : F	M : F	M : F	M : F
Snake bite	2 : 1	3 : 1	2 : 1	2 : 1	2 : 1

Occupational Incidence

It is a well known fact that farmers are the most common victims of snake bite with envenomation. Death rate is also highest among the farmers. They are mostly bitten at work in the paddy fields since the venomous snake (viper) inhabits these lands and paddy fields. Among the snake bite victims with envenomation, farmers top the list (Table 5).

TABLE 5
Occupation of snake bite victims

Occupation	Percentage
Farmers	85%
Others	15%

Seasonal Incidence

Though snake bite is perennial, the incidence varies from month to month. Table 6 shows the seasonal variation of snake bite incidence.

TABLE 6.
Seasonal Incidence of snake bite in Burma (1966 — 68).

Month	Incidence = %	Death = %
January	178 = 5.6	17 = 4.7
February	83 = 2.6	7 = 1.9
March	105 = 3.3	12 = 3.3
April	132 = 4.2	18 = 4.9
May	255 = 8.1	36 = 9.9
June	277 = 8.1	42 = 11.5
July	227 = 7.2	35 = 9.6
August	230 = 7.3	33 = 9.1
September	257 = 8.1	33 = 9.1
October	463 = 14.7	38 = 10.4
November	492 = 15.6	47 = 12.9
December	459 = 14.5	46 = 12.6
Total	3158 = 100	364 = 100

There are two peaks of incidence in a year. The smaller peak occurs in the month of June and the bigger and broader peak covers the months of October, November and December. The first peak coincides with the beginning of the rainy season when farmers start their preparatory field work and paddy planting, while the second peak coincides with paddy harvesting.

Snake Population

The incidence of snake bite can be expected to be highest at the time when snakes are most abundant. The Burma Pharmaceutical Industries purchase all kinds of venomous snakes available throughout the year. Table 7 shows the number of snakes purchased every month.

TABLE 7
Monthly Purchase of Snakes at the B.P.I.
(Average 1 yr.) (1969 — 73).

Month	Viper	Cobra	Krait
January	0.4	1.0	1.8
February	0.2	1.0	1.0
March	0.4	1.2	1.6
April	3.4	2.6	1.4
May	58.2	30.6	11.2
June	655.4	333.0	90.4
July	628.8	856.0	102.0
August	988.2	1,704.0	545.8
September	266.6	874.2	222.4
October	24.0	124.6	31.8
November	0.6	10.4	3.6
December	0.2	5.8	4.2
Total	2,636.4	3,944.4	1,017.2

The table reveals that June, July, August and September are the months during which the largest number of snakes are bought. This demonstrates the easy availability and also population of snakes in these months. The peak months of snake purchase do not coincide with the peaks of incidence of snake bites. Farmers are bitten and develop severe envenomation when they have to work in the paddy fields where snakes are present, though these are not the times when the snakes are most abundant.

Type of Snake Involved

The type of snake most commonly involved is seen in table 8. The table shows that Russell's viper is most commonly responsible for poisonous snake bites. The deaths in the group of unknown snake bites could possibly be due to vipers. If only the patients with severe envenomation or who died are analysed, Russell's viper will be probably responsible for more than 90% of cases. In fact, the snake bite problem in Burma is concerned mainly with *Vipera russelli.*

Regional Incidence of Snake bite

Snake bites are more common in certain parts of the country than others. Table 9 shows the incidence of snake bites in each division. The highest incidence of snake bite and deaths occur in the Sagaing division, followed by Pegu, Mandalay, Magwe, Irrawaddy and Rangoon divisions in descending order. This highlights the acuteness and gravity of the problem of snake bite in these areas.

TABLE 8
The Types of Snakes Involved in Snake bite Incidence
Burma 1966 — 68. (Dr. U Thaung)

Type	Incidence	M.R.
Russell's viper	71.3%	82.2%
Cobra	5.2%	5.5%
Krait	0.2%	0.3%
Sea snake	0.2%	—
Green snake	1.8%	—
Harmless snake	1.96%	—
Unknown's	19.34%	12.0%

TABLE 9.
Regional Incidence of Snake bite in Burma (1969 — 73)

Sr.No.	Division/States	1969	1970	1971	1972	1973
1.	Rangoon	883	794	694	819	739
2.	Sagaing	1469	1237	1509	1998	1590
3.	Mandalay	1052	1217	2091	2309	1793
4.	Magwe	951	1135	1236	1449	1066
5.	Pegu	1137	1619	1390	1596	2223
6.	Mon	249	343	273	377	108
7.	Tenessarim	26	35	24	36	47
8.	Irrawaddy	698	1041	831	996	1040
9.	Arakan	81	95	59	97	59
10.	Chin	20	30	95	61	12
11.	Kachin	50	65	95	60	120
12.	Shan	224	180	119	182	191
13.	Kayah	24	30	—	24	95
14.	karen	41	39	95	72	14
	Grand Total	6805	7860	8511	9976	9097

In fact there are 7 townships where the incidence of snake bite is more than 100 per 100,000 population. These townships are Myinmu, Budalin, Chang-U, Shwebo, Kyauktaga, Zigone and Phyu. (U Thaung, 1974).

According to available figures from the Medical Statistics Department, Rangoon, the incidence and deaths due to envenomation by snake bite, rank among the top ten single leading causes of death in the country.

To summarise from the foregoing figures presented, the total number of snake bites varies from 7000 to 9,000 a year of which the mortality ranges from 543 to 845; farmers of the 15 — 45 year age group are the most common victims; male dominates females by 3:1; the accidents occur in farm lands at the time of rice growing and harvesting; these peak incidences do not coincide with the high seasonal population of snakes. The venomous snake incriminated is almost always Russell's viper. Snake bite is one of the top ten single leading causes of death in Burma. Snake bite is avoidable. It afflicts farmers selectively in their farm lands while at work. So far, no organised preventive measures have been taken. Indeed, it clearly and unquestionably exists as an important national problem since the farmers are the bread-earners of the country.

Clinical Features And Management Of Russell's Viper Bite

The Russell's viper has the most efficient and well developed solenoglyphal apparatus ie. forward canalized mobile long fangs connected with large venom sacs. The viper bite is said to be more efficient than the injection with a hypodermic needle.

Russell's viper bite causes sharp pricking pain with slight burning sensation at the site. Sometimes the victim sees flashes of light and feels giddy. If a person knows that he has been bitten by a snake, venomous or not, he may become panicky and hysterical whereas the effects of envenomation usually take a few hours to manifest. Minimal envenomation produces only mild symptoms and slight local swelling. Local examination reveals two fangs marks of about 1.25 cm apart. The discoloration, blister formation and swelling will appear at the site of bite. In some cases the skin may slough off and form a shallow ulcer at a later date or if bitten on the finger, the digit may become gangrenous. There may be slight oozing of blood but profuse bleeding from the site is most unusual. Even with little or no local signs the victim can have severe systemic envenomation.

In a few hours, if envenomation is severe, the patient may develop haemorrhagic manifestations such as bleeding gums, epistaxis, haemoptysis, haematemesis and haematuria. Orbital oedema with subconjunctival haemorrhages also appear in severe cases. The victim may go into primary shock with obvious clinical features, and he may succumb to primary shock if envenomation is massive and also if adequate treatment is not instituted promptly.

But the usual clinical presentation is that the patient arrives with severe signs and symptoms since the victim reaches hospital about three to six hours after the bite; with initial treatment the condition often improves and the victim usually survives. The patient often complains of burning sensation in the epigastrium and sometimes in the chest. If the clotting time is measured it will be found that blood does not coagulate. Prothrombin time is very much prolonged and plasma fibrinogen level is extremely low. Fibrindex time is also increased. When adequate antivenin therapy has been administered the coagulation time comes back to normal within two to three hours. The platelet count begins to fall from the day after the snake bite and remains low for about a week to ten days. In the meantime, the patient becomes anuric or oliguric, though a fair amount of urine may have been passed on the day of snake bite before renal damage sets in. The urine may show frank haematuria or may be only slightly blood stained. Numerous red blood cells and granular casts are usually seen on direct microscopy of the urine, which forewarns the oncoming renal failure. Though the patient looks well initially, within three or four days he will show all the features of acute renal failure such as anuria, drowsiness, vomiting, hiccup, acidotic breathing (ie. rapid shallow respiration) and occasional convulsions.

On examination the patient now looks really ill and will have bilateral loin tenderness. He develops mild hypertension, the blood pressure ranges from 150/90 to 170/100, probably as a result of toxic nephropathy. In a week to ten days, spontaneous diuresis may develop and the patient may recover from acute renal failure without any long term residual renal dysfunction, or he may show a late haemorrhagic syndrome such as bleeding gums, epistaxis and melaena; later hypotension sets in, the clinical condition turns from bad to worse and the patient dies inspite of all the resuscitative measures. Hyperpyrexia and concurrent infection are often seen in these patients.

The postmortem findings in these patients are usually pituitary haemorrhage and swollen haemorrhagic kidneys. There are haemorrhages in the adrenal glands and other organs such as lungs, liver, stomach and other parts of gastrointestinal tract but they are never so severe or striking as in the pituitary gland or in the kidneys. The histology of kidney shows severe acute tubular necrosis and epithelial disintegration with widespread focal haemorrhages. The glomeruli and tubular basement membrane are usually intact.

This is the composite clinical picture reconstructed and compiled from personal experience obtained from managing 905 snake bite patients. Of course every individual patient may not manifest all these features described above.

Investigation

The investigation of snake bite is not for diagnosis but for assessment of severity of envenomation and progress of its sequela.

With severe envenomation the patient will look ill and show clinical features of serious envenomation as described above. At present there is no test to measure the amount of envenomation and the degree of poisoning in the victim. A technique that can simply measure the concentration of circulating plasma venom will be most useful.

In cases of significant envenomation, the clotting defect will appear within a few hours. If a patient comes immediately after the snake bite the blood clotting time will still be normal as clotting defect does not appear so fast. In such circumstances if clotting test is not repeated the medical officer can miss the case of severe envenomation until late. In such situation the doctor tends to be complacent and treat the patient less energetically. Therefore blood clotting time must be measured hourly for about six hours. If there is no coagulation defect discovered during that period then one can safely assume that either the offending snake is not Russell's viper or even if it is, there is no significant envenomation. Though the clotting test appears to be crude, it has the simplicity of being a bedside procedure and at once gives the information needed so urgently. The clotting time test tubes should then be placed in a rack for clot quality observation as serum will separate from cellular mass in an hour or two. The size and quality of the clot should be noted. The clot quality observation can only serve as a confirmatory test of coagulation process as serum separates slowly from the cells. Occasionally, a small flimsy clot formed initially would later disappear; this phenomenon perhaps represents fibrinoytic activity of the envenomed serum.

If facilities are available, prothrombin time, partial thromboplastin time, fibrindex time and fibrinogen level should be measured. These tests will show prolongation of the respective times and low fibrinogen level when blood is incoagulable. These levels returned to normal after an adequate dose of antivenin was given. These elaborate tests may be a little more sensitive than the simple clotting time measurement. But the facilities are not easy to acquire at remote rural places. The bleeding time measurement is rather painful particularly for repeated tests and also not more informative. The platelet count will gradually fall and remain thrombocytopoenic for about ten days to a fortnight. Very low platelet count may cause spontaneous secondary haemorrhage particularly where capillaries and small arterioles are partially damaged due to toxin, and the situation is aggravated by coexisting renal hypertension. There does not appear to be any real evidence of intravascular haemolysis though no specific searching investigation has been made in this study. Perhaps simple red cells fragility test may be useful. Even a mild clinical jaundice was rarely observed in these patients in the course of illness following snake bite.

Urine is routinely examined for haematuria, granular cast and albuminuria which reflect tubular necrosis and renal damage. The test for urobilinogen is usually negative even at the later phase of the illness. The daily urine output must be recorded accurately. A good urine output on the day of snake bite does not preclude incipient acute renal failure, as a large portion of urine might have been excreted prior to the onset of renal damage.

The urea and electrolytes estimation of blood and urine should be done daily. The U/P ratio is a good index of estimating renal function. The rising blood urea, low U/P ratio and decreasing urine output indicate onset of acute renal failure. After an effective Russell's viper bite resulting in severe envenomation, acute renal failure is very common; in fact it may be stated that if envenomation is severe there will be renal damage, and acute renal failure is certain to follow. It must be expected and prepared for. A good experience in acute renal failure treatment is really an advantage in the management of snake bite syndrome.

Treatment (as practised in Burma)

The treatment of snake bite patient may be divided into first aid treatment, rural health centre (RHC) treatment and hospital treatment.

The First Aid Treatment

This is an immediate treatment done by the patient himself or by someone nearby, often described and recommended in standard books for snake bite accident. Application of a tourniquet well above the site of bite just enough to impede venous return to prevent absorption, cleansing of the site with any available liquid or water, or wiping out the area with a piece of cloth are important first aid measures as these remove venom from the surface. Lancing the site and applying suction by means of a tube or a vacuum bottle are probably beneficial if done immediately. Direct suction using the mouth is not advisable as it is dangerous to the performer. Surgical excision of the site or amputation of the digit are too drastic and probably not necessary in view of the fact that about 80% of the victims in general are bitten by non-poisonous snakes, or in cases of poisonous snakes, no significant envenomation occurred. Perhaps the most important first aid treatment is to keep the part absolutely at rest; the person should not walk if he has been bitten on the leg. In most cases they are, and the victim should be carried to a nearby health centre or to a hospital. Delayed first aid treatment is valueless and adds injury to the site.

The Rural Health Centre Treatment

The health assistant or the nurse is the first health personnel whom the victim will likely meet for medical assistance. The health personnel should examine the site of bite for fang marks and local swellings. The blood pressure is recorded and the type of snake should, if possible, be identified. If it is a poisonous snake (in most cases it is Russell's viper), specific antivenin must be given. If the snake is not available and it is not known whether it is poisonous or not, then 20 ml of antiviper serum should be given if the accident occurred in the paddy field or along village tracks known to be infested with vipers. To dispel fear, the patient must be given a lot of reassurance. The patient must be referred immediately to the nearest hospital for further investigation and treatment. The patient must be sent along with a referral note containing information such as the time of bite, the site of bite, the fang marks, the place of accident, the type of snake (if known), the first aid measures done or not, the clinical findings and the treatment given at the particular time. If the offending (killed) snake was brought along, it must be sent for proper identification.

The Hospital Treatment

The snake bite victim usually arrives at the hospital a few hours after the accident. The medical officer should examine the patient immediately and assess the severity of envenomation. The clotting time should be measured at once. Usually the patient is found to be rather restless and frightened. But if there is no evidence of envenomation, placebo therapy, reassurance and moral encouragement would suffice. No antivenin therapy is needed and it should not be given indiscriminately. Locally, no special treatment is necessary. However, if the snake is definitely known to be Russell's viper and fang marks are evident, even in the absence of clinical signs, 20 ml of antivenin should be given as it cannot be harmful.

If the patient is found to have significant envenomation, 40 ml of antivenin is given intravenously as an initial dose after a test of hypersensitivity reaction. Then 20 ml of antivenin is administered by intravenous infusion. No antivenin was given locally in this study though its value cannot be denied especially if given soon after the bite. On an average, 60 ml of antivenin is sufficient though up to 160 ml had been given in few cases. If a patient comes in a state of shock, resuscitative treatment must be given promptly and energetically. Blood transfusion may be required in addition to other fluid therapy. Administration of high dose of cortisone appears to be beneficial. Antihistamine should be given and repeated if necessary to avoid allergic reaction and moreover it is believed that some manifestations in snake bite are probably due to histamine release.

In serious envenomation there will be renal damage as circulating venom is concentrated in the tubules, therefore it is considered appropriate to give diuretics such as mannitol or frusemide parenterally to promote immediate diuresis. The diuretic therapy will promote renal excretion, and dilute the venom concentration in the kidney thereby lessening the degree of damage. An initial good diuretic response to mannitol therapy, of course, does not necessarily prevent renal damage and preclude the onset of acute renal failure but hopefully reduces the severity of renal lesion. Therefore, a close watch on the daily urine output is essential. In fact, intravenous mannitol should be given everyday successively for two or three days as immediate initial response to diuretic therapy is often found to be good in a majority of patients and only one or two days later, the kidneys begin to pack up and fail to respond to diuretic therapy. In other words, if the urine output remains good even on the third or fourth day, it is very unlikely that the kidneys suffered any significant damage. Like antivenin therapy, the administration of diuretics cannot correct renal damage already sustained prior to treatment. It is believed that diuretic therapy reduces the severity of renal damage. The interval between the time of bite and the time of adequate antivenin therapy is of vital importance. It is logical that the larger the amount of venom injected and the longer the interval between the bite and antivenin therapy, the greater the organ damage and the worse the prognosis.

After initial antivenin therapy measurement of clotting time must be repeated hourly and if blood fails to clot two hours after initial therapy, another dose of 20 ml should be given. This regime should be carried on until clotting time returns to normal. It is a practical fact found by clinical experience that soon after neutralization of the venom. The coagulation defect disappears and the clotting process returns to normal. Once the clotting time has returned to normal it does not become abnormal again. It cannot be overstressed that though specific antivenin therapy is the mainstay of treatment, the therapeutic endeavour, indeed, should not end there. The damage already sustained by envenomation will certainly progress into a serious disease and manifest as a syndrome. It needs proper assessment and careful management throughout the course of illness.

As said above, the patient who survived serious envenomation may develop acute renal failure and other sequelae. Acute renal failure is a serious complication which demands early peritoneal dialysis and careful management. In this study 75 percent of patients with acute renal failure needed peritoneal dialysis.

Quite often these patients developed mild hypertension probably of renal origin. It is perhaps due to sustained release of renal angiotensin from the ischaemic kidney and also as a result of capsular constriction of swollen haemorrhagic kidneys. It is felt that high blood pressure should be treated with appropriate antihypertensive drugs to lower the blood pressure as it may induce spontaneous haemorrhages in various organs as the capillaries are already damaged by the venom. Antibiotics may be required to combat any infection. Sometimes high fever with delirium needs attention, and this hyperpyrexia appears to have grave prognostic significance. Its presence is viewed with great concern.

As regards hydrocortisone therapy, there is a feeling that cortisone therapy saved some of the patients and it was liberally given in massive doses in this study. It is regarded unethical to withhold the drug from these patients since post-mortem findings of pituitary and adrenal haemorrhages are so constant. The clinical picture of shock in snake bite victims appears somewhat similar to pituitary-adrenal crisis of other aetiology. Therefore, hydrocortisone therapy seems to be highly desirable. In fact, quite often, death is preceded by apoplectic hypotension with haemorrhagic manifestations. Massive doses of hydro-cortisone therapy appears to have a definite place in such a situation. The damaged capillaries of the organs with dangerously low platelet count, preconditions spontaneous haemorrhage and this catastrophe may be precipitated and aggravated by hypertension.

Knowing heparin's action of antithrombin like property, it can be expected to counteract the coagulant action of Russell's viper venom. It is also known experimentally that heparin prolongs the survival time of an animal after Russell's viper venom injection. Intravascular coagulation and widespread thrombosis as evidenced by consumption coagulopathy and progressive thrombocytopoenia, could possibly be prevented by early administration of heparin together with an adequate dose of specific antivenin. This is an attractive idea in theory, but in actual practice the happy marriage of an adequate dose of antivenin with heparin therapy is less easy. Firstly, with the present available method, an adequate dose of antivenin cannot be defined at the commencement of treatment since the injected amount of venom is always unknown. Secondly, the return of coagulation time marks the point of venom-antivenom neutralization, thereby representing the required dose of antivenin. By definition this is an adequate dose. In a similar manner the effectiveness and adequacy of heparin therapy is measured by prolongation of same coagulation time. Exactly the same method of measurement utilized for counter purposes is the real state of situation, in other words the parameter of the adequacy of one form of therapy is just the opposite of the others. In addition, heparin therapy has its own risks and complications; these may aggravate the already complicated haemorrhagic phenomenon of viper envenomation. Since these problems could not be overcome, heparin therapy was tried out only in few cases, before being discontinued because of the complications and its inherent difficulties.

Results

During the ten-year period from 1970 to 1979 a total of 905 snake bite patients were treated at the Insein Hospital, Rangoon. Among the 905 patients, 434 victims were bitten by Russell's viper. There were 151 deaths in the total of 905 snake bite victims, therefore, an average mortality rate of 16.7 percent; however among the Russell's viper bite the mortality rate is 33.41 percent. Russell's viper is responsible for 145 of the 151 deaths which account for 96%. Unlike other types of venomous snakes, Russell' s viper is effective, ie. the bite does inject venom and produce envenomation in 70 percent of the bites. In Burma, Russell's viper is responsible for 84.43 percent of venomous snake bites.

RESULTS OF SNAKE BITES (1970 — 79)

Non-Poisonous Snake Bites	391	43.20%
Poisonous Snake Bites	514	56.80%
(R.Viper Bites)	434	84.43%
(Other P.S. Bites)	80	15.56%
Total no. of Snake Bites	905	100.0%

FATAL CASES OF SNAKE BITE (1970 — 79)

Total No. of Snake Bites	905	
Total No. of Deaths	151	16.7%
R. Viper Bites Alone	145	96.0%
Common Cobra Bites	6	4.0%
R. Viper Bites Only (145 in 434)	—	33.41%

Among the victims mostly affected were farmers of 15 to 45 years age group, predominantly men. They are usually bitten on the legs, quite often below the ankle and the accidents happen in the paddy field while they are at work. Snake bite is seasonal though it occurs all year round; a majority of accidents happening at the beginning of the southwest monsoon when farmers start to prepare the ground for cultivation and during the months of paddy harvest ie. December — January.

Death can occur in the victims anytime after snake bite. But an analysis of 54 fatal cases in 1976 revealed that a large majority ie. about 80% of patients died within the first week though few patients survived for about a month and later died suddenly. Death within first 24 — 48 hours is certainly due to direct effects of severe envenomation. It is also true that up to the fourth day, the victims died directly as a result of envenomation or its delayed effect. But the victims who died after one week should be regarded as cases of complications, the most significant ones being acute renal failure, and late pituitary failure which often comes after the patient has recovered from acute renal failure.

In this study of 151 fatal cases, 27% died within 24 to 48 hours, 43% within first four days, 67% within a week and 33% after one week, out of which eleven patients survived for 20 to 51 days and died later.

Discussion

If there is a time interval between snake bite and neutralization of venom, there will be tissue destruction, the severity depending on the amount of venom and the duration of interval. Damage to the organs and tissues will progress gradually. This process is inevitable and cannot be stopped since there has been tissue destruction. The resuscitative measures will bring back the severely shocked patient to initial recovery. The specific antivenin therapy can neutralize only the free circulating venom and prevent further toxic action but understandably has no power to undo the damage already sustained.

Snake bite usually happens in the remote paddy fields and at the village tracks where immediate medical facilities are not available. If Russell's viper bite occurs, it is highly possible that there will be envenomation since venom delivery apparatus is so highly developed and the serpent bites the victim with tenacity. If envenomation occurs, there will be a time lapse between the bite and specific antivenin therapy, as immediate treatment is almost impossible. Therefore, if there is a snake bite patient admitted to the hospital, the victim usually presents a snake bite syndrome of varying severity. The medical personnel has to be prepared to meet this challenge and treat them accordingly.

Snake bite is preventable. There are suggested measures of prevention, such as wearing boots and gloves but these cannot be practiced easily for various reasons. Therefore prevention is still not successful. Eradication of the snakes is not practical; man has to coexist with them. Immunization against snake venom is a possible method but it is doubtful whether this prophylaxis will be practically effective. Immediate medical attention is easier said than done. Transport of unfortunate victims to the hospital is usually delayed as communication and transportation in rural areas is always difficult.

At present doctors have to be trained and they have to concentrate their effort on treating victims of snake bite. Although the snake bite syndrome is well defined, the basic mechanisms of venom action is far from complete. The investigation and assessment of severity of envenomation, the estimation of the dose of antivenin required, the prevention and treatment of complications such as acute renal failure and pituitary haemorrhage are still unsatisfactory. Why is there massive haemorrhage in the pituitary gland when the rest of the brain is almost unaffected? Is pituitary haemorrhage due to its peculiar arrangement of portal circulation of the organ? The mechanism of pituitary haemorrhage is still unknown and needs further study.

Green Pit Viper Bites

Green pit vipers belong to the genus *Trimeresurus* and are classified under the family Crotalidae. Like Russell's vipers, they have mobile canalized forward fangs (Solenoglypha) but are more akin to the Malayan pit viper *(Agkistrodon rhodostoma)*. Though the venom of the Green Snake is toxic it is not lethal. It produces coagulation defects in man as a result of hypofibrinogenaemia and thrombocytopoenia due to consumption coagulopathy. The coagulation defect often lasts for about a week despite the patient's feeling of being fit and well, and moreover there are no other significant systemic manifestations. Antivenin prepared with R. viper venom, has no effect and cannot neutralize or bring back the coagulation time. The local swelling at the site of bite lasts for a few days. There is no specific treatment and nothing needs to be done to the patient.

The clinical features and symptomatology of a case of Green Snake bite is illustrated here.

Saw T.T., a 40-year-old Burmese male was bitten by a Green Snake at about 8 pm. He was admitted to the hospital the next day, though he was feeling perfectly well. On admission his blood was found to be incoagulable and bleeding time was prolonged. Forty ml of antivenin (for R. viper) was given but there was no effect. A hundred ml of EACA (E-amino-caproic acid) and 100 ml of fibrinogen were given and again a bottle of EACA was administered the next day without any effect on the blood coagulation system. The coagulation defect lasted for 12 days without any untoward symptom. During the period, plasma fibrinogen levels and thrombocyte counts were very low. When their levels rose, the clotting time returned to normal.

The venom of the Green Snake does not appear to have any other effect except in producing coagulation defect. The only danger is that if the snake bite victim gets injured or needed an urgent operation, then the bleeding will not stop.

In this study of 20 patients bitten by Green Snake, 7 (35%) had signs of envenomation and 13 (65%) showed no clinical features. There was no fatality in this group. Among the 7 patients, 5 were bitten on lower extremities, one on the hand and another over the head. All had local swelling at the site of bite but no one had necrosis of ulceration.

Bites By Elapids

Common cobra (Naja naja), King cobra (Naja hannah) and Banded krait (Bungarus fasciatus) belong to the family of Elapidae. The venoms are usually neurotoxic and the site of action is peripheral ie. at the neuromuscular junction. It produces paralysis of motor muscles, preferentially muscles of deglutition and respiration. The cause of death is respiratory failure and death often occurs immediately. Specific antivenin therapy is the ideal treatment but in the author's experience, a cholinergic drug such as prostigmine, is found to be helpful and should be given since the depressant action of the venom at the neuromuscular junction is counteracted by the drug. Other measures, such as artificial respiration and tracheostomy may be required and it could be life saving.

Common Cobra

In the present study there were 25 cobra bites, of which only 8 (32%) victims showed signs of envenomation and 17 (68%) patients were asymptomatic. There was one fatality (4%) of the total number of cases or 12.5% of envenomed patients only. Among the 8 envenomed cases, 6 were bitten on the fingers, one on the foot and another on the thigh. Local swelling was present in all patients and severe necrosis which resulted in sloughing and ulceration was found in two patients.

Case history of a cobra bite:

Maung T.M., a 20-year old male was admitted to Insein Hospital within one hour of being bitten by a cobra on the inner side of thigh. In fact he was bitten while squatting to urinate in the field. On admission there was a black patch and gross swelling at the site of bite. Polyvalent serum, containing anti-viper-anti-cobra, was given intravenously on admission. On the next day the eye lids drooped and he developed signs of respiratory paralysis which demanded immediate tracheostomy and artificial respiration. He was again given antiserum with atropine and prostigmine with good response. The drugs were repeated as their actions had been only short lasting. The development of respiratory paralysis after an apparent recovery may indicate that there was a depot of venom at the site of bite from which it was absorbed slowly. This assumption may call for local infiltration. Locally there was extensive necrosis and ulceration requiring skin grafting at a later date.

King Cobra

King cobra bite is very rare and it is mostly a risk to professional snake charmers. Since the snake is huge and if the bite is effective, the victim has very little chance to survive long enough to get medical treatment. There are no authentic case histories of King Cobra bite. The venom needs a lot of toxinological studies.

Banded Krait

Banded Krait is a very docile snake and it does not bite man except on extreme provocation. The venom is neurotoxic. There were 5 patients in this study, which is less than 1% of the total snake bite patients. Among them only one had signs of envenomation.

Case history:

U.S.N. a 54-year-old male was bitten by a krait on his finger while he was holding the snake and trying to bite off its tail. Since the krait's tail is tough and stumpy he could not do it easily. Then with full intention he bit it hard and forcefully and while doing so the snake wriggled and slipped off his hand and bit his finger. He arrived at Insein hospital at about 10 pm, 1½ hours after the bite. On admission he was all right. However a polyvalent antiserum was given. Later he developed signs of respiratory paralysis. Lastly the respiratory movements were mainly of abdominal type. His mental state was clear and he understood the conversation though he could not speak. Tracheostomy was performed and he was on artificial respiration. Though polyvalent antiserum was given, the antivenin did not contain specific anti-krait antibodies. Prostigmine was not given in this case although it was felt that it might be helpful as in the case of cobra bite. He made a gradual recovery though he had dysphagia for some time.

Review of Research

Snake bite is a public health problem of great magnitude in Burma. It is in fact a national problem as it affects the farmers in a country with an agriculture based economy. About 10,000 snake bites occur and 1,000 lives are lost each year. The incidence and the mortality rate from snake bite have not declined appreciably in the last two decades. It still remains among the top ten single leading cause of mortality in the country.

Apparently, preventive measures against snake bites and public health education do not seem to be very effective as some of the measures suggested are not practical in the field, and also the cultural belief and the way of life among the farmers interfere with compliance of the protective measures against snake bite.

The Directorate of Medical Research Institute (DMRI) is doing research in snake bite on various aspects of the problem such as clinical, pathological and therapeutical. The progress has been made in collecting and analyzing the clinical data scientifically. The basic foundation of clinical research was done by the author (Aye, M.M., 1976).

DMRI Working Group had recently published the results of Active Immunization with venoid on human volunteers. It was concluded that the results were encouraging although some practical problems still exist in the field.

It is hopeful that in the near future, the incidence, morbidity and mortality from snake bite will be reduced by protective measures through public health education, prophylaxis by active immunization and prompt and adequate treatment of the envenomed victims with specific antivenom and the specialized management of the complications of snake bite patients.

Anti Snake Venom Serum
Cobra Only
(Purified Globulins)

Anti snake venom serum is a sterile solution of the specific antitoxic substances prepared from the serum or plasma of suitable animals immunised with the venoms obtained from Cobra *(Naja naja)* snakes.

One ampoule contains 10 ml antiserum which neutralises 10 mg of dried cobra venom.

It contains 0.15% para-chloro-meta-cresol as preservative.

For details of treatment and contraindications please see DIRECTIONS for use.

PRESENTATION:-

Boxes of 10 x 10 ml ampoules
STORE IN A DARK COOL PLACE
(Preferably at + 4° to 10°C temperature)
Manufactured in Burma
by
The Burma Pharmaceutical Industry,
Rangoon.

Anti Snake Venom Serum
Viper Only
(Purified Globulins)

Anti snake venom serum is a sterile solution of the specific antitoxic substances prepared from the serum or plasma of suitable animals immunised with the venoms obtained from viper *(Vipera russelli)* snakes.

One ampoule contains 10 ml antiserum which neutralises 20 mg of dried viper venom.

It contains 0.15% para-chloro-meta-cresol as preservative.

For details of treatment and contraindications please see DIRECTIONS for use.

Presentation:-

Boxes of 10 x 10 ml ampoules
Box of 1 x 10 ml ampoule or vial
STORE IN A DARK COOL PLACE
(Preferably at 4° to 10° C)
Manufactured in Burma
by
The Burma Pharmaceutical Industry,
Rangoon.

General

The three common species of snakes in Burma whose bites can be fatal to human are Cobra, the Krait and the Russell's viper. The symptoms of poisoning observed in human beings are as followed:-

1. **Cobra and Krait** — The venoms of cobra and Krait are neurotoxic and acts on the nervous system. There is pain at the site of bite which radiates along the limbs which is soon followed by numbness and weakness of muscles. The paralysis is ushered in by weakness of the limbs associated with staggering. The speech is slurred at this stage. The early symptoms of cobra and Krait bite closely resemble those of drunkenness. Later there may be ptosis, dribbling of saliva, dropping of the head, difficulty in swallowing, etc., as more muscles become paralysed. There may be giddiness and collapse with difficult breathing and cyanosis. Krait poisoning is characterised by intense pain in the abdomen in addition to the above symptoms.

2. **Russell's Viper** — The venom of viper is haemorrhagic and there is intense burning pain at the site of bite. There is marked swelling which may rapidly spread over the whole limb with ecchymosis. There may be bleeding from the fang wounds. The pulse is usually small and thready and the blood pressure low. There may be nausea and vomiting and collapse with the pupils dilated and insensitive to light. Spontaneous subcutaneous and submucous haemorrhages are common. Death as a rule is due to circulatory failure. Severe gangrene may supervene at the site of bite if the patient survives.

Treatment

First Aid — Main objective is to prevent the spread of toxin through the circulation and therefore tourniquet should be applied to prevent the venous flow towards the heart. If on the leg, apply the tourniquet on the thigh and if on the wrist or forearm, on the arm. To prevent gangrene it should be released after every half an hour for a minute or so and reapplied. This should be repeated until antivenom is available.

To reduce the concentration of venom, linear incisions should be made over the fang marks and bleeding encouraged.

The wound can be washed with a weak solution of potassium permanganate or even water to wash away the excess of venom. Crystals of potassium permanganate should not be used.

In cases of viperine bites it is advisable to infiltrate the surrounding area with antivenin; this will neutralise the excess venom locally and prevent necrotic change of the area.

Specific Serum Therapy — The antivenin is concentrated from the serum of horses immunized against the venoms of Cobra and Russell's viper. The antivenin should be administered immediately or as early as possible. 5 — 10 ml of the antivenin should be infiltrated into the tissues surrounding the bite either intramuscularly or subcutaneously. In case of severe toxic symptoms it can be given intravenously but very slowly with all the precautions that should be taken for intravenous serum therapy. If the symptoms are not severe the i.m. or s.c. injection should be undertaken. The dose recommended for concentrated serum by the i.v. route is 20 — 30 ml depending upon the severity of the symptoms and can be repeated every four hours if the symptoms persist.

If antivenin is given intramuscularly or subcutaneously the dosage should be increased by 2 or 3 times to that of the intravenous route.

If any allergic reactions are noted during injection, treatment must be discontinued and the injection of 1/1000 solution of Adrenalin be given immediately, and continue giving treatment for shock.

If the allergic reactions are neither subduced nor reduced by the Adrenalin or should either haematuria or anuria occur, either Hydrocortisone Sodium Succinate 100 mg or Beta-Methasone 1 mg should be given intravenously.

Reconstitution of Freeze-dried Serum

1. Draw 10 c.c. of distilled water, provided, in a sterile syringe.
2. Cut along the etched line of freeze-dried antivenom ampoule and break the neck.
3. Transfer distilled water from the syringe into freeze-dried antivenom ampoule.
4. Cover the opening of the ampoule with sterilized pad provided, gauze surface downwards, press it down with the thumb. Shake it vigorously for about one minute.
5. Let the ampoule stand for one minute. The reconstituted serum will then be clear and ready for injection. Froth and undissolved particles, if any, should be left in the ampoule, for which excess serum has been added.
6. For subsequent injections add 10 c.c. of distilled water into serum ampoule and rotate it between the palms of your hands until serum is fully dissolved and let the ampoule stand to clear.

Prevention of Snake Bite

In snake bite prevention the following methods should be considered.

1. Reduction and eradication of poisonous snakes
2. Prevention and protection from snake bite
3. Early treatment if accident happens

Reduction and Eradication

The aim should be set for an eradication of venomous snakes particularly the most common offender, the Russell's viper. From the knowledge of its natural habit and behaviour the vipers are most likely to be found in the paddy fields and the bushy area not far away from ponds and wet lands where rats and frogs dwell. Paddy fields are the Russell's viper's hunting ground for rats which competes with men in collection of grains. Terrestrial snakes like vipers dwell in the holes and crevices of the ground and also in bushy places. They come to the surface with the rains and floods; that is why professional snake catchers catch them in abundance during the early months of the rainy season ie. June, July and August though the snakes could be found all year round in their habitat.

The Burma Pharmaceutical Industry (B.P.I.) purchases poisonous snakes for venom extraction and by doing so it also aims to reduce the snake population although there has been no observable reduction in this population so far. Each year about 3000 vipers, 4000 cobras and 1000 kraits are bought. Although a few subcentres have been opened in lower Burma for the purchase of snakes in 1976, a large snake-aquarium should be built for venom extraction in upper Burma as well and in fact, a number of purchase centres should also be opened. B.P.I. has been exporting snakes through Myanma Export Import Corporation. All these marketing and exports should be encouraged.

Organised snake-hunts and round-ups by public could also be practiced at the beginning of the rainy season and just before harvesting, with due precaution against accidents. If competitions could be held and prizes given for the largest number, the biggest size and longest length of the snakes caught during these round-ups, then people will participate more eagerly in these activities. This sport, like any other sport is, of course, not without risk. Medical teams and Red Cross men must be in attendance for necessary assistance during these round-ups.

Many people eat snake meat; viper meat is said to be very tender and delicious. Such habit should be promoted. By doing so people will have more protein in their diet and at the same time the number of snakes will go down in that locality. A note of warning should be issued for indiscriminate killing of non-poisonous snakes since harmless snakes are useful to mankind in maintaining the ecology particularly against rats and other pests. In fact, indiscriminate killing, merchandizing of the snake skin, encroachment of human habitation and deforestation may result in some of the species of non-poisonous snakes approaching the danger of extinction.

Prevention of Snake bite

If the population of snakes can be effectively reduced, logically the incidence of snake bites will go down. In a similar manner, if people can avoid the snake-infested area there will be less accidents. But the farmers understandably cannot avoid the paddy fields though they are well aware that such land is the natural habitat of Russell's vipers. But the mere recognition of the risk of snake bite in the paddy field itself is a step towards precaution. It is known that in more than 80 percent of viper bites, the bite is on the foot and around the ankle. In the rest of the cases, fingers are the common sites. This means that if the feet and the hands are protected, the degree of envenomation will be greatly reduced. Therefore suitable foot-wear and gloves should be provided and it should be made compulsory for everyone to use them to cover their hands and feet when they go out to work in the fields. The foot-wear and gloves must be practical and appropriate for the field work. The superstition that the spirits do not like foot-wear in the fields has to be dispelled by education. Since the snakes are mostly nocturnal in habit, people should avoid as far as possible walking or working in late hours and at night in the paddy fields. The habit, behaviour and method of preying of the snakes as well as the precautionary measures should be taught to the farmers and to the people who are at risk.

It will be a great achievement if active immunization against venomous snakes especially against *Vipera russelli* could be carried out. At present the risks and side effects of active immunization are still formidable; moreover the immunity so obtained is only short-lasting. The process of detoxifying the venom also seems to destroy the antigenicity. Since Russell's viper venom contains a number of enzymes as well as complex antigens, the technique of safe and effective active immunization is still at its infancy. It is hoped that the method could be practical in the future with advancement of new biotechnological methods.

Early Treatment

No matter what measures are taken, anything short of eradication of snakes, which is not achievable, would still leave man confronting the venomous snake and thus the problem of snake bite will continue to exist. If a person has been bitten by a poisonous snake, treatment must be instituted immediately. First aid measures applied on the spot and the specific antivenin therapy adequately and promptly given at the earliest possible moment will minimize the degree of envenomation, and reduce the morbidity and mortality rate of snake bite. First aid measures should be taught to every villager.

The snake bite patient must be referred to hospital for necessary further treatment. No snake bite case should be treated as an outpatient. When it is definitely known that the offending snake is not poisonous or no envenomation has in fact occurred during the observation period, then only should the patient be discharged from hospital.

References

Aye, M.M. (1972). Some experience in management of snake bite. Bur. Med. Journal 20, 33-40.

Aye, M.M. (1976). "Snakes of Burma with Venomology and Envenomation". M.Sc. thesis submitted to Rangoon University.

Aye, M.M. (1978). Acute Renal Failure in Snake Bite (unpublished) — A paper presented at the 25th Burma Medical Conference, Rangoon, Burma.

Burma, DMR Working Group (1986). Human Immunization with venoid. Trans. of the Roy. Soc. of Trop. Med. and Hyg. 80, 423-425.

Biggs, R and Macfarlane, R.G. (1962). Human Blood Coagulation and its Disorders. Blackwell Scientific Publications, Oxford.

Boulenger, G.A. (1921). Vertebrate Fauna of the Malay Peninsula. Reptilia and Batrachia. First Edition, London : Taylor Francis, Ltd.

Deraniyagala, P.E.P. (1955). A coloured Atlas of some vertebrates from Ceylon, Vol III Serpentoid Reptilia, Ceylon : Government Press.

Ditmars, R.L. (1968). Snakes of the World, Seventeeth Printing New York : The Macmillan Company.

Gharpurey, K.G. (1962). Snakes of India and Pakistan. Fifth Edition. Bombay : Popular Prakashan.

Henriques, S.B. and Henriques, O.B. (1971). Pharmacology and Toxicology of Snake Venoms. Pergamon Press, Oxford.

Mason, Rev. F. (1882). Burma, Its People and Production. Vol. 1, Geology, mineralogy and zoology. First Edition, Hertford : Stephen Austin and Sons.

Master, R.W.P. and Rao, S.S. (1961). Identification of Enzymes and Toxins in venoms of Indian cobra and Russell's viper after starch gel electrophoresis. J. Bio. Chem., 236:1986.

Reid, H.A. (1956). Sea Snake Bites. Brit. Med. J. 2, 73-78.

Smith, M.A. (1962). Monograph of Sea Snakes (Hydrophiidae). First Edition — London: Taylor and Francis, Ltd.

Smith, M.A. (1943). The Fauna of British India, Ceylon and Burma, Reptilia and Amphibia Vol. III Serpentes London : Taylor and Francis, Ltd.

Stidworthy, J. (1969). Snakes of the World. London : The Hamlyn Publishing Group Ltd.

Tun-Pe, D.A. Warrell, Tin-Nu-Swe, et al (1987) "Acute and Chronic Pituitary Failure Resembling Sheehan's Syndrome Following Bite by Russell's Viper in Burma". The Lancet (1987). 763- 767.

Venomous Snakes of China

Ermi Zhao

(Chengdu Institute of Biology, Academia Sinica, Chengdu, PRC)

There are two hundred snake species known from China belonging to 62 genera and 8 families (table 1). Among them, 57 species, possessing fangs and poisonous glands, are venomous snakes:-

TABLE 1
Snakes of China.

Family	Number of Genera	Number of Species
Typhlopidae	2	4
Acrochordidae	1	1
Xenopeltidae	1	2
Anilidae	1	1
Boidae	2	3
Colubridae	37	144
Elapidae	13	24
Viperidae	5	21
Total 8	62	200

Solenoglypha — Family Viperidae

 Agkistrodon blomhoffii (Boie, 1826)
 A. intermedius (Strauch, 1868)
 A. monticola (Werner, 1922)
 A. saxatilis Emelianov, 1937
 A. shedaoensis Zhao, 1979
 A. strauchii (Bedriaga, 1912)
 A. ussuriensis Emelianov, 1929
 Azemiops feae Boulenger, 1888
 Deinagkistrodon acutus (Günther, 1888)
 Trimeresurus albolabris (Gray, 1842)
 T. gracilis Oshima, 1920
 T. jerdonii Günther, 1875
 T. medoensis Zhao, 1977
 T. monticola Günther, 1864
 T. mucrosquamatus (Cantor, 1839)
 T. stejnegeri Schmidt, 1925

T. tibetanus Huang, 1982
T. xiangchengensis Zhao, 1979
Vipera berus (Linnaeus, 1758)
V. russelli (Shaw and Nodder, 1797)
V. ursinii (Bonaparte, 1835)

Proteroglypha — Family Elapidae

Acalyptophis peronii (Duméril, 1853)
Bungarus fasciatus (Schneider, 1801)
B. lividus Cantor, 1839
B. multicinctus Blyth, 1860
B. niger Wall, 1908
Calliophis kelloggi (Pope, 1928)
C. macclellandi (Reinhardt, 1844)
C. sauteri (Steindachner, 1913)
Emydocephalus ijimae Stejneger, 1898
Hydrophis caerulescens (Shaw, 1802)
H. cyanocinctus Daudin, 1803
H. fasciatus (Schneider, 1799)
H. melanocephalus Gray, 1849
H. ornatus (Gray, 1842)
Kerilia jerdonii Gray, 1849
Lapemis hardwickii Gray, 1835
Laticauda colubrina (Schneider, 1799)
L. laticaudata (Linnaeus, 1758)
L. semifasciata (Reinwardt, 1837)
Microcephalophis gracilis (Shaw, 1802)
Naja naja (Linnaeus, 1758)
Ophiophagus hannah (Cantor, 1836)
Pelamis platurus (Linnaeus, 1766)
Praescutata viperina (Schmidt, 1852)

Opisthoglypha — Family Colubridae

Boiga cyanea (Duméril, Bibron, and Duméril, 1854)
B. kraepelini Stejneger, 1902
B. multomaculata (Reinwardt, 1827)
B. nigriceps (Günther, 1863)
Chrysopelea ornata (Shaw, 1802)
Dryophis prasinus Reinwardt, 1827
Enhydris bennettii (Gray, 1842)
E. chinensis (Gray, 1842)
E. enhydris (Schneider, 1799)
E. plumbea (Boie, 1827)
Psammodynastes pulverulentus (Boie, 1827)
Psammophis lineolatus (Brandt, 1838)

Ecological and Geographic Distribution of Chinese Venomous Snakes

Geographic relations (Fig 1)

In relation to latitudinal distribution, Chinese venomous snakes can be divided into three main groups:

A. Low latitude snakes. Ranges south of latitude 25°N, but can extend more north in eastern coastal region. Belonging to this group are: two *Trimeresurus* species *(albolabris, gracilis)*, *Vipera russelli*, three *Bungarus* species *(fasciatus, lividus, niger)*, *Calliophis sauteri*, *Ophiophagus hannah*, three *Boiga* species *(cyanea, multomaculata, nigriceps)*, *Chrysopelea ornata*, *Dryophis prasinus*, two *Enhydris* species *(bennetti, enhydris)* and *Psammodynastes pulverulentus*. *Ophiophagus hannah* has also been found in Yaluzangbo Valley, Xizang (Tibet) at a latitude about 29°N and in Anning River Valley, Sichuan at 27°N.

B. Moderate latitude snakes. It ranges between latitude 25°N and around 35°N. The typical moderate latitude snake is *Deinagkistrodon acutus*, although there was a record from Chapa, northern Vietnam. Two *Agkistrodon* species *(monticola* and *strauchii)* and three *Trimeresurus* species *(medoensis, tibetanus* and *xiangchengensis)* have also been found in this zone only.

C. High latitude snakes. It ranges north of around 35°N. Most *Agkistrodon* species *(intermedius, saxatilis, shedaoensis* and *ussuriensis)*, two northern species of *Vipera (berus* and *ursinii)* and *Psammophis lineolatus* belong to this group.

Ten species overlap the low and moderate zones. They are two *Trimeresurus* species *(monticola* and *mucrosquamatus)*, two *Calliophis* species *(kelloggi* and *macclellandi)*, two *Enhydris* species *(chinensis* and *plumbea)*, *Boiga kraepelini*, *Bungarus multicinctus*, *Naja naja* and *Azemiops feae*. Two species, *Agkistrodon blomhoffii brevicaudus* and *Trimeresurus jerdonii*, overlap the moderate and high zones. *Trimeresurus stejnegeri* widely ranges over low and moderate zones, and has also been found in Mt. Changbai, Jilin Province at 41°N. Therefore, it is the only one that overlaps three latitudinal zones.

Vertical distribution

Altitudinal distribution of Chinese venomous snakes is extensive, from coastal lowland to 4,000 metres in the Yunnan Plateau. Stratification is clear at lower and higher elevations, with diversions at middle levels not distinct. Six species *(Agkistrodon shedaoensis, Trimeresurus albolabris, Calliophis kelloggi, Boiga multomaculata, Enhydris chinensis* and *E. plumbea)* have not been found above 1,000 metres; three *(Vipera berus, Trimeresurus jerdonii* and *T. medoensis)* have not been found below 1,000 m; four *(Agkistrodon monticola, A. strauchii, Trimeresurus tibetanus* and *T. xiangchengensis)* have not been found below 2,700 m. Most species are known from low elevations to about 1,600 m (12 species) and around 2,000 m (9 species). The rest of eight species have no exact data available.

245

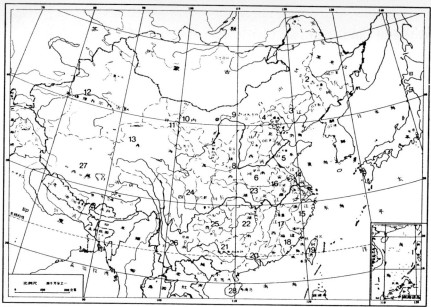

Figure 1
Provinces of China

Number on Map	Chinese	Pinyin Name
1	黑龙江	Heilongjiang
2	吉林	Jilin
3	辽宁	Liaoning
4	河北	Hebei
5	山东	Shandong
6	河南	Henan
7	山西	Shanxi
8	陕西	Shaanxi
9	内蒙古	Nei Menggu (Autonomous Region) (Inner Mongolia)
10	宁夏	Ningxia (Hui Autonomous Region)
11	甘肃	Gansu
12	新疆	Xinjiang (Uygur Autonomous Region)
13	青龙海	Qinghai
14	江苏	Jiangsu
15	浙江	Zhejiang
16	安徽	Anhui
17	江西	Jiangxi
18	福建	Fujian
19	台湾	Taiwan
20	广东	Guangdong
21	广西	Guangxi (Zhuang Autonomous Region)
22	湖南	Hunan
23	湖北	Hubei
24	四川	Sichuan
25	贵州	Guizhou
26	云南	Yunnan
27	西藏	Xizang (Autonomous Region) (Tibet)
28	海南	Hainan

Ecological distribution

Weaknesses in the ecological data exist. Chinese venomous snakes can be, ecologically, roughly divided as follows:

Aquatic

Fresh water : four *Enhydris* species.
Sea water : all fifteen sea snakes.

Terrestrial

Island : *Agkistrodon shedaoensis, Trimeresurus gracilis* and *Calliophis sauteri* have been found only on islands.

Mainland

a. Forest
 (i) Arboreal or climbing tendencies: *Trimeresurus mucrosquamatus, T. stejnegeri, Boiga kraepelini, Chrysopelea, ornata, Dryophis prasinus.*
 (ii) Ground: *Agkistrodon b. brevicaudus, Deinagkistrodon acutus, Trimeresurus jerdonii, T. medoensis, T. tibetanus, Vipera berus, Calliophis kelloggi, C. macclellandi, C. sauteri, Ophiophagus hannah, Psammodynastes pulverulentus.*
b. Scrub
 (i) Level or hilly open country: *Agkistrodon b. brevicaudus, A. ussuriensis, Trimeresurus albolabris, Vipera russelli, Bungarus fasciatus, Naja naja, Ophiophagus hannah, Boiga multomaculata.*
 (ii) Mountains: *Azemiops feae, Trimeresurus jerdonii, T. monticola, T. xiangchengensis.*
c. Steppe
 (i) High mountain steppe: *Agkistrodon monticola, A. strauchii.*
 (ii) Central Asia dry steppe: *Vipera ursinii.*
d. Deserts or semideserts: *Trimeresurus intermedius, Psammophis lineolatus*
e. Agricultural area: *Agkistrodon b. brevicaudus, Trimeresurus albolabris, T. mucrosquamatus, Vipera russellii, Bungarus multicinctus* and *Naja naja.*

Venomous Snakes of Medical Importance in China

It is known that the opisthoglyphous snakes are not dangerous. Of the fifteen sea snakes recorded along the coastal region of China, about half are common. Their bite is very rare. Among the rest of the thirty terrestrial elapids, viperids and crotalids, some are rare or very rare, and some inhabit high mountains or desolate and uninhabited deserts or semideserts. About ten species are often the cause of snakebite and are medically important venomous snakes. They can be recognized by external features using the following key.

1A. Head elliptic; no facial pit 2

1B. Head more or less triangular; with a facial pit on each side between nostril and eye 6

2A. Top of head covered by large shields 3

2B. Top of head covered by small keeled scales .... *Vipera russellii.*

3A. Body blackish brown, can spread a "hood" when alarmed by widening and flattening the neck 4

3B. Body black with prominent cross-band or rings; cannot spread a "hood" 5

4A. A "spectacle" marking on hood .... *Naja naja.*

4B. No "spectacle" marking on hood; an additional pair of large shields, occipitals, behind parietals .... *Ophiophagus hannah.*

5A. Back black with 30 to 50 narrow, white cross-bands; tail ending in a point .... *Bungarus multicinctus.*

5B. Body black with 22 to 30 wide, yellow rings; back with a vertebral ridge; tail ending bluntly .... *Bungarus fasciatus.*

6A. Top of head covered by large shields 7

6B. Top of head covered by small scales 8

7A. Body stout; head prominently triangular; snout with a pointed, upturned appendage .... *Deinagkistrodon acutus.*

7B. Body normal; head slightly triangular; no pointed, upturned appendage at the end of snout .... *Agkistrodon b. brevicaudus.*

8A. Body green in colour; eye red; tip of tail reddish 9

8B. Body colour not green 10

9A. Dark green above, a narrow, white, yellowish white or red and white line extends the length of body on each side; the first upper labial completely separated from the nasal .... *Trimeresurus stejnegeri.*

9B. Bright green above; without or with a narrow, whitish line on each side; the first upper labial partially separated from the nasal .... *Trimeresurus albolabris.*

10A. Body a little stout; back with a row of blackish brown battlement-like markings .... *Trimeresurus monticola.*

10B. Body not stout; back with a dark purplish wave-like longitudinal stripe .... *Trimeresurus mucrosquamatus.*

Bungarus fasciatus (Schneider)

Chinese name: Jin Huan She (Golden-banded Snake).
English name: Banded Krait.

Description

Entire length alternately banded with broad and yellow bands. These bands, 19 to 27 plus 3 to 5 in number, always completely encircle the body and tail. Black spots often in the yellow bands. Head black, with a lighter "∧" —shaped mark on the occiput. A prominent ridge along the vertebral line of back and tail, the cross-section of the body more or less triangular in shape. Head elliptic, less distinct from neck. Top of head with normal nine large shields. Pupil rounded; loreal absent; upper labials seven. Dorsal scales smooth, in fifteen rows throughout; vertebrals enlarged and pentagonal. End of tail blunt, sub-caudals in a single row.

Size

This medium snake, usually one metre long, reaches a maximum length of 1.71 m (male) and 1.36 m (female).

Biology

Inhabits plain or hilly region near water and well covered by plants, with an elevation from 180 metres up to 1,014 metres. Nocturnal. Snakes comprise its main diet. It occasionally eats lizards or other vertebrates. Oviparous, clutch size 8 to 12 eggs, laid from May to June, under dead leaves or in holes. Egg size 45 — 54 x 20 — 24 mm.

Distribution

Ranges generally south of 25°N in China, including Guangdong, Hainan, Guangxi, southern parts of Yunnan, Jiangxi and Fujian.

Disposition and venom

Inoffensive in disposition during daytime, bites occur only at night. Average venom yield from specimens kept on snake farms was 91.4 mg (= 27.5 mg dry venom) at one bite. LD_{50} to mouse i.c. is 2.4 mg/kg weight. Venom neurotoxic. The symptoms of victims caused by banded krait bite similar to those of many-banded krait. No pain or slight pain, surroundings of wound slightly red and swollen. Systemic symptoms, if occurring, develop slowly. General ache is much more serious, and appears as pain spasms.

Bungarus multicinctus Blyth

Chinese name: Yin Huan She (Silver-banded Snake)
English name: Many-banded Krait

Description

Black or bluish black above, with thirty to fifty narrow, white or creamy white, transverse bands throughout the entire length. Lower part of body white or dirty white. Head black, bluish black or dark brown above, sometimes a lighter "∧" — shaped mark on the occiput (Fig 2). Head elliptic, less distinct from neck. Top of head with normal nine large shields. Pupil rounded. Loreal absent; upper labials seven. Dorsal scales smooth, in fifteen rows throughout; vertebrals enlarged, pentagonal. Tail comparatively long, thin and tapering; subcaudals in a single row.

Size

This medium snake, usually one metre long, reaches a maximum length of 1.84 m (female).

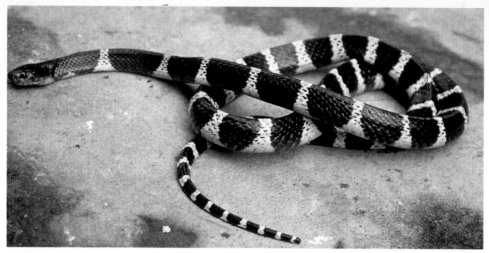

Figure 2
Bungarus multicinctus, Jingdezhen, Jiangxi

Biology

Inhabits from coastal low land up to 1,300 m, but is more common in low areas, especially in plains and hilly region. Active at night, generally staying near water, searching for frogs, fishes, eels, or snakes. During daytime, it hides under stones, or in holes. Appears from April and leaves for hibernation in November. Oviparous, deposits 3 to 15 (maximum 20) eggs in June. Egg size 29 x 16.5 to 52 x 19 mm. Hatching period about 1½ months. Hatchlings 20 to 27 cm in total length.

Distribution

Very common krait, ranges almost over most areas south of Chang Jiang (Yangtze River), including Taiwan and Hainan. It has also been found in southeastern Sichuan and southwestern Yunnan.

Disposition and venom

Inoffensive in disposition especially in daylight hours, but ready to bite at night if touched or interfered. Average venom yield from specimens kept on snake farms was 18.4 mg (= 4.6 mg dry venom) at one bite. Venom extremely virulent, LD_{50} is 0.09 mg/kg mouse weight i.c. Venom neurotoxic. The local symptoms of victims caused by many-banded krait bite are neither swelling, redness nor pain, the victims only feeling slightly itchy and numb. Systemic symptoms occur, in general, at the beginning of one to four hours after being bitten by this snake. The following symptoms may occur: chest uncomfortable, general ache, weak feeling in limbs, walking haltingly, glossolysis, loss of voice, swallowing paralysis, dim vision, blepharoptosis, palsy, difficult breathing. In case of serious poisoning, loss of breath may occur, leading to death. Fatalities have often been reported.

Infraspecific classification

Two subspecies are recognized. The nominate subspecies has less ventrals (203 — 221) and more white cross-bands (31 — 50 + 8 — 17); *Bungarus multicinctus wanghaotingii* Pope has more ventrals (213 — 231) and less white cross-bands (20 — 31 + 7 — 11), found in southern Yunnan only.

Naja naja (Linnaeus)

Chinese name: Yanjing She (Spectacle-marking Snake)
English name: Chinese Cobra or Taiwan Cobra

Description

Black, blackish brown or brown above, with or without narrow, light transverse lines at irregular intervals, which are especially prominent in juveniles. When disturbed, one third of the forebody is raised and the characteristic hood on the neck is expanded. There are mainly two types of whitish markings on the hood in Chinese specimens: 1) modified monocellate pattern or well known "spectacle" and its variations found in southeastern China, including Taiwan and Hainan specimens; 2) monocellate pattern, found in specimens from southwestern Guangxi, southwestern Yunnan and southwestern Sichuan. Pale white below, a broad blackish grey band under the hood with two black spots before it (Fig 3a). Head elliptic, less distinct from neck, with normal nine large shields on the top. Loreal absent; seven upper labials, the third being the largest, which is in contact with the nasal in front and entering eye posteriorly. A small scale on the border of lower lip inserts between the fourth and fifth lower labials. Dorsal scales smooth, in 25 (23-27)-21(19)-15 rows. Subcaudals in a double row.

Size

This medium snake, usually 1.2 m long, reaches a maximum length of 1.94 m (male) and 1.64 m (female).

Biology

Inhabits shrub, bamboo forest, banks of stream or pool, rice-field, road-side, urban area, and even in gardens or in house, of plain, hilly and mountainous regions from sea level up to 1,630 m. Found both in daylight hours and at night. Its food is composed of fishes, frogs, lizards, rodents, birds and their eggs, or other snakes. Appears from May and leaves for hibernation in November. Oviparous, mating in May to June, depositing 7 to 19 eggs from July to August. Egg size 42 — 54 x 26 — 31 mm. Hatching period about 50 days. Hatchlings about 20 cm in total length.

Distribution

Widely ranging over south of Chang Jiang (Yangtze River) from the coastal region in the east, westwards to Guizhou, Yunnan and southwestern Sichuan, and Taiwan and Hainan (Fig 3b).

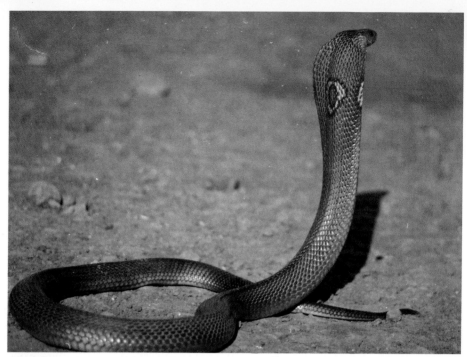

Figure 3a
Naja naja (monocellate), Miyi, Sichuan

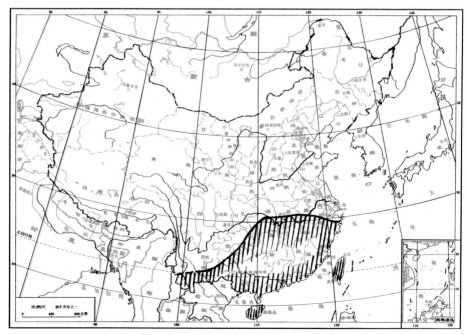

Figure 3b
Distribution of *Naja naja*, overlaps the low and moderate latitude zones.

252

Disposition and venom

Not aggressive but has a characteristic defensive behaviour, raising the forebody, inflating the hood, hissing and striking. The author saw a specimen in Guizhou Province spitting venom to a distance of two metres when captured. Average venom yield from specimens kept on snake farms at one bite was 250.8 mg (= 79.7 mg dry venom). LD_{50} to mouse i.c. is 0.53 mg/kg weight. Venom both haemotoxic and neurotoxic in property. Local symptoms of victims caused by Chinese cobra bite are: wound darkening, localised redness and swelling, pain, insensibility, and always accompanied by blisters and necrosis. Necrosis is a serious problem in case of bites by cobra as it may last a long period of many years after recovery of the victim. The following systemic symptoms may occur: chest uncomfortable, fever, sore-throat, difficulty in swallowing, glossolysis, loss of voice, weak feeling in limbs, walking haltingly, general ache, lockjaw, myosis, and difficult breathing, etc. Fatality occasionally occurs.

Taxonomic note

The Chinese Cobra was constantly recognized as subspecies *Naja naja atra*, which was described by Theodore Cantor in 1842 based on specimens from Chusan (Zhoushan Island), Zhejiang Province. The hood marking in specimens from southwestern China is distinctly different from specimens of southeastern part. The infraspecific classification of Chinese cobra needs to be settled.

Ophiophagus hannah (Cantor)

Chinese name: Yanjing Wang She (King spectacle-marking snake).
English name: King Cobra

Description

It is much more like the common cobra in defensive behaviour as well as in general features. The main differences from the common cobra are in: 1) larger size, usually three to four metres long, reaching a maximum length of about six metres on record; 2) an additional pair of large shields, occipitals as compared to the normal nine large shields on the top of head; 3) hood, when expanded, being narrow and extending farther down the neck than that of the common cobra, and without characteristic spectacle marking on its back; 4) dorsal scales smooth, in 19 — 15 — 15 rows, subcaudals partly in a single row. Dark brown or black with obscure banded markings above, whitish or greyish below. Throat and neck yellowish orange underneath. Back with thirty-four to forty-five buffs or white chevron-like bands encircling the body while young. (Fig 4a)

Biology

Inhabits from sea level up to an elevation of 1,800 m. Found in border of forest near water. Diurnal activity. Feeding mainly on other snakes, occasionally on lizards. Oviparous, depositing 20 to 40 eggs in nest made with dead leaves. We (Zhao, EM and SQ Li, 1983, Acta Herpetologica Sinica, Chengdu, 2(4): 44) reported an observation of a case, on first of August in 1983,

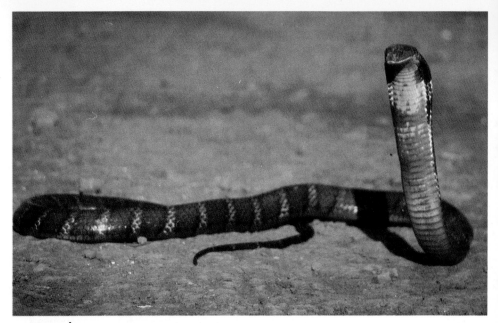

Figure 4a
Ophiophagus hannah, Miyi Sichuan

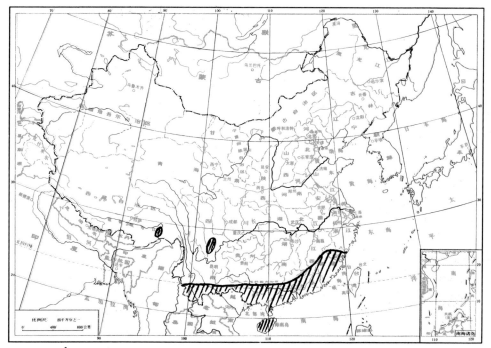

Figure 4b
Distribution of *Ophiophagus hannah.*

1983, of a female king cobra coiled on nest made by dead leaves with 25 eggs arranged in four layers underneath. Number of eggs in each layer was 5, 8, 8, and 4 from top to bottom. Eggs elliptical, diameters 65.5 x 33.2 mm. This is additional evidence for their habit of guarding eggs.

Distribution

It ranges, in general, south of about 25°N in China, including Fujian, Guangdong, Hainan, Guangxi and Guizhou, but there are some records indicating that it occurs further north; Qingyuan and Taishun Counties (about 27.5°N), Zhejiang in the east, Miyi County (near 27°N), Sichuan and Medog County (over 28°N), Xizang (Tibet) in the west (Fig 4b).

Disposition

Fast and agile, always attacks when guarding eggs. Average venom yield from specimens kept on snake farms was 384.2 mg (=101.9 mg dry venom) at one bite. LD_{50} to mouse i.c. is 0.34 mg/kg weight. Venom both haemotoxic and neurotoxic in property. The symptoms of king cobra bite are similar to those of the common cobra. It differs from the latter in rarely causing blisters and necrosis, but quickly developing serious systemic symptoms. Bites by king cobra should be treated accordingly. Fatal cases were often reported due to the large quantity of envenomation.

Vipera russelli (Shaw and Nodder)

Chinese name: Yuan Ban Kui (Rounded-spot viper)
English name: Russell's viper or Daboia

Description

Brown above, with three longitudinal, one median and two lateral, series of large rounded or oval spots. These spots are usually brown in the centre bordered with black and edged again with light yellow or white. Occasionally spots touch or fuse. A row of small black spots between median and lateral large spots. Dirty white or creamy below, uniform or marbled with semilunar black spots; small irregular black spots along both sides. Head subtriangular, snout rounded and broad; canthus rostalis prominent; nostrils large; rostronasal semilunar in shape. Top of head covered by many small, strongly keeled scales. Dorsal scales strongly keeled, in 31 — 29 (27 — 33) — 21 rows. Body stout, tail short.

Size

This is a medium sized snake, usually 0.9 — 1.2 m long, reaching a maximum length of 1.67 m.

Biology

Inhabits plains, hills or mountains, but prefers open country. Vertical distribution from coastal low land up to 2,100m. During harvest season, it has

255

often been found in rice-fields. It is quiet during daylight hours, but is more active in evenings and at night. It always produces, when disturbed, an unforgettable, very loud and deep hiss. Its food is composed of rodents, birds, lizards and frogs. Ovoviviparous, producing 20 to 40 (maximum 63 on record) living young from June to July.

Distribution
South of about latitude 25°, including Guangdong, Guangxi, Taiwan and southern Fujian.

Disposition and venom.
It is sluggish but ready to strike when the objects come into effective biting range. It is also known to hold on after striking. The young are more vicious than the adults. Average venom yield from specimens kept on snake farms at one bite was 191.9 mg (= 44.4 mg dry venom, Guangxi data) or 112 mg (= 30.4 mg dry venom, Fujian data.) LD_{50} to mouse i.c. is 1.6 mg/kg weight. Venom mainly haemotoxic in property. The symptoms of victims caused by Russell's viper bite are: localised strong causalgia, much more bleeding, swelling developing fast, many blisters and ecchymosis around wounds, necrosis, and serious ulceration, systemic symptoms occuring quickly and suddenly, and lasting a long period. It includes serious bleeding of subcutaneous tissues, viscerals and sense organs; earlier haematuria. In case of serious poisoning, haemolysis anaemia, jaundice, and acute renal failure may occur. Fatal cases have been known.

Infraspecific classification
There are two subspecies recorded from China. *Vipera russelli siamensis* Smith is distributed on mainland. On Taiwan island is another subspecies, *Vipera russelli formosensis* Maki. The latter subspecies differs from the former one, according to Maki's original description, in 1) having the additional series of spots interposed between the black rings of the dorsal series, or between the lateral series; 2) the dorsal additional spots being in contact with their fellows to form an X-shaped figure on the posterior portion of the body.

Agkistrodon blomhoffii brevicaudus Stejneger

Chinese name: Fu She (Short-tailed pit viper)
English name: Chinese mamushi

Description
Greyish brown, reddish brown, or blackish brown above, with large, dark edged, round blotches disposed in pairs, opposite or alternating. In reddish brown specimens, usually a reddish vertebral line exists. A broad, black stripe, bordered above by a narrow, white line, extending from snout, crossing the eye, to the angle of mouth. Upper lip uniform yellowish white. Greyish or yellowish below, more or less speckled or spotted with black. Tip of tail is yellowish. Head slightly triangular; facial pit present. Top of head covered with nine large

shields (Fig 5a). Internasal much broader than long, slightly curved, with its outer side pointed. Dorsal scales in 21 — 21 — 17 rows, strongly keeled; ventrals 134 — 150; subcaudals 29 — 45 pairs; ventrals plus subcaudals 167 — 189.

Size

A small snake, usually about 50 cm long, reaches a maximum length of 67 cm.

Biology

It has been found in various environment at different elevation, but it prefers plains and lower slopes of hills. It can be found among vegetation, under rocks, on road-side, or near residences in cultivated regions, in graveyards; it has also been found in gardens or parks in cities. Rodents, insectivores, frogs are its diet. It also eats lizards, fishes and birds. Ovoviviparous, producing 2 to 16 living young from August to September. Hatchlings 15.5 — 20.8 cm in total length.

Distribution

Widely distributed in Chinese Oriental Region except the most southern part about south of 25°N. It extends northward to southern Liaoning Province (about 41°N) in the east coastal region. (Fig 5b).

Disposition and venom

In general, it has a mild disposition. It takes, when disturbed, an alert attitude and faces the aggressor. It always vibrates the end of its tail when annoyed, or flattens the entire body. Average venom yield from specimens kept on snake farms at one bite was 126.7 mg (= 41.4 mg dry venom, southern Jiangsu data) or 69.7 mg (= 20.8 mg dry venom, Zhejiang data). LD_{50} to mouse i.c. is 2 mg/kg weight. Venom both haemotoxic and neurotoxic in property. The symptoms of victims caused by Chinese mamushi bite are: localised swelling, acanthesthesia, and becoming serious and extending outwards, and often accompanied by bleeding ecchymosis. Systemic symptoms occur, in general, at the beginning of one to six hours after being bitten by this snake. The following symptoms may occur: dim vision, double vision, blepharoptosis, movement obstruction of the bitten limb, agape with difficulty, neck rigidity, general ache, breathing with difficulty, uropenia or suppression of urine, dark reddish brown urine. Mortality due to mamushi bite is about 1%.

Deinagkistrodon acutus (Günther)

Chinese name: Jian Wen Fu (Pointed-snout pit viper)
English name: Hundred-pace pit viper, or Hundred pacer

Description

Back light brown or greyish brown, with a series of dark brown lateral triangles on each side. The two pointed tops of the two opposite triangles meet

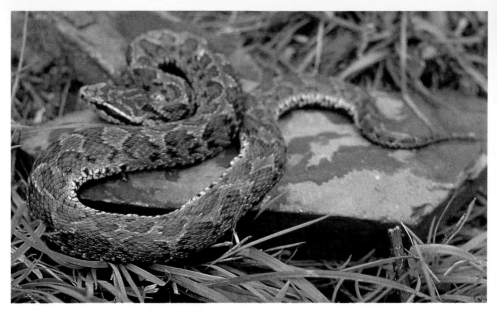

Figure 5a
Agkistrodon b. brevicaudus, Jingdezhen, Jiangxi

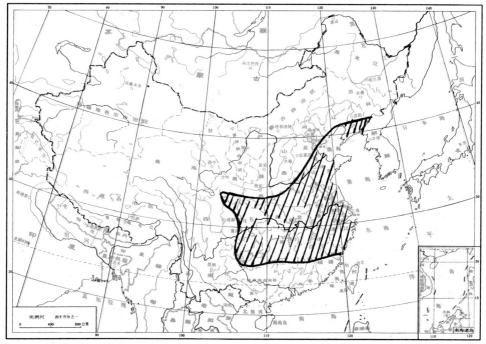

Figure 5b
Distribution of *Agkistrodon blomhoffii brevicaudus*, overlaps the moderate and high latitude zones.

each other at the mid line, forming a series of about twenty light brown, squarish blotches on back. A row of large black spots extends along each side near the belly. The top and upper sides of the head are uniformly black, with a black streak from the eye to the angle of mouth; yellowish below, spotted with dark brown. The young are much lighter than the adults with essentially the same pattern (Fig 6). Head large, triangular, with an upturned snout. Body very stout. Tail short, ending in a compressed, pointed slightly curved cornified scale. The top of head covered with nine large shields. Dorsal scales strongly and tubercularly keeled. Subcaudals mostly in pairs, some of the anterior ones single.

Size

This stout snake, usually 0.8 — 1.0 m long, reaches a maximum length of 1.57 m (male) and 1.41 m (female).

Biology

Inhabits high, forested mountains up to 1,350 m, but has also been found in low coastal region (100 m). It prefers lower mountain slopes or rocky hills with small valleys. It was generally discovered by day on rocks or among vegetation along banks of streams, or in firewood near houses, or even in houses. At night, it has always been observed attacking firelight. Frogs, toads, rats, birds and lizards form its diet. The author reported a specimen of a total length of 1.04 m and weighing 600 g having eaten a specimen of *Rattus rattus* of total length 51.5 cm and weight of 530 g. Oviparous, depositing 11 to 12 eggs from June to August. Egg size 40 — 56 x 20 — 31 mm. Hatching period about one month. Hatchlings have average total length of 21.7 cm.

Distribution

Ranges between latitudes of 25° and 31° east of longtitude about 104°E. Recorded from Anhui, Zhejiang, Jiangxi, Fujian, Taiwan, Hunan, Hubei, Guizhou, eastern Sichuan, northern Guangdong and Guangxi (Fig 7).

Disposition and venom

One of its common name in China is "lazy snake", indicating its sluggishness in the field, but it strikes and bites vigorously when aroused. It always remains in a coiled position, turning the head abruptly to face every nearby movement, and ready to strike at any time. Average venom yield from specimens kept on snake farms at one bite was 222.2 mg (= 59 mg dry venom, Guangxi data) or 688 mg (= 176.1 mg dry venom, Fujian data). The LD_{50} to mouse i.c. is 8.9 mg/kg weight. Venom haemotoxic, especially strongly haemorrhagic in property. Localised symptoms of victims caused by hundred-pace pit viper are: continuous severe causalgia, rare numbness, serious swelling and bleeding, more blisters, large and deep area of necrosis and ulceration. Systemic symptoms occur earlier and suddenly, including palpitation, uncomfortable chest feeling, dim vision, haematuria, haemoptysis, having blood in stool, purpura, and anuresis. Because of its body size and large hinged fangs which permit

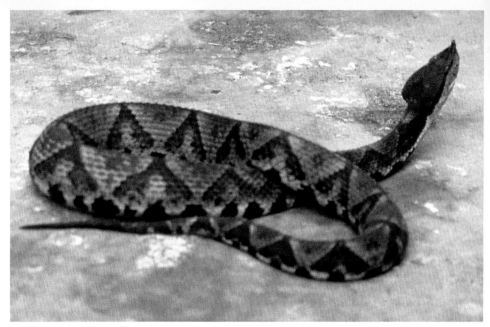

Figure 6
Deinagkistrodon acutus, Jingdezhen, Jiangxi

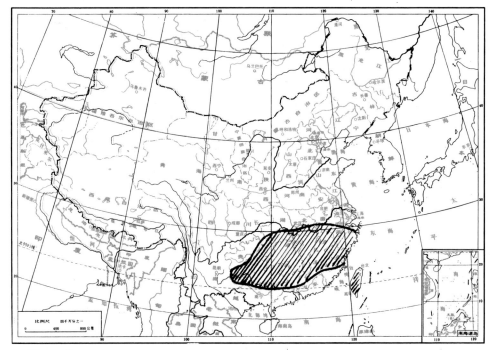

Figure 7
Distribution of *Deinagkistrodon acutus*, a typical moderate latitude snake.

260

effective delivery of large quantities of venom, victims bitten by this snake should be treated accordingly.

Trimeresurus albolabris (Gray)

Chinese name: Bai Chun Zhu Ye Qing (White-lipped green bamboo snake)
English name: White-lipped pit viper

Description

Uniformly bright green above, indistinct dark crossbands can be seen, especially in preserved specimens, in some individuals. Yellowish white below. Upper lip yellowish white. A narrow white longitudinal stripe along each side of the body on D_1 or absent in some females. Eye reddish. Tip and posterior part of upper surface of the tail brownish red. Head triangular, very distinct from the neck. Top of head covered by small scales, a pair of internasals are, except supraoculars, the large ones among them. Internasals in contact with each other or, occasionally, separated by one small scale. The first upper labial completely fused with, or partially separated from the nasal. Facial pit present. No small scale between nasal and prefoeval scale.

Size

This small snake, usually 600 mm long, reaches a maximum length of 915 mm.

Biology

Inhabits plains and hills, with an elevation from sea level up to 1,000 m. Nocturnal, sometimes found in daytime. Among vegetation or shrubs, occasionally entering residences in search of rats. Besides rodents, lizards and frogs are also composed of its diet. Ovoviviparous, producing 10 to 13 living young from late June to July. Hatchlings about 20 cm in total length.

Distribution

Very common in south of latitude 25°N. Reported from Guangdong, Hainan, Hong Kong, Guangxi, Taiwan, southern Fujian, Guizhou and Yunnan (Fig 8).

Disposition and venom

Beautiful small snake, looks gentle in disposition. Bites when touched or closely approached. Average venom yield from specimens just captured from the field of southern Yunnan at one bite was 10.43 mg dry venom, but from snakes after one month captivity, was only 5.17 mg. Venom predominantly haemotoxic. Most victims bitten by this snake only show localised symptoms, including oedema, discoloration and pain, etc. Occasional consequences include headache, palpitation and slow pulse. No fatal case recorded.

Trimeresurus stejnegeri Schmidt

Chinese name: Zhu Ye Qing or Qing Zhu She (Green bamboo snake)
English name: Green Bamboo Pit Viper

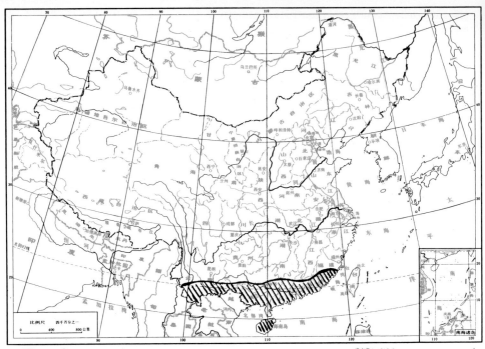

Figure 8
Distribution of *Trimeresurus albolabris,* a typical low latitude snake.

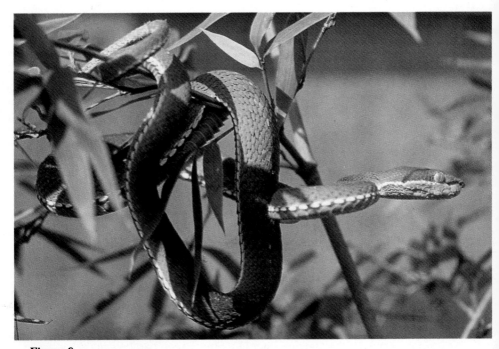

Figure 9
Trimeresurus stejnegeri, Sichuan

262

Description

It is much more like the white-lipped pit viper in general features. It differs from the latter in 1) dark green above, greenish yellow or yellowish white below; upper lip green; with a white, yellowish white, or red and white longitudinal stripe along each side of the body on D_1; 2) the first upper labial completely separating from the nasal; 3) one or two small scales between the nasal and prefoeval scale; 4) one to four small scales between internasals. (Fig 9)

Size

This small snake is usually 700 — 900 mm in total length.

Biology

Inhabits hilly and mountainous regions near water and well covered by plants, with an elevation from 150 to 2,300 m. Arboreal, always found on trees, bamboo, shrubs as well as on rocks along the banks of mountainous streams. Nocturnal. Feeding mainly on frogs and tadpoles, also on birds, rodents and lizards. Ovoviviparous, producing 3 to 15 living young from July to August.

Distribution

Widely ranges over south of Chang Jiang (Yangtze River), northwards to southwestern Gansu in the west, and southern Jiangsu in the east. A record from Mt. Changbai, southeastern Jilin Province, reported by the author poses a very interesting problem on zoogeography (Fig. 10).

Disposition and venom

Similar to the white-lipped pit viper, this snake is sluggish and seldom moves out of the way when approached. It remains quiet if an intruder is not too close, but is likely to strike when the intruder comes into its effective biting range. Due to these habits and also its good camouflage, a great majority of snake bite victims are attributed to these two snakes. Venom predominantly haemotoxic. The symptoms are similar to those caused by white-lipped pit viper bite. Fatality is very rare as far as the author knows, only one fatal case has been recorded where the victim was bitten on the head. Green bamboo pit viper and white-lipped pit viper, due to their common appearance, were always confused with each other by local people as well as medical persons. Thus, many cases of snakebite reported in Chinese journals caused by these two kinds of "green bamboo snakes" were grouped together.

Infraspecific classification

Two subspecies are recognized. The nominate subspecies has dorsal scales in 21 rows at midbody. Another subspecies, *Trimeresurus stejnegeri yunnanensis* Schmidt, has only 19 rows of dorsal scales at mid-body and distributed only in southern Yunnan and southwestern Sichuan.

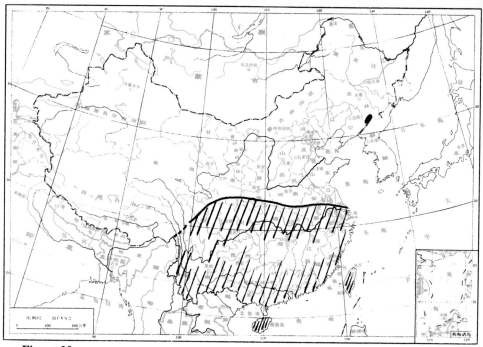

Figure 10
Distribution of *Trimeresurus stejnegeri*, overlaps all the three latitude zones.

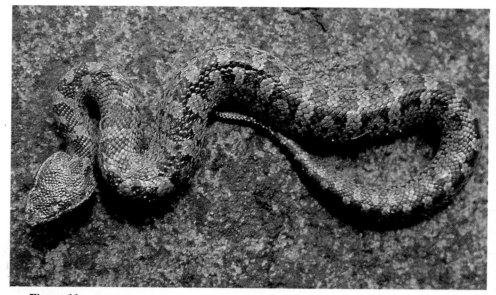

Figure 11
Trimeresurus monticola, Washan (Mt. Wa), Sichuan

264

Trimeresurus monticola Günther

Chinese name: Shan Laotie Tou (Mountain Iron-head Snake)
English name: Mountain pit viper

Description

Light or dark brown above, with one or two dorsal rows of large, squarish, dark brown or blackish patches; two rows of squarish patches may alternate and form battlements pattern; whitish below, spotted or powdered with brown. Head triangular, about as long as broad, distinct from the neck (Fig 11). Facial pit present. Internasals in contact with its fellow, or separated by one, rarely two, small scales; seven to ten scales on a line between the supraoculars. Dorsal scales in 23 (21 — 25) rows at mid-body, 9 — 19 median rows weakly keeled, the outer rows smooth.

Size

Stout-bodied snake, usually 60–80 cm long, can reach maximum length of 1.1 m (female).

Biology

Inhabits mountains or plateau with an elevation from coastal lowland up to more than 2,000 m. Found in tea-fields, cultivated areas, under shrubs, amongst vegetation, or near human habitation and sometimes in homes. Nocturnal. Eats rodents or insectivores. Oviparous, depositing 5 to 18 eggs from July to August. Egg size 34 — 42 x 23 — 24 mm, hatching in September. Hatchlings 18.3 — 19.5 cm in total length.

Distribution

Ranges widely over southern China from Himalayas in the west, eastward to coastal provinces. Records include Xizang (Tibet), Sichuan, Yunnan, Guizhou, Guangxi, Guangdong, Hainan, Hong Kong, Hunan, Fujian, Zhejiang and Taiwan.

Disposition and venom

Sluggish in disposition, but ready to bite when irritated, especially during the period when guarding eggs. Symptoms of victims bitten by this snake are similar to those of Chinese habu.

Trimeresurus mucrosquamatus (Cantor)

Chinese name: Laotie Tou (Iron-head snake)
English name: Chinese Habu or Taiwan Habu.

Description

Greyish brown above with a vertebral row of large, irregular, brown or purplish brown spots, each spot encircled by dark brown and edged with bright yellow; the spots sometimes joined antero-posteriorly forming a zigzag stripe.

Whitish below, marbled with brownish dots. Head brown with dark brown markings; sides light yellow, on each side with a narrow, blackish brown stripe from the eye to angle of mouth. Head large, longer than broad, typical triangular shape, very prominently distinct from the neck. Facial pit present. Two to six small scales separating the internasals; eleven to eighteen scales on a line between the supraoculars. Dorsal scales lanceolate, strongly keeled, in 25 (23 — 27) rows in mid-body.

Size

This slender figure snake, usually 0.8 — 1.0 m long, reaches a maximum length of 1.12 m (male) and 1.28 m (female).

Biology

Inhabits open area as well as forested regions with an elevation from coastal low land to 1,400 m. Found in bamboo forest, shrubs, banks of stream, tea-fields, agricultural area, or near residences. Nocturnal, but may be seen during the day. Eats birds, rodents and insectivores, frogs and snakes. Oviparous, depositing 5 to 13 eggs from July to August. Egg size 33 — 37 x 20 mm.

Distribution

Ranges widely over southern China, northward to southeastern Gansu in the west. Records include Sichuan, Yunnan, Guizhou, Anhui, Zhejiang, Jiangxi, Hunan, Fujian, Taiwan, Guangdong, Hainan, Guangxi, Shaanxi and Gansu.

Disposition and venom

It appears docile and sluggish, but ready to bite when irritated. Since it is often found around human habitations, or even inside houses, a large number of snake bite cases are caused by it. The localised symptoms of victims are swelling, strong causalgia, small blisters but less than those caused by green bamboo snake. Systemic symptoms, if occurring, are bleeding of sense organs and viscerals, and clouding of consciousness.

Medico-geographical Division of Snakebite in China

No statistical data on incidence of snakebite in China is available due to the country's size. According to the fragmentary materials from various places over the years since 1960, a general picture can be seen where the great majority of snakebite cases is caused by green bamboo snake (including both *Trimeresurus albolabris* and *stejnegeri)* and the Chinese mamushi, followed by many-banded krait and Chinese cobra. This is not surprising since these snakes are abundant and widely distributed. Based on data in combination with the geographical distribution of the snakes, a medico-geographical division of snakebite in China is given below (Fig 12).

(1) Serious Snakebite Region
The whole area south of 25°N. From southern Fujian of the eastern coast,

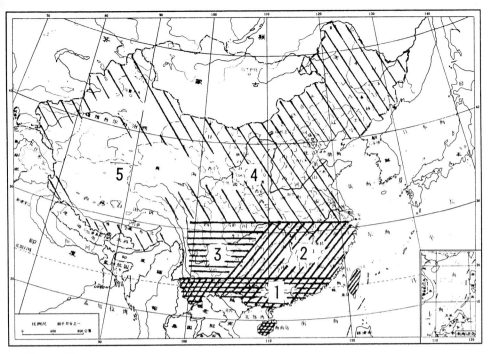

Figure 12

Map of medico-geographical division of snakebite in China.

1. Serious Snake bite region
2. Heavy Snake bite region
3. Moderate Snake bite region
4. Slight Snake bite region
5. Snakebite free region

the most part of Guangdong and Guangxi, towards southern Yunnan in the west, and Hainan Island. Almost all the medically important venomous snakes, except Chinese mamushi, range over this region. Snakebite cases in this region are caused mainly by *Naja naja*, *Bungarus multicinctus* and two kinds of green bamboo snakes. Bites of banded krait, king cobra and Russell's viper are also occurring in this region. For example, during the twelve years from 1973 to 1984, there was an average of 11.67 cases of snakebite per 100,000 population each year in Pingle County, Guangxi Zhuang Autonomous Region. These bites are caused by (in order of importance), *Naja naja*, *Bungarus multicinctus*, *Trimeresurus albolabris* and *stejnegeri*, *T. mucrosquamatus*, *Bungarus fasciatus* and *Ophiophagus hannah*. This, however, is a very incomplete estimation since many victims prefer to use folk remedy in treating snakebite and do not go to the hospital. Some fatal cases are recorded every year.

(2) Heavy Snakebite Region

Area between latitude of 25°N and 31°N east of longitude 105°E, including Taiwan Island. Medically important snakes in this region include *Naja naja* and *Bungarus multicinctus* of Elapidae, *Agkistrodon blomhoffii brevicaudus*,

Trimeresurus stejnegeri, T. monticola, T. mucrosquamatus and *Deinagkistrodon acutus* of Viperidae. The great majority of snakebite cases in this region are caused by Chinese mamushi and green bamboo snake, but hundred-pace pit viper bite is a serious problem in some places. For example, there are 9.7 cases of snakebite per 100,000 population in 1982 in Wujin County, Jiangsu Province. Chinese mamushi is the only venomous snake in Wujin and causes all the snakebites here. A few fatal cases are reported in this region every year.

(3) Moderate Snakebite Region

Southwest China. Yunnan-Guizhou Plateau and Sichuan Province belong to this region. Medically important species in this region belonging mainly to the genus *Trimeresurus*. The great majority of snakebite cases here are caused by *Trimeresurus stejnegeri, T. mucrosquamatus* and *T. monticola*. No data are available and fatal cases are rare.

(4) Slight Snakebite Region

The Palaearctic Region in China, except snakebite free area mentioned below. Although several venomous snake species range over this region, snakebite remains very rare.

(5) Snakebite Free Region

The whole Qinghai-Xizang Plateau, deserts and semideserts of northwestern China, South China Sea Islands and some other places. No venomous snake has been found in these areas.

Venomous Snake Bites and Snake Venom Research in China

Yuan-cong chen

Shanghai Institute of Biochemistry, Academia Sinica
320 Yue Yang Road, Shanghai, 200031, China

Introduction

It is well known that south and southeast Asia are inhabited by many species of snakes. China is located in east Asia adjacent to southeast Asia, has subtropical and warm temperate zones, and are abundant in snakes. In recent years, at least a million snakes were captured and killed in mainland China, as all parts of a snake can be used to make a good profit; such as venoms having prices higher than gold, skin for making art and craft, bile being used in traditional medicine, meat for making delicious dishes. In several southern Provinces in China, people have a habit of eating snake meat. Some snakes are used to make medicinal liquor by soaking the whole snake with some Chinese traditional herbs in alcohol, which is similar to the Japanese medicinal liquor, 'To-To Suh', believed to be effective against rheumatic pain and good for health and vitality.

Snake bite incidence, specially in the southern regions of China, is an important problem regarded by the Public Health Ministry of the Government due to the large number of peasants. Many research groups on snake and snake venom have been set up in medical universities and colleges in the southern provinces and have made important progress. The production of antivenins by Shanghai Institute of Biological Products supplies the whole country and it also provides widespread training on the knowledge of snake bite poisoning and treatment of snake bite to rural medical doctors. All of these should account for the sharp drop in snake bite fatality over recent years. Due to inconvenient transportation and communication in such a large rural area, no statistical data on snake bite each year is available. Nevertheless, the author has obtained data from some regions.

China has a rich source of snake venoms and research of snake venoms and application aroused the interest of scientists working on biochemistry, physiology, pharmacology and clinical surgery. In 1978 and 1981, symposiums on research of snake venoms and their application were organized by the Kunming Institute of Zoology at Kunming, Yunnan Province. In 1985 the First Conference of Research and Application of Toxin was held at Shaowu, Fujian Province, organized by the Special Committee of Toxinology of Chinese Biochemical Society where 102 participants from 20 cities and provinces involving 60 research groups made 142 presentations on animal, plant and microbial toxins, of which 60% were on snake venoms and snake bite poisoning.

All these activities have promoted the development of research on toxins in China.

Snake Venoms

Among 12 species of *Agkistrodon*, two species which are neurotoxic in China were discovered by Hsu's Snake Venom Research Group at the Shanghai Institute of Physiology. They are *Agkistrodon blomhoffii brevicaudus* from Zhejiang, (Chen et al, 1981), and *Agkistrodon intermedius* from Sinjiang Province (Zhang et al, 1985). The toxicities of the venoms of *Agkistrodons* in China are quite different from each other in their neurotoxin content. The LD_{50} of *A. intermedius* is the highest followed next by *A. b. brevicaudus* (Table 1).

TABLE 1.
Toxicity and Enzymatic activity of *Agkistrodon* Venoms

	Arginine esterase (USP unit/mg)	Protease (case in unit/mg)	Fibrinolytic activity	Toxicity LD_{50} i.p. in mice
Agkistrodon				
blomhoffii				
brevicaudus	180	29	1.0×10^3	0.525
A.b. ussuriensis	160	27	1.0×10^3	0.70
A.b. shedaoensis	190	16.5	0.82×10^3	0.735
A. saxatilis	220	18	0.82×10^3	2.064
A. strauchii	250	24.5	0.65×10^3	1.75
A. intermedius	450	11.5	1.1×10^3	0.285
A. acutus	78	62	1.1×10^3	2.95

Although *Agkistrodon acutus* is very aggressive, fatality caused by it is the lowest. The high content of haemorrhagic toxins and proteases causes serious localised necrosis which can be crippling. Snake bites by *Bungarus multicinctus* and *Ophiophagus hannah* are nearly 100% fatal due to their high content of neurotoxins (Table 2). Bungarotoxin activity is irreversible after binding with the receptors of synapses.

In the last 10 years in China, much progress has been made with many venom proteins purified and characterized. Some are strongly investigated, such as presynaptic neurotoxins, phospholipases A, thrombin-like enzyme, bradykinin releasing enzyme and bradykinin potentiating peptide (BPP) from the venom of *A.b. brevicaudus;* haemorrhagic toxins and hyaluronidase from *A. acutus;* neurotoxin from *Ophiophagus hannah;* platelet aggregation activator from *Trimeresurus mucrosquamatus;* cytotoxin from *Naja naja* (Table 3).

270

TABLE 2
Toxicity of Fatal Snake Venoms (Hu et al, 1979)

	Average amount delivered (mg)	LD_{50} mg/kg of mice
Naja naja	80	
Ophiophagus hannah	102	0.34
Bungarus multicinctus	5	0.09
Bungarus fasciatus	28	2.4
Vipera russelli	30 — 44	1.6
Trimeresurus stejnegeri	5	3.3
Agkistrodon halys	20 — 41	2.0
Agkistrodon acutus	59 — 176	8.9
Lapemis hardwickii	—	0.52
Trimeresurus mucrosquamatus	—	8.6 (Lee et al, 1962)

TABLE 3.
Venom Proteins Isolated and Characterized

Venom sources	Proteins
Agkistrodon blomhoffii brevicaudus	Presynaptic neurotoxin, phospholipases A_2, thrombin-like enzyme, bradykinin releasing enzyme, bradykinin potentiating peptide, phosphodiesterase.
Agkistrodon acutus	Haemorrhagic toxins, hyaluronidase.
Naja naja	Neurotoxin, cytotoxin, acetylcholine esterase, r-Glutamyl transpeptidase, alkaline phosphotase, A.
Ophiophagus hannah	Neurotoxin, L-Amino acid oxidase.
Vipera russelli	Phospholipase A.
Trimeresurus mucrosquamatus	Platelet aggregation activator.
Bungarus multicinctus	Neurotoxins.
Bungarus fasciatus	Carditoxin, neurotoxin.

Three types of phospholipases A_2 from the venom of *Agkistrodon blomhoffii brevicaudus* were identified (Table 4). Their isoelectric points are 4.5, 6.9 and 9.3 i.e. acidic, neutral and basic and they have similar molecular weights of nearly 14,000, but are different in lethal potency and biological activities (Wu et al, 1984).

TABLE 4.

Comparison of Properties of three Phospholipases A from the Venom of *Agkistrodon blomhoffii brevicaudus*

Property	Phospholipase A		
	Acidic	Neutral	Basic
Isoelectric point	4.5	6.9	9.3
Enzymatic activity	6.9	1.4	2.2
Lethal potency			
(LD$_{50}$ mg/kg mice)	300	0.055	20
Biological activity	Platelet aggregation inhibitor	Presynaptic neurotoxin	Haemolysin

Complete Amino Acid Sequence of Acidic Phospholipase A (Chen et al, 1987)

.10
Ser.Leu.Ile.Gln.Phe.Glu.Thr.Leu.Ile.Met.Lys.Val.Ala.Lys.Lys.Ser. Gly.Met.Phe.Trp
30
Tyr.Ser.Asn.Tyr.Gly.Cys.Tyr.Cys.Gly.Trp.Gly.Gly.Gln.Gly.Arg.Pro.Gln.Asp.Ala.Thr.
50
Asp.Arg.Cys.Cys.Phe.Val.His.Asp.Cys.Cys.Tyr.Gly.Lys.Val.Thr.Gly.Cys.Asp.Pro.Lys.
70
Met.Asp.Val.Tyr.Ser.Phe.Ser.Glu.Glu.Asn.Gly.Asp.Ile.Val.Cys.Gly.Gly.Asp.Asp.Pro.
90
Cys.Lys.Lys.Glu.Ile.Cys.Glu.Cys.Asp.Arg.Ala.Ala.Ala.Ile.Cys.Phe.Arg.Asp.Asn.Leu.
110
Thr.Leu.Tyr.Asn.Asp.Lys.Lys.Tyr.Trp.Ala.Phe.Gly.Ala.Lys.Asn.Cys.Pro.Gln.Glu.Glu.
124
Ser.lu.Pro.Cys.

Partial Amino Acid Sequences of Neutral and Basic Phospholipases A (Chen et al, 1987)

10
Neutral   Asn.Leu.Leu.Gln.Phe.Asn.Lys.Met.Ile.Lys.Glu.Glu.Thr. Gly.Lys.Asn.Ala.
Basic   Asn.Leu.Leu.Gln.Phe.Arg.Lys.Met.Ile.Lys.Lys.Met.Thr.Gly.Lys.Glu.—.

20.   30
Neutral   Ilu.Pro.Phe.—Tyr.Ala.Phe.Tyr.Gly.Cys.Tyr.Cys.Gly.Trp.Gly.Gly.Gln.
Basic   Val.Val.Trp.Tyr.Ala.Phe.Tyr.Gly.Cys.Tyr.Cys.Gly.—.Gly.—.Gly.

40.
Neutral   Gly.Lys.Pro.Lys.Asp.Gly.Thr.Asp.(R).Cys.Cys.Phe.Val.(H).Asp.Cys.Cys.
Lys.

53
Tyr.Gly.—

It should be pointed out that this presynaptic neurotoxin is a unique one like notexin from the Australian tiger snake venom, with a single polypeptide chain phospholipase A_2. Why these three phospholipases A_2 from the same venom have such diverse biological activities may be due to the structure and function relationship and studies on primary and spatial structure need to be conducted. Crystal structure is currently investigated by the research group in Institute of Biophysics in Beijing, using X-ray crystallography (Gui et al, 1987).

Bradykinin potentiating peptide (BPP) had been purified from the venom of *A. b. brevicaudus*. Interesting results on structure and function study by Edman degradation had been obtained (Wang et al, 1983). After removal of the N-terminal residue, pyroglutamyl, of this decapeptide BPP, the activity enhanced two-fold, then decreased gradually during the course of stepwise degradation. The final tripeptide, Ile.Pro.Pro. still retained 90% of the original activity. In the case of C-terminal dipeptide the activity disappeared abruptly. These data would be meaningful for the design of peptide drugs for disease of hypertension.

Pry-Glu.Gly.Arg.Pro.Gly.Pro.Pro.Ile.Pro.Pro.
1   5   10
BPP from the venom of *Agkistrodon blomhoffii brevicaudus*

Proteases in snake venoms involving haemorrhage and necrosis remain poorly understood. Xu et al (1981) had purified 5 components of haemorrhagic toxins from the venom of *Agkistrodon acutus*, which can be inhibited by the chemical reagent EDTA accompanying abolition of both proteolytic and haemorrhagic activities, shown to be metalloproteases. Chemical modification of haemorrhagic toxin 1 showed 3 of the 7 histidine residues being blocked and losing enzyme activities. The activity recovered after deblocking, showing that at least one histidine residue is essential for the enzymatic activity, but modification of tryptophane did not affect the activity, hence tryptophane residue is not essential (Xu et al, 1985).

Snake Bite Incidence in China

Nearly 80% of the population of China live in rural areas, especially in the southern regions, and face the danger of snake bite. Chinese traditional herbal medicine was used for treatment of snake bite, however, fatality remained high. In the 1950s a research group of the Department of Pharmacology, Zhongshan Medical College, engaged in the study of Chinese herbs used for treatment of snake bite. The results with experimental animals showed some protective effect but the mechanism is still not fully understood. Since 1960s, Shanghai Institute of Biological Products had produced antivenins. There are now six antivenins supplying the whole country (Table 5). Although antivenins are the best treatment, Chinese surgeons like to combine antivenins with Chinese herbal medicines for treatment of snake bite.

Antivenin against *A.b. brevicaudus* can be used for snake bite of all species of Agkistrodons. That against *A. acutus* and *brevicaudus* can be used for genus *Trimeresurus*, as they have crossed immunological reactions among the venom

273

TABLE 5.
Potency and Dosage of Antivenins Against Snake Venoms

Antivenins	Potency i.u./ampoule in 10 ml	Dosage	Treatment of snake bite
Agkistrodon halys	6,000	6,000-24,000	A.halys, Trimeresurus stejnegeri, T.macrosquamatus
A. acutus	2,000	4,000-8,000	A.acutus, T.stejnegeri T.mucrosquamatus
Bungarus multicinctus	8,000	8,000-16,000	B.multicinctus
B. fasciatus	5,000	5,000-10,000	B.fasciatus
Naja naja	1,000	2,000- 4,000	N.naja
V.russelli	5,000	5,000-10,000	V.russelli

(Protein concentration is about 15%, data from Shanghai Institute of Biological Products).

proteins. But the antivenins of Elapidae and Viperidae are very specific, so the accurate identification of species involved in snake bite is very important before using these antivenins. Two research groups, Guangsi Medical College and Anhui Chinese Traditional Medical College, had developed two fast test methods which need only about 15 minutes using a few ml of liquid from the wound.

Since the widespread use of antivenins to treat snake bite poisoning, fatality has dropped. It was estimated by Haining People's Hospital that fatality by pit viper bite of 5 — 8% has in recent years, dropped below 1. Haining County is located in Zhejiang plain with rice fields covering 681 square kilometres and has 592,000 people. *A.b. brevicaudus* is the only poisonous snake here. From 1973 to 1985, the Haining People's Hospital had received 1,427 snake bite poisoning patients. All recovered except one who died. The treatment was antivenin combined with Chinese traditional herbs (Yue et al, 1986).

Another data set of 120 cases of snake bite by five pace snake *(Agkistrodon acutus)* in the years from 1972 to 1986 treated with antivenin in Kaihua People's Hospital (Huang, 1986), was as follows:-

Fully recovered	87	
Died	2	
Disability	31	(necrosis 19, amputation 2, others 10)
Total	120	

Kaihua County is located in southwest Zhejiang Province which is a hilly region with warmer weather than Haining and contains many venomous snakes.

The snake bite by *Bungarus multicinctus* (silver krait) is usually easy to be ignored as no pain, redness or swelling of the wounds occur. A few hours later, difficulty in respiration can lead to respiratory arrest. Lee et al in Guangsi Medical College had successfully saved 11 out of 13 patients bitten by this snake. The shortest duration from arrest to automatic rerespiration was 10 hours and 45 minutes, the longest 864 hours, in which administration of antivenin and trypsin for local injection accompanying artifical respiration (Lee et al, 1981).

References

Chen, Y.C., Wu, X.F., Zhang, J.K., Jiang, M.S. and Hsu, K. (1981). Further purification and biochemical properties of presynaptic neurotoxin from the snake venom of *Agkistrodon halys pallas.* Acta Biochem. Biophys. Sin. 13, 205 (in Chinese).

Chen, Y.C. Maraganore, J.M., Readon, I. and Heinrikson, R.L. (1987). Characterization of the structure and function of three phospholipases A$_2$ from the venom of *Agkistrodon halys pallas.* Toxicon, 25, 401-409.

Gui. L.L., Bi, R.C., Lin, Z.J. and Chen, Y.C. (1987). The preliminary studies of crystallography of the neutral phospholipase A from the snake venom of *Agkistrodon halys pallas.* Ke Xus Tong Bao, 10, 776-777. (in Chinese).

Hu, S.Q. and Zhao, E.M. (1979). Venomous snake in China, 1. Major groups and distribution of venomous snakes, in book 'Venomous Snakes, Protection and Treatment of Snake Bite in China' edited by Chengdu Institute of Biology, Shanghai Natural Museum and Zhejiang Institute of Chinese Medicine.

Hu, X.R., Deng, C.R., Sun, J.J. Zeng, W.Y. Zhang, M.S. and Hong, X.J. (1979). Snake venoms, in book 'Venomous Snakes, Protection and Treatment of Snake Bite in China' pp. 117-175. (in Chinese).

Huang, D.G. (1986). Clinical obervation treatment with antivenins in 120 cases of snake bite incidence by five pace snakes. Rural Hospital, 2, 58 — 59. (in Chinese).

Lee, C.Y., Chang, C.C., Su, C. and Chen, Y.W. (1962). The toxicity and thermostability of Formosa snake venoms. J. Formosan Med. Assoc., 61, 239 in Tu, A. T. (ed) 'Venoms; Chemistry and Molecular Biology' John Wiley & Sons, Inc. p. 225.

Lee, H.P., Lin, K.K. and Liao, G.S. (1981). Emergent treatment of respiration arrest by snake bite of Chinese krait *(Bungarus multicinctus* Blyth). An analysis of artificial respiration of 13 cases. Zool. Res. 2, Supplement, 167-168. (in Chinese).

Wang, M.Y., Lo, S.S., Chi, C.W. (1983). Studies on the bradykinin potentiating peptide (BPP) from the venom of Zhejiang pit viper *(Agkistrodon halys pallas).* 9, 15 — 16 (in Chinese).

Wu, X.F., Jiang, Z.P. and Chen, Y.C. (1984). A comparison of three phospholipase A$_2$ from the venom of *Agkistrodon halys pallas.* Acta, Biochim, Biophys. Sin. 16, 664-671. (in Chinese).

Xu, X., Wang, C., Liu, J. and Lu, Z. (1981). Purification and characterization of haemorrhagic components from *Agkistrodon acutus* (hundred pace snake) venom. Toxicon, 19, 633.

Xu, X., Zhu, Y.H., Wang, Y.Z., Ma, Y. and Lu, Z.X. (1985). Studies on the chemical modification of haemorrhagic toxin 1 from five pace snake *(Agkistrodon acutus)* venom. Toxicon, 23, 283 — 288.

Zhang, J.K., Xu, K., Yu, J.B., Liu, H. and Ren, J. (1985). Presynaptic toxins from *Agkistrodon intermedius* venom. Acta Herpet. Sin. 4, 291-295. (in Chinese).

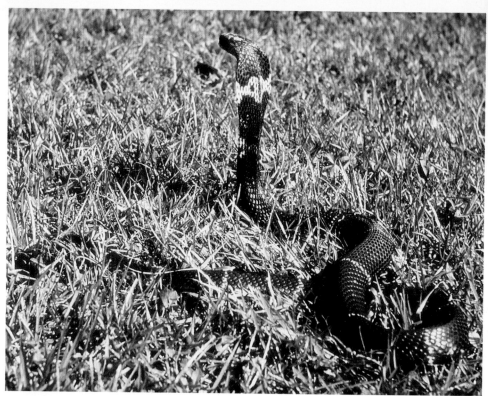

Figure 1
Naja naja atra

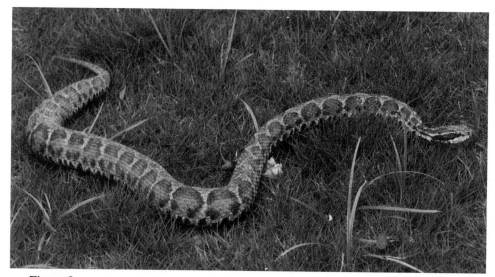

Figure 2
Agkistrodon halys (pit viper)

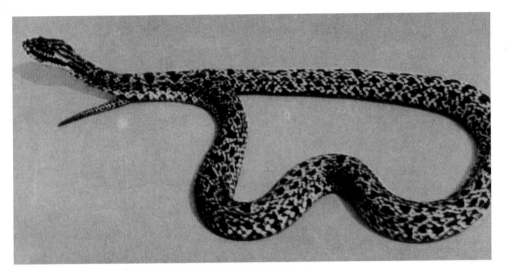

Figure 3
Trimeresurus jerdonii

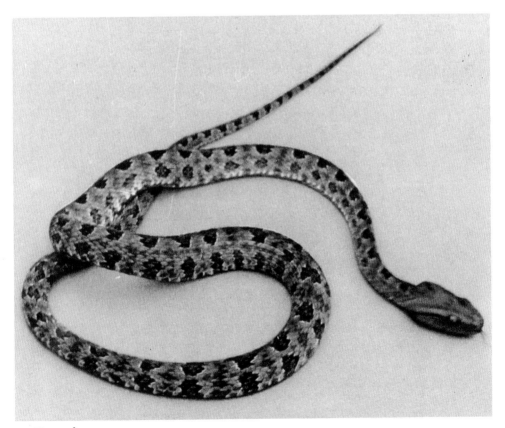

Figure 4
Trimeresurus mucrosquamatus (Flat iron head)

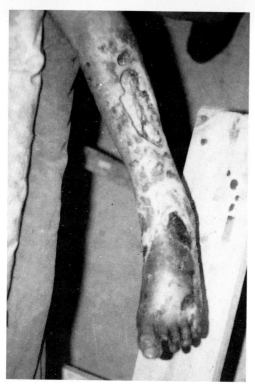

Figure 5
Necrosis by snakebite *Agkistrodon acutus*

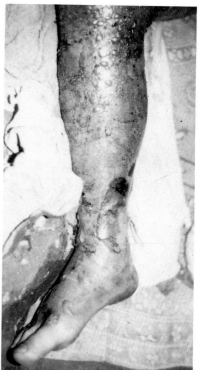

Figure 6
Necrosis by snake bite, by *Agkistrodon acutus* (Five pace snake), offered by Institute of Snakebite in Qimen, Anhui Province.

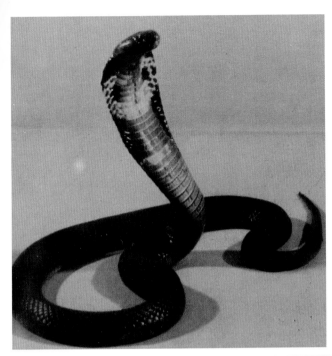

Figure 7
Naja naja (cobra)

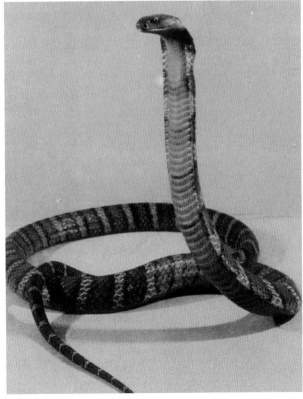

Figure 8
Ophiophagus hannah
(King Cobra)

Venomous Snakes Of Medical Importance In India (Part A)

T.S.N. Murthy
Zoological Survey of India, India.

Introduction

India lies in the southern peninsula of the Asian continent between latitudes 8°4'N and 37°6'N and longitudes 68°7'E and 97°25'E. Its land area, including the main land mass, the Bay Islands (the Andamans and the Nicobars), and the Lakshadweep in the Arabian Sea, exceeds 3 million km². As one might expect, a vast country like India varies enormously both physically and climatically. Its physiography falls into three well-defined regions: first, the great Himalayan mountain system; second, the Indo-Gangetic plain, and third, the Deccan plateau. The average rainfall varies from 100 mm in the Thar desert of Rajasthan, to about 5000 mm in Cherapunji in Meghalaya. The temperature also varies greatly, shooting up to 49°C in some places and dropping to zero in other places. The vegetation changes from tropical evergreen forests to arid desert tracts.

Concentration of the Snake Fauna

In India, as elsewhere in the tropics, man and snakes coexist and confront each other in sudden and unexpected encounters. The snakes fauna of India, like the other animal groups, consists of the principal elements — the oriental, the palaerctic, and the Ethiopian.

Snakes live in a variety of habitats: human dwellings, dilapidated buildings, marshy lands, lakes, estuaries, agricultural areas, forests and even in mountains up to elevations of 5000 m.

Cultivated areas abounding in manure heaps, refuse pits, garden beds and plantations hold an undeniable attraction for snakes. Rice fields in particular are a haven for insects and frogs which in turn provide better feeding conditions for snakes. A wall of loose stones in an ill-constructed farm building serves as a good hiding place for snakes of all kinds.

The heavy concentration of venomous snakes can be found in the cultivated areas of the States like West Bengal, Orissa, Andhra Pradesh, Tamil Nadu, and Kerala.

Snakebite as a Medical Problem in India

An accurate estimate of the mortality from snakebite in India, is almost impossible owing to the insuperable difficulties of recording them. However, a more recent figure is 10,000 to 15,000 deaths per annum. A record number of deaths occur in West Bengal. A number of people die due to snakebite in the

States of Maharastra, Gujarat, Kerala, Andhra Pradesh, Madhya Pradesh, Uttar Pradesh, Bihar, and Orissa as well.

Throughout India the frequency of snakebite is at its peak in the rainy season which coincides with increased agricultural operations. The flooded paddy fields and low lands with their teeming populations of fish, frogs, and lizards provide a favourable feeding and breeding ground for snakes. It is during this season that the eggs of the cobras and kraits hatch. The inadequately clad farmers and agricultural labourers working barefooted suffer heavy casualties. The catastrophic floods, apart from the devastation they cause, bring human beings and snakes closer. Thus snakebite in India is mainly a rural and occupational hazard. Farmers and their families, therefore, are the main victims. Most snakebites occur during the evening or at night. The Indian krait is implicated in a majority of the fatal snakebites that occur during this time. It is said to bite those sleeping on the floor. The cobra sees better at night and strikes with a determination and the intent to hold on to the victim.

Sawai et al. (1975) collected the information on snakebite deaths recorded in some major States of India, based on the cases reported to the hospitals:

State	Number of deaths
West Bengal	384
Maharastra	100
Kerala	97
Madhya Pradesh	90
Uttar Pradesh	68
Rajasthan	62
Karnataka	36
Jammu and Kashmir	33
Tamil Nadu	31
Orissa	27
Andhra Pradesh	23
Bihar	21

List of very Common Venomous Snakes of India

There are fewer than 240 species of snakes in India. Of these, some 50 species including 20 living in the sea are venomous. But there are only four venomous snakes which are very common and are of medical importance. Leading the list would be the cobra *(Naja naja)*, followed by the common krait *(Bungarus caeruleus)*, the Russell's viper *(Vipera russelli)* and the Saw-scaled viper *(Echis carinatus)*. The other venomous snakes either are not toxic enough to be dangerous to man, or rarely encountered. Bites by pit vipers of the genera *Agkistrodon, Hypnale,* and *Trimeresurus* seldom produce fatalities. Deaths due to sea snakes are not recorded. The king cobra is an insignificant cause of death because it is a very uncommon snake in India. Coral snake bites are exceedingly rare. The four dangerously venomous snakes, however, live in cohabitation with men. They share his fields, his gardens or the scrub and rubble near his home.

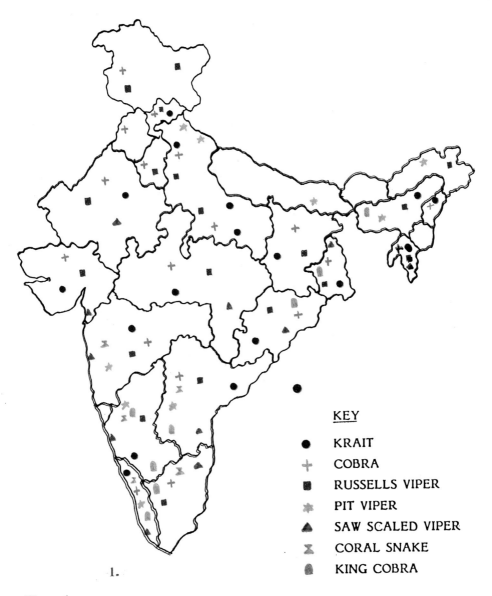

KEY

● KRAIT
✝ COBRA
▣ RUSSELLS VIPER
✳ PIT VIPER
▲ SAW SCALED VIPER
✕ CORAL SNAKE
⬮ KING COBRA

Figure 1
Distribution of Venomous Snakes in India (Khaire etal).

The very common venomous snakes of India may be classified as follows:

REPTILIA
Order SQUAMATA
    Suborder Serpentes (Ophidia)
        Family Elapidae
            Genus *Bungarus* Daudin
                Bungarus caeruleus (Schneider)
            Genus *Naja* Laurcnti
                Naja naja (Linn.)
        Family Viperidae
            Genus *Vipers* Laurenti
                Vipera russelli (Shaw)
            Genus *Echis* Merrem
                Echis carinatus (Schneider)

Description of the Common Venomous Snakes of India

Bungarus caeruleus (Schneider)

English names

Common Indian krait; Blue krait.

Vernacular names

Bengali Kalaz, Domna Chitti: *Hindi* Manner or kariat; *Kannada* kadambale; *Malayalam* Vella pambu; *Marathi* Manyar; *Tamil* Kattu viriyan; *Telugu* Katla pamu.

Description

Head flat. Neck hardly evident. Body rather cylindrical, tapering towards the tail. Tail short, rounded. Eye rather small, with a rounded pupil, indistinguishable in life. Head shields normal, no loreal; four shields along the margin of the lower lip; 3rd and 4th supraoculars touching the eye. Scales highly polished, in 15-17 rows; the vertebral row distinctly enlarged and hexagonal. Ventrals 185-225. caudals 37-50, entire.

Colour and pattern (Fig. 2)

Generally black or bluish black, with about 40 thin, white crossbars which may be indistinct or absent anteriorly. The pattern however, is complete and well defined in the young which are marked with conspicuous crossbars even anteriorly; in old individuals the narrow white lines may be found as a series of connected spots, with a prominent spot on the vertebral region. A white preocular spot may be present: upper lips and the belly white.

Size

Adults range in length from 1 m to 1.75 m. Males are longer with proportionately longer tails.

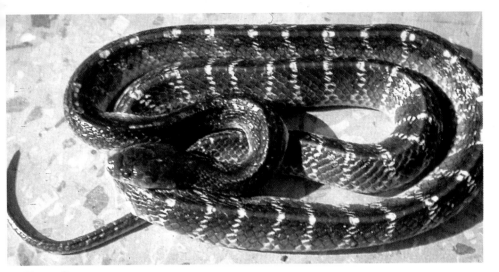

Figure 2
Common Indian Krait (*Bungarus caeruleus*) (T.S.N. Murthy)

Habitat and Habits

The common krait is essentially a plains snake and is usually found in the open country, cultivated areas, and scrub jungles at low altitudes. It seems to avoid a very rocky and sandy terrain. Its favourite dwelling places are the termite mounds, rat holes and bushes of other rodents, heaps of rubbish, manure or brick in the open country and the gardens, roofs of houses and forsaken buildings and other secluded or cool spots in or near the human buildings. It is fond of water. Like the common cobra, it enters the human dwellings frequently.

The krait is strictly nocturnal in its habits and is not seen usually during the day. It becomes active at night and moves quickly. It sometimes turns cannibalistic and feeds exclusively on snakes including its own kind. It also feeds on small mammals, lizards, frogs and toads. The krait is remarkably quiet and inoffensive in disposition, biting only under severe provocation. When alarmed in the wild, it makes no attempt to escape or defend but lies quietly and conceals the head in the coils of its body. The female krait lays from 6 to 12 eggs which are deposited in holes in the ground, or under leaves and stays with the clutch till the young emerge.

May be confused with

The harmless wolf snakes *Lycodon aulicus*, with the crossbars on the back superficially resembles the common krait. Not only does the wolf snake prefer human habitations but it also is nocturnal in its habits. However, the snakes can be easily told apart by a close examination of the colour pattern: the white-lines across the back appear very near the head in the wolf snakes whereas they appear beyond the neck and extend up to the end of the tail in the krait.

Distribution

India, Pakistan, and Sri Lanka.

Venom

The krait's venom is more toxic, perhaps six to eight times, than that of the cobra. Its fangs are short and the venom yield is 8-12 mgm, of which very little, probably 2-3 mgm may be considered as a lethal dose for a human adult.

Naja naja naja (Linn.)

English names

Common cobra; Indian cobra.

Vernacular names

Bengali Gokhura; *Hindi* Nag; *Kannada* Nagara havu; *Malayalam* Moorkan; *Marathi* Nag.

Tamil Nalla pambu; Naga pambu; *Telugu* Thrachu pamu; Nagu pamu.

Description

Snout rounded, short. Head depressed, not very distinct from neck; neck wide, dilatable to form a hood (in life); nostril large, between the nasals; 1 preocular, in contact with the internasals; loreal absent; 7 supralabials, 3rd largest, 3rd and 4th touching the eye; a tiny angular shield called 'cuneate' present between the fourth and fifth infralabials. Eye moderate, pupil round. Body dorsoventrally flattened and subcylindrical behind. Scales smooth, strongly oblique, in 21-25 rows. Ventrals 176-200, caudals 48-75, paired.

Colour and pattern

The usual colouration is dark brown or black to yellowish white above and white or yellowish below. Apart from the well-defined "spectacle" mark on the expanded hood, a cobra can be distinguished from other land snakes by the presence of a dark spot on either side of the underside of the hood and two or more broad black crossbands further below. (Figs. 3 & 4).

Size

Adults average from 1 m to 2 m in length. Males are longer.

Habitat and Habits

The most distinctive and impressive characteristic is the hood which is formed by raising the anterior portion of the body and spreading some of the ribs in the neck region when the snake is annoyed or frightened. While displaying the hood, the common cobra can erect itself from one quarter to more than two-thirds of its total length. We are so familar with the pictures of them displaying their hoods that some of us do not realise that the cobra looks like any other snake when it is not displaying its hood.

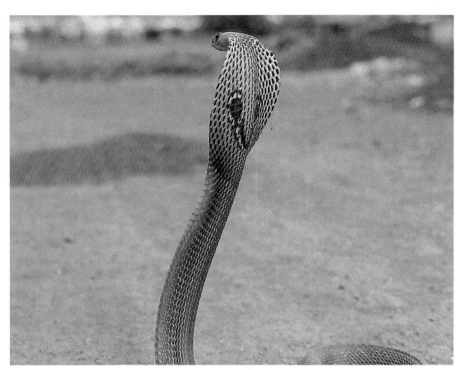

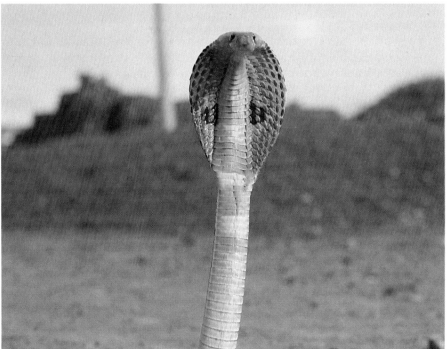

Figures 3 & 4
Dorsal and ventral views of the hood of the common cobra (N. Khaire)

287

Cobras are remarkably adaptable snakes and found in all types of country; plains, jungles, open fields, and even in the regions heavily populated by man. Their favourite haunts are the holes in embankments, hollows of trees, old termite mounds, ruined buildings, rock-piles, and dens of small mammals. They are fond of water and prefer the late afternoon and early evening hours for moving about and seeking food. It is said that their vision is quite good and that they can see moving objects situated at a distance up to 3 m.

Cobras feed chiefly on rats, mice, toads and frogs but birds, eggs, and other snakes are also eaten. Females usually lay from 10 to 30 eggs in rat holes or termite mounds and the young when hatched are exact replicas of the parents. Cobras have strong parental instincts as the pair tend to remain together from the time of mating till when the young hatch.

Cobras are not aggressive snakes and tend to escape when encountered in the wild. They strike only when accidentally stepped on or are under extreme provocation. When cornered, they spread the hood, hiss, sway the body from side to side, and strike repeatedly. The cobra's strike is said to be ineffective during the day but is considered much more severe and a determined one at night when the snake sees better. Young cobras are much more aggressive than adults. The young, less than 30 cm long, are capable of rearing up, spreading their hoods and are ready to follow up the intimidatory gesture with a venomous bite. It is on record that the bite of a 5-day old cobra caused the death of a guinea pig 22 minutes later.

Others varieties

Two varieties are recognised: the one with a white circle round a black spot on the hood *(Naja naja kaouthia)* (Fig. 5) is a found in Bengal and Orissa and the other with a plain hood *(Naja naja oxiana)* is common in parts of Gujarat, Rajasthan, Punjab, and Kashmir. The king cobra (Fig. 6) *(Ophiophagus hannah)*, despite all the stories about its aggressive temperament, is an uncommon snake in India.

May be confused with

The common cobra is often confused with the large sized (3 m) and equally aggressive rat snake *(Ptyas mucosus)* but the narrow neck and the thin head of a rat snake establishes its identity.

Distribution

Throughout the Indian subcontinent and Sri Lanka.

Venom

The average discharge of venom at bite is about 211 mg and the poison is mainly neurotoxic. The adult cobra's fangs are about 7 mm in length. According to Gharpurey (1935) a man bitten by a cobra will usually die within 2 to 6 hours of the bite and some cases in which death occurred within half an hour have been reported.

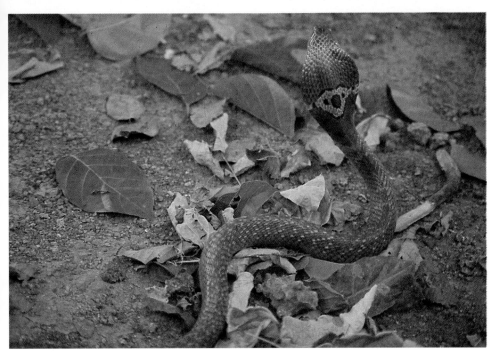

Figure 5
Naja naja kaouthia (N. Khaire)

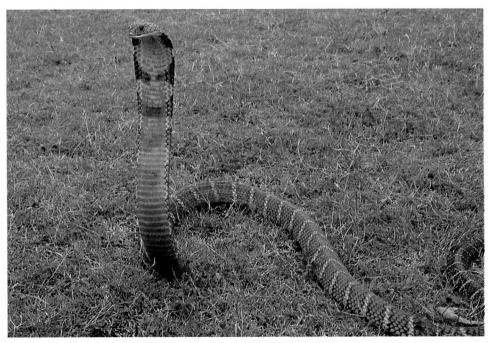

Figure 6
King Cobra *(Ophiophagus hannah)* (N. Khaire)

Family Viperidae

Vipera russelli (Shaw)

English names

Russell's viper.

Vernacular names

Bengali Chandra bora: *Gujarati* Chitra: *Hindi* Daboia: *Kannada* Mandalatha havu: *Malayalam* Mandali: *Marathi* Ghonas: *Sindhi* Koraile: *Tamil* Kannadi viriyan: *Telugu* Raktha pinjara: Katukarekula poda.

Description

Head flat, triangular, and covered with small scales; snout short and bluntly pointed; nostril large, crescent shaped. Eye large, with vertical pupil. Body stout, short, and flattened dorsoventrally. Scales strongly keeled and arranged in 17-23 rows. Ventrals 153-180, caudals 41-64, paired. Tail short.

Colour and pattern

Light-brown above with a bold and distinct pattern consisting of three rows of large, dark oval spots: head with two large black spots at base and a light V-shaped mark with its apex on top of snout; lower parts yellowish white or marbled with brown (Figs. 7 & 8).

Size

1 m — 1.85 m.

Habitat and habits

The Russell's viper is found both in the plains and hills even at elevations up to 3000 m. It is partial to open country, where it is found in the bushy areas, grasslands, farmlands, cultivated fields, and rocky areas. It avoids the hot weather during summer by hiding in the termite mounds and rat holes.

The Russsell's viper is a sluggish and quiet snake during most of the day although it remains alert always. It becomes active in the evening and at night when it wanders about in a slow, crawling motion. It does not move away quickly when disturbed but holds the ground and emits a loud hiss to indicate its annoyance. Although it does not strike readily, the Russell's viper can bite with force and determination if injured or provoked with its highly efficient biting mechanism and large fangs. The young are more aggressive than the adults.

The Russell's viper feeds chiefly upon small mammals but lizards, birds, and frogs are also taken occasionally.

May be confused with

Three harmless snakes namely the Indian Python *(Python molurus)*, the Common Sand Boa *(Eryx conicus)* and the Royal Snake *(Sparelosophis*

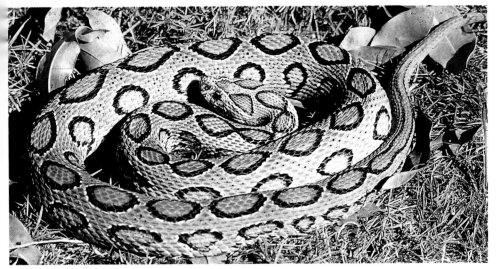

Figure 7
Russell's Viper *(Vipera russelli)* (T.S.N. Murthy)

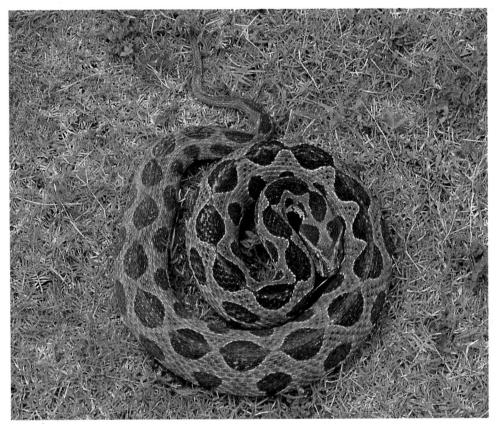

Figure 8
Russell's Viper *(Vipera russelli)* (N. Khaire)

diadema) resemble the Russell's viper superficially. But they all lack the broad belly plates, the minute scales on the head, the chain-like black spots on the body and the divided subcaudals which are characteristic of the Russell's viper.

Venom
The venom discharged at a bite may be about 145 mgm.

Echis carinatus (Schneider)
English names
Saw-scaled viper; The Little Indian Viper.

Vernacular names
Bengali Bankoray; *Gujarati* Taracha; *Hindi* Afai; *Kannada* Kallu havu; *Malayalam* Churuta; *Marathi* Phoorsa; *Tamil* Suruttai pambu.

Description
Head triangular, very distinct from neck. Eye with vertical pupil. Scales keeled, in 27-37 rows, the laterals serrated. Ventrals 132-185, caudals 23-39. Tail short.

Colour and pattern
It is usually brown, buff, sandy or greenish above and white below, speckled with brown or black. The usual pattern comprises a pale sinuous white line running down the back. Head with a characteristic white cross-like mark which appears like the imprint of a bird's foot (Figs. 9 & 10)

Size
30 cm — 80 cm.

Habitat and Habits
The Saw-scaled viper is partial to semi-arid tracts, preferring the sandy soil, sans jungles or thick vegetation. Its favourite haunts are small hills and scrub jungles. It seems to be fond of basking in the scorching heat of the midday sun. When alarmed, it throws itself into a double coil somewhat looking like figure 8 and rubs the sides of the body, producing a violent rustling sound. It is a very nervous snake, and quick to strike at the slightest provocation. It is said that this little viper flings itself about 30 cm or so in the air to deliver the bite. Despite its small size, this viper's habit of lying in the sand with only the head exposed poses a threat to the inhabitants of the desert area.

May be confused with
The rear-fanged colubrid *Boiga trigonata* is mistaken for the saw-scaled viper owing to their superficial resemblance. However, the presence of the minute scales on the head of the viper distinguishes it easily from the cat snake which has shields on the head.

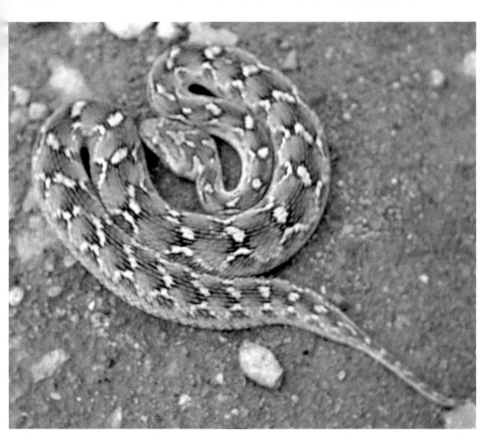

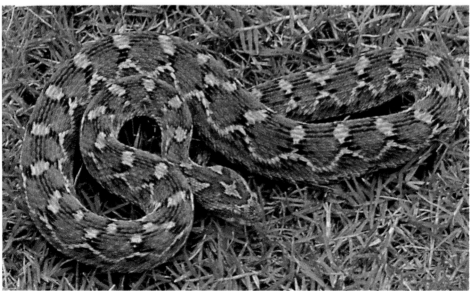

Figures 9 & 10
Saw-Scaled Viper *(Echis carinatus)* showing colour variation (Murthy & Khaire)

Distribution

The Saw-scaled viper is found in the whole of India south of the Ganges, except Bengal. As it is partial to the dry country, it is especially abundant on the coramondel coast. It is very common in the States of Maharastra, Tamil, Nadu, and Andhra Pradesh.

Venom

The venom of this viper is said to be five times as toxic as cobra venom and sixteen times as toxic as Russell's viper venom. Despite its size, the fangs are remarkably long; a 380 mm long specimen having fangs 5 mm in length. The lethal dose for a human adult is estimated to be 5 mg and the average venom yield varies from 18 mg to 72 mg. According to Gharpurey *(op. cit.)*, death may occur within 24 hours or even after 2 to 20 days following the bite and that nearly 10 to 20 percent of the victims bitten by this viper die.

A Simplified Key to the Identification of the Common Venomous Snakes of India

1. Head with small scales between the eyes 2
   Head with small shields between the eyes ....,...................... 3
2. Dorsal scales oblong; size large; chain-like black spots in three series on the back; size large .... *Vipera russelli*
   (Russell's viper)

   Dorsal scales serrated at the sides; a zigzag like sinuous white line on the sides of the body; size small .... *Echis carinatus*
   (Saw-scaled viper)
3. Back with a middle row of scales enlarged and almost hexagonal; fourth lower labial largest. Neck not dilatable (in life) ....:..... *Bungarus caeruleus*
   (Common krait)

   Back without hexagonal scales; third supralabial largest; neck dilatable into a hood (in life) .... *Naja naja*
   (Indian cobra)

Snake Venom Research in India: A Review

The earliest reference to Indian snakes available might be credited to Dr. Patrick Russell who may rightly be called the 'Father of Indian Ophiology'. The credit for distinguishing the venomous from the non-venomous snakes goes to him. It was he who focussed attention on the viper *Vipera russelli*, which was appropriately named after him. He has extensively studied the dentition of the harmless and dangerous species and based his conclusions after conducting a series of experiments on the toxicity of their venoms when injected into other animals. Russell's original work (1796) was made good use of by the latter workers like Boulenger (1890) and Smith (1943). Sir J.B. Fayrer (1873, 1892) was another physician cum surgeon turned ophiologist. Availing himself of the leisure he could afford from his strenous duties, he wrote a book entitled 'Thantoophidia of India' in 1874. He had carried out detailed investigations on the physiology of venoms of Indian snakes. Joseph Ewart's (1878) book on the poisonous snakes of India was also an invaluable publication. Col. Frank Wall's (1908) services in the cause of Indian ophiology will never be forgotten because it was he more than any other ophiologist who strived hard to add to our knowledge of the habits and distribution of Indian snakes. His work entitled 'The Poisonous Terrestrial Snakes of our British Indian Dominions and How to Recognise them' bears his stamp of authority on the subject. Dr. Malcolm Smith's (1943) celebrated volume on snakes in the Fauna of British India series continues to be the standard digest of literature.

It was Colonel Gharpurey (1935), a medical man turned ophiologist, who first attempted to dispel the ignorance and superstition woven around the Indian snakes, both venomous and non-venomous. His book entitled 'Snakes of India' (1935), written in semi-technical language, is a mine of information on the venomous snakes. Several medical personnel have conducted investigations on the venomous snakes of India and the properties of their venoms. The list of such workers is long and exhaustive but the reader is referred to the admirable work by Russell and Scharffenberg (1964) which contained all the citations. Nevertheless mention should be made of the pioneering work carried out in recent times by Ahuja and Gurkripal Singh (1954), Deoras (1963, 1965, 1968, 1971) and Whitaker (1978). Daniel (1983) has given detailed facts and figures in respect of the venom of the common venomous snakes. Murthy (1985) discussed the common venomous snakes of India and also gave an account of these snakes (1986) for the benefit of the layman. The review of the progress of snakes venom research in India will be incomplete without paying our tributes to the services rendered by the three famous institutes namely (1) the Haffkine Institute for Training, Research & Testing, (2) the Haffkine Bio-Pharmaceutical Corporation Ltd, and (3) the Central Research Institute which served as catalysts for the dissemination of knowledge related to the venomous snakes of India and their venoms, preparation of anti-snake venom sera, and treatment of snakebite etc.

Treatment

The antivenin is prepared at the Haffkin Bio-Pharmaceutical Corporation Ltd., Bombay and Central Research Institute, Kassuli, by hyperimmunising horses against the venom of the four very common venomous snakes discussed in the present paper. Dr. R.C. Kankonkar, General Manager, Haffkine Bio-Pharmaceutical Corporation Ltd writes: "There is no fixed potency as such of the snake venom used in immunization of horses . . . . . the quantity of venom administratered for hyperimmunization depends upon horse's response, route of administration of injection, antigenicity of venom, etc".

Acknowledgements

I am grateful to Dr. P. Gopalakrishnakone, Department of Anatomy, Faculty of Medicine, National University of Singapore, Singapore for the suggestion that I write a chapter on the venomous snakes of India and for his continued encouragement in preparation of this paper. I am also thankful to the Assistant

Director, Haffkine Institute for training, research and testing, Bombay, General Manager, Haffkine Bio-pharmaceutical Corporation Ltd., Bombay and the Director, Central Research Institute, Kasauli for furnishing valuable information pertaining to the manufacture of antivenin and details of treatment of the snakebite in India. Finally, I reserve my special thanks to the Director, Zoological Survey of India, Calcutta for his keen interest in my work.

References

Ahuja, M.L. and Gurkripal Singh, 1954. Snakebite in India. *Indian J. Med. Res.* 42: 664-680.

Boulenger, G.A. 1980. *The Fauna of British India, including Ceylon and Burma.* Reptilia and Batrachia. London. 541 pp., text-figs.

Daniel, J.C. 1983. *The Book of Indian Reptiles.* (A Bombay Natural History Society's Publication).

Deoras, P.J. 1963. Studies on Bombay Snakes: Snake Farm Venom Yield Records and their probable significance. *in* H.L. Keegan and W.V. Macfarlane eds., Venomous and Poisonous Animals of the Pacific Region: 337-349. (Oxford: Pergamon Press, Inc.)

Deoras, P.J. 1965 *Snakes of India.* xiii + 156 pp. New Delhi (National Book Trust).

Deoras, P.J. 1968. Toxicity of salivary secretions in some Indian snakes. *Proceed.* 11th *Pan Pacific Congress,* Tokyo 8: 22.

Deoras, P.J. 1971. The story of some Indian poisonous snakes *in Venomous Animals and their Venom,* 2: 19-34. (New York: Academic Press).

Ewart, J. 1878. *The Poisonous Snakes of India.* 64 pp., Col. pls. (New Delhi: The English Book Store).

Fayrer, J. 1873. Snake-poisoning in India. *Med. Times Gaz.* 1: 601.

Fayrer, J. 1892. The venomous snakes of India and the mortality caused by them. *B.M.J. J.:* 620.

Gharpurey, K.G. 1935. *The Snakes of India* (Popular). 165 pp. (Bombay: Popular Prakashan.)

Murthy, T.S.N. 1985. The common venomous snakes of India. *Everyday Science* 30(1-4): 31-36.

Murthy, T.S.N. 1986. *The Snake Book of India.* (Dehra Dun: The International Book Distributors).

Russell, F.E. and Richard S. Scharffenberg. 1964. Bibliography of snake venoms and venomous snakes. viii + 220 pp. (California: Bibliographic Associates, Inc.).

Russell, Patrick, 1796. An account of Indian Serpents collected on the coast of coramandel; containing descriptions and drawings of each species, together with experiments and remarks on their several poisons. London. 90 pp & 44 coloured pls.

Sawai, Yoshio and Manabu Homma. 1975. Snakebites in India. *The Snake* 7 (1): 1-16.

Smith, M.A. 1943. *The Fauna of British India. Reptilia and Amphibia.* Vol III. *Serpentes.* (London: Taylor and Francis).

Vidal, G.W. 1890. A list of the venomous snakes of North Kanara, with remarks as to the imperfections of existing records of the distribution of snakes and facts and statistics showing the influence of *Echis carinata* on the death-rate of the Bombay Presidency. *J. Bombay Nat. Hist. Soc.* 5:64-71.

Wall, F. 1908. The poisonous terrestrial snakes of our British Dominions (including Ceylon) and how to recognise them, with symptoms of snake poisoning and treatment. Bombay.

Whitaker, R. 1978. *Common Indian Snakes: A Field Guide.* (New Delhi: Macmillan & Co.).

Venomous Snakes of Medical Importance in India (Part B) — Clinical Aspects.

Anil Khaire[1], Neelimkumar Khaire[2] and D.N. Joshi[3]

1. Indian Herpetological Society, Poona — INDIA.
2. Poona Snake Park, Poona, INDIA.
3. B.J. Medical College, Poona — INDIA.

Introduction

India has been known as the land of snakes. It is bestowed with a rich flora and fauna. It is bounded to the north by the majestic Himalayan ranges. The Arabian Sea, The Bay of Bengal and the Indian Ocean form its coastal boundary. India with its diversified habitats, creates suitable ecological niches which are home for several kinds of snakes, both the venomous and non-venomous kinds (Murthy, 1983).

Clinical Features of Snake Bites

In a predominantly agricultural country like India with its rich ophio-fauna, the encounter between man and snake is a frequent occurrence. Snake bite victims form a significant group in the hospital practice. Documented reports are few. About 2,000,000 persons are bitten by snakes every year in India, of which about 15,000 are fatal (Swaroop and Grab, 1954). Sawai and Honma (1976) have collected the statistical data on snake bite cases. The total number of patients visiting government hospitals and dispensaries in 1969 was 24,000 of which 1100 (4.6%) cases were fatal. This documented data only indicates the tip of the iceberg of the total number of snake bite cases. This incidence is definitely phenomenally higher in comparison to any other country in the world.

Unfortunately various unscientific methods of treating snake bite victims like worshipping of God Hanuman, herbal medicines, traditional faith healers are still common in India. Transport facilities are still poor in the hilly regions and it is often very difficult to seek medical aid in time. This unfortunate delay in treatment causes fatal outcome in otherwise positively curable patients.

As it is difficult to identify the offending snake in many cases, clinical features of snake bite are conveniently classified as vasculotoxic and neuroparalytic groups.

Clinical Features in Vasculotoxic Group

Patients bitten by Russells Viper *(Vipera russelli)*, Saw Scaled Viper *(Echis carinatus)* and Bamboo Pit Viper *(Trimeresurus graminius)* present with vasculotoxic manifestations.

Apart from the general symptoms of snake bite like fright, apprehension, pain, local swelling, cellulitis, patients present the following vasculotoxic manifestations.

1. Haemorrhagic bleb at the site of bite,
2. Uncontrolled bleeding from the site of bite,
3. Bleeding diathesis. Within 2 to 24 hours of bite features like generalised ecchymosis, haemotomas and purpura appear.
4. Features suggestive of Schwartzman like phenomenon, painful large ecchymosis and purpura, gangrene of lips, tip of nose, fingers and toes,
5. Frank or microscopic haematuria,
6. Haemoptysis,
7. Gingival bleeding,
8. Haematemesis and malena,
9. Cerebral haemorrhage,
10. Acute renal shut down,
11. Shock and evidence of hepatocellular damage,
12. Gangrene of the part bitten by the snake.

The bleeding and clotting abnormalities are due to thrombocytopenia, hypofibrinogenaemia with secondary deficiency of other plasma clotting factors. Haemolysis is not commonly reported in Indian literature.

Clinical Features in Neuroparalytic Group

Patients bitten by Cobra, Krait, Sea snakes present neurotoxic symptoms which appear within 20 minutes to 15 hours of bite.

Apart from the general symptoms, the following features are seen,

1. Ptosis,
2. Diplopia,
3. Ophthalmoplegia,
4. Palatal and pharyngeal paralysis with dysphagia,
5. Dysphonia,
6. Flaccid limb paralysis,
7. Respiratory paralysis,
8. Features of anoxaemia like drowsiness, semicoma,
9. Convulsions, coma,
10. Cardiotoxic symptoms like hypotension, cardiac arrhythmia and cardiac arrest.

Neuroparalysis is seen due to either blockade of the post junctional membrane of the motor end plate as seen with cobrotoxin, alpha-bungarotoxin and erabutoxin or a presynaptic block as seen with beta-bungarotoxin (Khaire, 1987).

The d.tubocurarine like neuromuscular block produced by alpha bungarotoxin, cobrotoxin and erabutoxin is easily reversed with neostigmine while the presynaptic block produced by beta bungarotoxin resembles botulinum toxin and is not reversed by neostigmine.

Review of The Snake Bites.

After screening case histories of 700 patients of snake bite cases getting admitted in Sassoon General Hospital, Pune, from Jan. 1986 to Dec. 1986, we found venomous effects in 79 patients. Fifty patients had vasculotoxic manifestations and 29 patients showed neuroparalytic features. Clinical features were noted as shown in Tables 1 and 2 respectively.

From the Sassoon General Hospital studies (Joshi, et. al. 1987) it was seen that the early rainy season showed maximum incidence. Adult males were frequent victims, nocturnal bites were mostly neuroparalytic. Acute renal failure and acute respiratory failure were major complications. Hypotension and abnormal liver functions tests carried grave prognosis.

Management of Snake Bite Victims in India.

Apart from general supportive care, administration of Polyvalent antivenom is the mainstem of treatment of snake bite. Neostigmine with atropine to reverse the neuroparalysis is used. Ventilatory support is essential in many neuroparalytic cases. Fresh blood transfusions, transfusion of fibrinogen along with heparin is used to correct bleeding diathesis. Conservative management of acute renal failure along with active intervenation in the form of either peritoneal dialysis or haemodialysis is used to treat acute renal failure. Surgical debridement or amputation are performed whenever required.

Status of Antivenoms

The treatment of venomous snake bites in India conventionally includes the use of polyvalent antisnake venom serum. The serum is acquired through the hyperimmunization of horses with a mixture of the venoms of the four important species, namely Indian Cobra (*N. naja naja*), Common Krait (*B. caeruleus*), Russell's Viper (*V. russelli*) and Saw Scaled Viper (*E. carinatus*), is being used to process and manufacture the polyvalent antivenom. This polyvalent antivenom is presently manufactured in India by (1) Haffkine Institute, Bombay, (Fig 11) (2) Central Research Institute, Kasauli, (3) Bengal Laboratories, Calcutta, (4) King's Institute, Guindy and (5) Serum Institute of India, Poona (Fig 12).

A track record and study of snake bites in South India elaborately reveals the fact that the number of viper bites exceed the number of elapid bites. Therefore, Serum Institute has come up with a bivalent antivenom as its research product. The report of the test for estimating the efficacy of this bivalent antivenom by The Incorporated Liverpool School of Tropical Medicine, a W.H.O. Collaborative Centre for the Control of Antivenoms clearly states that although the efficacy of the bivalent antivenom in neutralisation of *E. carinatus* venom is almost similar to that of the polyvalent antivenom, it is statistically proved to be much more effective in neutralising *V. russelli* venom.

The bivalent antivenom to be launched in the Indian market is to be priced at Rs.85/- per vial of 10 ml. This costing would prove to be economically viable (Jadhav, 1987) as compared to the prices of polyvalent antivenom available in the market. At present the polyvalent antivenom vials manufactured by Serum Institute cost Rs.118/- while those manufactured by Haffkine Institute cost Rs.124/-. Therefore it is hoped that the use of bivalent and monovalent antivenom in future would be functionally and economically advantageous.

Acknowledgement

The authors wish to sum up here their immense and many sided indebtedness to Dr. D.B. Kadam of B. J. Medical College, Pune and Mr. Ajit Peshave of Indian Herpetological Society for reviewing this manuscript. We wish to express our special gratitude to Dr. S. S. Jadhav of Serum Institute for his valuable suggestions for finalising the contents of this manuscript.

References

Banerjee, R. N.   (1978)   Poisonous Snakes of India, their Venoms, Symptomatology & Treatment of Envenomation, *Progress in Clinical Medicine In India* (Second Series), *ed.* M. M. S. Ahuja *Arnold Heinemann*, 136-179.

Deoras, P.J.   (1965)   *Snakes of India, National Book Trust*, New Delhi.

Jadhav S. S.   (1987)   (Personal Communication)

Joshi, D. N. Kadam, D. B. Khaire, A. Khaire, N. and Mitra, P. D.
     (1987)   Clinical Profile of cases of Venomous Snake Bite in Sasoon General Hospitals, Pune, INDIA. Presented at *First Asia Pacific Congress on Animal Plant and Microbial Toxins* Singapore, 24-27 June 1987.

Khaire, A.   (1987)   The Snake Venom, *Times of Science & Technology*, November 7 - 10 New Delhi.

Mahendra, B. C.   (1984)   *Handbook of the Snakes of India, Ceylon, Burma, Bangla Desh and Pakistan* Academy of Zoology.

Murthy, T. S. N.   (1981)   Reptiles of the Silent Valley and New Amarambalam Area, Kerala, *The Snake* Vol. 13, 42-52.

Murthy, T. S. N.   (1983)   A Historical Resume and Bibliography of the Snakes of India, *The Snake* Vol. 15, 113-135.

Sawai, Y. and Honma, M.   (1976)   Snakes Bites in India, *Animal Plant and Microbial Toxins Vol.2.* Eds. A. Ohsaka, K. Hayashi and Y. Sawai, Plenum Press N. Y. 451-460.

Swaroop, S. and Grab, B.   (1954)   Snake bite mortality in world. *Bull W.H.O.* 10,35.

TABLE 1
Clinical features in 50 cases of vasculotoxic bites in our study (1987) Safdarjang Hospital Study of Banerjee & Siddiqui (1978).

Symptoms	Sasson General Hospital Study (Pune) Jan 1986 — Dec 1986	Safdarjang Hospital Study (New Delhi) (1971 — 1975)	
Total Cases	50	53	
Bleeding from site	Not mentioned	48	90.5%
Bleeding from gums	Not mentioned	9	16.9%
Ecchymosis, Haematoma & Purpura	29 — 58%	40	75.4%
Purpura fulminans	- - - -	16	30.1%
Haematuria	17 — 34%	47	88.7%
Acute renal failure	11 — 22%	9	16.9%
Haematemesis	Not mentioned	7	13.2%
Malena	Not mentioned	6	11.1%
Haemoptysis	Not mentioned	11	20.7%
Cerebral haemorrhage	0	6	11.1%

TABLE 2
Clinical features in 29 patients of neuroparalytic bites in our study (1987) & Safdarjang Hospital study by Banergee & Siddiqui (1976).

Symptoms	Sassoon General Hospital Study (Pune) Jan 1986 — Dec 1986		Safdarjang Hospital Study (New Delhi) (1971 — 1975)	
Total Cases	29		42	
Ptosis	22	75.8%	36	85.7%
Ophthalmoplegia	16	55.1%	18	42.9%
Palatal paralysis	8	27.5%	16	38.09%
Pharyngeal Paralysis	13	44.8%	16	38.09%
Flaccid limb paralysis	18	62%	11	26.2%
Convulsions	3	10.3%	8	19.05%
Nec Weakness	19	65.5%	Not mentioned	
Coma	8	27.5%	11	26.2%
Local pain	4	13.7%	Not mentioned	
Epigastric pain	1	3.4%	Not mentioned	
Clotting abnormality	4	13.7%	Not mentioned	
Ventilatory care	14	48.2%	Not mentioned	

Figure 11

HAFFKINE INSTITUTE POLYVALENT SERUM INFORMATION

(The printed leaflet carrying directions for use of polyvalent antivenin and the label of a vial.)

HAFFKINE BIO - PHARMACEUTICAL CORPORATION LTD. Parel, Bombay-400 012. LYOPHILISED POLYVALENT ANTI-SNAKE-VENOM SERUM DIRECTIONS OF USE

This anti-snake-venom serum is prepared by hyperimmunizing horses against the venoms of the four common poisonous snakes of India, namely, (1) Cobra (Naja naja), (2) Common Krait (Bungarus caeruleus) (3) Russell's Viper (Vipera russelli) and (4) Saw-scaled Viper (Echis carinatus). Plasma obtained from the hyperimmunized horses is enzyme refined, purified and concentrated. Each ml. of the serum neutralizes not less than the following quantities of dried venoms when the serum is injected mixed with the venoms intravenously into white mice; Cobra—0.6 mg; Common Krait—0.45 mg; Russell's Viper—0.6 mg. and Saw-scaled Viper—0.45mg.

The serum is lyophilsed by drying it from the frozen state under high vacuum. The drying process is continued until the moisture content is reduced to less than 1 percent. The dried serum, however, retains its affinity for water to the fullest extent and therefore, dissolves on addition of water. This property is maintained by the dried serum even after storage for many years.

TREATMENT OF SNAKE-BITE
I. FIRST-AID

Snake-bites should be treated immediately. The measures to meet the emergency should be quick and positive. The following first aid measures have definitely proved their value—

1. Remove the patient to a well-ventilated and quiet place. Assure the patient that there is no reason to be nervous or frightened. Try to gain his confidence. Institute measures to combat shock which has a major psychological element in it.

2. Ligation — A ligature of some type should be bound a moderate distance above the bitten part, to prevent the venom being absorbed into the upper part of the limb. The ligature may consist of a strip of cloth, a large handkerchief, or even a piece of heavy cord. A rubber ligature is by far the best. It is necessary to make the ligature sufficiently tight to cause a stoppage of venom circulation. Ligation should not continue for over half an hour and even than should always be slackened at regular intervals of ten minutes during this time. Ligature should not be applied if an hour or more has elapsed after the bite.

3. Treat the wound in the usual surgical way. Clean the bitten part and apply antiseptic dressings without rubbing. Immobilize the bitten part as per fracture.

II SPECIFIC SERUM TREATMENT

Once the venom has got into the circulation, it is only the anti-snake-venom serum that can neutralize it, and in order to derive the greatest benefit out of serum treatment, the serum should be injected as soon as possible, after the bite. As a first dose, at least 20ml. of the reconstituted serum (see below) should be injected intravenously very slowly (not over 1 ml. per minute). The second dose should be repeated two hours after the first dose or even earlier, if symptoms persist. If the symptoms, which vary with different venoms, indicate persistence of venom action, further doses should be repeated every six hours until the symptoms completely disappear. In case of a viper bite some serum should also be injected around the site of the bite to prevent gangrene which otherwise results owing to the very destructive effect of localized viper venom on tissue.

In cases of Cobra and Krait poisoning constitutional symptoms are more prominent than local pain and swelling. General intoxication is soon followed by a sense of creeping paralysis beginning in the legs and ascending to the head by way of trunk. Paralysis of the muscles of eyelids, staggering gait, inco-ordination of speech, paralysis of the limbs, drooping of the head and complete paralysis of all voluntary muscles develop. Nausea and vomitting frequently occur. Breathing gets more and more difficult and finally stops. In case of Krait poisoning, in addition there are convulsions and violent abdominal pains due to internal harmorrhages.

In cases of Russell's and Saw-scaled Viper poisonings the local symptoms are prominent and severe. There is a great and persistent pain and intensive swelling. There is constant and incessant oozing of blood from the punctures. Sloughing occurs permitting other infections. The constitutional symptoms are characterised by haemorrhages, both external and internal. Haemorrhages in the abdomen are responsible for pain tenderness and vomitting. Death is due to death failure, there is no paralysis.

The venoms of Cobra and Krait act very rapidly if a large amount of venom is absorbed into the circulation. Hence, it must be understood, that unless the absorption of the venom into the circulation is retarded by ligation, the anti-snake-venom serum does not get a fair chance to neutralize the venom and save the victim. First-aid treatment should, therefore, never be relaxed even when the serum is administered.

Intravenous injection of serum in horse-serum-sensitive subjects can produce very severe serum reaction and even acute anaphylaxis. Every care should be taken to prevent these reactions (see below).

Intramuscular or subcutaneous injections of the anti-snake-venom serum are not as effective as intravenous injections. But if expert medical aid is not available, the serum may be administered by the subcutaneous or the intramuscular route.

III ASSOCIATED TREATMENT

In case of Russell's and Saw-scaled Viper poisonings, sedatives, such as small doses of barbiturate and/or analgesics (e.g. aspirin) may be given to relieve nervousness and pain. For collapse, strychnine, pituitrin or other general stimulants like coramine are of special value. The use of Corticosteriods helps to minimise serum reaction and minor allergic reactions. Antibiotics may also be given to combat local sepsis. In all severely poisoned persons, great relief is likely to be experienced from the infusion of a large amount of physiological saline, or still better transfusion of blood or plasma, the effect of which may be life-saving in border-line cases. Respiratory paralysis should be treated by tracheostomy and artificial respiration.

RECONSTITUTION OF LYOPHILISED SERUM

1. Draw 10 ml. of the distilled water in a sterile syringe.
2. Cut a line with the file about half way round the neck of the ampoule of lyophilised serum, and gently break open the neck.
3. Transfer the water from the syringe to the serum ampoule.
4. Cover the opening of the ampoule with the sterilized pad of handyplast, gauze surface downwards, press it down with the thumb, and holding the ampoule in the hand shake it vigorously for about one minute.
5. Now let the ampoule stand for one minute for the serum to clear. The reconstituted serum will become crystal-clear and ready for Injection. Froth and undissolved particles, if any, should be left in the ampoule.
6. For the second and subsequent injections, you will have more time to dissolve the lyophilised serum. For these add 10 ml. distilled water to the serum ampoule and rotate it between the palms of your hands until the serum is fully dissolved, and let the ampoule stand for serum to clear.

STORAGE

Liquid serum is very unstable at room temp. It requires storage at 0^0 to 4^0C. Even then it deteriorates, and 2 years from the date of manufacture, the serum becomes unfit for use. In India, proper coldstorage facilities are not freely available and therefore liquid serum only be stored at the risk of very rapid deterioration. Lyophilised serum obviates this difficulty. It is many times more stable than liquid serum. It should retain its potency for 5 years even if stored in any cool dark place. Thus anti-snake-venom serum can be made available for use far away from cold-storage facilities. It can be safely kept at rural dispensaries even carried in a haversack on one's back if an occasion demands it. However, it is preferable to store it in a refrigerator if one is available.

PREVENTION OF SERUM REACTION

Before injection of anti-venom serum it is necessary to enquire from the patient:

(1) whether he has had injections of serum (e.g. anti-tetanus or anti-diphtheria serum) before.

(2) whether there is personal or familial history of allergy, i.e. asthma, eczema or drug allergy.

The sensitivity of the patient to serum is tested by injecting subcutaneously 0.1 ml. of serum diluted 1:10. The patient should be observed for 30 minutes for local and general reactions. If the test dose shows either local reaction such as wheal and flare or general anaphylactic reaction such as pallor, sweating, nausea and vomitting, urticaria and fall of blood pressure, these should be countered immediately by intramuscular injection of 1 ml. of 1:1000 adrenaline and with corticosteroids which should be always kept handy.

In allergic or sensitive patients, it is better to inject the anti-snake-venom serum under cover of anti-histamines. This is done by injecting anti-histamine such as antistine (100 mg.) and hydrocortisone (100 mg.) intramuscularly 15 to 30 minutes before the administration of anti-venom. The administration of adrenaline and hydrocortisone may be repeated, if necessary.

When symptoms of snake-bite are severe, it may not be advisable to wait for 30 minutes to observe reactions to test dose of serum. In such cases it may be better to inject 1 ml. of 1:100 adrenaline intramuscularly at the same time as the serum in order, to lesson the risk of anaphylaxis. Half the dose of adrenaline may be repeated 15 minutes later, if necessary.

LYOPHILISED POLYVALENT
ANTI-SNAKE VENOM SERUM
ENZYME REFINED

Contains equivalent of 10 ml of purified globulins, 1 ml of reconstituted serum neutralizes 0.6 mg. of dried Cobra (Naja-naja) venom, 0.45 mg. dried Krait (Bungarus caeruleus) venom, 0.6 mg. of dried Russell's Viper (Vipera russelli). Venom, 0.45 mg. of dried Saw-scaled Viper (Echis carinatus) Venom. Phenol I.P. (preservative) 0.25%.

HAFFKINE BIO-PHARMACEUTICAL CORPORATION LTD.
(A Govt. of Maharashtra Undertaking)
Parel. Bombay 400 012 Made in India.

Mfg. Lic. No. 91   Date of Exp.   Batch No.   Date of Mfg.

Figure 12

ANTISNAKE-VENOM SERUM FROM SERUM INSTITUTE OF INDIA AND THE
DIRECTIONS OF USE.

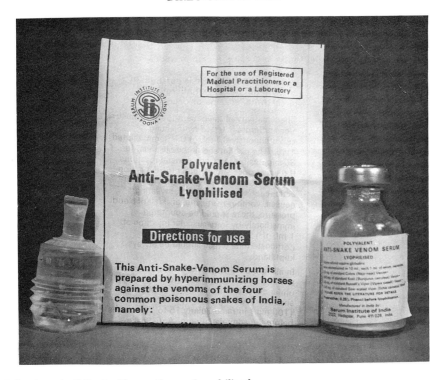

Polyvalent Anti-Snake-Venom Serum Lyophilised

DIRECTIONS OF USE

This Anti-Snake-Venom Serum
is prepared by hyperimmunizing horses against the
venoms of the four common
poisonous snakes of India,
namely:

- Cobra (Naja naja)
- Common Krait (Bungarus
  caereuleus)
- Russell's Viper (Vipera
  russelli) &
- Saw-scaled Viper (Echis
  carinatus)

Plasma obtained from the
hyperimmunized horses is
enzyme refined, purified and
concentrated. Each ml. of the
reconstituted Anti-Snake-
Venom Serum neutralizes not
less than the following
quantities of standard venoms

when tested in white mice:
Cobra — 0.6 mg (10 Mcg)
Common Krait — 0.45 mg (3
Mcg)
Russell's Viper — 0.6 mg. (10
Mcg)
Saw-scaled Viper 0.45 mg. (12
Mcg)

Treatment of Snake-Bite
I. First-Aid

Snake-bite should be
treated immediately. The
measures to meet the
emergency should be quick
and positive. The following
first-aid measures have
definitely proved their value:

1. Remove the patient to
a well-ventilated and quiet
place. Assure the patient that
there is no reason to be

nervous or frightened. Try to
gain his confidence. Institute
measures to combat shock
which has a major
psychological element in it.

2. Ligation. A ligature of
some type should be bound a
moderate distance above the
bitten part, to prevent the
venom being absorbed into the
upper part of the limb. The
ligature may consist of a strip
of cloth, a large handkerchief,
or even a piece of heavy cord.
A rubber ligature is by far the
best. It is necessary to make
the ligature sufficiently tight
to cause a stoppage of venom
circulation. Ligation should
not continue for over half an
hour and even then should
always be slackened at regular

intervals of ten minutes during this time. Ligature should not be applied if an hour or more has elapsed after the bite.

3. Treat the wound in the usual surgical way. Clean the bitten part and apply antiseptic dressings without rubbing. Immobilize the bitten part as in fracture cases.

II. Specific Serum Treatment

Once the venom has got into the circulation, it is only the Anti-Snake-Venom Serum that can neutralize it.

In order to derive the greatest benefit out of serum treatment, the serum should be injected as soon as possible, after the bite. As a first dose, at least 20 ml. of the reconstituted serum (see below) should be injected *intravenously* very slowly (not over 1 ml. per minute). The second dose should be repeated two hours after the first dose or even earlier, if symptoms persist. If the symptoms, which vary with different venoms, indicate persistence of venom action, further doses should be repeated every six hours until the symptoms completely disappear. In case of a viper bite some serum should also be injected around the site of the bite to prevent gangrene which otherwise results owing to the very destructive effect of localized viper venom on tissue.

In cases of Cobra and Krait poisoning, constitutional symptoms are more prominent than local pain and swelling. General intoxication is soon followed by a sense of creeping paralysis beginning in the legs and ascending to the head by way of trunk. Paralysis of the muscles of the eyelids, staggering gait, inco-ordination of speech, paralysis of the limbs, drooping of the head and completely paralysis of all voluntary muscles develop. Nausea and vomitting frequently occur. Breathing gets more and more difficult and finally stops. In the case of Krait poisoning, in addition there are convulsions and violent abdominal pains due to internal haemorrhages.

In case of Russell's and Saw-scaled Viper poisonings the local symptoms are prominent and severe. There is great and persistent pain and intensive swelling at the site of the bite. There is constant and incessant oozing of blood from the punctures. Sloughing occurs permitting other infections. The constitutional symptoms are characterised by haemorrhages, both external and internal. Haemorrhages in the abdomen are responsible for pain, tenderness and vomitting. Death is due to heart failure; there is no paralysis.

The venoms of Cobra and Krait act very rapidly if a large amount of venom is absorbed into the circulation. Hence, it must be understood, that unless the absorption of the venom into the circulation is retarded by ligation, the anti-snake-venom serum does not get a fair chance to neutralize the venom, and save the victim.

First-aid treatment should, therefore, never be relaxed even when the serum is administrered.

Intravenous injection of a serum in horse-serum-sensitive subjects can produce very severe serum reaction and even acute anaphylaxis. Every care should be taken to prevent these reactions (see below).

Intramuscular or sub-cutaneous injections of the anti-snake-venom serum are not as effective as intravenous injections. But if expert medical aid is not available, the serum may be administered by the subcutaneous or the intramuscular route.

Intravenous injections should always be given very slowly. It is of great advantage to dilute the serum 5 to 10 times with normal or glucose saline and to administer it very slowly, if possible, as a slow drip.

III. Associated Treatment

In case of Russell's and Saw-scaled Viper poisonings, sedatives, such as small doses of barbiturate and/or analgesics (eg. aspirin) may be given to relieve nervousness and pain. For collapse, strychnine, pituitrin or other general stimulants like coramine are of special value. The use of corticosteroids helps to minimise serum reaction and minor allergic reactions. Antibiotics may also be given to combat local sepsis. In all severely poisoned persons, great relief is likely to be experienced from the infusion of a large amount of physiological saline, or still better, transfusion of blood or plasma, the effect of which may be life-saving in border-line cases. Respiratory paralysis should be treated by tracheostomy and artifical respiration.

Reconstitution of Lyophilised Serum

1. Draw 10 ml. of Water for Injection in a sterile syringe.

2. Transfer the water from the syringe to the serum vial and shake well till the contents dissolve.
3. Let the vial stand for one minute for the serum to clear. The reconstituted will become crystal-clear and ready for injection. Froth and undissolved particles, if any, should be left in the vial.
4. For the second and subsequent injections, you will have more time to dissolve the lyophilised serum. For these add 10 ml. Water for Injection to the serum vial and rotate it between the palms of your hands until the serum is fully dissolved, and let the vial stand for serum to clear.

Storage:

Liquid serum is very unstable at room temperature. It requires storage at 0° to 4°C. Even then it deteriorates, and 2 years from the date of manufacture, the serum becomes unfit for use. In India, proper cold-storage facilities are not freely available and, therefore, liquid serum may only be stored at the risk of very rapid deterioration. Lyophilised serum obviates this difficulty. It is many times more stable than liquid serum. It should retain its potency for 5 years even if stored in any cool dark place. Thus Anti-Snake-Venom Serum can be made available for use far away from cold-storage facilities. It can be safely kept at rural dispensaries and even carried in a haversack if an occasion demands it. However, it is preferable to store it in a refrigerator if one is available.

Prevention of Serum Reaction

Before injection of Anti-Snake-Venom Serum it is necessary to enquire from the patient:

(1) whether he has had injections of serum (e.g. anti-tetanus or anti-diphtheria serum) before.

(2) whether there is personal or familial history of allergy, i.e. asthma, eczema or drug allergy.

The sensitivity of the patient to Anti-Snake-Venom-Serum is tested by injecting subcutaneously 0.1 ml. of this serum diluted 1:10. The patient should be observed for 30 minutes for local and general reactions. If the test dose shows either local reaction such as wheal or flare or general anaphylactic reaction such as pallor, sweating, nausea, vomiting, urticaria, and fall of blood pressure, these should be countered immediately by intramuscular injection of 1 ml. of 1:1000 adrenaline and with corticosteroids which should be always kept handy.

In allergic or sensitive patients, it is better to inject the Anti-Snake-Venom Serum under cover of anti-histamine such as antistine (100 mg.) and hydrocortisone (100 mg.) intramuscularly 15 to 30 minutes before the administration of Anti-Snake-Venom Serum. The administration of adrenaline and hydrocortisone may be repeated if necessary.

When symptoms of snake-bite are severe it may not be advisable to wait for 30 minutes to observe reactions to test dose of serum. In such cases it may be better to inject 1 ml. of 1:1000 adrenaline intramuscularly at the same time as the serum in order to lessen the risk of anaphylaxis. Half the dose of adrenaline may be repeated 15 minutes later if necessary.

Packing — *One dose vial of lyophilised Anti-Snake-Venom Serum with 10 ml. ampoule of Water for Injection.*

Manufactured in India by:
Serum Institute of India.
Office: 283, Mahatma Gandhi Road, Poona-1.

Venomous Snakes of Israel

by Elazar Kochva*

Department of Zoology, George S. Wise Faculty of Life Sciences,
Tel Aviv University, Tel Aviv.

Introduction

Israel is a small country, with a variety of climatic and topographic regions. Venomous snakes are found in two main areas: (1) the Mediterranean area, that extends along the coast from the north, down to the town of Beer-Sheba in the south, and (2) the Desert, which extends southwards to the Red Sea and eastwards to the Dead Sea region. Some venomous and non-venomous desert snakes penetrate northwards along the Jordan Valley, as far as Mount Gilboa, just south-west of the Sea of Galilee. Of the 35 or more snake species of Israel, 8 are venomous and belong to three families: Viperidae with six species, *Vipera palaestinae*, *Vipera bornmuelleri*, *Echis coloratus*, *Pseudocerastes fieldi*, *Cerastes cerastes*, *Cerastes vipera;* Elapidae, with one species, *Walterinnesia aegyptia;* Atractaspididae with one species, *Atractaspis engaddensis*.

The biology of the venomous snakes described here is based on life-long observations diligently collected by Prof. H. Mendelssohn (1963; 1965; 1977).

Description:

Vipera palaestinae (Fig. 1.) is the clinically most important venomous snake of Israel. Its distribution covers the entire Mediterranean region, a region which is also the most densely populated and agriculturally developed. Between 100 to 300 bites are caused by this species each year, with 0-2 fatalities.

Vipera palaestinae is a predominantly nocturnal snake, which may be seen also during the day. It usually avoids humans and bites occur when the snake is stepped on, or otherwise threatened and has no possibility of fleeing. Before specific antivenom was available, mortality rates reached 6-10% (Hadar and Gitter, 1959), but then dropped to 2-3% and since 1960 very few to zero lethal cases per year have been recorded.

Vipera palaestinae is a heavyset snake that may attain a maximum length of more than 1.3 metres and a weight of 1.5 kg. As in other vipers, the tail is rather short, less than 15% of the body length. *V. palaestinae* has a triangular head with an anteriorly pointing V-shaped mark. The coloration is grey to ochre with a dorsal zig-zag pattern of reddish-brown colour. This pattern may break up into separate rhomboid blotches, with intermediate patterns being found in the same or in different specimens. In addition, there is a series of

---

*Incumbent: The Rose and Norman Lederer Chair in Experimental Biology

brown spots along the sides of the body. The variation in colour pattern could not be connected with sex, age, distribution or habitat of the snake.

Vipera palaestinae feeds mainly on rodents and is commonly found near and in agricultural settlements. During the month of August, 20 or more eggs are laid which take about 45 days to hatch, at 30 degrees C. When laid, the eggs already contain well-developed embryos (Kochva, 1965). Hatchlings are about 200 mm in length and have a well-developed venom apparatus. The toxicity of their venom has not been compared to that of the adults. The venom secretion of *Vipera palaestinae* has been studied in detail (see Kochva, 1987 for review). The venom glands of large specimens may contain as much as 0.5-1.0 gm of venom (about 120-150 mg protein), of which 10% will be injected on the average. About 20% of the bites may carry no envenomation, while doses as high as 200-250 mg have been injected by vipers in experiments conducted with mice and rats. There is a dispute in the literature on whether there is a difference in the amount of venom injected during a "feeding bite" (into mice) and a "defensive bite" (into humans). However, "blank" bites (no venom injected) are known in humans and a rough calculation shows that doses higher than 70 mg may be injected and are probably fatal, when no specific treatment is given (Kochva, 1978). In mice, the i.v. LD_{50} of the venom is about 0.3 $\mu g/gm$. On acrylamide gel isoelectrofocusing, the venom can be resolved into approximately 30 bands, 16 of which may be identified as specific enzymes and toxins (Oron and Bdolah, 1978; Oron *et al.* 1978). Amongst the enzymes, there are L-amino acid oxidases, phosphodiesterases, proteases and phospholipases A_2. The latter two enzymes are related to toxins: proteases to hemorrhagins, whilst phospholipase A_2 forms part of the so-called two-component toxin, of which the other component is a non-enzymatic protein. The two-component toxin was first assumed to be a neurotoxin (Moroz *et al.*, 1966) but was later proven not to have neurotoxic activity; it causes hypotension and other circulatory difficulties (Lee *et al.*, unpublished). It is a highly lethal toxin, of an approximate combined molecular weight of 30,000 (Ovadia et al., 1977), which is probably responsible for the human fatalities caused by *Vipera palaestinae* bites.

The clinical picture of envenomation of this and of other species has been summarised by Efrati (1979), Gitter and de Vries (1968), Mann (1976) and Mann and Gunders (1977). The clinical evolution of *V. palaestinae* envenomation in severe cases, before specific antivenom was available, could be characterised by severe pain at the site of the bite (15-20 minutes after the bite), weakness and restlessness, vomitting, profuse perspiration and abdominal pain. Diarrhoea is frequent and severe peripheral circulatory failure is observed. Hypotension is present, the blood pressure cannot be measured, the pulse is not palpable and the heart rate is rapid. Angioneurotic edema of the upper lip may be found and the face and tongue may be swollen. Local changes include swelling of the bitten extremity, which is tender and painful to palpation. The swelling increases and spreads centripetally and may extend up to the trunk and pass over to the opposite side of the body. Several hours later, ascending lymphagitis and lymphadenitis may appear on the affected

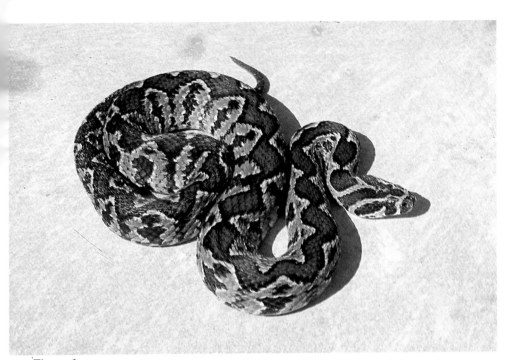

Figure 1
Vipera palaestinae

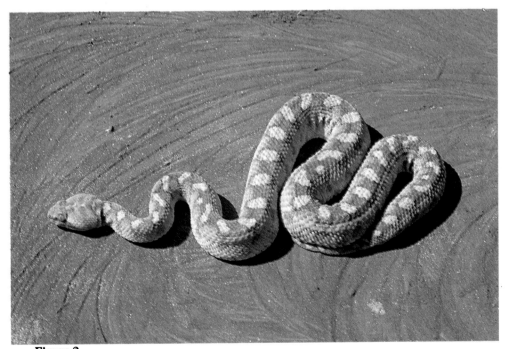

Figure 2
Echis coloratus

extremity, followed by reddening of the skin and blister formation. The swelling usually clears after one to two weeks.

The primary circulatory failure may pass over to hypovolemic shock caused by extravasation, and severe anemia and bleeding into some internal organs may follow. Circulatory failure or bleeding is the frequent cause of death.

The available monospecific antivenom against *Vipera palaestinae* bites (Fig. 7) is most efficient and, as mentioned above, death is now very rare in Israel.

The following treatment is recommended (Efrati, 1979; Bernstein, pers. comm.).

I. First Aid
    Reassurance of the victim.
    Immobilisation of the bitten extremity.
    Transport to a medical facility (preferably central hospital -EK).
    Identification of snake, if available (usually not important in cases of *V. palaestinae* bites, since its distribution very rarely overlaps that of other venomous snakes - EK).

II. Hospital
    Installation of intravenous drop infusion set.
    Intracutaneous sensitivity test to horse serum.
    Alleviation of pain with Dipyrone sol. or a small amount of Pethidine but *not* Morphine.
    Intravenous drop infusion of physiological solution with or without vasopressor drugs until hypotension is overcome.
    Intravenous administration of specific antivenom in adequate quantities (50-60 ml for *V. palaestinae* bites).
    Tetanus toxoid as indicated with other infected wounds.
    Transfer to ward.
    Monitoring blood pressure, blood count, coagulation, observation of edema.
    Blood transfusion, if anemia develops.
    Surgery is sometimes necessary, when a necrotic area appears.

Vipera bornmuelleri is a brownish snake of a maximum length of 75 cm, a weight of 400 gm and a restricted distribution. It is viviparous, with about 10 young per litter.

The only bite known was uneventful and caused only a very slight local swelling.

Echis coloratus (Fig. 2) is responsible for about 40 bites with at least one fatal case that has been reported recently.

Echis coloratus is found in the desert area, mainly in rocky environments and extends further north along the Jordan Valley to Mount Gilboa, about 35 km south-west of the Sea of Galilee. It is a rather small and slender snake, attaining a maximum length of 80 cm and a weight of 200 gm. The head is distinctly triangular and the tail is short. When threatened, rather than hissing, the snake produces a warning noise by rubbing its lateral scales, which are keeled; this behaviour is considered as a water saving adaptation to arid environments by this and by some other desert snakes. About 9 eggs are laid in August and the young hatch after 50 days at 30 degrees C.

Echis coloratus appears in several colour patterns. The most common colouration is a yellowish or light brownish grey, with a row of greyish-white elongated rhomboid blotches or crossbands along the back. Dark blotches, sometimes accompanied by light bands above, are found along the sides of the body. Some marking is usually found on the head and a brownish-grey band with a light stripe above it passes along the sides of the head, from the nostril to the corner of the mouth. In some areas, such as the mountains near Elat with their coloured rocks, reddish-brown specimens are found, with white to ash-grey or bluish-grey dorsal blotches.

Echis coloratus venom is known mainly to affect the blood circulatory system, causing widespread haemorrhage, afibrinogenemia and severe thrombocytopenia. Severe alterations in the blood clotting mechanism of patients were observed and a reported death case was due to renal failure caused by acute interstitial nephritis. Local symptoms include pain, swelling, subcutaneous haemorrhage and necrosis (Rechnic *et al.*, 1962, in Lee 1979; 1976; Schulchynska-Castel *et al.*, 1986).

A monospecific antivenom is available (Fig. 7).

Pseudocerastes fieldi (Fig. 3) has variably been considered as a subspecies Pseudocerastes persicus or together with it, as belonging to the genus *Vipera*. However at least from the toxinological point of view, the genus *Pseudocerastes* should retained and *Pseudocerastes fieldi* should be considered as a separate species. It venom has recently been shown to differ markedly from vipers in general and from Pseudocerastes persicus in particular (Bdolah, 1986).

Pseudocerastes fieldi is a heavyset snake of a maximum known length of 80 cm and weight of 500 gm. It has a prominent triangular head with horn-like projections above the eyes. Its background colour is yellowish-grey with brownish blotches on the back and sides of the body. The head has some irregular small blotches and a light brown stripe extends from the eyes to the corner of the mouth. The tail is short with a black tip.

Pseudocerastes fieldi is a desert snake that prefers biotopes that contain some vegetation. It feeds on birds and mice and also accepts dead food. It lays 15-20 eggs, which already contain well-developed embryos. Incubation lasts about 30 days at 30 degrees C. The venom of *Pseudocerastes fieldi* is colourless: it has relatively few components and no L-amino acid oxidase nor hemorrhagic activities. Its main toxic fraction is a two-component presynaptic neurotoxin, component of which is phospholipase A_2 (Bdolah *et al.*, 1985; Shabo-Shina and Bdolah, 1987).

The very few clinical cases showed only local symptoms and all survived.

There is no antivenom against this species and the anti-*Pseudocerastes* product is obviously not efficient (see Bdolah, 1986).

Cerastes cerastes (Fig. 4) is a heavyset snake that inhabits sandy areas of the desert. It usually stays burrowed in the sand with only the eyes and nostrils

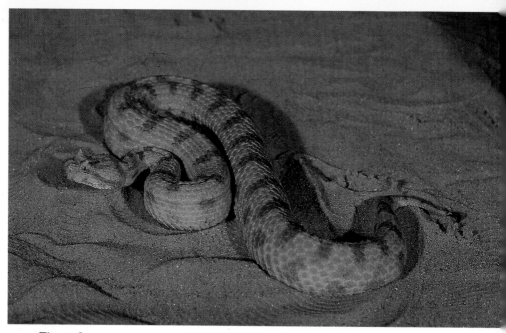

Figure 3
Pseudocerastes fieldi

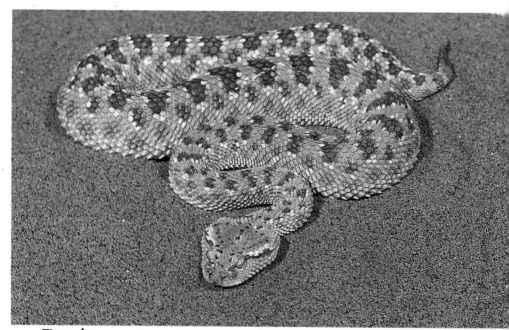

Figure 4
Cerastes cerastes

barely visible above ground. It is a sidewinder and a scale-rubbing snake. Specimens in Israel have no horns above the eyes.

Cerastes cerastes lays up to 20 eggs, which take about 9 weeks to hatch. This species may attain 75 cm in length and a weight of 400 gm. It is of a general colouration, with darker brown, white-edged blotches on the back and sides of the body. Its well distinguished triangular head bears two lateral brown and grey stripes along its sides. The venom of *Cerastes cerastes* is strongly hemorrhagic and cases with marked local reactions have been described. Blood clotting and kidney function were also affected. In one case, systemic manifestations were observed, including nausea, vomiting and abdominal pain (Shulzinska *et al* 1978; Schulchynska-Castel, pers. comm.).

Local antivenom is not yet available and other products only partially and insufficiently neutralise the venom. Recent taxonomical studies show significant differences between the Israeli population from the Arava region of the Negev and those of Sinai and north-eastern Africa (Y.L. Werner, pers. comm.).

Cerastes vipera is a small snake that attains a length of 30 cm and a weight of 50 gm. It is of a general yellowish colour with brown spots along the body. It is found mainly in the sands of the north-western part of the Negev Desert. *Cerastes vipera* feeds mainly on lizards and lays 2-8 eggs which hatch immediately (ovoviviparous). Several bites are known (A. Keynan, pers. comm.).

Walterinnesia aegyptia (Fig. 5) is the only elapid snake found in Israel. It is of a uniform black to brownish-black shiny colour, which to the uninitiated may resemble the non-venomous colubrid "black snake" *(Coluber jugularis)*. Fortunately the distribution of these two overlaps only slightly in the northern Negev and Judean Deserts, *Walterinnesia* being a desert snake that does not enter the Mediterranean area. In addition, subadult "black snakes" up to 130-140 cm long are not black at all; this length already exceeds *Walterinnesia aegyptia* which is only about 100 cm long and weighs 700 gm. *Walterinnesia* lays about 12 eggs, which take 5-6 weeks to hatch. It feeds on toads, lizards, birds and mice and will also accept dead food. It is frequently found near human habitations.

The venom of *Walterinnesia aegyptia* has postsynaptic neurotoxins but no presynaptic ones and no cardiotoxins (Lee *et al.*, 1976). However, each of its three phospholipases, when combined with the *Vipera palaestinae* venom non-enzymatic component, becomes markedly toxic. Several *Walterinnesia* bites have been recorded thus far, none with any serious systemic signs. In one case, considerable swelling of the entire bitten area developed (A. Yayon, E. Sikular and A. Keynan, in press).

A monospecific antivenom has been prepared in goats (Fig. 7).

Atractaspis engaddensis (Fig. 6) is a rather slender, black, burrowing snake, that reaches a maximum of 80 cm and about 140 gm. After intensive deliberations in the literature, it has recently been suggested to resurrect a separate family for this monotypic genus, which differs from all other

317

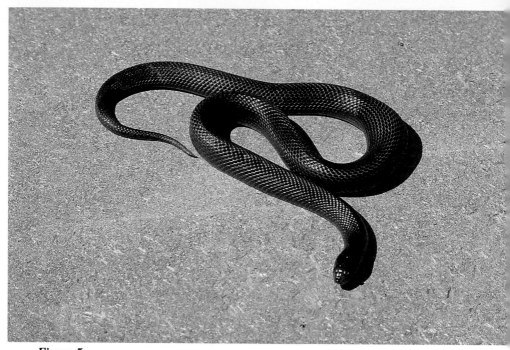

Figure 5
Walterinnesia aegyptia

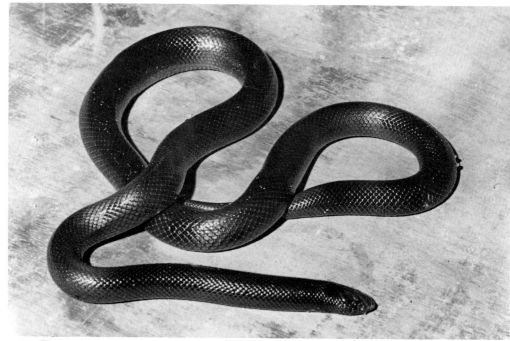

Figure 6
Atractaspis engaddensis

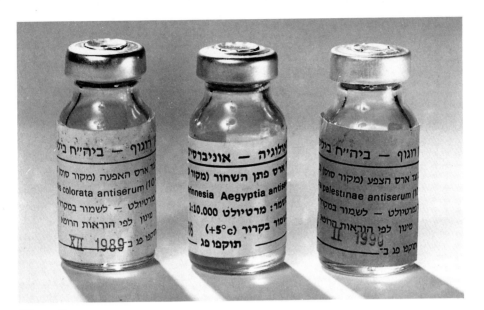

Figure 7
Monospecific antivenoms

venomous snakes in many respects, starting with the morphology of the head and body down to the composition of its venom and the primary chemical structure of its strongly cardiotoxic components (Underwood and Kochva, 1989; Takasaki *et al.*, 1988).

Atractaspis engaddensis is a desert snake, the distribution of which, however, extends along the Jordan Valley east of the water divide and up to Mount Gilboa (south-west of the Sea of Galilee). In nature, *Atractaspis* probably feeds on lacertilians; during September-November, 2-3 eggs are laid, which take more than 3 months to hatch.

The number of bites by *Atractaspis* seems to be on the rise, as people usually mistake it for non-venomous and try to pick it up by hand. It has a peculiar biting behaviour involving a lateral-downward movement of the head, with one fang only being erected and the mouth remaining essentially closed (Golani and Kochva, 1988). Owing to the highly toxic venom, the not so severe consequences of its bites can be explained by the rather small amount of venom injected.

The i.v. LD_{50} of the venom in mice is about 0.07 $\mu g/gm$ and of the cardiotoxic components - 0.015 $\mu g/gm$, which makes it one of the most lethal snake toxins. The venom is also hemorrhagic and may cause significant local symptoms (Kochva *et al.*, 1982; Ovadia, 1987). However, the most important clinical effects could be attributed to the cardiotoxic components, several of which were recently characterised and sequenced and found to be polypeptides of about 2000 MW, which differ markedly from the elapid cardiotoxins (Takasaki *et al.*, 1988; Wollberg *et al.*, 1988). Each of these toxins, as well as the whole venom, causes immediate and severe coronary vasoconstriction and marked changes in the ECG in mice, consisting primarily of a transient slope elevation of the S-T segment with a diminution of the S-wave and increased amplitudes of the R and T waves. A severe A-V block develops and leads to complete cardiac arrest. Interestingly enough, some of these changes were also observed in human victims, but were considered to be secondary to the other symptoms (see below).

There are no neurotoxic components in *Atractaspis engaddensis* venom. Cases of envenomation by *Atractaspis* are characterised by pain and numbness at the site of the bite, swelling and necrosis, that in one case progressed to gangrene necessitating amputation of a thumb. Systemic symptoms involve nausea, vomiting, abdominal pain, diarrhoea, sweating, profuse salivation, loss of occular accommodation, loss of consciousness, liver damage and dyspnoea (Mann, 1976).

In one case, a patient was admitted with respiratory failure; he had lost consciousness and was cyanotic and examination of arterial blood revealed hypoxia and hypercapnia. ECG alteration of the S-T segment and the T wave were also found, but were considered secondary to the other symptoms (Mann, 1976). It is now evident that the cardiotoxic symptoms are most probably of primary origin and are caused by the sarafotoxins found in *Atractaspis* venom (Wollberg *et al.*, 1988 Takasaki *et al.*, 1989).

Antivenom is not available against any species of *Atractaspis*.

In conclusion it should be pointed out that the most dangerous snake of Israel is *Vipera palaestinae;* it is responsible for most of the bites and almost all of the deaths. Monospecific antivenoms (Fig. 7) are available against *Vipera palaestinae* and *Echis coloratus* (Rogoff-Wellcome Institute) and against *Walterinnesia aegyptia* (Department of Zoology, Tel Aviv University).

References

Bdolah, A. (1986) Comparison of venoms from two subspecies of the False Horned Viper *(Pseudocerastes persicus)*. Toxicon, *24:* 726.

Bdolah, A., Kinamon, S. and Batzri-Izraeli, R. (1985) The neurotoxic complex from the venom of *Pseudocerastes fieldi.* Contribution of the nontoxic subunit. Biochem. Intern., *11:*627.

Efrati, P. (1979) Symptomatology, pathology and treatment of the bites of viperid snakes, p. 956. *In:* Snake Venoms, C.Y. Lee, Ed., Springer Verlag, Berlin, Heidelberg, New York.

Gitter, S. and de Vries, A. (1968) Symptomatology, pathology and treatment of bites by Near Eastern, European and North African snakes, p. 359. *In:* Venomous Animals and their Venoms, Vol. I, W. Bucherl, E.E. Buckley and V. Deulofeu, Eds., Academic Press, New York.

Golani, I. and Kochva. E. (1988) Striking and other offensive and defensive behavior patterns in *Atractaspis engaddensis* (Ophidia, Atractaspididae). Copeia, 1988:792.

Hadar, H. and Gitter, S. (1959) The results of treatment with Pasteur antiserum in cases of snake bite. Harefuah, *56:*1 (in Hebrew).

Kochva, E. (1965) Development of the venom gland and trigeminal muscles in *Vipera palaestinae*. Acta Anat., *52*:49.

Kochva, E. (1978) Evolution and secretion of venom and its antidotes in snakes. Period. Biol., *80* (Suppl. l):11.

Kochva, E. (1987) The origin of snakes and evolution of the venom apparatus. Toxicon, *25*:65.

Kochva, E., Viljoen, C.C. and Botes, D.P. (1982) A new type of toxin in the venom of snakes of the genus *Atractaspis* (Atractaspidinae). Toxicon, *20*:581.

Lee, C.Y. (1979) Snake venoms. Springer Verlag, Berlin, Heidelberg, New York.

Lee, C.Y., Chen, Y.M. and Mebs, D. (1976) Chromatographic separation of the venom of Egyptian black snake *(Walterinnesia aeqyptia)* and pharmacological characterization of its components. Toxicon, *14*:275.

Mann, G. (1976) Snake bites in Israel. MD — thesis, Hebrew University of Jerusalem (in Hebrew).

Mann, G. and Gunders, A.E. (1977) Epidemiology of snake-bites in Israel. The Family Physician, *7*:12 (in Hebrew).

Mendelssohn, H. (1963) On the biology of the venomous snakes of Israel. I. Israel J. Zool., *12*:143.

Mendelssohn, H. (1965) On the biology of the venomous snakes of Israel. II. Israel. J. Zool., *14*:185.

Mendelssohn, H. (1977) On the biology of the venomous snakes of Israel. The Family Physician, *7*:29 (in Hebrew).

Moroz, C., de Vries, A. and Goldblum, N. (1966) Preparation of antivenin against *Vipera palaestinae* venom with high antineurotoxic potency. Toxicon, *4*:205.

Oron, U. and Bdolah, A. (1978) Intracellular transport of proteins in active and resting secretory cells of the venom gland of *Vipera palaestinae* J. Cell. Biol., *78*:488.

Oron, U., Kinamon, S. and Bdolah, A. (1978) Asynchrony in the synthesis of secretory proteins in the venom gland of the snake *Vipera palaestinae*. Biochem. J., *174*:733a.

Ovadia, M., Kochva, E. and Moav, B. (1977) Purification and partial characterization of lethal synergistic components from the venom of *Vipera palaestinae*. Toxicon, *15*:549.

Ovadia, M. (1987) Isolation and characterization of a hemorrhagic factor from the venom of the snake *Atractaspis engaddensis* (Atractaspididae). Toxicon, *25*:621.

Schulchynska-Castel, H., Dvilansky, A. and Keynan, A. (1986) *Echis colorata* bites: Clinical evaluation of 42 patients. A retrospective study. Israel J. Med. Sci., *22*:880.

Shabo-Shina, R. and Bdolah, A. (1987) Interactions of the neurotoxic complex from the venom of the False Horned Viper *(Pseudocerastes fieldi)* with rat striatal synaptosomes. Toxicon, *25*:253.

Shulzinska, H., Keynan, A. and Dvilansky, A. (1978) Effect of *Cerastes cerastes* snake bite on coagulation. Harefuah, *90:* 323 (in Hebrew).

Takasaki, C., Tamiya, N., Bdolah, A., Wollberg, Z. and Kochva, E. (1988) Sarafotoxins S_6: Several isotoxins from *Atractaspis* venom that affect the heart. Toxicon, *26*:543.

Underwood, G. and Kochva, E. (1988) On the affinities of the Burrowings Asps (Serpentes, Ophidia). (In preparation).

Wollberg, Z., Shabo-Shina, R., Intrator, N., Bdolah, A., Kochva, E., Shavit, G., Oron, Y., Vidne, B.A. and Gitter, S. (1988) A novel cardiotoxic polypeptide from *Atractaspis engaddensis* venom: Cardiac effects in mice and isolated rat and human heart preparations. Toxicon, *26*:525.

Yayon, E., Sikular, E. and Keynan, A. Desert black snake *(Walterinnesia aegyptia)* bites: A presentation of four cases. Harefuah (in Hebrew). (In press).

Venomous Snakes of Medical Importance in Japan

by M. Toriba and Y. Sawai

Japan Snake Institute

Introduction

Japan is composed of four major islands with small islands (Japan proper) (Fig. 1) and Southwestern Islands (Ryukyu Archipelago) (Fig. 2). They are situated at the northwestern corner of the Pacific Ocean. The Japan proper is separated from the Asian Continent by the Sea of Japan, while the Ryukyu Arch. is separated from the continent by East China Sea. There are three areas which are close to the continent in Japan: northern Hokkaido is related to the continent via Sakhalin; northern Kyushu is close to Korean Peninsula; and Yaeyama Islands, western-most islands in Ryukyu Archipelago, is related to China proper via Taiwan. Among them, the Kyushu-Korean line is important in the spread of the animals from the continent to Japan proper, and the fauna of Ryukyu is close to southern China via Yaeyama-Taiwan line. On the other hand, the presence of numerous endemic species in Japan suggests the long time separation from the continent.

Zoogeographically, Japan is divided into two parts by Watase line which is drawn between Osumi and Tokara Islands. The fauna of northern part (Japan proper) is palearctic, while that of southwestern (Ryukyu Arch.) is oriental. In the distribution of venomous snakes, the southwestern part is further subdivided into two: Tokara, Amami and Okinawa Islands on one hand and Yaeyama Islands the other.

List Of The Venomous Snakes In Japan

Japan proper
    Natricinae
        Rhabdophis tigrinus (Boie)
    Crotalinae
        Agkistrodon blomhoffii blomhoffii (Boie)

Ryukyu Archipelago (northeastern part)
    Elapinae
        Calliophis japonicus Gunther (including two subspecies)
    Crotalinae
        Trimeresurus tokarensis Nagai
        Trimeresurus flavoviridis (Hallowell)
        Trimeresurus okinavensis Boulenger

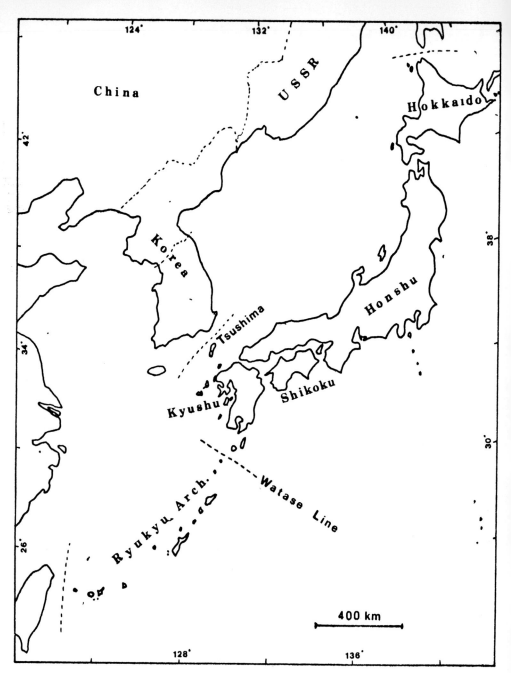

Figure 1.
Map of Japan and adjacent regions.

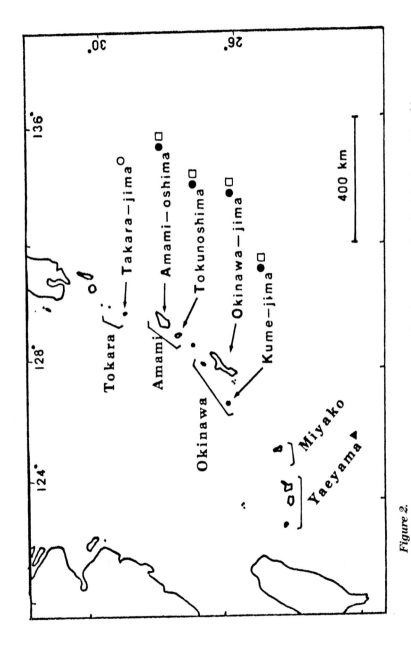

Figure 2.
Map of Ryukyu Archipelago, showing the islands groups and major islands mentioned in the text. Symbols indicate the presence of each species of the genus *Trimeresurus:* Hollow circle, *T. tokarensis;* solid circles, *T.flavoviridis;* square, *T. okinavensis;* triangle, *T, elegans.*

Ryukyu Arch. (Yaeyama Islands)
    Elapinae
        Calliophis macclellandi iwasakii Maki
    Crotalinae
        Trimeresurus elegans (Gray)

In this list, sea snakes are not included. Among the species listed above, two species of the genus *Calliophis* are not responsible for fatal snake bite cases in Japan, and are not treated in the following account.

Species Account

Rhabdophis tigrinus (Boie) . . . . Yamakagashi

Tropidonotus tigrinus Boie, 1826 Isis (T. typ.: Japan).
Natrix tigrina Stejneger, 1907, Maki, 1931.
Rhabdophis tigrina Malnate, 1960.
Rhabdophis tigrina Nakamura and Ueno, 1963; Mori, 1982.

Description:

A pair of enlarged posteriormost maxillary teeth, with sharp lateral ridges, without anterior grooves; nine symmetrical shields on heads; one loreal, two pre- and 3-4 postoculars; temporals 1+2; seven upper labials, 3rd and 4th enter the orbit; 9-10 lower labials; dorsal scales strongly keeled with a pair of apical pits, 21-19-17 rows; ventrals 150-170, anal divided, subcaudals 55-86 pairs; about 20 pairs of nuchal glands on mid-dorsal part of neck region; length about 1 m in females, less in males.

Coloration:

There is geographical variation in addition to some individual variation. Three populations with typical colorations were recognised by Goris (1971). Fundamentally, there are five longitudinal rows of dark blotches on dorsum. Among them, the mid-dorsal and both lateral ones are larger and conspicuous, while remaining two rows of dorso-lateral blotches, arranged alternatively with other ones, are small and sometimes obscure in darkness especially on posterior body. In neck region, however, the dorso-lateral blotches are large and conspicuous. The intervening area of the blotches is reddish especially on anterior body, but in some specimens, reddish colour is absent. The ground color is light greenish brown to greenish gray. Two typical colorations are shown in figures. (Figs. 3 & 4)

Habits and habitat:

This is one of the commonest snakes in Japan. Its habitat varies from paddy field to mountain forests. It feeds on frogs, occasionally toads and fishes (Fukada, 1959; Moriguchi and Naito, 1982). Copulation occurs at autumn, rarely at spring. Eggs (2-41) are laid in June through August, mainly July (Fukada, 1965; Moriguchi and Toriba, 1986). If cornered, it flattens the anterior

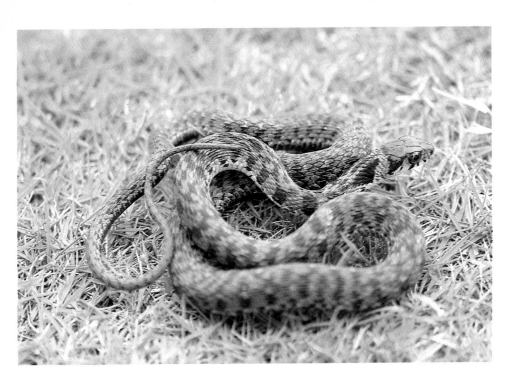

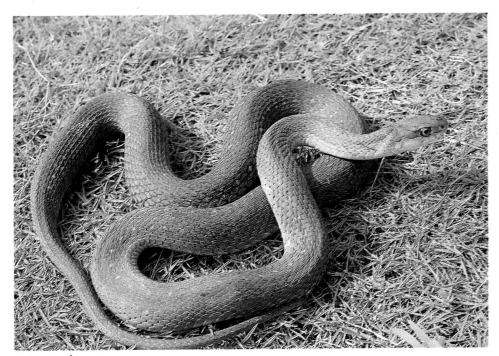

Figure 4.
Rhabdophis tigrinus in west-central Honshu.

body with arched neck. This behaviour seems to be connected with the presence of nuchal glands.

Distribution:

Honshu, Shikoku, Kyushu and some smaller islands. Absent in Hokkaido. Outside Japan — Korea, Southern Primorsky of USSR and China including Taiwan.

Remarks:

On the subspecific division of this species, there have been several opinions among workers (Nakamura and Ueno, 1963). Although we do not recognise any subspecies in this article, recent workers, especially in China, tend to recognise the following three subspecies based on the coloration. *R. t. tigrinus* in Japan, *R. t. lateralis* in the continent and *R. t. formosanus* in Taiwan. On this problem, future study is needed.

Agkistrodon blomhoffii blomhoffii (Boie) . . . . . Mamushi

Trigonocephalus blomhoffii Boie, 1826 Isis (T. typ.: Japan).
Agkistrodon blomhoffii blomhoffii Stejneger, 1907.
Agkistrodon halys blomhoffii Maki, 1931.
Agkistrodon halys (part) Nakamura and Ueno, 1963.
Agkistrodon blomhoffi blomhoffi Mori, 1982.
Agkistrodon blomhoffii ?affinis Stejneger, 1907.
Gloydius blomhoffii blomhoffii Hoge and Romano-Hoge, 1981.
Gloydius halys affinis Hoge and Romano-Hoge, 1981.

Description:

Nine symmetrical shields typical in many colubrids on head; a pair of loreal pits; a loreal and a prefoveal; three preoculars, one postocular and an elongate subocular; 7 upper labials, 3rd and 4th largest; lower temporals large; pupil elliptical and vertical; dorsal scales keeled, 21-21-17 rows; ventrals 132-151, anal undivided and subcaudals 43-56 pairs; length about 40-60 cm.

Coloration:

Brownish with a pair of longitudinal rows of dark oval blotches which have darker margin, light inner area and dark spot in centre. Lower lateral side whitish with a series of dark spots and venter has numerous dark flecks (Fig 5). Labial whitish and a dark postocular stripe extends from preocular to posterior jaw with light stripe on its upper edge. Tail tip reddish in young specimens.

Habits and habitat:

It is most common in and around forests and feeds on a variety of vertebrates, of which frogs are common (Fukada, 1959; Mitsui and Higashizono, 1986). It is the only viviparous snake in Japan proper and 5-6 young on average are produced in autumn (Fukada, 1962).

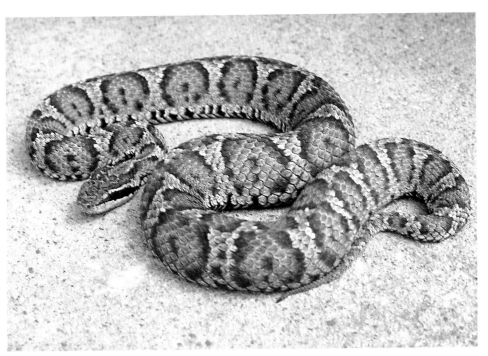

Figure 5.
Agkistrodon b. blomhoffii in west-central Honshu.

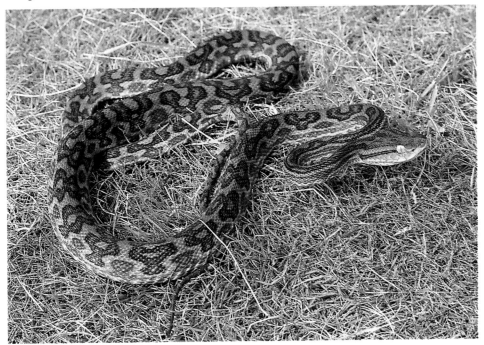

Figure 6.
Trimeresurus flavoviridis from Tokunoshima Is.

Distribution:

Hokkaido, Honshu, Shikoku, Kyushu and some smaller islands. *Agkistrodon* is absent in Ryukyu Arch., south of Watase line.

Remarks:

The name of mamushi is well known as dangerous by the people. However, there are many persons who confuse young *Elaphe climacophora* which has blotched pattern, with mamushi. *E. climacophora* can be distinguished from mamushi by the presence of the round pupil.

The population of *Agkistrodon* in Tsushima Is., Japan has been considered as *A. b. blomhoffii.* However, a recent study by Isogawa et al. (1987) indicated that the population in Tsushima has intermediate characters between *A. caliginosus (A. ussuriensis)* in Korea and Japanese *A. b. blomhoffii.* The taxonomic status of this population would be determined by future study.

Hoge and Romano-Hoge (1981) proposed a new genus *Gloydius* for Asian *Agkistrodon* (sensu lato) based on the cranial osteology. As for the validity of their new name, we are still studying it. At present we use the older, more commonly accepted name.

Trimeresurus flavoviridis (Hallowell) . . . . Habu

Bothrops flavoviridis Hallowell, 1860 Proc. Phila. Acad. (T. typ.: "Amakarima" Island = Kerama Islands, Okinawa group).

Trimeresurus riukiuanus Hilgendorf, 1880.

Trimeresurus flavoviridis Stejneger, 1907; Hoge and Romano-Hoge, 1981; Mori, 1982.

Trimeresurus flavoviridis flavoviridis Maki, 1931; Nakamura and Ueno, 1963.

Trimeresurus flavoviridis tinkhami Gloyd, 1955.

Description:

Top of head covered by small scales except a pair of large supraoculars; canthals also slightly larger than other scales; 10-14 scales between supraoculars; upper labials 7-10, usually separated from eye by one or two rows of small scales and elongated subocular ; eye large with vertically elliptical pupil; scale rows at midbody 35 or 36, with the range of variation 31-39, ventrals 217-239, anal entire and subcaudals 72-95 pairs; the duplication of transverse rows of dorsal scales occurs, and the number of scales along vertebral line do not correspond to the number of vertebrae (similar condition occurs in *T. tokarensis;* Toriba, 1985); largest snake of the genus, more than 1 m, rarely exceeds 2 m.

Coloration:

Both individual and geographic variation occur. The ground color is yellowish brown, olive, reddish brown or light brown, on which some irregular darker patterns are present. These patterns can vary, but in general it is composed of a pair of rows of elongate blotches with lighter inner areas, which are united to form a row of large blotches especially in posterior part of the body or sometimes become longitudinal stripes mainly in anterior part (Figs 6 & 7). In general, the population in Amami Islands has more clear patterns, while in Okinawa Islands the pattern is obscured by numerous lighter spots. The venter is whitish with dark flecks.

Habits and habitat:

This dangerous pit viper inhabits various areas including mountain forests, woods along seashore, cultivated and residential areas. It is abundant in cultivated fields and their vicinity, especially in cycad woods, rough stone walls and old tombs. It is a good climber and active at night. It feeds mainly on rats and other vertebrates. Fifty-four species of vertebrates have been recorded as the prey of Habu (Koba, 1971). The mature size is about 120 cm in length and 3-17 eggs are laid during July to August. They hatch about 40 days after oviposition. The ecology and the behaviour of Habu have been reviewed by Tanaka and Wada (1977).

Distribution:

Amami and Okinawa Islands, where 25 islands including Amami-oshima, Tokunoshima and Okinawa Is. are known to be inhabited by this pit viper (Takara, 1962).

Remarks:

Some specimens in Kume-jima Is. show characteristic color pattern, in which the dark blotches are restricted to vertebral area to form longitudinal stripe, which markedly differs from other forms in appearance. Although Gloyd (1955) described this form as distinct subspecies, *T. f. tinkhami*, Takara (1962) indicated that this color pattern is seen only in some individuals of the population in Kume-jima and placed the name *tinkhami* as a synonym of *T. flavoviridis*.

Trimeresurus tokarensis **Nagai . . . . Tokara-habu**

Trimeresurus tokarensis Nagai, 1928 Kagoshima-ken Hakubutsu Chosa (T. typ.: Takara-jima Is.); Koba and Kikukawa, 1971; Mori, 1984.
Trimeresurus flavoviridis tokarensis Maki, 1931; Nakamura and Ueno, 1963.

Description:

In general, similar to *T. flavoviridis*. Scales between supraoculars 11-13; supralabials 8 with the range of 7-9; scale rows at midbody 31 with the range of 31-33; ventrals 199-210, subcaudals 72-84; length about 1 m or less, the largest 1.5 m, smaller than *T. flavoviridis*.

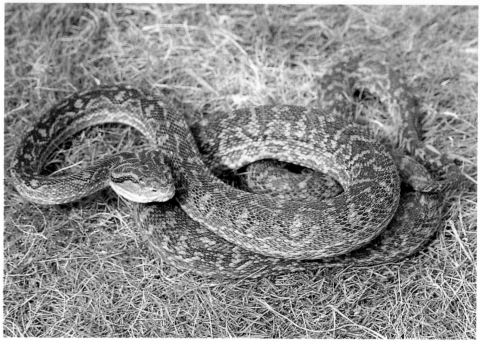

Figure 7.
Trimeresurus flavoviridis from Okinawa-jima Is.

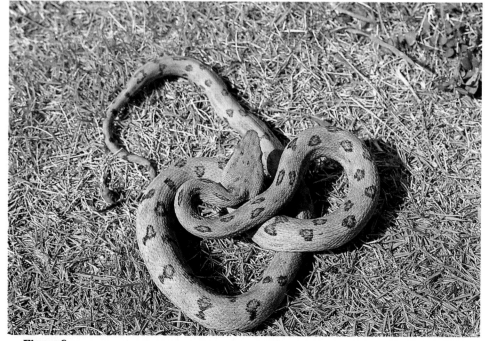

Figure 8.
T. tokarensis, light brown color phase.

Coloration:

There are two markedly different color types in this species. The greyish brown color type has the ground color of greyish brown with a longitudinal series of a pair of small dark blotches (Fig 8). The blackish brown color type is blackish brown on whole body (Fig 9). The former type is abundant.

Habits and habitat:

The two islands inhabited by this species are small and their fauna are also simple. Some lizards and rodents are its prey. Eggs (2-7) are laid in July through August (Koba et al., 1970a).

Distribution:

Takara-jima and Kodakara-jama Is., Tokara Islands.

Remarks:

Although some workers recognise this species as a subspecies of *T. flavoviridis* due to their similarities, there are marked differences in scutelation and the toxicity of venom.

Trimeresurus okinavensis Boulenger . . . . . . Hime-habu

> *Trimeresurus okinavensis* Boulenger, 1892 Ann. Mag. Nat. Hist (T. typ.: Okinawa); Stejneger, 1907; Maki, 1931; Nakamura and Ueno, 1963; Mori, 1982.
> *Ovophis okinavensis* Hoge and Romano-Hoge, 1981.

Description:

Canthus rostralis prominent; the scales between supraoculars 6-9; supralabials 8 with the range of 7-9, separated from eye by two rows of scales and 2-3 suboculars; dorsal scale rows at midbody 23 with the range of 21-25; ventrals 126-135, anal entire and subcaudals 36-55 pairs; short, stout snake with length between 40 to 70 cm.

Coloration:

The ground color is light brown or grayish brown, on which dark square blotches are present along vertebral line. Another series of smaller blotches is present lateral to the major blotches. There are additional blackish blotches along the border of the ventrals and dorsal scales. Venter is slightly dark. Top of head is uniformly brownish with postocular dark stripes, which are bordered by whitish streaks on their lower edges (Fig. 10).

Habits and habitat:

This pit viper lives in mountain forests and feeds mainly on frogs, although some reptiles, rodents and birds are also eaten (Mishima, 1966). It lays 3-14 eggs during August to September. The young hatch in the same day of

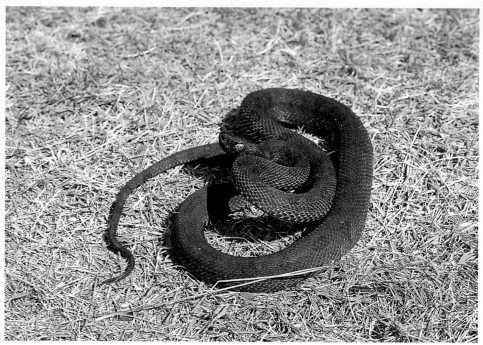

Figure 9.
T. *tokarensis*, dark brown color phase.

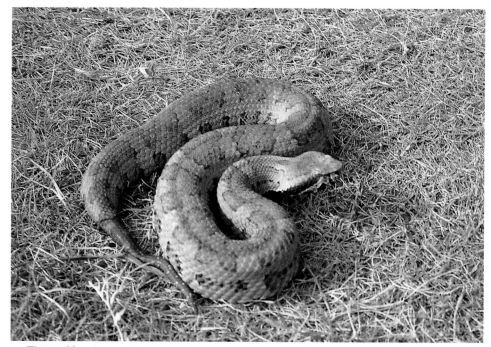

Figure 10.
T. *okinavensis*, from Amami Islands.

oviposition or in most cases the next day. Egg shells are relatively thin (Koba et al., 1970b). This reproductive habit may be considered as intermediate between oviparous and viviparous ones.

Distribution:
Amami and Okinawa Islands, and similar to *T. flavoviridis*, though some islands have only one species of the genus *Trimeresurus*.

Remarks:
This species is closely related to *T. monticola* in China and Southeast Asia. Burger (1971) proposed a new genus, *Ovophis*, for them based on the skull characters, which was followed by Hoge and Romano-Hoge. We are working on the validity of this genus and retain the older name in this account.

Trimeresurus elegans (Gray) . . . . . Sakishima-habu
Craspedocephalus elegans Gray, 1849 Catalogue of the specimens of snakes in the collection of the British Museum. (T. typ.: West coast of America, in error, probably Ishigaki-jima Is.)
Trimeresurus luteus Boettger, 1895
Trimeresurus elegans Stejneger, 1907; Maki, 1931; Nakamura and Ueno, 1963; Mori, 1984.

Description:
The scales between supraoculars 11-15; supralabials 8 with the range of 7-9, separated from eye by a row of scales and elongate subocular; dorsal scales keeled with a single apical pit, 23-25 rows at midbody; ventrals 182-196, anal entire and subcaudals 64-76 pairs; length about 1 m.

Coloration:
The ground color varies from light brown, yellowish brown to dark brown. There are dark blotches along the vetebral line, which are diamond in shape or connected to each other to form a zigzag pattern. Along lower lateral side, additional rows of blotches are present. Venter is greyish white (Fig 11).

Habits and habitat:
It lives in various habitat, and feeds on reptiles, frogs and rodents (Araki and Mitsui, 1984).

Distribution:
Yaeyama Islands.

Remarks:
This species is closely related to *T. mucrosquamatus* in Taiwan and Southern China. The former has smaller number of scales.

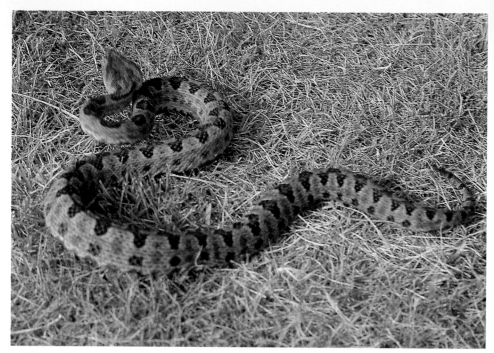

Figure 11.
T. elegans from Ishigaki-jima, Yaeyama Islands

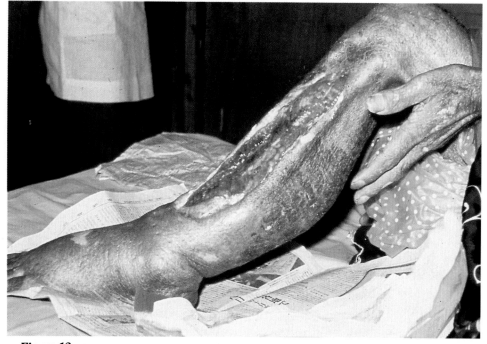

Figure 12.
Severe necrosis occurred on the left lower leg by habu bite.

Epidemiological aspects of the bites

Habu (*Trimeresurus flavoviridis*).

Epidemiological studies on habu bites have been extensively carried out by several workers (Sasa et al., 1959; Sawai et al., 1967b, 1976; Sawai and Kawamura, 1983a,b, 1984a,b, 1985a,b, 1986). The average annual number of the bites on the Amami and Okinawa Islands during 14 years from 1971 to 1984 was 467 in which 2.5(0.54%) were fatal cases. Morbidity and mortality rates per 1,000 population were 2.4 and 0.26, respectively.

During warmer months from March to October, more than 80% of the total bites occurred, in which two peak months are June and October. Eighty-seven percent of the total bites occurred in the age group from teens to sixties in which higher number of bites occurred in the ages of forties and fifties. Bites in males were 2.5 times as frequent as those in females. Forty-four percent of the total bites occurred in agricultural fields whereas 23% occurred in residences. Thus, the habu bites are a hazard to human life. Although habu is nocturnal, 70% of the total bites occurred in daylight hours during from 6 am to 6 pm and the majority of the bites occurred in agricultural fields, whereas 30% of the bites occurred after sunset from 6 pm to 6 am in residential areas and on roads.

Sakishima-habu (*Trimeresurus elegans*).

The annual number of bites is smaller than that of habu, because the area of occurrence of the bite is limited to Yaeyama Islands. Thus, the average annual number of bites during 14 years from 1971 to 1984 is 60, and average morbidity rate per 1,000 population is 1.27. Death due to the bites is very rare. Marked difference is not seen in monthly incidence, because the weather of the islands is warmer than those in Amami and Okinawa. Frequency of bite by age and sex, location and time of the day of bite is similar to habu bite.

Hime-habu (*Trimeresurus okinavensis*) and Tokara-habu (*T. tokarensis*).

The bites by hime-habu occurred in Amami and Okinawa Islands in 5 to 10% of the habu bites and the bites by tokara-habu are limited to Takara and Kodakara Is. Because of the small population of less than 1,000 the bites are not frequent.

Mamushi (*Agkistrodon b. blomhoffii*).

It is estimated that the annual number of the bites is more than 500. Fatality rate is 0.9%. More than 80% of the total bite occurred among the age group from teens to fifties. Seventy percent of the bites occurred in males and 30% in females. Sixty percent of the bites occurred on fingers and hands, and 19% on feet. Most of the bites occurred during the day (Tateno et al., 1963).

Yamakagashi (*Rhabdophis tigrinus*).

Severe bites by this snake is not frequent, although the snake is very common in Japan.

Toxicity of the Venoms

The yield and toxicity of venoms of habu, mamushi and yamakagashi are listed in Table 1. The lethal toxicity of the venoms represented by LD_{50} (50% dose) and MLD (minimum lethal dose) is different according to the route of injection and species of animal used. Thus, LD_{50} and MLD of habu venom in mice by intraperitoneal (i.p.) injection are 80 and 300 μg (Mitsuhashi et al., 1961). As shown in Table 1, minimum haemorrhagic dose (MHD) is represented as a macular haemorrhage of 1 cm of diameter which is induced by intracutaneous (i.c.) injection in depilated rabbit (Kondo et al., 1960). MLD is also calculated by intramuscular (i.m.) injection into the leg of mice (Sawai et al., 1967c,d) or subcutaneous (s.c.) injection into the sole of mice (Seu and Sawai, 1981). Studies on the quantitative determination of swelling, haemorrhage and necrosis of muscle induced by the injection of venom into *M. vastus lateralis* of the leg of rabbit was also reported (Fukami, 1978; Fukami and Hattori, 1982).

Biological activity of factors separated from the venoms
Haemorrhagic factors.

Two haemorrhagic principles (HR1 and HR2) were separated from habu venom by gel filtration and column chromatography (Ohsaka et al., 1960) MHD of HR1 was 0.0058 μg which was 43 times higher than that of crude venom. MHDs of both HR2a and HR2b which were further separated from HR2 were 0.066 μg (Takahashi and Ohsaka, 1970).

Two haemorrhagic principles were also separated from mamushi venom. The HR1 from mamushi venom showed proteinase activity. It is interesting to note that the two haemorrhagic principles induced different type lesions by i.v. injection into mice, HR1 induced intraperitoneal haemorrhage and HR2 did subcutaneous haemorrhage (Suzuki, 1970).

TABLE 1
Lethal and haemorrhagic toxicity of venoms.

Snakes	Yield of venom (mg)	LD_{50} (μg)	MLD (μg)	MHD (μg)
T. flavoviridis[1]	300.0	80(i.p.)		0.6
T. tokarensis[2]	32.9		300(i.m.)	2.0
T. elegans[1]	124.0	95(i.p.)		1.8
T. okinavensis[1]	22.2	300(i.p.)		8.6
A. b. blomhoffii[3]	15.0	19.5(i.v.)		2.5
R. tigrinus[4]	8.5	5.3(i.v.)		

1) Mitsuhashi et al. (1961).   3) Kosuge (1968).
2) Sawai et al. (1967c).   4) Sakai et al. (1983).

338

Necrotic activity of habu venom.

Two necrotic principles, one heat-labile and the other heat-stable were separated from habu venom. The former showed proteinase activity. Further, it was elucidated that the necrotic activity was accelerated by phospholipase (Maeno et al., 1962; Kurashige et al., 1966). On the other hand, a necrotic factor (Chinzei, 1974) and necrosis inducing phospholipase A_2 were separated from habu venom (Kihara et al., 1986). It is also reported that proteinase participates in the necrotic activity of habu venom (Seu and Sawai, 1981).

Factor inducing swelling.

A study on the quantitative determination of a swelling factor without haemorrhage, separated from sakishima-habu venom has been reported (Yamakawa et al., 1976).

Factor inducing coagulant activity of blood.

A thrombin-like enzyme which converts fibrinogen to fibrin is separated from mamushi venom (Sato et al., 1965).

Venom extracted from Duvernoy's glands of yamakagashi (*R. tigrinus)* showed potent activation of prothrombin (F II) which converts prothrombin to thrombin, and the thrombin in turn converts fibrinogen to fibrin. Prolonged coagulation, hypofibrinogenemia and systemic haemorrhage occurred in the envenomated mice due to the cooperative action of haemorrhagic factor and the prothrombin activator in the venom (Sakai et al., 1983).

Immunogenicity of Snake Venoms
Production of antivenom against habu, mamushi and yamakagashi venoms.

Purified and freeze-dried habu antivenom were prepared in 1959 (Sawai et al., 1961). Horses were injected intramuscularly with 10 mg of habu venom dissolved in 2.5 ml saline added to the same amount of Freund's adjuvant as basic immunization. One month after the injection, 1 mg of the venom dissolved in 5 ml alone was injected intramuscularly as booster shot at an interval of one week, and the amount of venom was increased to 20 mg as final dose. The crude antivenom obtained from immunized horses was fractionated by 30 and 50 % of saturated ammonium sulphate. The final product contained 0.9% NaCl and 5% phenol. Four percent glycine was added before freeze-drying to increase solubility. The anti-lethal and anti-haemorrhagic effect of the antivenom was tested by i.m. injection of 0.1 ml of antivenom mixed with the venom dilutions into mice. Twenty-four hours after the injection, survival or death and local lesion in mice were inspected. Thus, 0.1 ml of the antivenom neutralized 300 μg venom (2 MLDs and 150 MHDs).

It was also elucidated that the antivenom injected by i.v. route within one hour after the envenomation is effective to protect rabbits from lethal and local effect of the venom as compared with those given by i.m. route.

Later, the anti-lethal and anti-haemorrhagic potency of the antivenom was decided to indicate as a unit of anti-HR1 and anti-HR2 antibody separated from habu venom (Kondo et al., 1971a). The antivenom freeze-dried and purified by ammonium sulphate and pepsin digestion (20 ml vial) is commercially produced by Laboratory of Chemotherapy and Serotherapy, Kumamoto, Japan. One ml of the antivenom contained 6000 u. of anti-HR1 and anti-HR2 antibody. Anti-mamushi antivenom is also available commercially at Chiba Prefectural Serum Laboratory, Konodai, Chiba, Japan.

Studies on the production of purified and freeze-dried anti-yamakagashi antivenom were carried out in Japan Snake Institute. Both formalin vaccine and crude venom extracted from Duvernoy's glands of yamakagashi were used for the immunizing antigen in rabbits and goats. The antivenom obtained from immunized rabbits was fractionated by Na_2SO_4 whereas method of $(NH_4)_2SO_4$ and pepsin digestion was applied for goat antivenom. The results of the neutralization test indicated that LD_{50}s of 0.1 ml of the purified rabbit antivenom and venom control were 115 μg and 4.3μg, respectively, and the same amount of antivenom neutralized 26.9 MLDs of the venom (Kawamura et al., 1986).

Habu toxoid for prophylactic immunization.

Application of antivenom for the patient is limited, because the envenomation occurs in remote areas and the transportation of the patient to hospital is usually delayed. Local necrosis developed shortly after the bite. In such a situation, the habu toxoid may decrease the reactions to severe bite due to habu. The results that the habu venom treated by dihydrothioctic acid (DHTA) have proven to be a good antigenic for experimental animals suggested the possibility of immunizing human beings against habu venom by the toxoid venom (Sawai et al., 1969).

During a 3-year period from 1965 to 1967, the field trial of prophylactic vaccination with DHTA-toxoid was undertaken in Amami and Okinawa Islands, and it was elucidated that the toxoid was effective to decrease severe local necrosis of the patients (Sawai et al., 1969a, 1973, 1979).

Studies on purification and inactivation of the toxoid have been carried out by several workers (Okonogi and Hattori, 1968; Sadahiro, 1971b, Kondo et al., 1971b, Sawai et al., 1972). In the mean time, the minimum requirement for the habu toxoid was determined. The potency test of the toxoid was performed by immunizing guinea pigs with the toxoid to be tested and a reference toxoid, and the titration of the circulating antibody of the immunized guinea pigs was tested for anti-HR1 and HR2. The potency of the toxoid was represented as relative value of reference toxoid (Kondo et al., 1971b). Thus, mixed-toxoid of HR1 and HR2 (Sadahiro, 1971a,b; Kondo et al., 1971b) and APF toxoid fractionated by ethanol and inactivated by formalin (Sawai et al., 1972) were used in another field trial to investigate the circulating antivenom and side reaction due to the vaccination (Someya et al., 1972). Surveillance of the prognosis of the patients who received toxoid was also carried out (Fukushima et al., 1976; Murata and Fukushima, 1981).

Hypersensitive reaction caused by habu venom.

The reaction was induced in persons while balancing the dried habu or mamushi venom. The main symptoms were sneezing, serous rhinorrhea, conjunctival itch, difficulty in breathing like asthma and nettle rash. It is suggested that sensitization occurred by repeated inhalation of particles of dried venom (Sawai et al., 1967a).

A delayed type of hypersensitive reaction of erythema like wheal appeared following intracutaneous injection of habu toxoid in persons previously received the veccination (Sawai et al., 1969a).

Clinical Aspects of the Bites

Habu bites.

More frequent bites occurred in the upper extremities in which bites on fingers and hands were common, whereas lower legs were the main site of bite in the lower extremities. Severe bites including fatal cases and necrosis of muscle tissue are decreasing because of successful antivenom treatment. Intense pain and swelling develop around the bite wound accompanied not infrequently by vesicles and subcutaneous haemorrhage. When the venom penetrates into the muscle layer, haemorrhagic necrosis of muscle tissue occurs. In fatal cases, systemic signs and symptoms such as hypotension, feeble pulse, cyanosis, fever, vomiting and diarrhea occurs and the patient expires within 24 hr.

Most of the patients visit hospital and dispensary within one hr after the bite and are treated by i.v. drip of 20 to 40 ml of antivenom by fluid transfusion. Vasopressor drug is necessary to recover from hypotension. Administration of steroid and anti-histamine is also effective for systemic symptoms. Incision of the wound is indicated only to accelerate the drainage of intense swelling which might lead to severe necrosis of muscle tissues. Necrosis occurring in fingers or hand induced in high rate a certain motor disturbance after the wound had healed. On the other hand, bites occurring at lateral aspect below the knee caused severe necrosis of *M. tibialis anterior* and ankylosis of foot joint (Fig. 12).

Mamushi-bites.

Intense swelling and subcutaneous haemorrhage occur, although necrosis of muscle tissue is not frequent as compared with that of habu bite. Systemic symptoms such as fever, vomiting and diplopia occur in severe bites. Acute renal failure is the main cause of death due to the bite, which occurs within 3 to 9 days (Tateno et al., 1963). Antivenom therapy is indispensable to prevent such a complication.

Yamakagashi-bites.

Severe bites rarely occur, although the mild cases without intoxication are more frequent. Several hours after the bites, patients visit hospital complaining of ceaseless bleeding from the bite wound. Gum bleeding, haematuria and systemic ecchymosis of the body follow marked coagulation abnormality in blood such as prolonged bleeding time, hypofibrinogenemia and increase of FDP. Brain haemorrhage is reported in fatal bites (Ogawa and Sawai, 1986). Acute renal failure following the bite is also reported (Mori et al., 1983). Antivenom therapy is effective to recover the haemorrhagic diathesis of the patient (Wakamatsu et al, 1986).

Serum sickness.

Hypersensitive reaction to horse serum is reported in ten percent of the patients treated by antivenom. Immediate type of serum sickness occurs during or immediately after the injection of antivenom and delayed type occurs around 7 days. Hypotension, dyspnea and urticarial rash occur in immediate type, whereas urticarial rash, fever, lymphadenopathy and arthralgia occur in delayed type.

Anti-histamine, steroid, noradrenalin and fluid transfusion are used for the treatment. Steroid added to the antivenom is effective to prevent serum sickness.

The Nuchal Glands Secretion of Yamakagashi

The nuchal glands have no duct. The skin which covers the glands is relatively thin and easily broken on pressure to release the secretion.

There have been several reports on corneal disturbances caused by the secretion of the nuchal glands of yamakagashi (Kawashima, 1957, 1959; Suzuki, 1960). As clinical symptoms, disturbances of vision, anesthesia, cloudiness of cornea, miosis, and in some cases mydriasis were recognised. Asahi et al. (1985) experimentally investigated the damage caused by crude venom from nuchal glands of yamakagashi using rabbits and dogs. They observed fugitive corneal epithelial detachment and strong miosis in pupil which occurred within 60 min of instillation.

The component of the venom from nuchal glands was analysed by Akizawa et al., (1985a, b) and Azuma et al., (1986). They found ten kinds of poly-hydroxylated cardiotonic steroids, bufadienolides, and riboflavine in the secretion. Among the bufadienolides found in the secretion, one is identical with gamabufotalin from the parotoid glands of toads, *Bufo* spp. These bufadienolides showed the positive inotropic action in guinea pig papillary muscle and inhibition of the activity of $(Na^+ + K^+)$ATPase.

References

Akizawa, T., Yasuhara, T., Kano, R. and Nakajima, T. (1985a). Novel polyhydroxylated cardiac steroids in the nuchal glands of the snake, *Rhabdophis tigrinus*. Biomedical Research, 6:437-441.

Akizawa, T., Yasuhara, T., Azuma, H. and Nakajima, T. (1985b). Chemical structures and biological activities of bufadienolides in the nucho-dorsal glands of Japanese snakes, *Rhabdophis tigrinus*. Journal of Pharmacobio-dynamics, 8:s-60.

Araki, Y. and Mitsui, K. (1984). Food habits of *Trimeresurus flavoviridis* and *T. elegans*. Reports of ecological researches to diminish habu-bites in Okinawa Prefecture, 7:59-65. (in Japanese).

Asahi, H., Kohtari, Y., Chiba, K. and Mishima, A (1985). Effect of the nucho-dorsal gland venom of the yamakagashi snake on the eye. Folia Ophthalmologica Japonica, 36:379-383. (in Japanese with English summary).

Azuma, H., Sekizaki, S., Akizawa, T., Yasuhara, T. and Nakajima, T. (1986). Activities of novel polyhydroxylated cardiotonic steroids purified from nuchal glands of the snake, *Rhabdophis tigrinus*. Journal of Pharmacy and Pharmacology, 38:388-390.

Chinzei, H. (1974). Isolation of myonecrotic factor from the venom of habu (*Trimeresurus flavoviridis*). Japanese Journal of Tropical Medicine & Hygine, 2:111-112.

Fukada, H. (1959). Biological studies on the snakes. V. Food habits in the fields. Bulletin of Kyoto Gakugei University, B. 14:22-28.

Fukada, H. (1962). Biological studies on the snakes. IX. Breeding habits of *Agkistrodon halys blomhoffii*. Ibid., 20:12-17.

Fukada, H. (1965). Breeding habits of some Japanese reptiles (critical review). Ibid., 27:65-82.

Fukami, M. (1978). A quantitative study of local lesions in experimental snake envenomation. 1. Studies on composite lesions of muscular tissue caused by the venom of habu (*Trimeresurus flavoviridis*), Sakishima-habu (*Trimeresurus elegans*) and hime-habu (*Trimeresurus okinavensis*). The Snake, 10:114-130. (in Japanese with English summary).

Fukami, M. and Hattori, Z. (1982). Study on quantitative determination of local lesions induced by snake venom. Ibid. 14:23-34.

Fukushima, H., Minakami, K., Koga, S., Higashi, K., Kawabata, H., Yamashita, S., Katsuki, Y. and Sakamoto, M. (1976). Study on prevention of habu snake (*Trimeresurus flavoviridis*) bites by using habu toxoid. Medical Journal of Kagoshima University, 28:1005-1024.

Gloyd, H.K. (1955). A new crotalid snake from Kume Shima, Riu Kiu Islands. Bulletin of Chicago Academy of Sciences, 10:123-134.

Goris, R.C. (1971) Geographic variation in color and pattern of *Rhabdophis tigrinus* (Boie). The Snake, 3:57-59.

Hoge, A.R. and Romano-Hoge, S.A.R.W.L. (1981). Poisonous snakes of the world. Part 1. Check list of the pit-vipers (Viperoidea, Viperidae, Crotalinae). Memorias do Instituto Butantan, 42/43:179-309.

Isogawa, K., Moriya, A., Higashizono, S. and Okada, T. (1987). The taxonomic status of the mamushi, genus *Agkistrodon*, from Tsushima Island. Japanese Journal of Herpetology, 12:77-78. (in Japanese)

Kawamura, Y., Sakai, A. and Sawai, Y. (1986). Studies on the pathogenesis of envenomation of the Japanese colubrid snake, yamakagashi, *Rhabdophis tigrinus* (Boie). 3. Preparation of anti-yamakagashi antivenom. The Snake, 18:1-3.

Kawashima, J. (1957). Disturbance of the eye by snake venom (*Natrix tigrina*). Ganka Rinsho Iho, 50:837-839. (in Japanese).

Kawashima, J. (1959). Disturbance of the eye by snake venom (*Natrix tigrina*), II Ibid., 53-834-837. (in Japanese).

Kihara, H., Terashi, S., Ohno, M., and Hashimura, S. (1986). Induction of myonecrosis by phospholipase A_2 from habu (*Trimeresurus flavoviridis*) venom. The Snake, 18:84-91.

Koba, K. (1971). Natural history of the habu, *Trimeresurus flavoviridis* (Hallowell). Ibid., 3:75-96. (in Japanese with English summary).

Koba, K. and Kikukawa, D. (1971). A taxonomic study of the tokara-habu, *Trimeresurus tokarensis* Nagai. Ibid., 3:39-52. (in Japanese with English summary).

Koba, K. and Kikukawa, D. (1976). The morphology of *Trimeresurus elegans* (Serpentes: Viperidae). Bulletin of Ginkyo College of Medical Technology, 1:19-32. (in Japanese with English summary).

Koba, K., Tanaka, K., Nakamoto, E. and Morimoto, H. (1970a). The eggs of the tokara-habu (*Trimeresurus tokarensis*): Condition in the oviduct, laying and hatching. The Snake, 2:32-38. (in Japanese with English summary).

Koba, K., Tanaka, K., Yoshizaki, K. and Nakamoto, E. (1970b). Eggs and hatching of the hime-habu, *Trimeresurus okinavensis* Boulenger. Ibid., 2:111-121. (in Japanese with English summary).

Kondo, H., Kondo, S., Ikezawa, H., Murata, R. and Ohsaka, A. (1960). Studies on the quantitative method for determination of haemorrhagic activity of habu snake venom. Japanese Journal of Medical Science and Biology, 13:43-51.

Kondo, H., Kondo, S., Sadahiro, S., Yamauchi, K. and Murata, R. (1971a). Standardization of *Trimeresurus flavoviridis* (habu) antivenin. Ibid., 24:323-327.

Kondo, H., Sadahiro, S., Yamauchi, K., Kondo, S. and Murata, R. (1971b). Preparation and standardization of toxoid from the venom of *Trimeresurus flavoviridis* (habu). Ibid., 24:281-294.

Kosuge, T. (1968). Biological toxicity of mamushi-snake venom (*Agkistrodon halys*) and morphological changes caused by the venom. Kitakanto Medical Journal, 18:353-379. (in Japanese with English summary).

Kurashige, S., Hara, Y., Kawakami, M. and Mitsuhashi, S. (1966). Studies on habu snake venom. VII. Heat stable myolitic factor and development of its activity by addition of phospholipase A. Japanese Journal of Microbiology, 10:23-31.

Maeno, H., Mitsuhashi, S., Okonogi, T., Hoshi, S. and Honma, M. (1962). Studies on habu snake venom. V. Myolysis caused by phospholipase A in habu snake venom. Japanese Journal of Experimental Medicine, 32:55-64.

Maki, M. (1931). A monograph of the snakes of Japan. Dai-ichi Shobo, Tokyo.

Mishima, S. (1966). Studies on the feeding habits of *Trimeresurus okinavensis* on the Amami Island. Acta Herpetologica Japonica, 1:67-74. (in Japanese with English summary).

Mitsuhashi, S., Maeno, H., Sato, I., Tanaka, T., Kawakami, M., Yagi, S., Sawai, Y., Okonogi, T., Ono, T. and Matsushita, N. (1961). Studies on habu snake venom. 1b. Comparative studies of several biological activity of snake venoms belong to *Trimeresurus*. Japanese Journal of Bacteriology, 16:904-908. (in Japanese with English summary).

Mitsui, S., and Higashizono, S. (1986). Food items of mamushi, *Agkistrodon b. blomhoffii*, in nature. Acta Herpetologica Sinica, 5(1): 49.

Mori, K., Hisa, S., Suzuki, S., Sugai, K., Sakai, H., Kikuchi, T., Hiwatashi, N., Shishido, H. and Yoro, Y. (1983). A case of severe defibrination syndrome due to snake (*Rhabdophis tigrinus*) bite. Japanese Journal of Clinical Haematology, 24:256-262. (in Japanese with English summary).

Mori, M. (1982). Japans Schlangen. Band 1. Igaku-Shoin, Tokyo.

Mori, M. (1984). Japans Schlangen. Band 2. Igaku-Shoin, Tokyo.

Moriguchi, H. and Naito, S. (1982). Activities and food habits of *Amphiesma vibakari* (Boie) and *Rhabdophis tigrinus* (Boie). The Snake, 14:136-142. (in Japanese with English summary).

Moriguchi, H. and Toriba, M. (1986). Note on the number of eggs in oviduct of *Rhabdophis tigrinus*. Ibid., 17:144-147.

Murata, R. and Fukushima, H. (1981). Immune response of man to habu venom toxoid. Japanese Journal of Medical Science and Biology, 34:197-212.

Nakamura, K. and Ueno, S. -I.(1963). Japanese reptiles and amphibians in colour. Hoikushu, Osaka. (in Japanese).

Ogawa, H. and Sawai, Y. (1986). Fatal bite of yamakagashi (*Rhabdophis tigrinus*). The Snake, 18:53-54.

Ohsaka, A., Ikezawa, H., Kondo, H., Kondo, S. and Uchida, N. (1960). Haemorrhagic activities of habu snake venom, and their relations to lethal toxicity, proteolytic activities and other pathological activities. British Journal of Experimental Pathology, 41:478-486.

Okonogi, T. and Hattori, Z. (1968). Attenuation of habu snake (*Trimeresurus flavoviridis*) venom treated with alcohol and its effect as immunizing antigen. Japanese Journal of Bacteriology, 23:137-144. (in Japanese with English summary).

Sadahiro, S. (1971a). Studies on toxoid from the venom of habu (*Trimeresurus flavoviridis*),a crotalid. I. Detoxification of habu venom with formalin. Ibid., 26:214-221. (in Japanese with English summary).

Sadahiro, S. (1971b). Studies on toxoid from the venom of habu (*Trimeresurus flavoviridis*),a crotalid. II. Immunogenicity of toxoids derived from main toxic principles separated from habu venom. Ibid., 26:319-324. (in Japanese with English summary).

Sakai, A., Honma, M. and Sawai, Y. (1983). Studies on the pathogenesis of envenomation of the Japanese colubrid snake, Yamakagashi, *Rhabdophis tigrinus* (Boie). 1. Study on the toxicity of the venom. The Snake, 15:7-13.

Sasa, M., Teruya, K., Uchiyama, H. and Imai, S. (1959). Epidemiology of the poisonous snakebite in the Amami and the Ryukyu Islands. Japanese Journal of Experimental Medicine, 29:417-444.

Sato, T., Iwanaga, S., Mizushima, Y, and Suzuki, T. (1965). Studies on snake venom. XV. Separation of argininester hydrolase of *Agkistrodon halys blomhoffii* venom with three enzymatic entities: "Bradykinin releasing ", "clotting" and "permeability increasing". Journal of Biochemistry, 57:380-391.

Sawai, Y. (1979). Vaccination against snake bite poisoning. In : Handbook of Experimental Pharmacology, Vol. 52, "Snake Venoms" (Ed. by C.-Y. Lee), pp. 881-897. Springer-Verlag.

Sawai, Y., Chinzei, H., Kawamura, Y., Fukuyama, T. and Okonogi, T. (1972). Studies on the improvement of treatment of habu (*Trimeresurus flavoviridis*) bite. 9. Studies on the immunogenicity of the purified habu venom toxoid by alcohol precipitation. Japanese Journal of Experimental Medicine, 42:283-307.

Sawai, Y., Fukuyama, T., Kato, K., Kawamura, Y. and Honma, M. (1967a). Case report on hypersensitivity to habu (*Trimeresurus flavoviridis*) venom. Japanese Journal of Bacteriology, 22:58-60. (in Japanese with English summary).

Sawai, Y. and Kawamura, Y. (1983a) Habu (*Trimeresurus flavoviridis*) bites on the Amami Islands of Japan in 1977. The Snake, 15:1-6.

Sawai, Y. and Kawamura, Y. (1983b). Habu (*Trimeresurus flavoviridis*) bites on the Amami Islands of Japan in 1978. Ibid., 15:75-80.

Sawai, Y. and Kawamura, Y. (1984a). Habu (*Trimeresurus flavoviridis*) bites on the Amami Islands of Japan in 1979. Ibid., 16:1-6.

Sawai, Y. and Kawamura, Y. (1984b). Habu (*Trimeresurus flavoviridis*) bites on the Amami Islands of Japan in 1980. Ibid., 16:85-89.

Sawai, Y. and Kawamura, Y. (1985a). Habu (*Trimeresurus flavoviridis*) bites on the Amami Islands of Japan in 1981. Ibid., 17:1-5.

Sawai, Y. and Kawamura, Y. (1985b). Habu (*Trimeresurus flavoviridis*) bites on the Amami Islands of Japan in 1982. Ibid. 17:91-95.

Sawai, Y. and Kawamura, Y. (1986). Habu (*Trimeresurus flavoviridis*) bites on the Amami Islands of Japan in 1983. Ibid., 18:65-69.

Sawai, Y., Kawamura, Y., Ebisawa, I., Okonogi, T., Hokama, Z. and Yamakawa, M. (1967b). Studies on the improvement of treatment of habu (*Trimeresurus flavoviridis*) bites. 6. Habu bites on the Amami and Ryukyu Islands in 1964. Japan J.Exp. Med., 37:51-59.

Sawai, Y., Kawamura, Y., Fukuyama, T. and Keegan, H.L. (1967d). Studies on the inactivation of snake venom by dihydrothioctic acid. Ibid., 37:121-128.

Sawai, Y., Kawamura, Y., Fukuyama, T. and Okonogi, T. (1969a). Studies on the improvement of treatment of habu (*Trimeresurus flavoviridis*) bites. Experimental study on the habu venom toxoid by dihydrothioctic acid. Ibid., 39:109-117.

Sawai, Y., Kawamura, Y., Fukuyama, T. Okonogi, T. and Ebisawa, I. (1969b). Studies on the improvement of treatment of habu (*Trimeresurus flavoviridis*) bites. 8. A field trial of the prophylactic inoculation of the habu venom toxoid. Ibid., 39:197-203.

Sawai, Y., Kawamura, Y., Fukuyama, T. Okonogi, T. and Ebisawa, I. (1973). A study on the vaccination against snake venom poisoning. In : "Toxins of Animal and Plant Origin, Vol. 3" (Ed. by A. DeVries and E. Kochva). pp.877-889. Goldon and Breach, New York.

Sawai, Y., Kawamura, Y., Fukuyama, T., Shimizu, T., Lin, T. and Okonogi, T. (1967c). Studies on the snake venom of *Trimeresurus tokarensis* (Tokara-habu) and on the snake bite in Tokara Islands. Japan J. Bacteriology, 22:21-24. (in Japanese with English summary).

Sawai, Y., Makino, M., Kawamura, Y., Chinzei, H., Okonogi, T., Hokama, Z. and Yamakawa, M. (1976). Epidemiological study of habu bites on the Amami and Okinawa Islands of Japan. In: "Animal, Plant and Microbial Toxins (Ed. by A. Ohsaka et al.), Vol. 2" pp. 439-450. Plenum Press, New York.

Sawai, Y., Makino, M., Miyazaki, S., Kato, K., Adachi, H., Mitsuhashi, S. and Okonogi, T. (1961). Studies on the improvement of treatment of habu snake (*Trimeresurus flavoviridis*) bites. 1. Studies on the improvement of habu snake antivenin. Japanese Journal of Experimental Medicine, 31:137-150.

Seu, J.-H. and Sawai, Y. (1981). The effect of proteinase inhibitory substance (ISV) on oedema, haemorrhage and necrosis of habu (*Trimeresurus flavoviridis*) venom. The Snake, 13:99-103.

Someya, S., Murata, R., Sawai, Y., Kondo, H. and Ishii, A. (1972). Active immunization of man with toxoid of habu (*Trimeresurus flavoviridis*) venom. Japanese Journal of Medical Science and Biology, 25:47-51.

Stejneger, L. (1907). Herpetology of Japan and adjacent territory. Bulletin of U.S. National Museum, 58:1-577.

Suzuki, R. (1960). Disturbance of the eye by snake venom (*Natrix tigrina*) (Boie). Journal of Clinical Ophthalmology, 14:1384-1387. (in Japanese with English summary).

Suzuki, T. (1970). Studies on snake venom enzymes, centering around *Agkistrodon halys blomhoffii* venom. The Snake, 2:75-94. (in Japanese with English summary).

Takahashi, T. and Ohsaka, A. (1970). Purification and some properties of two haemorrhagic principles (HR2a and HR2b) in the venom of *Trimeresurus flavoviridis;* complete separation of the principles from proteolytic activity. Biochimica et Biophysica Acta, 207:65-75.

Takara, T. (1962). Studies on the terrestrial snakes in the Ryukyu Archipelago. Science Bulletin of Division of Agriculture, Home Economics and Engineering, University of Ryukyus, 9:1-202. (in Japanese with English summary).

Tanaka, H. and Wada, Y. (1977). Venomous snakes. In : "Animals of Medical Importance in the Nansei Islands in Japan, (Ed. by M. Sasa et. al.)", pp. 29-71. Shinjuku Shobo, Tokyo.

Tateno, I., Sawai, Y. and Makino, M. (1963). Current status of mamushi snake (*Agkistrodon halys*) bites in Japan with special reference to severe and fatal cases. Japanese Journal of Experimental Medicine, 33:331-346.

Toriba, M. (1985). Note on dermal-vertebral relationship in the crotaline snakes, *Trimeresurus flavoviridis* and *T. tokarensis*. The Snake, 17:79-81.

Wakamatsu, M., Kawamura, Y. and Sawai, Y. (1986). A successful trial of yamakagashi antivenom. Ibid., 18:4-5.

Yamakawa, M., Nozaki, M. and Hokama, Z. (1976). Fractionation of Sakishima-habu (*Trimeresurus elegans*) venom and lethal, haemorrhagic and oedema-forming activities of the fractions. In : "Animal, Plant and Microbial Toxins (Ed. by A. Ohsaka et al.), Vol. 1" pp. 97-109. Plenum Press, New York.

Venomous Snakes In Jordan

Ahmad M Disi
Department of Biological Sciences
Faculty of Science
The University of Jordan, Amman — Jordan

Introduction

The location which Jordan occupies between the three zoogeographical regions: the Palaearctic, Afrotropical, and Oriental, favours and allows the expansion range of some venomous snakes from the three herpetofauna (European, Asian and African) to be interconnected in Jordan through Syria, Syrian Desert (eastern desert) and Sinai respectively. The presence of four different biotopes in a restricted area such as Jordan is of prime significance as it adds a wide range of diverse habitats. According to Al-Eisawi (1985) the four biogeographical regions are:

1. The Mediterranean region which extends from northern border of Jordan with Syria down to Ras El-Nagab, which is characterised by high mountains. The mean annual rainfall is usually above 300 mm. The soil type here is the terra rosa and the rendzina which are the richest in Jordan and supports the best vegetation: *Pinus halepensis*, *Qurecus calliprinus*, *Q. ithaburenisis*, *Ceratonia*, *Pistacia* and *Juniperus phoenicea*. In this region, representatives of the Palaearctic fauna is found, e.g. *Vipera palaestinae*.

2. The Irano-Turanian region which forms a narrow strip surrounding the Mediterranean region except at the north. It may interrupt the Mediterranean region in certain depressions that is, Wadi Mujeb and Wadi-Al-Hasa. The mean annual rainfall is usually over 150 mm. The soil type here is mostly poor, eroded, and the dominant soil type is the calcareous or loess. The vegetation is mainly small shrubs and bushes, i.e., *Retama reatum*, *Artemisia herba-alba* and *Anabasis syriaca*. In this region poisonous snakes of the Afrotropical and Oriental origin are found, example, *Walterinnesia aegyptia* and *Pseudocerastes persicus fieldi*.

3. The Saharo-Arabian region: It borders the Irano-Turanian region from the east which comprises the majority of Jordan and links with the Arabian Desert at the borders of three Arab countries, Saudi Arabia, Iraq and Syria from the south, east and north respectively. The mean annual rainfall is usually over 50 mm. The soil type is very poor, mostly of the hammada types with some sandy hammadas, saline soil or mud flats. The vegetation is very poor and sparse. Most of the plant cover is mainly found in the wadies depressions where the water is collected after rain. The most dominant plants are *Artemisia herba-alba*, *Astragalus*, *Stipa*, etc. The poisonous

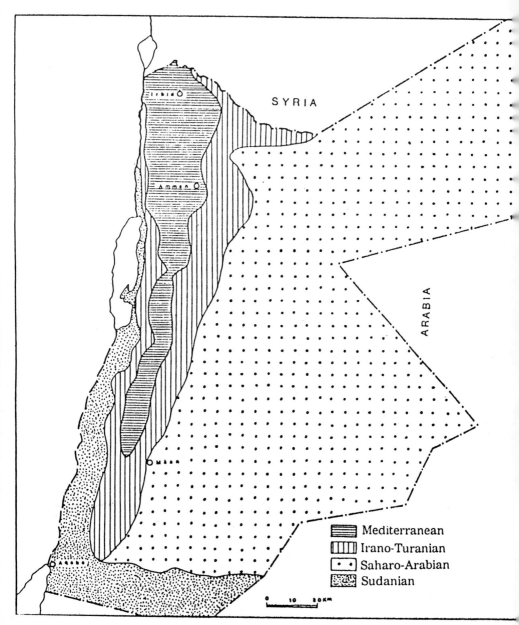

The four biogeographical regions in Jordan (Al-Eisawi, 1985)

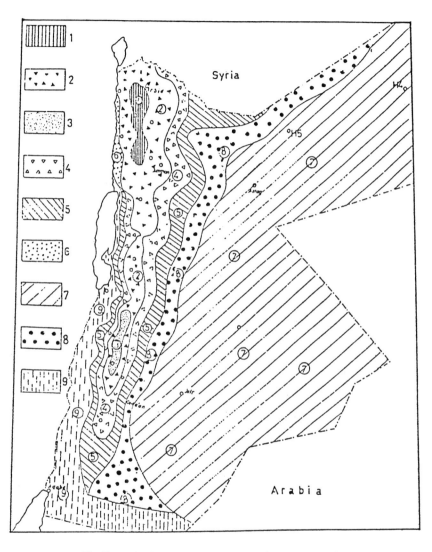

Bioclimatological map of Jordan (Al-Eisawi, 1985)

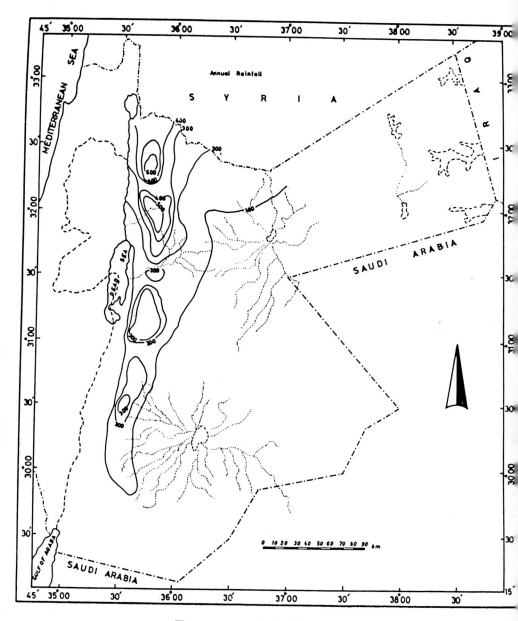

The mean annual rainfall in Jordan.

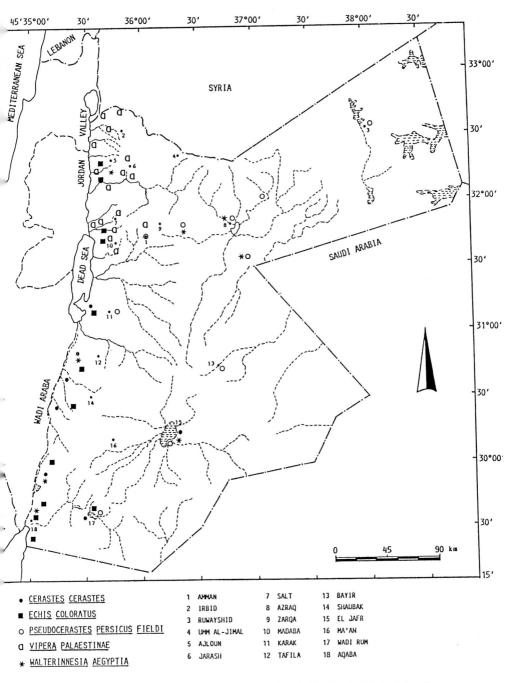

•	CERASTES CERASTES	1 AMMAN	7 SALT	13 BAYIR
■	ECHIS COLORATUS	2 IRBID	8 AZRAQ	14 SHAUBAK
○	PSEUDOCERASTES PERSICUS FIELDI	3 RUWAYSHID	9 ZARQA	15 EL JAFR
◘	VIPERA PALAESTINAE	4 UMM AL-JIMAL	10 MADABA	16 MA'AN
		5 AJLOUN	11 KARAK	17 WADI RUM
✱	WALTERINNESIA AEGYPTIA	6 JARASH	12 TAFILA	18 AQABA

Recent distribution of the venomous snakes in Jordan (Disi *et al*, 1988)

353

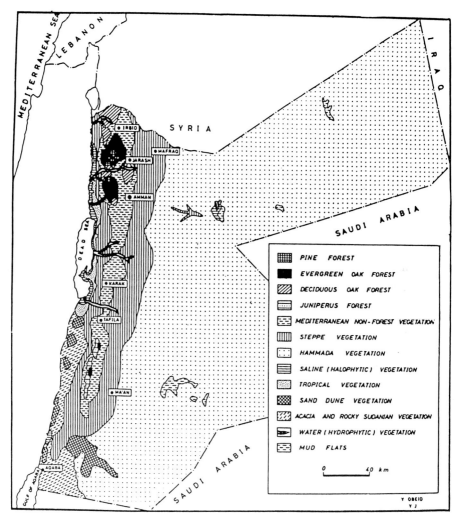

Vegetation types in Jordan. (Al-Eisawi, 1985)

snakes found in this region belong to the Afrotropical and Oriental regions, example, *Walterinnesia aegyptia* and *Pseudocerastes persicus fieldi*.

4. The Sudanian Region: This region comprises the Rift Valley, including the Southern Jordan Valley, the Dead Sea, Wadi Araba, Wadi Rum and Aqaba area. The mean annual rainfall is usually less than 50 mm. This region is the warmest of all four regions as temperature may reach 48° C during the hot Summer. The soil is mostly sandy or sandy hammada, some granite fragments and saline soils. The vegetation here is related to tropical variety, that is *Acacia* spp., *Haloxylon persicum*, etc. Certain flora and fauna of the African origin are restricted to this biotope. This region has the highest number of viper populations, mainly of Afrotropical origins example, *Cerastes cerastes, Echis coloratus* and *Walterinnesia aegyptia*. Moreover, *Vipera palaestinae* penetrates the northern part of this region in association with the expansion of agriculture and human settlements.

Five different species of venomous snake are so far recorded from Jordan (Disi, 1983). Four of them belong to the family Viperidae: *Vipera palaestinae, Echis coloratus, Cerastes cerastes* and *Pseudocerastes persicus fieldi* — while the fifth one *Walterinnesia aegyptia* belongs to family Elapidae.

Amr and Amr (1983) reported that during a nine-year period (1970-1972 and 1975-1980), 112 cases of snakebites were officially reported with seven fatal cases. During the period 1982-1986, official statistics of the Ministry of Health indicated that sixty-five cases of snakebites have occurred (Disi, *et al.*, 1988.b.). The previous authors believe that the actual number of snakebites is much higher than the above figures. Since snakebites were treated with folklore medications, remote areas and military personnel were not included in the official records.

Disi *et al*, (1988.b.) found that the highest incidence of snakebites happened in 21.5%) and the lowest incidence occurred in October (1.5%). July (35.4%) followed by June. Moreover, the highest incidence of snakebites (1982-1986), which is about 76% occurred in the northern part of the country, due to the fact that this region is mostly part of the Mediterranean biotope. The northern part is followed by Jordan Valley and Madaba. Mostly, the bites would be attributed to *Vipera palaestinae* which flourishes in the northern Jordan and occupies different habitats. Moreover, it is the most dominant viper in the Mediterranean biotope, and is abundant in and around human habitations, new settlements and irrigated farms (Mendelssohn 1963; Disi, 1983). According to the records (1982-1986), snakebites in males which is around 72.3%, was 2.5 folds greater than females (27.7%., Disi *et al.*, 1988.b.). In countries where several species of venomous snakes are present, it is difficult to obtain reliable data concerning snakebites of one species especially for vipers where only on few occasions were specimens available for identification.

Antivenins: Two polyvalent antivenins have been used in Jordan during the last nine years. The imported antivenins cost Jordan about 60,000 dollars in the period 1982-1986 (Ministry of Health Statistics). One of them is Pasteur anti-*Bitis, Echis, Naja* (Isper Africa). None of the snakes which were used to develop this antivenin are present in Jordan. The other antivenin is Behringwerke (Near and Middle East), with only *C. cerastes* present in Jordan (Disi *et al.*, 1988.b.).

Behringwerke antivenin has a higher titer of neutralization antibodies against the crude venom of *C. cerastes* and *V. palaestinae* than Pasteur antivenin. However, Pasteur antivenin provided no protection against *P. p. fieldi*, while Behringwerke antivenin provided a partial protection against this viper.

Both antivenins provided full protection against 10 LD_{50} of *W. aegyptia* venoms, but no protection was provided at higher doses (Disi *et al.*, 1988.b.).

Disi *et al.* (1988.b.) indicated that both imported antivenins were inefficient to protect against most of the snakebites in Jordan, because of venom variations in different species of vipers and even within the same species over its wide range of distribution. Therefore, the national health authorities in the countries concerned, should be encouraged and assessed by WHO to develop its own antivenin (WHO, 1971).

The problem of snakebites in Jordan is a noteworthy one which deserves more attention, (Amr and Amr, 1983). Especially with the recent expansion of the cultivated landscape and human settlements in the Jordan Valley, Wadi Araba and eastern desert where most of the venomous snakes are present. It is indicated that the number and occurrence of venomous snakes have tremendously increased in association with the range of *Bufo viridis* which forms mostly part of the diet of *W. aegyptia* and *E. coloratus*. It is also found that *V. palaestinae* expanded its range of distribution into the Jordan Valley in correlation with the expansion of the irrigated farms (Mendelssohn 1963, Disi 1983). Moreover, a positive relationship exists between densities of *P. p. fieldi* and vegetation densities, where shrubs and bushes are found (Disi 1983). In Shaumari Wildlife Reserve area, two wild animals, Syrian wild ass and an ostrich, were bitten by the latter viper. There is no doubt that these vipers may create a problem to the farmers and settled bedouins.

A Simplified Key For The Venomous Snakes Of Jordan

1. A. Colour of snake shiny black. 2
   B. Colour of snake not black (viper) 3
2. Adults uniformly shiny black, a moderately stout snake with short tail and small head not distinct from neck, crown with large shields ....
   .... *Walterinnesia aegyptia*
3. A. Head with distinct marking 4
   B. Head without distinct markings 8
4. A. A horn-like projection with small imbricate scales above the eye 5
   B. V-shaped band of dark brown coloration on the head 6
   C. Head with or without marking 7
5. Head broad and triangular very distinct from neck, tip of the tail black, found mainly in the eastern part of Jordan ....
   .... *Pseudocerastes persicus fieldi*

6. Head large, triangular, rather long and distinct from neck, often associated with forests and cultivated regions; the distance between the marks of the two fangs is one cm .... *Vipera palestinae*

7. Head broad, flattened, triangular, very distinct from neck; always associated with sandy or near sandy areas (some vipers from Wadi Rum may have spine-like scale above the eye) The distance between the marks of the two fangs is more than 10 mm .... *Cerastes cerastes*

8. Head without distinctive marks, not clearly distinct from neck, usually inhabits rocky hillsides of the mountains with hard ground and covered by rocks; the gap between the two fangs is less than 10 mm .. *Echis coloratus*

Vipera palaestinae
Palestine viper

The coloration of all specimens examined agrees with Mendelssohn's (1963) descriptions, including the variations demonstrated by his large collection. The background colour of the dorsum varies from grey to orche irrespective of the colour of the soil where the vipers inhabit. Moreover, variations of the colour among the members of this species were noticed in the same area. The dorsal blotches have a brown or red colour which forms a dorsal zig zag stripe or interconnected row of rhomboid blotches or a combination of both. In addition, there is a lateral row of spots which may be connected with the dorsal band. Head is large, with dark brown markings. The pattern of the head coloration is constant in all vipers examined. Also, the head is triangular, rather long, distinct from neck, body stout, tail tapers abruptly behind cloaca. These vipers grow to a length of almost 1.3 m (Mendelssohn 1963).

It mainly inhabits the Mediterranean biotope which is rich in avifauna and rodents. Also, it is found in a large number in the Jordan Valley in association with farms and agricultural settlements as well as in dense vegetation. Its diversified habitat include forests, rocky hills, plains, farms, marshy areas and around villages and human settlements. There is a considerable increase in the number of this viper in the Jordan Valley in correlation with the expansion of cultivated land and irrigated citrus and banana farms. The reason for this expansion is the abundance of small rodents especially mice and rats. Also, these places offer the moisture needed by this viper for drinking and humid oviposition sites, which form an appropriate habitat for *V. palaestinae*.

Food and Feeding Habits:

The Palestine viper feeds on small mammals and birds. It drinks readily if water is available. It is also able to make use of dew by sucking up drops while using normal drinking movements (Mendelssohn 1963). This viper is a nocturnal animal. In spring, it may be found during the day time, but in summer, it is usually active after sunset.

This is an arboreal viper, and usually found in trees high above the ground. In other cases it may be found to inhabit hollows of trees (Mendelssohn 1963). Moreover, it is collected from caves and underneath large rocks. This viper shows positive correlation with temperature and humidity parameters.

However, its distribution was not affected by the type of soil or vegetation (Disi, 1987).

In defence, this viper hisses and contracts the forepart of the body to an S-shape in preparation to strike. But if the snake retreats, hissing generally stops. If excitation is high, then the forepart of the body is raised and flattened by spreading of the ribs. However, if the snake flees after showing this behaviour, it generally continues to keep the anterior part of the body above the ground with continuous hissing and spreading the forepart of the body (Mendelssohn 1963).

Many cases of snake bites happen at night, when farmers irrigate their trees, when they open the water canals, stepping on the snake accidentally, or when they clean the large pipes and water canals by hand. Also, people were bitten when they inserted their hands in to dark holes where vipers usually hide.

The venom of *V. palaestinae* was found to be composed of six fractions. The haemorrhagic activity of this venom was fraction A_3, and about 80% of the lethal activity was due to this fraction (Gitter *et al*, 1957). Moreover, by ion exchange chromatography, it was demonstrated that *V. palaestinae* venom consisted of five fractions, each fraction with one or more activity (Kochwa *et al*, 1960). Moroz *et al* (1966) isolated a homogeneous protein (Viperotoxin) with a molecular weight of 11,600 daltons, which had neurotoxic activity. In addition, a large acidic protein from the venom of this snake was isolated and had both haemorrhagic and proteolytic activities. The molecular weight of this protein was 44,000. Spherocytosis following the intravenous administration of lethal and sublethal doses of this viper venom into rabbits was demonstrated by Danon *et al* (1961). Ovadia (1978) reported three haemorrhagic fractions in the venom of *V. palaestinae*, these fractions were devoid of any proteolytic activities.

The extravasation of blood under mucous membranes and the parenchymatous organs was observed following venom administration. In more severe envenomation, widespread haemorrhage in internal organs was noticed. Also, disk-sphere transformation and decrease in sedimentation rate of the erythrocytes were demonstrated after treatment of human blood with *V. palaestinae* venom. The spherical form of the erythrocytes could be reversed by washing the cells with normal plasma or addition of albumin (Gitter *et al*, 1959; Danon *et al*, 1961; Condrea *et al*, 1961; and DeVries *et al*, 1962).

DeVries and Gitter (1957), indicated that both coagulant and anticoagulant activities were present in the venom of *V. palaestinae*. The latter activity was manifested only at high concentrations of this venom. Aloof *et al* (1962) reported the absence of fibrinogenolytic factor in the venom of *V. palaestinae*.

DeVries *et al* (1962) showed that phospholipase A from *V. palaestinae* venom produced spherocytosis five minutes after intravenous injection into rabbits. The same authors assumed the presence of another unknown factor which was responsible for haemolysis. This latter assumption was supported recently by Sosa *et al* (1979), who observed very high haemolysis.

Efrati and Reif (1953) treated sixty five cases envenomated by *V.*

palaestinae. Those patients did not receive specific antivenin, but only supportive treatment was given. The following is the summary of the prominent symptoms and signs.

Symptoms of envenomation may appear after half an hour or less which depends on the amount of injected venom and the activities performed by the bitten patient. At the beginning, the patients felt pain at the site of envenomation accompanied by general weakness, restlessness and a pale face. Usually, the fangs mark appear as two bluish puncture marks. In rare cases they may appear as one spot, or as four spots if the viper repeatedly bites the victim, also scratch marks may be seen. The distance between the marks of the two fangs is one centimetre, and one would notice blue discoloration around the marks. The patient may vomit repeatedly, perspire profusely, have abdominal pain, diarrhoea and severe hemoconcentration may develop with severe peripheral circulatory failure resulting in primary anaphylactoid shock. Also, widespread haemorrhage develops on the bitten part accompanied by an extension of swelling which increases and spreads centripetally and toward the trunk as time passes. The skin in the bitten area becomes tender and painful to pressure. One can notice ascending lymphangitis and lymphadenitis several hours after the local swelling appears on the bitten limb. Also, skin changes in colour accompanied by extensive haemorrhage and blister formations. Moreover, secondary hypovolemic, shock, extravasation of plasma and blood, anemia, thrombocytopenia and late sequela may appear. Efrati (1979) indicated that drastic changes in the pattern of the course of envenomation will appear if a specific antivenin is administered to patients who have similar clinical features.

Amr and Amr (1983) reported a case believed to be caused by *V. palaestinae*, in which the victim (a farmer, 30 years old) had been bitten on his right hand. The patient had developed melena, haematuria with marked swelling and bleeding at the site of bite. Blood clotting time was 160 minutes (normal clotting time is 9 — 15 minutes). The patient required blood transfusion and his prothrombin time (PT) was 300 seconds while that of normal individuals is 12 seconds. The patient developed hypofrinogenemia of 90 mgs/dl (normal 150 — 300 mgs/dl). The patient was in hospital for 12 days.

The above mentioned symptoms vary from patient to patient which may be attributed to several factors, age and weight of the victim and the patient's sensitivity to the venom, site of bite, and depth of penetration of the fangs, the number of bites and the amount of the venom injected into the victim, the species and size of the snake, and the state of the venom glands and fangs at the time of bite. The psychological state of the viper and the bitten person should also be considered. The patient should remain calm, with minimum movements, especially of the bitten part. If the time interval between the snake bite and hospital treatment is minimized, then the case would be less severe. Another factor to consider, is whether the patient had received on site first aid treatment and if specific antivenin is applied.

Efrati (1979) indicated that the bite may cause complications later after the patient has recovered from acute envenomation. One patient had intermittent claudication in the bitten limb, and the peripheral pulse could not be felt in the bitten limb even after one year of the accident. Moreover, problems in the hand of the patients who had been envenomated by *V. palaestinae* were stiffness of the metacarpophalangeal joints, sensory disturbances and adduction contracture of the thumb.

Pathological changes:

Efrati Reif (1953) stated that four envenomated patients died following *V. palaestinae* bite and showed that the anatomical and histopathological changes in all four cases were similar. The prominent features were swelling and haemorrhages. Sanguineous fluid infiltrate the muscles, the skin, and the subcutaneous tissues in areas closer to the site of bite as well as far from it. Haemorrhage and great distention of the lymph vessels and nodes especially in the envenomated region was well seen. Extensive haemorrhage was also seen in the internal organs, ie. under the endocardium of the left ventricle, in the septum and papillary muscles and in the lung. Petechiae may be seen in various parts of the internal organs such as the kidney and urinary bladder. Blood did not clot after death and remained fluid in the blood vessels many hours after death.

The microscopic histopathologic changes were haemorrhages and acute stasis. There were marked changed in the walls of arterioles and capillaries. In the kidneys. the blood vessels were distended both in the cortex and medulla. Also, the capillaries of the glomeruli were filled with RBC. In the intestine, the capillaries of the mucous lining were dilated with blood. However, the changes in the parenchymatous organ were slight except for the liver which showed a mild proliferation of cells and infiltration into the sinuses which were enlarged.

It is clear that circulatory failure or bleeding is the frequent cause of death.

Echis coloratus
Carpet viper

In Jordan its colour varies from one area to another and blends with the background. The background of the dorsum is yellowish grey or brownish grey. In areas such as the south of Wadi Araba where the granite red stone colour of the ground is dominant, the ground colour of this viper is reddish or reddish brown. The colour of this viper is in accordance with the description of Mendelssohn (1965). Along the dorsum, a row of dark greyish white rhomboid blotches or crossbands are found. The light dorsal blotches may have a narrow dark border. The pattern of orientation of the blotches and crossbands varies even on the same animal. On the side of the body, a row of brownish blotches is positioned. Along both sides of the head, a brownish band, with a lighter stripe above it, starts at the nostril and passes below the eye reaching the end of the jaw. Markings on top of the head varies, and generally are formed of a dark colour internally surrounded by a light colour on its periphery or vice versa. The colouring pattern and scales of this viper help to camouflage it so effectively with the surrounding where it lives.

In Jordan this viper is abundant in the dry rocky hill-sides of the mountains which surround Jordan Valley, Wadi Araba and Wadi Rum. It favours hard ground covered by rocks with widely scattered vegetation dominated by the following plants: *Retama ratam, Salvia graveolens,* and *Urginea maritima* (Disi, 1983).

This species shows a positive correlation with temperature parameters and negative correlation with humidity (Warburg, 1964; Mendelssohn, 1965 and Disi, 1987). In early spring, this viper is found close to the surface of the ground under rocks or logs. As the season becomes hotter in the summer, vipers retract deeper into their burrows (Disi, 1987).

Mendelssohn (1965) indicated that this species feeds on arthropods, lizards, frogs and birds as well as small rodents.

Males are usually slightly larger than females and some specimens may exceed a length of 80 cm. (Mendelssohn, 1965).

E. coloratus uses sidewinding, rectilinear, serpentine types of locomotion or combinations of these. The carpet viper always starts rubbing its scales, moves rapidly and immediately strikes with great speed in all directions with the head raised upward in an S-shape.

Aloof *et al* (1962) reported the presence of fibrinogenolytic factor in the venom of *E. coloratus.* Moreover, Rechnic *et al* (1962); Djaldetti *et al* (1964) observed that intravenous administration of *E. coloratus* venom of lethal doses produced acute afibrinogenemia in dogs, rabbits and guinea pigs. Rechnic *et al* (1962) also reported hypofibrinogenemia, factor V deficiency and thrombocytopenia following intravenous administration of the whole venom or its fractions in dogs. They also found that a dose of 400 ug caused severe thrombocytopenia (platelet count, 10,000 to 20,000 per mm^3). An early intravascular clotting, and fibrin deposition in the glomeruli, were also observed following injections of lethal doses. Furthermore, the venom of *E. coloratus,* contains two agents phospholipase A and a procoagulant. Both factors caused marked drop in the platelet count. The thrombocytopenia produced by the procoagulant component was more prolonged and similar to that caused by the whole venom (Joshua *et al*, 1964). Moreover, phospholipase A and B were found in the venom of *E. coloratus* (Mohammad *et al*, 1969a). Barzilary *et al* (1978) stated that the action of phospholipase A is catalyzed by Ca^{2+}. Hydrolysis of glycophosphatides of both intact and ghost red blood cells failed in the absence of Ca^{2+}. Phospholipase A attacked the beta-acyl bond in phosphatids, producing free fatty acid and lysolecithin from phosphatidylcholine (Lecithin). Lysolecithin is the factor responsible for the destruction of red blood cells. Phospholipase B attacked the alpha-acyl bond in lysophosphatides (Klibansky and DeVries, 1963; Condrea and DeVries, 1965). Roy (1945) demonstrated the absence of lecithin in the erythrocytes membrane of ox, sheep and goat. In these three species, erythrocyte were insensitive to phospholipase A. Klibansky and DeVries (1963) noted that various stages in the haemolytic process depend upon the amount of lysolecithin produced from the available lecithin encountered in the process of phospholipase A activity. In addition, crenation, spherocytosis of the RBC and the hydrolysis of the plasma lecithin have been reported following intravenous administration of *E.*

coloratus. Also, the attachment of lysolecithin to the RBC membrane, which caused increases in osmotic and mechanical fragilities, was reported. In their investigations, on the *E. coloratus* venom, Klibansky *et al* (1966) demonstrated intravascular haemolysis and increase in plasma haemoglobin, following intravenous administration of a lethal dose of this venom in dogs. Plasma lysolecithin increased while plasma lecithin decreased. In mice, Gitter *et al* (1960) showed that the leakage of RBC cells was through diapedesis, following a lethal dose of this viper. Rechnic *et al* (1962) noticed in guinea pigs that intravenous lethal dose of *E. coloratus* venom, was of the major role in producing haemorrhage in the internal organs. Homma *et al* (1967) found that the response to venom was both concentration and time-dependent. Djaldettti *et al* (1967) reported the effects of *E. coloratus* venom on the circulating lymphocytes and lymph nodes. Marked lymphopaenia developed in guinea pigs, following intraperitoneal administration of lethal dose. The electron microscopic observation of these investigators revealed severe destruction to the lymphocyte nucleus, and other organelles like mitochondria and endoplasmic reticulum. Mohamed *et al* (1963) described hyperglycemia in rabbits following subcutaneous administration of sublethal doses of *E. coloratus* venom. They found that the maximum rise in blood glucose was reached two hours after injection of venom. In addition, a drop in liver and muscle glycogen was also observed. It was suggested that the venom might inhibit the activity of glycokinase or stimulate the release of adrenalin.

The effect of *E. coloratus* venom on the internal organs was observed following intraperitoneal administration of a dose corresponding to 2 LD_{50} in mice, haemorrhages in the abdominal wall muscles, peritoneum and the diaphragm, were noticed two hours after the injection (Gitter *et al* 1960). A relatively higher dose corresponding to 3 LD_{50} which was intravenously administered caused severe haemorrhage in the lungs and heart in one hour, in addition to the above pathologic abnormalities.

Sandbank and Djaldetti (1966) reported the destruction of blood brain barrier following lethal intravenous dose of *E. coloratus* venom into dogs and guinea pigs. However, paralysis and epistaxis of envenomated animals were demonstrated following intravenous injections of 100 ug *E. coloratus* venom and 10 mg horse radish peroxidase into the mice (Sandbank *et al* 1974). Mendelssohn (1965) reported that the venom of *E. coloratus* in man lowers the level of fibrinogen in the blood and may cause profuse bleeding. In a case by carpet viper bite, bleeding reached a dangerous state and needed several blood transfusions. This was stopped successfully by administration of *E. coloratus* antivenin (Zinner, 1976). Efrati (1979) also reported a case of envenomation by carpet viper. At the beginning, no general or severe local symptoms were observed. Meanwhile, the number of platelets was 150,000/mm^3, while the haemoglobin concentration was normal. Fibrinogen concentration was found to be 50 mg and prothrombin activity decreases by ¼ of normal value. Minor gingival haemorrhage appeared one hour later. Dropping in fibrinogen concentration continues without any activity detected for prothrombin after two hours of bite. The blood did not clot. The number of platelets was within the normal count. However, irrespective of the application of blood transfusion and E-amino caproic acid, the blood values did not return to normal. When the patient received 50 ml of specific antivenin i.v. (around 35 hours after the bite), the haemorrhagic tendency stopped after two hours. The prothrombin activity and all other blood values started to return to normal values on the second day.

Zinner (1976) indicated that the venom of this viper can be fatal for children if they do not receive prompt medical treatment. The venom also reduces the level of fibrinogen and induces general weakness and malaise which stays for several days in adults. The patients are usually released from the hospitals only after few days, whether or not they receive the antidote.

Efrati (1979) indicated that in most envenomation cases caused by *E. coloratus*, no drastic general manifestation were present. However, in some patients, mild hypotension, renal failure and vomiting may appear. The patients showed swelling of the bitten extremity, a remarkable phenomena in most of the reported cases was of the absence of important clinical manifestations but the observation of the drastic changes in the clotting mechanism.

Studies have indicated that the toxicity of the venom varies from one viper to another, and that is really true in all geographical regions of its range of distribution. Flower (1933) stated that three persons were killed by *E. coloratus*, while Mendelssohn (1965) indicated that none of *E. coloratus* bites were fatal. Zinner (1976) indicated that the danger of *E. coloratus* bites is usually exaggerated and of the ten persons bitten, only one died.

Efrati (1979) mentioned that the cause of death (44 year-old man) who died 24 hours after the bite from *E. coloratus*, was acute renal failure, due to severe interstitial nephritis. Other pathological changes observed on post mortem were skin necrosis at the site of bite and serosanguineous swelling at various areas of the body such as skin, subendocardial tissues and retroperitoneum.

The highest percentages of victims were hikers, communications and road workers, farmers, bedouins and soldiers. Expansion of arid agricultural projects with new human settlements into the usual habitat of *E. coloratus*, allows for more contact with this viper. In addition, its distribution and time of activity increase the chance resulting in a considerable percentage of bites (Zinner, 1976). Moreover, the carpet viper blends with the surrounding and if anyone comes close to it, it starts rubbing its scales, moves rapidly and immediately strikes with great speed in all directions including upwards. This viper should be considered seriously and must be avoided at all cost. Bites by *E. coloratus* can be distinguished from other vipers by measuring the gap between the marks of the two fangs, which is less than 10 mm. Also, by knowing the region where the accident occurred will provide valuable information about the type of viper.

Cerastes cerastes

Sand Vipers

The background colour of the dorsum is sandy yellow, pinkish or light brown in young vipers, while in large old animals becomes paler. The vertebral area is covered with alternate square blotches that may fuse into cross bands of dark brown and grey colours. These blotches extend from the head to the tip of the tail. There are two series of dark brownish blotches on the sides of the body. Moreover, the dorsal and lateral sides of the body are spotted with irregular brown spots. The ventrum is uniformly white. Head is triangular, wide flattened and clearly distinct from neck. Head covered with small irregular tubercularly-keeled scales. *C. cerastes* is characterized by a thick body and short tail. The above description agrees with that of Flower (1933) and Moore (1980).

In Jordan, this species inhabits the area east of the Dead Sea, Wadi Araba and Wadi Rum, which is characterized by sand dunes. This area is considered the warmest part of Jordan. The annual mean daily temperature is around 22 — 24° and the difference between the mean temperature of the warmest and coldest month is considered the lowest in Jordon (Meteorological Dept., Ministry of Transport, Climatic Atlas of Jordan, 1971). Vegetation that occur in this area have subtropical affinities and are dominated by the following plants: *Haloxylon persicum*, *Anabasis articulata* and *Acacia* sp. Hass (1957) reported that out of 23 specimens from Saudi Arabia only five of them were horned. In Sinai, too, both horned and horn-less specimens have been found (Hass and Werner, 1969; Disi, 1983). A horned specimen is collected form Wadi Rum. (Disi *et al*, 1988.a.)

C. cerastes shows a positive correlation with temperature parameters and a negative correlation with humidity (Warburg, 1964 and Disi, 1987). This species is limited to sand-dune areas. It is nocturnal and feeds mainly on small rodents. It was also observed hiding in rodent borrows. *C. cerastes* is very noisy when irritated, and emits a loud puffing-hissing sound from the mouth and a rasping hissing sound by rapidly rubbing the scales of the inflated loops of its body over each other.

C. cerastes uses sidewinding type of locomotion on both sand-dunes and on hard soil. During their investigation on *C. cerastes* and other Egyptian snake venom, Mohamed *et al* (1969b) isolated phospholipases A and B. Some of their activities were determined on lecithin and lysolecithin as substrates. The maximal activity of phospholipase A was at the pH range 7.0 to 9.0 and it was activated by Ca^{2+} and Mg^{2+}, but inhibited by EDTA. Labib *et al* (1981a) investigated the proteolytic activities of *C. cerastes* and *C. vipera* on casein, gelatin and haemoglobin. In both venoms, pool A contained the major proteolytic activities, besides L-amino acid oxidase and phosphodiesterase activities. This pool may cause lethality through the haemorrhagic activities. Moreover, Mohamed *et al* (1969b) reported variations in specific activities of different batches of venom. The differences were mainly due to the age of the snake, seasonal variations, and the length of the captivity period. In their work on *C. cerastes* venom, they also demonstrated a remarkable effect on the blood coagulation mechanism, fifteen minutes after an intravenous lethal dose administration in dogs and rabbits. The blood was incoagulable due to a deficiency in plasma fibrinogen, factor V and VIII. Moreover, in their studies, on the effect of the viper snake venoms on blood coagulation disturbances, Labib *et al* (1981.b.) reported that both *C. cerastes* and *C. vipera* venoms, showed procoagulant activities at low concentrations. However, at high concentrations, the venom showed anticoagulant activity. Two anticoagulant and three procoagulant fractions, were isolated from the above venoms. The anticoagulant fractions had direct or indirect proteolytic activities on plasma fibrinogen, causing hypofibrinogenemia. The procoagulant components have different sites of action on blood coagulation levels. Mohamed and El-Damarawy (1974) administered lethal doses of *C. cerastes* venom intravenously into rabbits and noticed strong fibrinolytic activity in vitro and weak fibrinolytic activity in vivo.

The haemostatic changes in rabbits, following intraperitoneal injection of venom was studied. There was an initial rise in erythrocyte count 15 minutes after injection of venom, followed by a marked decline. Significant leucopenia and thrombocytopenia also developed. Erythroid hyperplasia of the bone marrow was noticed after 3 to 4 hours of venom administration (Mohamed *et al*, 1977). The latter authors also noted that *C. cerastes* venom did not produce any histological changes in the spinal cords of rabbits injected i.p.. However, these investigators described respiratory failure followed by death after intrathecal injection of a dose corresponding to 0.2 LD$_{50}$. Also, haemorrhages in the spinal cord, spinal ganglia and meninges were observed. In addition, binucleation of the spinal cord and spinal ganglion cells, were noticed after repeated sublethal intraperitoneal injections of *C. cerastes* venom. Mohamed and Khaled (1966) showed that *C. cerastes* venom blocked the conductance of the nerve, followed by block of the muscle contraction when the venom was applied to the isolated nerve compartment. In addition, Mohamed et al (1969b) investigated the inhibition of oxygen uptake by isolated brain slices treated with *C. cerastes* venom. On the other hand there was no inhibition to the oxygen uptake by the cardiac, skeletal and plain muscles in vitro experiments. Shakhanbeh (1985) studied the effect of i.p. administration of *C. cerastes* venom in white mice and found that the pathogenicity of this venom was mainly vasculotoxic. The venom acted promptly on the vascular endothelium, resulting in the extravasation of the RBC. It also caused severe degeneration of the parenchymatous cells forming the internal organs and damage to the muscular tissue. It was evident that the kidneys and liver, were highly damaged, while the brain was the least affected. The intraglomerular coagulation showed may be regarded as the major cause of renal failure. Al-Khalil (1985) studied the effect of i.p. repeated small doses of *C. cerastes* venom in white mice. He found that proximal tubules and glomeruli were the most sensitive components of the kidney. Perivascular inflammation was the common lesion observed in the liver. Thickening of alveolar septa, haemorrhage and inflammation were seen in the lung. Also, focal degeneration, karyopyknosis and periauricular hyalinization were found in the heart. Ultrastructural alterations included dilation of sarcoplasmic reticulum, cisternae, vacuolation, sarcolemmal damage, mitochondria deterioration, nuclear changes and highly damaged fibers.

Moore (1980) recorded some bites caused by *C. cerastes*, but mortalities were rare. Zinner (1976) reported that cases of bites were also recorded in Palestine but were not fatal. However, the results of the bite can be unpleasant such as severe necrosis and shortening of the tendons and muscles resulting in the crippling of limbs.

Efrati (1979) described seven cases of envenomation caused by *C. cerastes* which showed symptoms similar to the clinical picture of mild envenomation caused by *V. palaestinae*. One case ended by amputation of the bitten finger as a result of gangrene developed from necrotic lesion. Also, the envenomated person usually showed swelling of the bitten parts, with very mild general manifestations. In addition, nausea, vomiting, haemorrhages in the skin and haematuria may be observed. Moreover, disturbances in blood clotting were seen as in those bites caused by *E. coloratus*, but less severe. There was a fall in fibrinogen concentration and decrease in prothrombin activity. In one case a mild DIC was noticed.

In Wadi Araba, an old man was bitten in the abdominal region. Local necrosis at the site of bite was developed. This man had received medical treatment two days after the bite. Bites by *C. cerastes* can be distinguished from other vipers bite by the following: the distance between the marks of the two fangs is usually more than 10 mm, also the area of accident gives us clear information about the type of viper. If bites occurred in a sandy region the snake is most likely to be *C. cerastes*.

Pseudocerastes persicus fieldi
Field's horned viper

Its colour blends with the background. In the lava desert where it lives, it tends to be dark grey with numerous black spots. In the eastern desert, the dorsal side is yellowish grey. Dorsally two rows of transverse rhomboid blotches in varying shades of brown may fuse to form brown crossbands. On the lateral side of the body is a row of smaller brown blotches which alternate with the dorsal blotches. In the large specimens these lateral blotches become smaller in size and may become unclear. Along the sides of the head, oblique brown bars extend from the eye to the lower labials. Brown spots with irregular shapes and with varying densities from one habitat to another may occur on the dorsal side of the head. Tip of tail is black in all the examined specimens irrespective of sex, age or distribution. The ventral side is uniformly white. On both sides above the eye, there are erect horn-like projections formed of several small imbricate scales. Head is triangular, wide, very distinct from neck, nostrils are dorsolaterally positioned and valves are present. Head is covered dorsally with small imbricate scales. The above description is similar to that of both Schmidt (1930) and Mendelssohn (1965).

This viper inhabits most of the basalt and limestone deserts of the northern and eastern parts of Jordan. Type of soil in the indicated regions vary from sandy to bared mud flats but never in true sand dunes, with sparse mosaics of *Artemisia* and annual grasses or with no vegetation. Moreover, this viper inhabits rolling steppes with volcanic outcrops and dense scattering of rocks and boulders. It was collected from Jawa on the borders between Jordan and Syria at an altitude of 1,000 m. It is nocturnal, and rarely found in or under shrubs during the day. It was also encountered on almost flat desert, living in crevices of rodent burrows in association with higher densities of plants closer to the wadi sytems near Qasr Amra (eastern desert) and east of El-Kark (mid-south of Jordan) (Disi, 1983). The largest number of specimens was collected from Shaumari Wildlife Reserve which is characterized by high densities of plants, avifauna and other small rodents. This made Shaumari Reserve a suitable habitat for *P. p. fieldi.*

Bdolah (1986) indicated that the venom of *P. p. persicus* showed around 30 protein bands while *P. p. fieldi* revealed a simple pattern with very few protein bands. Moreover, molecular sieve chromatography, of *P. p. fieldi* had no haemorrhagin or 1-amino oxidase, and the high molecular weight protein was absent. However, the venom of *P. p. persicus* showed a typical elution profile of viperid venom with haemorrhagic activity and 1-amino acid oxidase activity confined to the high molecular weight peak of protein.

Batzri-Izraeli & Bdolah (1982) isolated and characterized the main fractions from the venom *P. p. fieldi.* Most of the protein and lethality of the venom were eluted in a main symmetrical peak (C). The lethality of this peak was due to a basic protein fraction which consisted of two proteins. The first one CbII possessed phospholipase A activity in addition to direct haemolytic activity. The other protein may act as a specifier which potentiates the toxicity of the phospholipase A at the target cells, since it did not show any known biological activity.

A major toxic component (fraction Cb) was isolated and characterized from the venom of *P. p. fieldi.* This protein had neurotoxic activities and consisted of two protein subunits, which act synergistically on the presynaptic membrane. Tsai *et al* (1983) demonstrated the mode of blocking action of the above neurotoxic component at the chick biventer crevicis nerve muscle preparations, and in isolated phrenic nerve-diaphragm preparations. Initially, the neurotoxic component, caused increase in quantal contents of the end plate potentials, followed by gradual decrease until complete neuromuscular blockage. The electron microscopic studies on the mouse diaphragm treated with the above neurotoxin, revealed the swelling of the mitochondria and the synaptic vesicles in the motor end plate.

Shabo-Shina and Bdolah (1987), studied the interaction of the toxin with nerve endings in rat striatal synaptosomes. They showed that very high lethal potent neurotoxic complex (Cb) from the venom of *P. p. fieldi* acts on the central nervous system. Also, CbII enhanced the release of acetylcholine from synaptosomes.

Gitter *et al* (1962) noticed congestion in the liver blood vessels following intraperitoneal administration of this venom in mice. Also, degeneration of the hepatic cells and necrotic foci were commonly noticed. The venom also caused congestion in the lung but without haemorrhage up to three hours.

Zinner (1976) indicated that there were no reports of bites of *P. p. fieldi.* in nature. Our records show a captive viper having bitten a teacher without serious results. Also, a dog was bitten on the nose, resulting in swelling for several days but without complications. It is advisable that the bitten person especially children should be hospitalized.

P. p. fieldi venom is highly toxic, but usually produces local tissue damage. This viper should be regarded as dangerous (Moore, 1980).

Concerning the two imported antivenins into Jordan, Behringwerke antivenin provided a partial protection against *P. p. fieldi*, while Pasteur antivenin provided no protection (Disi *et al*, 1988.b.).

Walterinnesia aegyptia
Black Desert Cobra

The snake has a uniform shiny black colour dorsally and is bluish black ventrally. It is a proteroglyphous snake, the fixed grooved fangs are positioned near the front corner of the mouth under each nostril and in front of the eye. It is a stout snake with a small head not clearly distinct from neck, with large shields dorsally, and a short tail. The largest mature specimen measured is about 1.3 m long. It does not stretch the skin of the neck as in *Naja naja* or other related species. Similar observations were reported earlier (Gasperetti, 1974, 1976; Reed and Marx, 1959; Marx, 1953).

In the last few years a considerable increase in the number of the black desert snake were encountered. This increase is associated with the expansion of agricultural settlements in the eastern desert and Wadi Araba. These newly irrigated establishments resulted in an increase in number and range of distribution of *Bufo viridis* (green toad). In the area of Shaumari Wildlife Reserve, *W. aegyptia* feeds on *Bufo viridis*. Also, a considerable number of this black snake was caught from an irrigated farm where vegetables, and olive tree grew at Qasr Al-Habalat area, in the eastern desert of Jordan. Similar observations were reported by Zinner (1976). Anderson (1963) collected *W. aegyptia* from Iran, in and around gardens in the housing area. In Jordan its range of distribution extends into the foothills of the vegetated Mediterranean biotope, N.E. Salt, which is characterized by a lower winter temperature and a higher annual rainfall ranging from 300 — 400 mm. Similar observations were made by Reed and Marx (1959) in northeastern Iraq.

Zinner (1971) indicated that *W. aegyptia* might have a very poor vision, so it is probable that it sometimes misses its prey when it strikes. It usually hisses loudly, strikes sideways, often with the mouth closed, at the intruder. The body of the snake swells, and shrinks by inflating the lungs.

W. aegyptia feeds on all kinds of lizards, skinks, geckoes, agamids and snakes. It prefers and always accepts *Bufo viridis* rather than any other species. Occasionally, it feeds on mice and birds (Zinner, 1971).

W. aegyptia, depends on its sense of smell and sight (although weak) when finding its prey. The black desert snake *(W. aegyptia)* will not envenomate its prey with open mouth as in other vipers. It usually bites its prey only at short distance and usually sideways. It can also, constrict and suffocate its prey (Zinner, 1971). There is a noticeable decrease in the activity attained by this snake, when it hibernates during December and January. Also, this species spends all of its activity on the surface of the ground and is not subterranean (Zinner, 1971).

In spite of the enormous increase in the population of *W. aegyptia*, its confrontation with man is little due to their time of activity, which is usually around midnight. Its venom is highly potent (Moore, 1980; Zinner, 1976) but the yielded quantity is much less than that obtained from the Indian cobra. However, this snake is not the most dangerous and it is not very aggressive. If stepped upon, it will try to flee, and does not promptly strike out. Zinner (1976) reported that only one known case of death resulting from this snake, when a young Bedouin female sat on the snake at night. She did not receive any medical care and died after twenty hours. It ejects its venom by a chewing movement. The venom is not injected as it bites, but a few seconds after the chewing movement. Moore (1980) mentioned that there is no antivenin available for the venom of this snake, and it is advisable to stay away from this snake. In Wadi Araba, Bedouins do not kill the black desert snake and let it escape even if it enters their houses or tents. This is the only snake which is not killed by Bedouins. Similar observations were made in Saudi Arabia by Gasperetti (1974 and 1976) who indicated that the black desert snake was highly feared by the Bedouins and many stories were reported about the supernatural powers of this snake and its possession by "Jinnis".

Gitter *et al* (1962) demonstrated that following intraperitoneal injection of a lethal dose of *W. aegyptia* venom into mice, severe congestion in the central veins and the sinusoids of the liver occur. They also noticed patchy necrosis and vacuolation of the liver hepatocytes after injection of fraction I of this venom. However, low doses caused leuckocytic infiltration, mainly neutrophils in the periportal areas. Congestion of the blood vessels and leuckocytic infiltration in the lung also occurred.

Treatment

The following references cover this topic: Andrews *et al*, 1968; McCollugh and Gennaro, 1970; Warrell *et al*. 1975; Huang *et al*, 1978; Watt, 1978; Clement and Pietrusko, 1979; Efrati, 1979; Moore, 1980; and Saxena, 1987.

First Aid Treatment

1. Move away from the snake, since there is a chance of being bitten more than once by the same snake. Identify the snake if possible. In case you can't identify it, it is preferable to bring the dead snake to the hospital. Be careful not to hold the freshy killed snake by the mouth opening. On two occasions in Jordan, persons were bitten by a freshly killed viper.
2. The bitten person should be calm and avoid excitation to facilitate the necessary first aid.
3. Immobilize the bitten part, by applying a splint and keep this part in case of limbs, horizontal. The bitten person should not walk in order to decrease the spread of the venom.
4. A tourniquet should be applied above the bitten area. The tourniquet should not be too tight, so that a finger can pass under the tourniquet. It is advisable not to release it periodically before seeing the physicians if less than one and a half hours from the medical centre. However, in case of deep envenomation,

the application of a tourniquet will not prevent the spreading of the venom (Moore, 1980). Efrati (1979) indicated that the application of tourniquet is one of the issues of intense debate, especially both arterial and venous tourniquets which may lead to undesired complications. In addition the lymphatic tourniquet does not exist.

5. Saxena (1987) indicated that it is advantageous to infiltrate the area around the bitten site with antivenin. This may help to fix the venom locally to some extent as well as to prevent necrotic changes of the area which is characteristic of viperine venoms. Antivenin should never be administered into a finger or toe. However, McCollugh & Gennaro (1970), and Efrati (1979) indicated that antivenin should not be administered intramuscularly nor around the site of the bite, especially when that antivenin will not counteract appreciable amounts of venom. Moreover, the tissues at the site of bite are not capable of absorbing antivenin as a result of the rapid local action of the venom.

6. It is absolutely not recommended to use any form of cryotherapy.

Early Hospital Treatment

1. The physician should be with the patient in the emergency room and should seek prompt advice from experts if needed.

2. Identify the offending snake if possible, or check the exact region from which the patient was bitten since venomous snakes prefer certain habitats. The patients should be observed closely for at least the first hour and in certain bites, may need more time of close observation. Signs and symptoms of the patient are very helpful in determining the poisonous, nature of the snake. Observe pain, swelling, ecchymosis or belbs. In some cases there may be dizziness, nausea, vomiting, diarrhea, tachycardia, weakness, numbness of the bitten part of the body, cold and clammy skin. Hypotension and shock-like state may ensue. If the patient had a dangerous snakebite, place an 18-gauge plastic line in the vein, then administer the specific antivenin (or polyvenin) intravenously before releasing the tourniquet.

Do not postpone giving the antivenin, especially in a case of viper snake poisoning, the antivenin should be given without delay. In this case it is preferable to start giving an aqueous epinephrine (1:1,000 dilution) as a premedication. Watt, (1978) indicated that the recommended dose is 0.01 ml/kg body weight to total of 0.3 ml in a small child and 0.5 ml in a larger child or adult.

Check for history of allergy and have aqueous epinephrine (1:1,000) readily available in a syringe in case of severe allergic reaction. Glucose and lactated Ringer's solution 5% should be given i.v.

A skin test or eye test for hypersensitivity to horse serum should be done before giving the antivenin. If the allergic test is negative, cautiously administer the antivenin i.v. But in the hypersensitivity test, antivenin should be given slowly following the instructions accompanying the antivenin.

The serum may be administered subcutaneously, but it is highly effective intravenously, which should be the route of choice in spite of the attendant risk. Intravenous administration of the antivenin may produce severe serum sickness or even acute anaphylaxis in patients allergic to horse serum. In severe cases of snake bite, the route of choice is i.v. If the antivenin is being given i.m. or s.c., two or three times of the recommended dosage should be administered. Moreover, if any anaphylactic reaction happens, it is much easier to control it if the antivenin is administered i.v. than i.m.

If problems arise during the infusion, administration of the antivenin is stopped, usually temporarily, and anaphylaxis or serum sickness is controlled by further doses of epinephrine or by levarterenol bitartrate 0.2% infusion (in 500 ml of saline solutions) as indicated by Watt (1978).

In areas where snake bites are common and far from the main hospitals, clinics should keep enough units of antivenin on hand at all times.

By continuous checking of complete coagulogram, blood pressure, pulse rate, respiration rate, urine output, pain, slowing down of swelling, detection of improvement in vital signs can be made, at which time the physician should discontinue giving the antivenin. It is difficult to determine the necessary amount of antivenin to be given. Generally bites on digits require more antivenin than those on other parts of the body. Also, bites in children may require 50% more antivenin as indicated by Watt (1978). In case of persistent hypotension from anaphylaxis crystalloid, colloids or vasopressors may be useful in addition to epinephrine in treatment of anaphylaxis.

Watt (1978) and Efrati (1979) mentioned that it is totally impractical to use corticosteroids in the primary treatment of venomous bites without using antivenin. Moreover, most of the patients receiving antivenin require steroids to allay the ensuring serum sickness, which can be dangerous. Watt (1978) recommended giving 80 mg of prednisone daily in divided dosages, from the fourth day after the bite to the 12th day. This dosage should be increased if the serum sickness worsens, and should be adjusted for children.

Laboratory Studies

Immediately after the arrival of the bitten person at the hospital, the following laboratory studies as indicated by Andrews *et al* (1968), should be made:

1. Drawing of blood, about 50 cc, for baseline studies:
    A. Complete blood cell count, typing and crossmatching should be done promptly. As time passes it becomes difficult to perform crossmatching, since they are influenced by haemolysis.
    B. Complete coagulograms, includes: bleeding time, clotting time, platelet count, clot reaction time, prothrombin, time, fibrinogen level and thromboplastin level.
    C. Electrolyte package, essential tests for the effects of venom on various tissues and organs such as: BUN, transaminase, LDH, blood sugar, alkaline phosphatase, protein and electrophoretic studies to check the effect of the venom on different proteins.

These studies should be repeated almost every 6 hours during the first day and daily after that.

An adequate intravenous route should be kept ready for the purpose of medications as well as blood replacement. Four to six units of fresh blood should be kept available.

In case of neurotoxic envenomation, intubation and ventilatory support are essential, and sometimes, tracheostomy may be needed.

Toxicities of Poisonous Snakes Venoms in Mice.

Venom	Route of injection	LD_{50} mg/kg	References
Vipera palaestinae	i.p.	2.53 mg/kg	Gitter *et al* 1957
	i.p.	1.90 mg/kg	Krupnick *et al* 1968
	i.p.	1.90 mg/kg	Disi *et al* 1988
	i.v.	0.18 mg/kg	Minton 1974
	s.c.	9.40 mg/kg	Minton 1974
Echis coloratus	i.p.	1.55 mg/kg	Gitter *et al* 1960
	i.p.	1.75 mg/kg	Rechnic *et al* 1962
	i.v.	0.575 mg/kg	Gitter *et al* 1960
	i.v.	0.25 mg/kg	Ovadia & Kochva 1977
	s.c.	3.875 mg/kg	Gitter *et al* 1960
Cerastes cerestes	i.p.	1.35 mg/kg	Mohamed *et al* 1980
	i.p.	1.75 mg/kg	Shakhanbeh 1985
	i.p.	1.75 mg/kg	Disi *et al* 1988
	i.v.	0.45 mg/kg	Hassan & Hawary 1975
	s.c.	15.0 mg/kg	Minton 1974
Pseudocerastes persicus fieldi	i.p.	1.00 mg/kg	Gitter *et al* 1962
	i.p.	0.675 mg/kg	Disi *et al* 1988
	i.v.	0.30 mg/kg	Ovadia & Kochva 1977
	i.v.	0.25 mg/kg	Batzri-Izraeli and Bdolah 1982
Walterinnesia aegyptia	i.p.	0.30 mg/kg	Gitter *et al* 1962
	i.p.	0.285 mg/kg	Mohamed *et al* 1980
	i.p.	0.45 mg/kg	Disi *et al* 1988
	i.v.	0.30 mg/kg	Ovadia & Kochva 1977

References

Al-Eisawi, D.M. (1985). Vegetation in Jordan. In: Studies in the History and Archeology of Jordan. A. Hadidi, ed.: Vol. 1, 45-47, Dept. of Antiquities, Amman.

Al-Khalil, M. (1985). the Effect of Repeated Small Doses of *Cerastes cerastes* Snake Venom on Certain Tissues of Mice. M.Sc. Thesis. The University of Jordan, Amman, XI, 82 pp. and 69 Plates.

Aloof, S., Kirschmann, C. and DeVries, A. (1962). Action of near eastern Viperidae venoms on human platelets in vitro. Arch. Int. Pharmacodyn., 142(1-2), 216-227.

Amr, Z.S. and Amr, S.S. (1983). Snakebites in Jordan. The Snake, 15, 81-85.

Anderson, S.C. (1963). Amphibians and reptiles from Iran. Proc. Calif. Acad. Sci., 31(16), 417-498.

Andrews, C.E., Dees, J.E., Edwards, R.D., Jackson, K.W., Synder, C.C., Moseley, T., Gennaro, J.F.Jr. and Gehres, G.W. (1968). Venomous snakebites in Florida. J. Florida. Med. Assoc., 55(4), 308-316.

Barzilay, M., Kaminsky, E. and Condrea, E. (1978). Exposure of human red blood cell membrane phospholipids to snake venom phospholipases. A-II. Hydrolysis of substrates in intact and released cells by phospholipases from rhinghals *(Hemachatus hemachatus)* venom: Effect of calcium ions. Toxicon, 16, 153-161.

Batzri-Izraeli, R. and Bdolah, A. (1982). Isolation and characterization of the main toxic fraction from the venom of the false horned viper *(Pseudocerastes fieldi)*. Toxicon, 20(5), 867-875.

Bdolah, A. (1986). Comparison of venoms from two subspecies of the false horned viper *(Pseudocerastes persicus)*. Toxicon, 24(7), 726-729.

Clement, J.F. and Pietrusko, R.G. (1979). Pit viper snakebite envenomation in the United States. Clinical Toxicology, 14(5), 515-538.

Condrea, E. and DeVries, A. (1965). Venom phospholipase A : A review. Toxicon, 2, 261-273.

Condrea, E., Livni, E., Berwald, J. and DeVries, A. (1961). Changes in red blood cell fragilities due to the action of phospholipase and lipoprotein lipase on human blood in vitro. Arch. Int. Pharmacodyn., 3(4), 368-379.

Danon, D., Gitter, S. and Rosen, M. (1961). Deformation of red cell shape induced by *Vipera palaestinae* venom in vitro. Nature. 189, 320-321.

DeVries, A., Condrea, E., Klibansky, C., Rechnic, J., Moroz, C. and Kirschmann, C. (1962). Haematological effects of the venom of two near eastern snakes: *Vipera palaestinae* and *Echis colorata*. New Istanbul. Contrib. Clin. Sci., 5, 151-169.

DeVries, A. and Gitter, S. (1957). The action of *Vipera xanthina palaestinae* venom on blood coagulation in vitro. Brit. J. Haemat., 3., 379-386.

Disi, A.M. (1983). A contribution to the herpetofauna of Jordan, 1. Venomous snakes. Dirasat, 10(2), 167-180.

Disi, A.M. (1985). A contribution to the herpetofauna of Jordan, 2. New records and a systematic list of snakes from Jordan. The Snake, 17, 31-42.

Disi, A.M. (1987). Environmental factors affecting snake distribution in Jordan. Proceedings of the Symposium on the Fauna and Zoogeography of the Middle East, Mainz 1985. F. Krupp, W., Schneider and R. Kinzelbach, eds. Beihefte zum TAVO A 28, 296 + 310, Wiesbaden.

Disi, A.M.; Amr, Z.S. Defosse, D. (1988.a.). Contribution to the herpetofauna of Jordan, III. Snakes of Jordan. The Snake, 20(1), 40-51.

Disi, A., Gharaibeh, M. and Salhab, A. (1988.b.). Comparative potency of two polyvalent antivenins in mice and recent incidents of snakebites in Jordan. The Snake, 20 (2), 144-150.

Djaldetti, M., Joshua, H., Bessler, H., Rosen, M., Gutglas, H. and DeVries, A. (1964). Coagulation disturbances in the dog following *Echis coloratus* venom inoculation. Hemostase, 4, 423-432.

Djaldetti, M., Sandbank, U. and Dannon, D. (1967). Effect of *Echis colorata* envenomation on circulating lymphocytes and lymph nodes of the guinea pig. An electron microscopic study. Rev. Franc. Etudes. Clin. Et. Biol., 12, 55-63.

Efrati, P. (1979). Symptomatology, Pathology and Treatment of the Bites of Viperid Snakes. In: Handbook of Experimental Pharmacology, Lee, C (ed). Chapter 26, 52, 956-977.

Efrati, P. and Reif, L. (1953). Clinical and pathological observation on sixty-five cases of viper bite in Israel. Am. J. Trop. Med. Hyg. 2(6), 1085-1108.

Flower, S.S. (1933). Notes on the recent reptiles and amphibians of Egypt, with a list of the species recorded from that Kingdom. Proc. Zool. Soc. London, 19(3), 735-853.

Gasperetti, J. (1974). A preliminary sketch of the snakes of the Arabian Peninsula. J. Saudi Arab. Nat. Hist. Soc. 12, 1-72.

Gasperetti, J. (1976). *Walterinnesia aegyptia* Lataste a rare black snake. J. Saudi Arab. Nat. Hist. Soc. 16, 2-8.

Gitter, S., Kochwa, S., Danon, D. and DeVries, A. (1959). Discksphere transformation and inhibition of rouleau formation and sedimentation of human red blood cells induced by *Vipera xanthina palaestinae* venom. Arch. Int. Pharmacodyn., 18(3-4), 350-357.

Gitter, S., Kochwa, S., DeVries, A. and Leffkowitz, M. (1957). Studies on electrophoretic fractions of *Vipera xanthina palaestinae* venom. Am. J. Trop. Med. Hyg. 6, 180-189.

Gitter, S., Levi, G., Kochwa, S., DeVries, A., Rechnic, J. and Casper, J. (1960). Studies on the venom of *Echis colorata*. Am. J. Trop. Med. Hyg., 9, 391-399.

Gitter, S., Moroz-Perimutter, C.H., Boss, J.H., Livini, E., Rechnic, J., Goldblum, N. and DeVries, A. (1962). Studies on the Near East *Walterinnesia aegyptia* and *pseudocerastes fieldi*. Am. J. Trop. Med. Hyg., 11, 861-868.

Hass, G. (1957). Some amphibians and reptiles from Arabia. Proc. Calif.Acad. Sci., Ser. 4, 29, 47-86.

Hass, G. and Werner, Y.H. (1969). Lizards and snakes from south-western Asia, collected by Henry Field, Bull, Mus. Comp. Zool. Hrv., 138, 327-406.

Hassan, F. and El-Hawary, M.F.S. (1975). Immunological properties of antivenins. I. Bivalent *Cerastes cerastes* and *Cerastes vipera* antivenin. Amer. J. Trop. Hyg., 24, 1031-1034.

Homma, M., Kosoge, T., Okonogi, T.m, Hattori, Z. and Sawi, Y. (1967). A histopathological study on arterial lesions caused by habu *(Trimeresurus flavoviridis)* venom. Japan J. Exp. Med., 37(4), 323-335.

Huang, T.T., Lewis, S.R. and Lucas, B.S. (1978). Venomous snakes. In: Dangerous Plants, Snakes, Arthropods and Marine Life: Toxicity and Treatment. Ellis, M.D. (ed.). Drug Intelligence Publication, Inc. Hamilton, Illinois.

Joshua, H., Djaldetti, M., Ozcan, E., Bessler, H., Rosen, M. and DeVries, A. (1964). Mechanism of Thrombocytopenia in the dog and the guinea pig following *Echis colorata* venom inoculation. Hemostase, 4, 333-340.

Klibansky, C. and DeVries, A. (1963). Quantitative study of erythrocyte-lysolecithin interaction. Biochem. Biophys. Acta., 76, 176-187.

Klibansky, C., Ozcan, E., Joshua, H., Djaldetti, M., Bessler, H. and DeVries, A. (1966). Intravascular haemolysis in dogs induced by *Echis colorata* venom. Toxicon, 3, 213-221.

Kochwa, S., Perimutter, C., Gitter, S., Rechnic, J. and DeVries, A. (1960). Studies on *Vipera palaestinae* venom. Fractionation by ion exchange chromatography. Am. J. Trop. Med. Hyg. 9, 374-380.

Krupnick, J., Bichner, H.I. and Gitter, S. (1968). Central neurotoxic effects of the venoms of *Naja naja* and *Vipera palaestinae*. Toxicon, 6, 11.

Labib, R., Awad, E.R. and Farag, N.W. (1981.a.). Proteases of *Cerastes cerastes* (Egyptian sand viper) and *Cerastes vipera* (Sahara sand viper) snake venoms. Toxicon, 19, 73-83.

Labib, S.R. Azab, H.M. and Farag, N.W. (1981.b.). Effects of *Cerastes cerastes* (Egyptian sand viper) and *Cerastes vipera* (Sahara and viper) snake venoms on blood coagulation: separation of coagulant and anticoagulant factors and their correlation with organine esterase and protease activities. Toxicon, 19, 85-94.

Marx, H. (1953). The Elapid genus of snakes *Walterinnesia* Fieldiana (Zool.), 34(16), 189-196.

McCollugh, N.C. and Gennaro, J.F. (1970). Treatment of venomous snakebite in the United States. Clinical Toxicology, 3(3), 483-500.

Mendelssohn, H. (1963). On the biology of the venomous snakes of Israel. I — Is. Jour. Zool., 12, 143-170.

Mendelssohn, H. (1965). On the biology of the venomous snakes of Israel. II — Is. Jour. Zool., 14, 185-212.

Minton, S.A. (1974). Venom Diseases, Charles, C. Thomas, Springfield, Ill., U.S.A.

Mohamed, A.H., Abdel-Baset, A. and Hassan, A. (1980) Immunological studies on monovalent and bivalent *Cerastes* antivenin. Toxicon, 18, 384-387.

Mohamed, A.H. and El-Damarawy, A.N. (1974). The role of the fibrinolytic enzyme system in the haemostatic defects following snake envenomation. Toxicon, 12, 467-475.

Mohamed, A.H., El-Serougi, M. and Hanna, M.M. (1969a).Observations on the effect of *Echis carinatus* venom on blood clotting. Toxicon, 6, 215-219.

Mohamed, A.H., El-Serougi, M. and Kamel, A. (1963). Effect of *Echis carinatus* venom on blood glucose and liver and muscle glycogen concentrations. Toxicon, 1. 243-244.

Mohamed, A.H., El-Serougi, M. and Khaled, Z.L. (1969b). Effects of *Cerastes cerastes* venom on blood coagulation mechanisms. Toxicon, 7, 181-184.

Mohamed, A.H. and Khaled, Z.L. (1966). Effects of the venom of *Cerastes cerastes* on nerve tissue and skeletal muscle. Toxicon, 3, 223-224.

Mohamed, A.H., Saleh, A.M., Ahmed, S and El-Maghraby, M. (1977). Effects of *Cerastes cerastes* snakes venom on blood and bone marrow cells. Toxicon, 15, 35-40.

Moore, G.M. (ed.), (1980). Poisonous Snakes of the World. Castle House Publications, Ltd. London, 212 pp.

Moroz, C., DeVries, A. and Sela, M. (1966). Isolation and characterization of a neurotoxin from *Vipera palaestinae* venom. Biophys. Acta., 124, 136-146.

Ovadia, M. (1978). Isolation and characterization of three haemorrhagic factors from the venom of *Vipera palaestinae*. Toxicon, 16, 479-487.

Ovadia, M. and Kochva, E. (1977). Neutralization of Viperidae and Elapidae snake venoms by sera of different animals. Toxicon, 15, 541-547.

Rechnic, J., Trachtenberg, P., Casper, J., Moroz, C. and DeVries, A. (1962). A fibrinogenemia and thrombocytopenia in guinea pigs following injection of *Echis coloratus* venom. Blood, 20, 735-749.

Reed, C.A. and Marx, H. (1959). A herpetological collection from northeastern Iraq. Trans. Kansas Acad. Sci. 62, 91-122.

Roy, A.C. (1945). Lecithin and venom haemolysis. Nature, 55, 696-697.

Sandbank, U. and Djaldetti, M. (1966). Effects of *Echis colorata* venom inoculation on the nervous system of the dog and guinea pig. Acta Neuropathologica, 6, 61-69.

Sandbank, U., Jerushalmy, Z., Ben-David, E. and DeVries, A. (1974). Effects of *Echis coloratus* venom on brain vessels. Toxicon, 12, 267-271.

Saxena, S.N. (1987). Central Research Institute, Kasauli (Punjab, India). C.R.I., 62, 104, and 112 (special publications).

Schmidt, K.P. (1930). Reptiles of Marshall Field North Arabian Desert Expedition. Field Mus. Nat. Hist. Zool. Ser., 17(6), 223-230.

Shabo-Shina, R. and Bdolah, A. (1987). Interactions of the neurotoxic complex from the venom of the false horned viper *(Pseudocerastes fieldi)* with rat striatal synaptosomes. Toxicon, 25(3), 253-266.

Shakhanbeh, J.M. (1985). histological and Ultrastructural Alterations in Some Mice Tissues Induced by *Cerastes cerastes* venom. M.Sc. Thesis. The University of Jordan, Amman, VIII, 98 pp., + 43 plates, 4 Tables, 1 Figure and 5 Appendices.

Sosa, B.P., Alagon, A.C., Possani, L.D. and Julia, J.Z. (1979). Comparison of phospholipase activity with direct and indirect lytic affects of animal venoms. Compt. Bioch. Physiol. B: 648: 231-234.

Tsai, M.C., Lee, C.Y. and Bdolah, A. (1983). Mode of neuromuscular blocking action of a toxic phospholipase A_2 from *Pseudocerastes fieldi* (Field's horned viper) snake venom. Toxicon, 21(4), 527-534.

Warburg, M.R. (1964). Observations on the microclimate in habitats of some desert vipers in the Negev, Arava and Dead Sea region. Vie et Millieu, 15, 1017-1041.

Warrell, D.A., Ormerod, L.D. and Davidson, N.McD. (1975). Bites by puff-adder *(Bitis arietans)* in Nigeria and Value of antivenin. British Medical Journal, 4, 697-700.

Watt, C.H. Jr. (1978). Poisonous snakebite treatment in the United States. JAMA, 240(7), 654-686.

World Health Organization. (1971). Requirements for snake antivenins (Requirements for Biological Substances, No.21). WHO Tech. Rep. Ser. No. 463, 27-44.

Zinner, H. (1971). On ecology and the significance of semantic coloration in the nocturnal desert-Elapid *Walterinnesia aegyptia* Lataste (Reptiles, Ophidia). Oecologia, 7, 267-275.

Zinner, H. (1976). Six venomous snakes of southern Israel. Isr. Land and Nature, 1(4), 140-146.

Venomous Snakes of Medical Importance in Korea

M. Toriba

Introduction

Korea is composed of Korean Peninsula and some nearby islands and separated from Northeastern region of China by Yalu river and Tumen river. It has a small contact with USSR. At present, Korea is politically divided into two, Republic of Korea (South Korea) and Democratic People's Republic of Korea (North Korea). Because there is only few information on the venomous snakes and snake bite cases in North Korea, mainly those of South Korea are described here. The snakes of North Korea were recently reviewed by Szyndlar and O (1987) who also briefly mentioned on the snakes of South Korea.

There are 14 species of land snakes in Korea (both North and South). Among them, 5 species are regarded as venomous, which are one natricine, one viperine and three crotaline snakes. A key for the venomous snakes in Korea is as follows:

1. Top of head covered by nine symmetrical shields 2
1a. Top of head with many small scales on anterior part ... *Vipera berus berus*
2. Loreal pit absent 3
2a. Loreal pit present 4
3. Scales strongly keeled, in 19 rows; more than 152 ventrals; colour greenish with transverse dark bands or spots, ventrals dark. .. *Rhabdophis tigrinus*
3a. Not as above .... non-venomous snakes
4. Scales in 21 rows 5
4a. Scales in 23 rows; post-ocular dark stripe not bordered above by light line; dorsal pattern dark crossbands .... *Agkistrodon saxatilis saxatilis*
5. Dorsal pattern dark around blotches; tongue black; tail tip yellowish in adult .... *Agkistrodon blomhoffi brevicaudus*
5a. Dorsal pattern dark squarish blotches; tongue pink; tail tip dark in adult ... . *Agkistrodon ussuriensis*

Species Account

Natricinae

Rhabdophis tigrinus (Boie)
> *Tropidonotus tigrinus* Boie, 1826 Isis (T. typ.: Japan).
> *Natrix tigrina tigrina* Slevin, 1925,
> *Natrix tigrina lateralis* Stejneger, 1907; Maki 1931; Tanner, 1953; Steward, 1954; Shannon, 1956; Dixon, 1956; Hahn, 1960; Kang and Yoon, 1975.

Rhabdophis tigrina lateralis Webb et al., 1962.
Rhabdophis tigrina tigrina Paik, 1982.
Rhabdophis tigrina Szyndlar, 1984; Szyndlar and O, 1987.

Remarks

Although there are several reports of severe bite cases by this snake including two fatal cases in Japan (see account by Toriba and Sawai in this book), there are no reports of envenomation by this snake in Korea. The reason for this difference is not clear. The difference in size of the snake may account for it. The largest known specimen in Korea is 991 mm in total length and less than 1 m (Szyndlar and O, 1987), while in Japan, specimens exceeding 1 m are not rare (Moriguchi, 1985; Moriguchi and Toriba, 1985). Such a difference in size is important in the degree of envenomation. According to Szyndlar and O (1987), the people of North Korea are familiar with the potential danger from this snake's bite. This evidence suggests that some cases of mild envenomation occur without official records.

Many previous workers recognised this snake as a valid subspecies, *lateralis*. However, recent workers found that there are no marked separation in ventral and subcaudal counts between the populations in the continent and Japan and did not recognize subspecies *lateralis* (Nakamura and Ueno, 1963; Paik, 1982). Because there is a geographic variation in coloration, a photograph of a specimen from South Korea is shown (Figure 1). The toxicity of the venom of this snake in the continent including Korea is not known.

Viperinae

   Vipera berus berus (Linnaeus)
      Coluber berus Linnaeus, 1758, Syst. Nat. 10 ed., (T. typ.: Upsala, Sweden).
      Vipera berus sachalinensis Maki, 1931; Shannon, 1956; Kang and Yoon, 1975; Paik, 1982.
      Vipera berus berus Szyndlar and O, 1987.

Distribution:

Restricted to northern part of North Korea in Korea and extends to Northeastern China. Other population has large range across the Eurasian Continent.

Remarks:

Due to its rarity and restricted range, it seems to be not a very important venomous snake in Korea. On its taxonomic status, many workers followed Maki (1931) in considering it as subspecies *sachalinensis*. Recently Szyndlar and O (1987) pointed out that the head scutellation of this snake in Korea is similar to nominate subspecies instead of *sachalinensis*. Thus they tentatively placed it in nominate subspecies, and actual taxonomic status is under study by Nilson, Andren and Szyndlar. It lives in high mountains and feeds on frogs, birds and birds' eggs (Szyndlar and O, 1987). The toxicity of the venom of this snake in Korea is not known.

Crotalinae

Agkistrodon saxatilis saxatilis (Emelianov)
> *Ancistrodon saxatilis* Emelianov, 1937, Bull Far East. Branch Acad. Sci. USSR (T. typ.: Vladivostok, USSR).
> *Agkistrodon blomhoffii intermedius* Stejneger, 1907 (part).
> *Agkistrodon blomhoffii brevicaudus* Slevin, 1925 (part).
> *Agkistrodon halys intermedius* Maki, 1931 (part).
> *Agkistrodon halys* Kang and Yoon, 1975 (part).
> *Agkistrodon saxatilis* Gloyd, 1972; Paik et al., 1979; Paik, 1982; Szyndlar, 1984; Szyndlar and O, 1987.
> *Agkistrodon intermedius saxatilis* Gloyd and Conant, 1982.
> *Agkistrodon saxatilis saxatilis* Ji, 1987.

Description:

In general, this species, is larger and more robust than the other two species of *Agkistrodon* in Korea, and extends to about 80 cm in total length. Dorsal scales keeled, 23 rows at midbody, rarely 21. Head distinct from neck. 2 preoculars, and 2 or 3 postoculars, 7 or 8 supralabials, last 3 very low, infralabials 10 or 11. Ventrals 147-164 in males, 148-165 in females, subcaudals 37-48 in males, 33-48 in females.

Coloration:

Ground color is light grey to light brown, with 29-54 transverse dark bands, which is sometimes separated at dorso-lateral region. Post ocular dark stripe is not bordered dorsally by clear light line (Figure 2).

Habits and habitat:

Because three species of *Agkistrodon* in Korea were confused under the name *A. halys* till recently, the statement in older literature cannot be applicable to any species. Therefore the descriptions on the same species in Northeast China or Far Eastern region of USSR are quoted here from Ji (1987) or Emelianov (1929, 1937). This pit-viper lives mainly in mountain region with rocky piles and grassy bushes. It feeds on small rodents and occasionally on frogs. It is not aggressive in captivity. In China, it appears from hibernation in early May and starts the hibernation in late September. 5-8 young are born in September, each more than 20 cm in total length. Mating occurs in late May.

Distribution:

North and South Korea except Cheju-do Is. Northeast China and Far Eastern region of USSR.

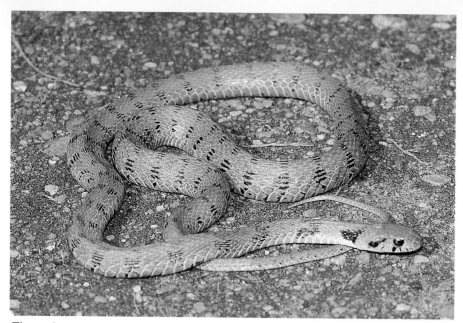

Figure 1.
Rhabdophis tigrinus from Taegu, South Korea.

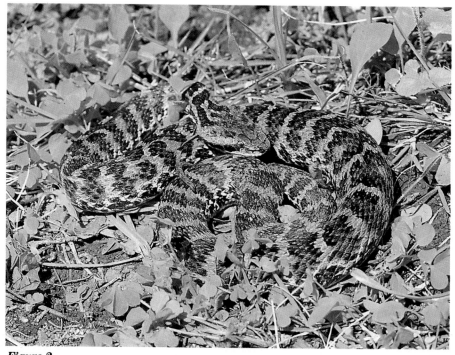

Figure 2.
Agkistrodon s. saxatilis from Taegu, South Korea.

Remarks:

The name *saxatilis* was long been ignored by the workers till Gloyd (1972) revived and applied it to one of three sympatric species in Korea. Although Gloyd and Conant (1982) regarded this species as a subspecies of *A. intermedius*, I do not consider that they are conspecific and reject their combination. A detailed discussion will be given elsewhere. Here I consider that *A. shedaoensis* Zhao is subspecies of *A. saxatilis* and treat it as nominate subspecies. The coloration of this species seems to be more dark in South Korea than in the Northern area of the continent.

Agkistrodon ussuriensis (Emelianov)

Ancistrodon blomhoffii ussuriensis Emelianov, 1929, Zap. Vladivost. Otd. Gos. Russk. Geor. Obsch. (T. typ.: Suchan River, USSR).

Agkistrodon blomhoffii brevicaudus Stejneger, 1907 (part); Slevin, 1925 (part).

Agkistrodon halys brevicaudius Stewart, 1954; Webb et al., 1962 (part).

Ancistrodon halys brevicaudus Shannon, 1956 (part); Dixon, 1956.

Agkistrodon halys Kang and Yoon, 1975 (part).

Agkistrodon caliginosus Gloyd, 1972; Gloyd and Conant, 1982; Paik et al., 1979; Paik, 1982; Szyndlar, 1984; Szyndlar and O, 1987.

Agkistrodon ussuriensis Toriba, 1988.

Description:

This is a relatively slender snake among the three species of *Agkistrodon* in Korea, and less than 70 cm in total length. Dorsal scales moderately keeled with pair of inconspicuous apical pits, 21 rows at midbody. Head distinct from neck. 2 preoculars, 2 postoculars, 7 supralabials and 10 infralabials with some exceptions. Ventrals 139-153 in males, 141-159 in females, subcaudals 40-52 in males, 30-48 in females.

Coloration:

General color is highly variable, usually dark brown or dark grey, sometimes orange, blackish grey. There are a series of darker blotches on both sides of dorsal body, which are mainly rectangular in shape sometimes forming broad dark crossbands in Korea. However, these blotches are round in some specimens of Korea and many of China and USSR. The blotches have lighter center with or without dark central spots. Number of blotches is about 22-33 (Figure 3). Semicircular light spots present on lower labial margin. Tongue is pink. Tail tip is dark in adults.

Habits and habitat:

It lives in low mountains, hills, edge of forests, grassy areas near stream, marshy areas near paddy fields, etc. If feeds on mainly mice and frogs, occasionally fishes, lizards and snakes, and eggs of ants are also recorded as food in China. 2-10 young are born in late August through middle September.

Distribution:

South and North Korea including Cheju-do Is, extending to Northeastern China and Far Eastern region of USSR. Similar to *A. saxatilis* in distribution.

Remarks:

Since Gloyd (1972) described it as new species, *A. caliginosus*, most workers followed him and treated it as *A. caliginosus*. However, Toriba (1988) indicated it as synonymous with *A. b. ussuriensis* and the latter is a full species distinct from *A. blomhoffii* based on morphological and karyological study.

Agkistrodon blomhoffi brevicaudus Stejneger
    Agkistrodon blomhoffii brevicaudus Stejnger, 1907, Bull. U.S. Nat. Mus. (T. typ.: Fusan, South Korea); Slevin, 1925 (part); Gloyd, 1972; Paik et al., 1979; Paik, 1982; Szyndlar, 1984; Szyndlar and 0, 1987.
    Agkistrodon halys brevicaudus Maki, 1931 (part); Hahn, 1960; Webb et al., 1962.
    Ancistrodon halys brevicaudus Shannon, 1956 (part).
    Agkistrodon halys Kang and Yoon, 1975 (part).

Description:

This is intermediate among the three species of Korean *Agkistrodon* in body configuration. The largest one exceeds 70 cm in total length. Dorsal scales keeled with a pair of small apical pits, 21 rows at midbody. Head distinct from neck. Two preoculars, 2 or 3 postoculars, 7 rarely 8 supralabials, and 10 (occasionally 9 or 11) infralabials. Ventrals 135–151 in males, 134–159 in females, subcaudals 32–52 in males, 27–47 in females.

Coloration:

Ground color is light brown or grey with a series of dark round blotches with lighter center. In general, the markings of this species are clearer than those of *A. ussuriensis*. Venter has conspicuous dark markings also. Tail tip is yellowish and not dark in adults (Figure 4). Tongue is black.

Habits and habitat:

The habitat of this species is not markedly different from that of *A. ussuriensis*. It lives in grassy areas of valleys, hillside and paddy fields. It feeds on mice and frogs. 2–14 young are born in September.

Distribution:

North and South Korea including Cheju-do Is. extending to southern part of Northeastern China. If the populations in the continent are considered as single subspecies (Chen et al., 1984; Toriba, 1988), then it extends to central part of China. The nominate subspecies is in Japan.

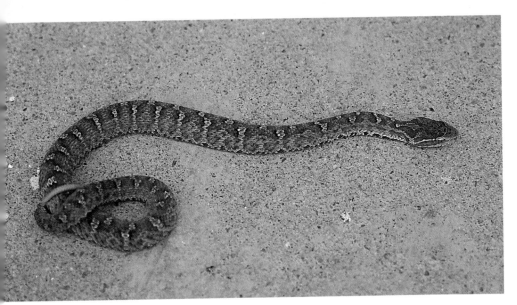

Figure 3.
A. *ussuriensis* from Taegu, South Korea, young.

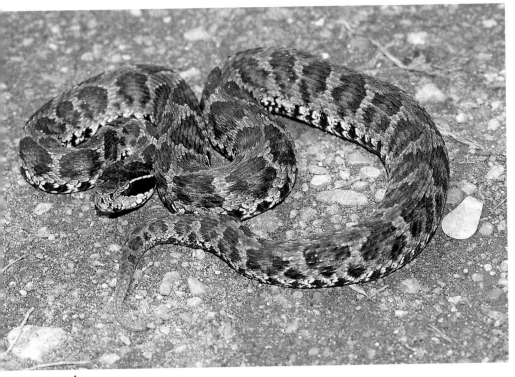

Figure 4.
A. *b. brevicaudus* from Taegu, South Korea.

Snake bite cases

There are only two reports on the venomous snake bites in South Korea by Sawai and Lah (1978) and Sho et al. (1978). The former reported 82 cases at Wonju Union Christian Hospital, Wonju during 15 years from 1959 to 1973. The latter reported 126 cases from 5 hospitals in Seoul, Jeounju, Wonju, Gwangju and Incheon during two years of 1976 and 1977. All the cases were due to *Agkistrodon*. However, the snake species reponsible for bites were not identified in most cases due to poor information. Sawai and Lah (1978) identified 13 cases as *A. ussuriensis*, 12 cases as *A. b. brevicaudus*, and 3 cases as *A. saxatilis*. Sho et al. (1978) did not identify the snake and suspected that the majority of the cases is due to *A. ussuriensis*.

Majority of the cases occurs during warmer months from May through September with the peak of August. The bites in males were more than twice as frequent as in females. Major occurrence was distributed among the ages of 10–59, although there is a slight difference in pattern between the two studies. Most of the bites occur in open fields including vegetable gardens, then in mountains, and a few in residences. In the day, bites occur from 6:00 to 23:59, most frequently during 12:00 to 17:59. Majority of bites occur at both upper and lower extremities with fingers and feet most frequent. Among 82 cases reported by Sawai and Lah (1978), 4 cases were fatal, while Sho et al. (1978) reported no fatal cases.

As local symptoms and signs, pain, swelling, bleeding from wound, petecheal hemorrhage, necrosis, bulla and lymphadenpathy were recorded. Sawai and Lah (1978) mentioned severe necrosis due to prolonged tourniquet.

As systemic symptoms and signs, ptosis of eyelids, blurred vision, vomiting, dizziness, chest discomfort, drowsiness, dyspnea, abdominal pain, diplopia, fever etc. were recorded. Ptosis of eyelids and blurred vision suggest the presence of neurotoxic factors in the venom of Korean *Agkistrodon* species. In the four fatal cases, state of shock, cardiac arrest, and pulmonary edema caused death.

Many of the patients were treated symptomatically by fluid transfusion, vitamin K, and antibiotics. Although Wyeth Polyvalent Antivenin were applied in certain cases, the effectiveness of the antivenin was uncertain.

The venoms

The values of LD_{50} in mice and MHD of the venoms of three *Agkistrodon* species are summarized in Table 1, in which the study on the snakes in China by Zhao et al. (1979) is also included. There are only slight differences in the toxicities of them. The venom of *A. ussuriensis* is most toxic and that of *A. s. saxatilis* is least toxic. Considering the difference in size of the snakes, their potential danger seems to be similar.

Studies on the components of the venoms were made by several workers. Two thrombin-like enzymes were purified from the venom of *A. ussuriensis* by Suzuki and Takahashi (1984). From this venom a capillary permeability-increasing enzyme was also purified and studied by Ohtani and Takahashi (1983) and Ohtani et al. (1985). On the other hand, Seu and Yi (1979) discovered a microbial inhibitory substance to snake venom proteinases from *Penicillium* sp. and the study on the proteinase and hemorrhagic factor of *A. b. brevicaudus* was made using this substance by Seu and Kwon (1986). As suggested by clinical symptoms, neurotoxins were found from the venom of *A. b. brevicaudus* (Jiangsu and Zhejiang, China) and *A. ussuriensis* (Jilin, China) by Zhang (1988).

TABLE 1

Toxicities of the venom of three species of *Agkistrodon*

Snakes	LD$_{50}$(μg/g)	MHD (mice) (im, μg)	MHD (rabbits) (ic, μg)
A. s. saxatilis[1]	0.83 (ip)		
A. ussuriensis[2]	1.14 (iv)	0.5	0.5
A. ussuriensis[1]	0.33 (ip)		
A. b. brevicaudus[2]	2.04 (iv)	0.5	0.5
A. b. brevicaudus[1]	0.49 (i.p.)		

1) Zhao et al. (1979), localities are Jilin, Jilin and Zhejiang, respectively.
2) Kawamura (1974) localities are South Korea.

References

Chen, Y., Wu, X. and Zhao, E. (1984) Classification of *Agkistrodon* species in China. Toxicon, 22: 53-61.

Dixon, J.R. (1956) A collection of amphibians and reptiles from West Central Korea. Herpetologica, 12:50-56.

Emelianov, A.A. (1929) Snakes of the Far Eastern District. Zapiski Vladivostokskogo Otdela Russkogo Geograficheskogo Obschesta, 3:1-208. (in Russian with English resume).

Emelianov, A.A. (1937) On a new species of *Ancistrodon* (Ophidia) in the Far East. Bulletin of the Far Eastern Branch of the Academy of Sciences of USSR, 24: 19-40. (in Russian with English summary).

Gloyd, H. K. (1972) The Korean snakes of the genus *Agkistrodon* (Crotalinae). Proceedings of the Biological Society of Washington, 85: 557-558.

Gloyd, H.K. and Conant, R (1982) The classification of the *Agkistrodon halys* complex. Japanese Journal of Herpetology, 9: 75-78.

Hahn, D.E. (1960) Collecting notes on Central Korean reptiles and amphibians. Journal of Ohio Herpetological Society, 2: 16-24.

Ji, D. (1987) Serpentiformes. In "Fauna Liaoningica. Amphibia Reptilia. Ed. by D. Ji et al." Liaoning Science and Technology Press, Shenyang, p. 89-139. (in Chinese)

Kang, Y.-S. and Yoon, I-B (1975) Illustrated encyclopedia of fauna and flora of Korea. vol. 17. Amphibia — Reptilia. Ministry of Education, Seoul, 191 pp. (in Korean)

Kawamura, Y. (1974) Study of the immunological relationships between venom of six Asiatic Agkistrodons. The Snake, 6: 19-26. (in Japanese with English summary)

Maki, M. (1931) A monograph of the snakes of Japan. Dai-ich Shobo, Tokyo, 240 pp.

Moriguchi, H. (1985) Body size differences between two populations of *Rhabdophis tigrinus*. The Snake, 17: 140-143.

Moriguchi, H. and Toriba, M. (1985) Note on the number of eggs in oviduct of *Rhabdophis tigrinus* (Boie). The Snake, 7: 144-147.

Nakamura, K. and Ueno, S.I. (1963) Japanese reptiles and amphibians in colour. Hoikusha, Osaka, 214 pp. (in Japanese)

Ohtani, Y. and Takahashi, H. (1983) Purification of a capillary permeability increasing-enzyme from the venom of *Agkistrodon caliginosus* (kankoku-mamushi). Toxicon, 21: 871-878.

Ohtani, Y., Suda, T. and Takahashi, H. (1985) Capillary permeability-increasing enzyme from the venom of *Agkistrodon caliginosus* (kankoku-mamushi): activity due to the release of peptide material from a protein in bovine plasma. Toxicon, 23: 53-61.

Paik, N.-K. (1982) Systematic studies on the suborder Serpentes (Reptilia) in Korea. Ph. D. Dissertation, Sungkyunkwan University, 86 pp. (in Korean with English abstract)

Paik, N.-K., Kim, Y.-J. and Yang, S.-Y. (1979) Biochemical variation and systematic status of the genus *Agkistrodon* (Crotalidae) in Korea. Korean Journal of Zoology, 22: 153-164.

Sawai, Y. and Lah, K.-Y. (1978) Snakebites in the South Korea. The Snake, 9: 39-47.

Seu, J.-H. and Kwon, G.-S. (1986) Studies on the proteinase and hemorrhagic factor of *Agkistrodon blomhoffii brevicaudus*. The Snake, 18: 47-52.

Seu, J.-H. and Yi, D.-H.(1979) A microbial inhibitory substance to snake venoms. The Snake, 11: 184-198.

Shannon, F.A. (1956) The reptiles and amphibians of Korea. Herpetologica, 12: 22-49.

Sho, C.-T., Min, H.-K., Bae, S.-K., Im, S.-C. and Kim, C.-K. (1978) Current status of snakebite in Korea. Yonsei Reports on Tropical Medicine, 9: 48-56.

Slevin, J.R. (1952) Contributions to Oriental Herpetology. II. Korea or Chosen. Proceedings of the California Academy of Sciences, 4th series, 14: 89-100.

Stejneger, L. (1907) Herpetology of Japan and adjacent territory. Bulletin of the U.S. National Museum, 58: 1-577.

Steward, G.D. (1954) A small collection of reptiles from Central Korea. Copeia, 1954: 65-67.

Suzuki, T. and Takahashi, H. (1984) Purification of two thrombin-like enzymes from the venom of *Agkistrodon caliginosus* (kankoku-mamushi). Toxicon, 22: 29-38

Szyndlar, Z. (1984) A description of a small collection of amphibians and reptiles from the People's Republic of Korea with notes on the distribution of the herpetofauna in that country. Acta Zoologica Cracoviensia, 27: 3-18.

Szyndlar, Z. and O, H.-D. (1987) Reptiles of the Democratic People's Republic of Korea. Part I. Serpentes. Chinese Herpetological Research, 1987: 22-59.

Tanner, V.M. (1953) Pacific islands herpetology. no. VIII. Korea. Great Basin Naturalist, 13: 67-73.

Toriba, M. (1988) Taxonomic status of *Agkistrodon caliginosus* Gloyd and *A. blomhoffii ussuriensis* (Emelianov). The Snake, 20: 30-39.

Webb, R.G., Jones, J.K., Jr., and Byers, G.W. (1962) Some reptiles and amphibians from Korea. University of Kansas Publications, Museum of Natural History, 15: 149-173.

Zhao, E., Wu, G. and Yang, W. (1979) Comparisons of toxicity and neutralization test among Pallas' pit-viper, Snake-island pit-viper and black eye-brow pit-viper. Acta Herpetologica Sinica, 1(3): 1-6. (in Chinese with English summary)

Zhang, J. (1988) Neurotoxins from the venoms of Crotalidae snakes collected in China. Abstract of papers presented to Second Japan-China Herpetological Symposium, Kyoto. p. 14.

Venomous Land Snakes Of Malaysia

Lim Boo Liat
Kuala Lumpur, Malaysia

Most snakes are harmless to human beings and may be considered as non-venomous. Only snakes which have a venom gland, a duct to carry the venom from it and a specialised grooved to tubular tooth, called the fang (fig 1) to inject that venom, are considered as venomous. In Malaysia, 17 of 105 strictly land snakes are venomous and are dangerous to man. These venomous snakes comprise two families, the Elapidae and the Viperidae, the former with nine and the latter with eight species respectively. Most other land snakes are practically harmless to man, though some may be mildly venomous, like the Mangrove Snake, *Boiga dendrophila* (fig 2) and the Red-necked Keelback, *Rhabdophis subminiatus* (fig 3). All 14 species of fresh-water snakes are harmless, but all the 22 species of sea-snakes are venomous, and this latter group is dealt separately.

Almost all of the Malaysian venomous land snakes are brightly coloured; they can be individually recognised by the coloration and behaviour, and based on these, a key is made for identification of these poisonous snakes.

Key To The Identification

1. Top of head covered with small irregularly arranged scales (fig 4) ....
   Trimeresurus 2
   — Top of head covered with symmetrically arranged scales (fig 5) 8
2. Scales on top of the head, between the eyes, strongly keeled; green with small red and white spots (young), black spotted and banded with green and yellow (adult) (fig 6) *Trimeresurus wagleri*
   — Scales between the eyes, smooth or bluntly keeled; colour green, brown or blackish 3
3. Body wholly or predominantly green 4
   — Body predominantly brown or blackish 6
4. Without markings, green above, pale green below, head coloured as the body; tail red, entirely or towards the tip (adult); a white stripe bordered below with red, along the lowest row of dorsals (young) (fig 7) ....
   Trimeresurus popeiorum
   — Without markings 5
5. Head green with a pale streak behind the eye; a white line running along the lowest two rows of dorsals bordering below with the same shade of green as the body (fig 8) .... *Trimeresurus sumatranus*
   — Head green with a pinkish streak behind the eye; a white line running along the lowest two rows of dorsals bordered by a dark line or series of dark spots (fig 9) .... *Trimeresurus hageni*

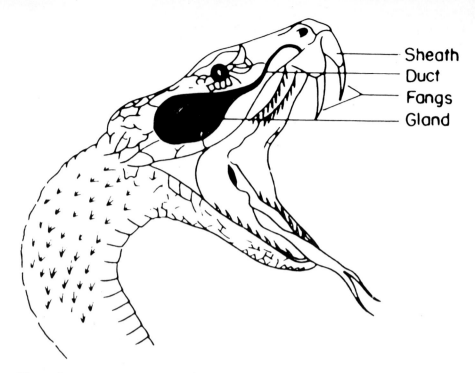

Figure 1
Illustrated drawing of head of viper showing poison gland & fang.

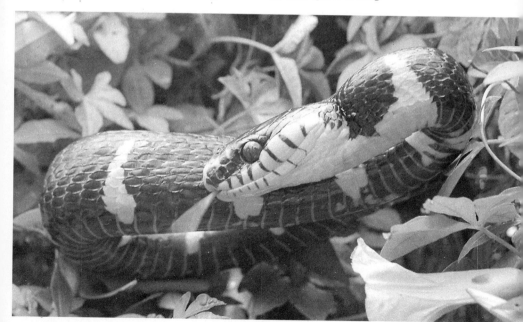

Figure 2
Boiga dendrophila.

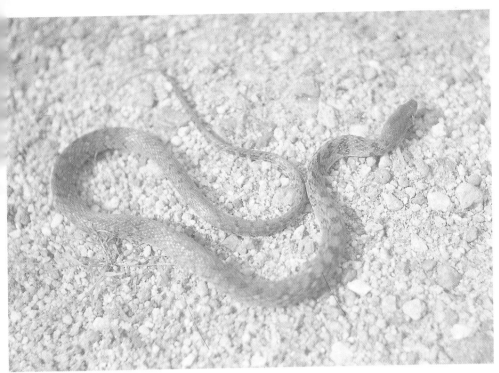

Figure 3
Rhabdophis subminiatus.

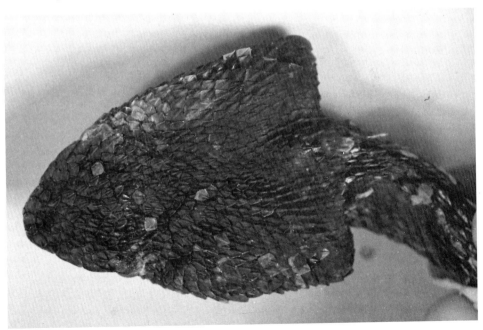

Figure 4
Viper head showing head with irregularly arranged scales.

6. Snout projected and flat (fig 10) .... *Trimeresurus puniceus*
   — Snout not flatly projected 7
7. Body brown with a series of large square black spots along each side of the back (fig 11) .... *Trimeresurus monticola*
   — Body light brown or yellowish, with darkish markings on the back (fig 12) .... *Trimeresurus purpureomaculatus*
8. Side of head with a pit between the eye and nostril (fig 13 & 14) .... *Calloselasma rhodostoma*
   — Side of head without a pit between the eye and nostril 9
9. Third upper labial large, and touching both the eye and nostril (fig 15) 10
   — Third upper labial normal, and not touching both the eye and nostril (fig 16) 11
10. A pair of occipital shields in contact with each other behind the parietals (fig 17 & 18) .... *Ophiophagus hannah*
    — No occipital shield behind the parietals (fig 19) .... *Naja naja*
11. Subcaudals of underside of tail, single anteriorly and paired posteriorly (fig 20), or wholly single throughout (fig 21) 12
    — Subcaudals of underside of tail paired throughout (fig 22) 14
12. Subcaudals single behind the anus, paired posteriorly; body is bluish black with the head, neck and tail bright red (fig 23) .... *Bungarus flaviceps*
    — Subcaudals single throughout 13
13. Body is banded with alternate black and white bands; the black bands encircling the body; tail with blunt end (fig 24) .... *Bungarus fasciatus*
    — Body is banded with alternate black and white bands; the black bands confined to back and sides; tail tapering to a point (fig 25) .... *Bungarus candidus*
14. Body brightly coloured with a series of blackish spots .... *Callophis* 15
    — Body brightly coloured with bold longitudinal coloured stripes *Maticora* 16
15. Belly is banded with black and white patterns (fig 26) .... *Callophis gracilis*
    — Belly is uniformly red (fig 27) .... *Callophis maculiceps*
16. Body is dark blue or bluish black with a pale blue band on each side. Belly, head and tail are red (fig 28) .... *Maticora bivirgata*
    — Body is striped with red and orange stripes enclosed between two black lines and white stripes below each side. Belly is banded with alternate black and white pattern (fig 29) .... *Maticora intestinalis*

Family: Viperidae

This is a very distinct group of snakes whose most obvious feature distinguishing them from all other snakes, is the triangular-shaped head with a pit situated between the eye and the nostril (fig 13), and have long poison fangs (fig 1). The pit according to Tweedie and Reid (1956) acts as a thermosensitive organ, capable of detecting radiant heat in minute amounts, and is probably used by the snakes for locating warm-blooded prey. The family consists of two genera, *Agkistrodon* with a single species, and *Trimeresurus* with seven species.

Marbled Pit Viper (fig 14)
Malay name: Ular Kapak bodoh
Calloselasma rhodostoma (Boie)

Description:

The Marbled or Malayan Pit Viper is reddish or purplish brown in colour with a series of large brown triangular spots on each side of the back. The head is dark brown above with a lighter patch on the nape and on each side a pinkish brown streak running from the eye to the corner of the mouth. The belly is uniformly pinkish or purplish. It grows to about 0.6 — 1 m long.

Occurrence:

In Malaysia, this viper is found very commonly in the northern states of Kedah and Perlis in Peninsular Malaysia only. It occurs also in Continental Asia, Java and southern Sumatra. It is a terrestrial form found in lowland forest and cultivated areas, such as rubber estates and rice fields mainly during harvesting periods. This species is largely nocturnal, but also active diurnally. It is oviparous and guards the eggs until the young are hatched.

Disposition and venom:

This viper may not appear to be aggressive, but will strike and bite readily if disturbed. The venom of this snake contains a substance that promotes defibrination of the blood which prevents clotting for a period of a week or more following the bite. Reid & Chan (1968) found that the anti-coagulant in the venom of this snake might be separated and used as a specific agent against thrombosis (Arvin).

Temple Pit Viper (fig 6)
Malay name: Ular Kapak tokong
Trimeresurus wagleri (Boie)

Description:

The Temple or Wagler's Pit Viper is green with the scale black-edged and with yellow crossbands on the back. The belly is yellowish. Young green with regularly spaced spots, each of which is partly white, partly red running along the length of the body. The snake grows to about 1 — 1.3 m long.

Occurrence:

This species is widely distributed throughout Malaysia. It occurs also in Sumatra and Kalimantan of Indonesia. It is arboreal, found in lowland forest up to 600 m elevation. It is largely nocturnal.

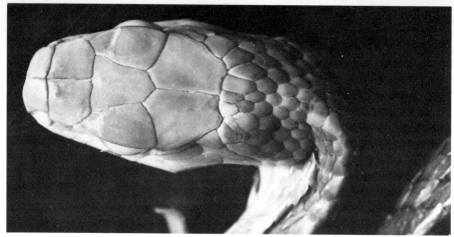

Figure 5
Head with symmetrically arranged scales.

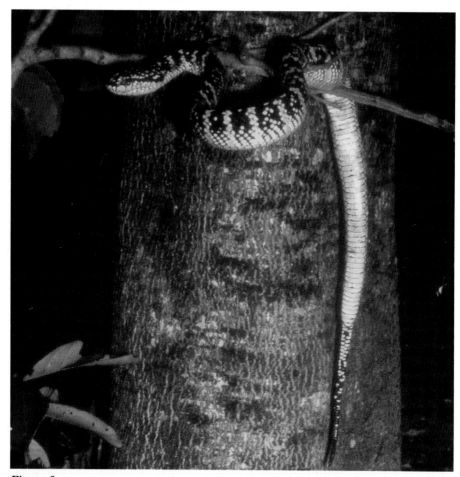

Figure 6
Trimeresurus wagleri.

Disposition and venom:

During the day this snake is sluggish and docile. Nothing is known of its venom, but a bite from it may cause quite severe pain and swelling. It is viviparous. One captive specimen gave birth to 41 young. This snake is commonly exhibited in the Snake Temple of Penang, Malaysia.

Pope's Pit Viper (fig 7)
Malay name: Ular kapak ekor merah
Trimeresurus popeiorum Smith

Description:

The Pope's Pit Viper or Red-tailed Pit Viper is uniformly green with a reddish tail. Young has a white stripe running along the lowest row of dorsals bordered below with red. It grows to about 1 m long.

Occurrence:

In Malaysia, this viper is confined to montane forest above 1,000 m throughout the country. It occurs also in Sumatra and Kalimantan of Indonesia. It is largely nocturnal.

Disposition and venom:

This viper is semi-arboreal, seen climbing in low bushes nearby forest streams. It is viviparous. Nothing is known of its venom, but there is no report of snake bite by this snake.

Sumatran Pit Viper (fig 8)
Malay name: Ular Kapak sumatra
Trimeresurus sumatranus (Raffles)

Description:

The Sumatran Pit Viper is bright green with dark crossbands at intervals of 4 to 5 scales along the body. A white line running along the lowest two rows of dorsals bordered below with the same shade of green as the body; tail green with brown spots, wholly brown in posterior half. The belly is yellowish green. It is the largest of the Malaysian Pit Vipers, growing to about 1.6 m long.

Occurrence:

In Malaysia this species is widely distributed in lowland forest. It occurs also in Sumatra and Kalimantan of Indonesia. It is largely nocturnal.

Disposition and venom:

This viper is arboreal, confining to the lower canopy of the forest. In Sabah, it is also found in cocoa and pepper plantations adjacent to fringes of the forest. It is very aggressive and will strike at the slightest of movements. Reports

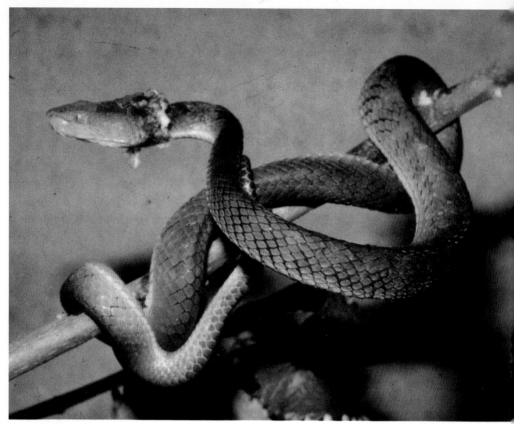

Figure 7
Trimeresurus popeiorum.

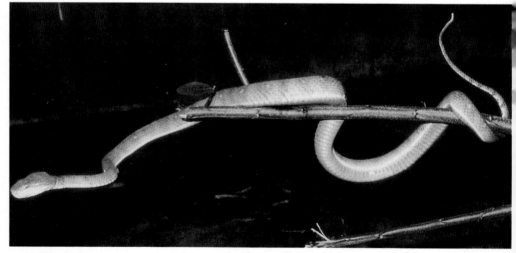

Figure 8
Trimeresurus sumatranus.

of snake bites by this snake is quite dangerous causing very severe pain and swelling, however, nothing is known of is venom.

Hagen's Pit Viper (fig 9)
Malay name: Ular Kapak hijau
Trimeresurus hageni (Lidth de Jeude)

Description:

This viper is green, the scales narrowly edged with black, the latter does not form crossbands. A row of rather widely spaced pinkish spots on each side of the back. A white line running along the lowest two rows of dorsal, bordered below by a dark line or series of dark spots. Head with a pink streak behind the eye. Tail green banded with pinkish bands and entirely pinkish posteriorly. In the past, this snake is confused with that of the Sumatran Pit Viper, but the colour pattern affords more reliable separation characters (Grandison 1972). Adult specimen measures averagely 1.1 m long.

Occurrence:

This viper is distributed throughout Peninsular Malaysia and is common in lowland forest in inland localities. It occurs also in Sumatra.

Disposition and venom:

It is an arboreal snake usually found in the lower canopy of the forest. An aggressive snake which attacks readily, but there is no report of snake bite by this snake. Nothing is known of its venom.

Flat-nosed Pit Viper (fig 10)
Malay name: Ular Kapak hidong pipeh
Trimeresurus puniceus (Boie)

Description:

The Flat-nosed Pit Viper is light brown with darker markings on the body. A light dark-edged streak behind each eye. Tail and lower surface mottled brown, darker than the upper surface. It grows to about 1 m long.

Occurrence:

In Malaysia, this snake is more restricted in its distribution confining to lowland forest. It occurs also in Kalimantan, Sumatra and Java of Indonesia. It is the rarest of the *Trimeresurus* spp. So far only a few records of this species is noted by Grandison (1972) and by Lim (1964).

Disposition and venom:

It is strictly an arboreal snake and is usually found as high as 20 m above ground level in primary forest. A captive specimen lived for 7 years and fed on rats, birds and lizards. It is a very sluggish snake. There is no report of snake bite by this snake and nothing is known of its venom.

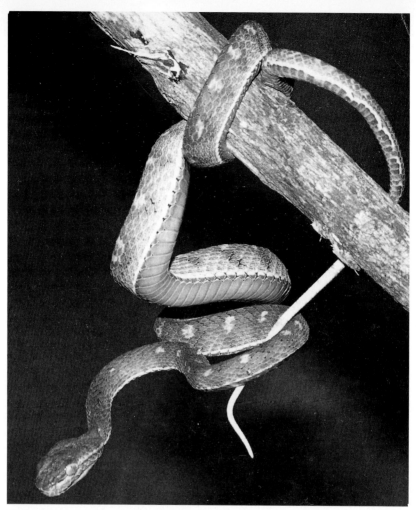

Figure 9
Trimeresurus hageni.

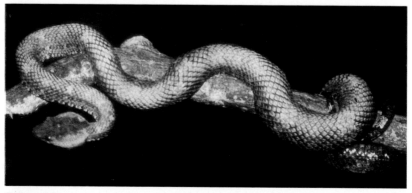

Figure 10
Trimeresurus puniceus.

396

Mountain Pit Viper (fig 11)
Malay name: Ular Kapak gunung
Trimeresurus monticola Gunther

Description:

The Mountain Pit Viper is brown in colour with rows of large, square-shaped spots on the body. The head is dark brown and the belly brownish. Tail coloured as the body. It grows to about 0.6 — 1 m long.

Occurrence:

This species is restricted to montane forest above 1,000 m in Peninsular Malaysia. It also occurs in Continental Asia.

Disposition and venom:

It is semi-arboreal, but more commonly found on the forest floor near stream areas. It is one of the exception among the *Trimeresurus* spp. that is oviparous instead of producing its young alive. A captive specimen lived for more than 8 years and fed on rats, lizards and rats. There is no report of snake bite by this species and nothing is known of its venom.

Shore Pit Viper (fig 12)
Malay name: Ular Kapak bakau
Trimeresurus purpureomaculatus (Gray)

Description:

The Mangrove or Shore Pit Viper is purplish brown or yellowish-brown, sometimes with a white line along each side of the body. The belly is brown and the head is the same colour as the body. It grows to about 1 m long.

Occurrence:

This species is widely distributed along the coastal regions in mangrove and swampy forests in Peninsular Malaysia. It also occurs in Continental Asia and in Sumatra of Indonesia.

Disposition and venom:

It is quite an aggressive snake and bites from this species are common. The bite causes very severe local symptoms accompanied by dizziness and nausea, with recovery after about ten days (Frith 1975). Venom of this snake is known to be quite potent. An arboreal snake which stays on the lower canopy of the forest.

Family: Elapidae

The only obvious character distinguishing this family of snakes from the other non-poisonous land snakes is the presence of the enlarged poison fangs at the front of each upper jaw. The family includes a large proportion of the

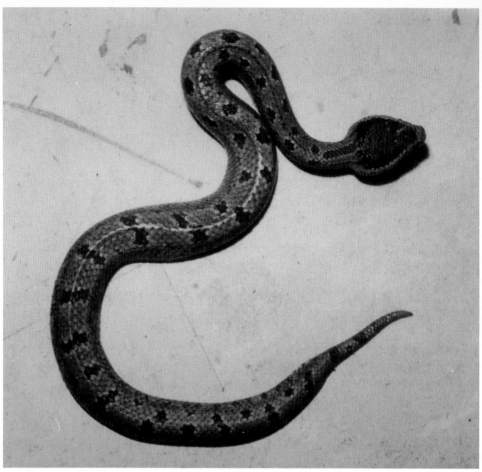

Figure 11
Trimeresurus monticola.

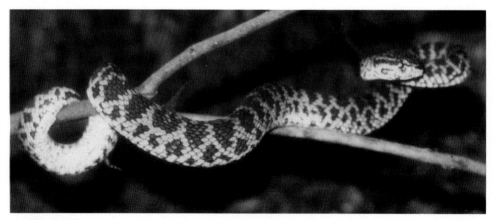

Figure 12
Trimeresurus purpureomaculatus.

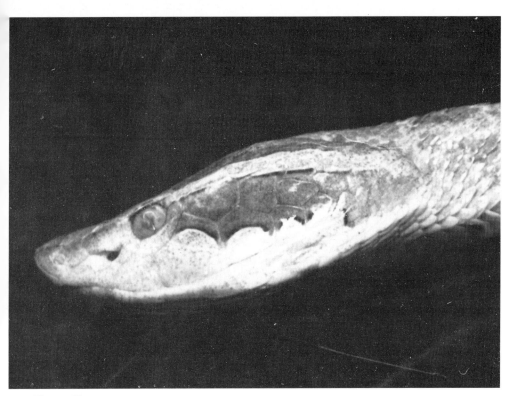

Figure 13
Head of *Ancistrodon rhodostoma* showing a nasal pit.

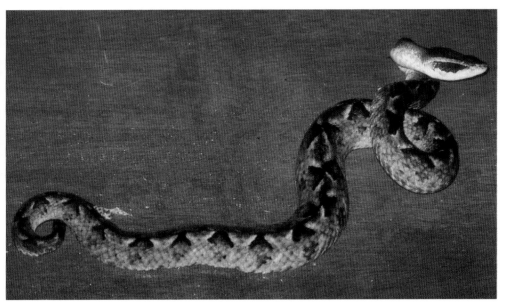

Figure 14
Calloselasma rhodostoma.

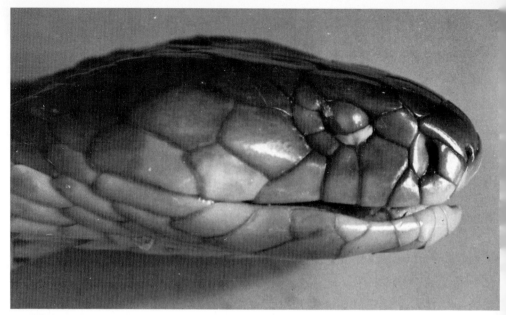

Figure 15
King Cobra's head showing the enlarged third upper labial.

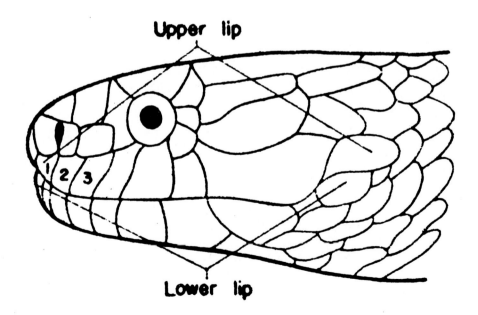

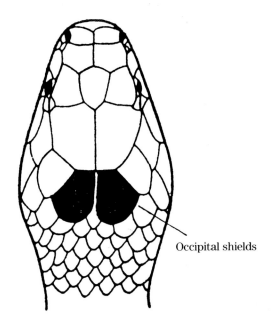

Figure 17
Illustrated drawing showing the occipital shield of King Cobra.

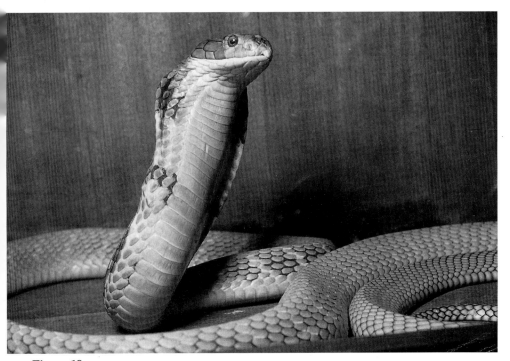

Figure 18
Ophiophagus hannah.

world's venomous snakes and all the really dangerous land snakes found in Malaysia belong to this family. In Malaysia, the elapid snakes consist of five genera represented by nine species. These are the cobras, kraits and the coral snakes.

King Cobra or Hamadryad (fig 18)
Malay name: Ular Tedung Selar
Ophiophagus hannah (Cantor)

Description:

The King Cobra is uniformly brown above, the scales dark-edged especially on the tail and hind part of the body. Head coloured as the body, belly greyish brown. Young is black with narrow white and yellow cross-bars and the belly is whitish. The King Cobra is the largest poisonous snake in the world and may exceed 6 m long.

Occurrence:

The King Cobra is widely distributed throughout Malaysia in forests and invades fields adjacent to human habitations. It also occurs in Continental Asia, Kalimantan, Sumatra and Java of Indonesia.

Disposition and venom:

The King Cobra is strictly a terrestrial snake. It is largely nocturnal but also active in the day. When confronted accidentally, it stands up with its expanded hood as high as 1.8 m. In forests, this snake is seen near forest streams. It is not an aggressive snake as otherwise believed. The bite is usually severe and is likely to be rapidly fatal (Tweedie & Reid 1956; Lim & Bakar 1970). The venom is highly potent.

The Common Cobra (fig 19)
Malay name: Ular sendok
Naja naja (Linnaeus)

Descriptions:

The Common Cobra is black with bluish grey belly. There are some markings on the throat. Like the King Cobra, the most distinguishing feature is the spreading of the hood and its hissing sound when confronted. In Malaysia two forms are present. In northern part of Malaysia the non-spitting form *(N. naja kaouthia* is abundant. In other parts of the country the spitting form *(N. naja sputatrix)* is common. It grows to about 1.3 — 1.6 m long.

Occurrence:

Naja naja sputatrix is widely distributed and *N. naja kaouthia* is more confined to the northern parts of Malaysia. They are found in all kinds of habitats, from forests to fields and human surroundings. It also occurs in Continental Asia, Kalimantan, Sumatra and Java of Indonesia.

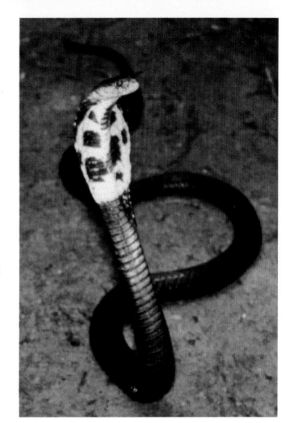

Figure 19
Naja naja sputatrix.

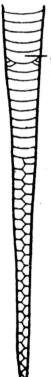

Anus
entire

Figure 20
Illustration showing subcaudals of underside of tail,
single anteriorly and double posteriorly.

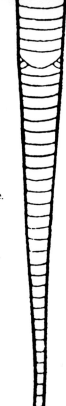

Figure 21
Illustration showing subcaudals of underside of tail, wholly single.

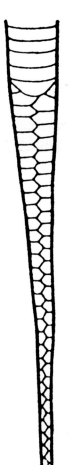

Figure 22
Illustration showing subcaudals of underside of tail, wholly double.

Disposition and venom:

The cobra is not an aggressive snake and will nearly always avoid encounters with humans by making for cover. *N. naja sputatrix* spits venom when provoked and if the venom comes in contact with an open wound or the eye, it can be very dangerous and may cause permanent injury. The venom of the cobra is very potent. Death due to the bite of this cobra, which depends on the volume of the venom injected, varies from 2 to 48 hours. An average cobra can secrete enough venom to kill 15 persons.

Both the Common and King Cobra are oviparous. The eggs, from 20 to 40 in number, are guarded by the female usually. Brooding females of these snakes are more dangerous than the males.

Red-headed Krait (fig 23)
Malay name: Ular Katang kepala merah
Bungarus flaviceps (Reinhardt)

Description:

The Red-headed Krait is blue black with the head, neck and tail bright red. Young with white stripe along the lowest dorsals on each side and a vertebral row of white dots. Belly is black. It grows to about 1.6 m long.

Occurrence:

It is distributed throughout Malaysia, confined to forested habitats. Most specimens were found in mountain or foothill forests, but one was recovered from sea level near the coast of Perak (Tweedie 1983). It also occurs in Continental Asia and Kalimantan, Sumatra and Java of Indonesia.

Disposition and venom:

It is nocturnal and strictly terrestrial. A slow moving snake, but when provoked, raises its red head and wags its tail slowly. It is the rarest of the Kraits and is oviparous. There is no report of snakebite by this species, and nothing is known of its venom.

Banded Krait (fig 24)
Malay name: Ular Katong belang
Bungarus fasciatus Schneider

Description:

The Banded Krait is marked with alternate black and pale yellow or white crossbands. The black bands are complete and encircle the body. The tip of the tail is peculiar in being blunt, not tapering to a point. The belly is coloured as the body. It grows to about 1.6 m long.

Occurrence:

It is well distributed throughout Malaysia in lowland forest, and is very

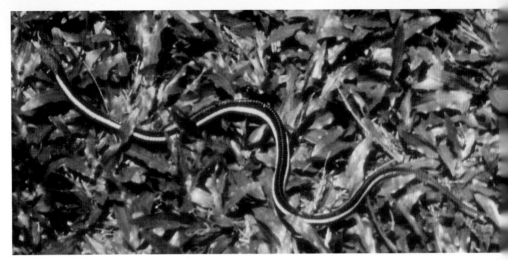

Figure 23
Bungarus flaviceps.

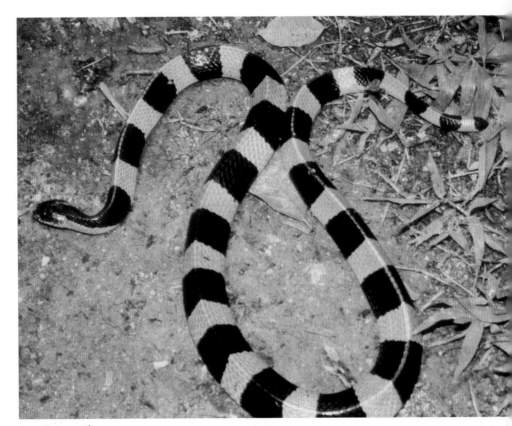

Figure 24
Bungarus fasciatus.

common in the northern parts along the coastal regions and also in human habitations in Peninsular Malaysia. It also occurs in Continental Asia and Kalimantan, Sumatra and Java of Indonesia.

Disposition and venom:

It is nocturnal, a very slow moving snake and extremely inoffensive in disposition, flinching convulsively and hiding its head in its coil if molested. Snake bites by this snake is fairly common. It is a highly venomous and deadly snake, its venom being estimated to be 16 times as powerful as that of the cobra (Gharpurey 1935).

Malayan Krait (fig 25)
Malay name: Ular Katang tebu
Bungarus candidus Linnaeus

Description:

The Malayan Krait is black with white crossbands on the body and tail. The black bands do not encircle the body but stop at the flanks. The white bands are speckled with brownish spots. The tail tapers to a point. It grows to 1.6 m long.

Occurrence:

This snake is well distributed throughout Malaysia in lowland forest, and seldom found in human habitations. It is not as common as the Banded Krait. It also occurs in Continental Asia, and Sumatra and Java of Indonesia.

Disposition and venom:

It is nocturnal, and a very timid snake. It avoids moving about in daytime. It becomes active at dusk and goes about at night in search of food. Very few snake bite cases by this snake have been reported. The signs and symptoms in krait poisoning are similar to those of cobras. The venom of this krait was shown to be as virulent as that of the cobra (Lim & Abu Bakar 1970).

Spotted Coral Snake (fig 26)
Malay name: Ular Pantai bintik
Callophis gracilis Gray

Description:

The Spotted Coral snake is brown, the scales dark-edged. A black vertebral stripe at the body which connects a series of small spots. At each side of the body there are large black spots alternating in position with smaller ones. A dark streak runs from the mouth back through the eye. The belly is banded with alternate black and white. It grows to over 30 cm long.

Occurrence:

This snake is found in foothill country up to 900 m in Peninsular Malaysia, but is nowhere common. It also occurs in Sumatra of Indonesia.

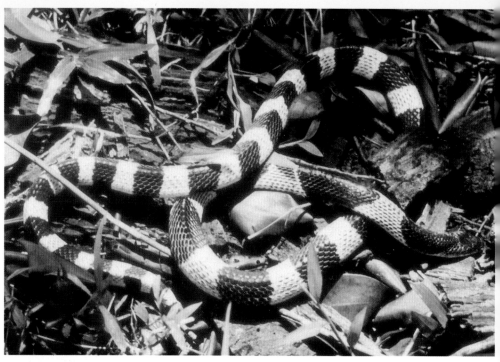

Figure 25
Bungarus candidus.

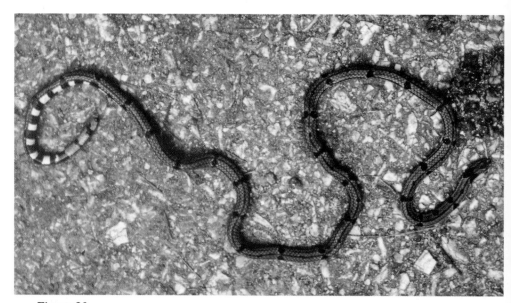

Figure 26
Callophis gracilis.

Disposition and venom:

It is oviparous, a very sluggish snake and extremely inoffensive. Captive specimens lived for more than 2 years, fed on smaller snakes, lizards and small skinks. Nothing is known of its venom.

Small Spotted Coral Snake (fig 27)
Malay name: Ular Pantai bintik kechil
Callophis maculiceps (Gunther)

Description:

This snake is light brown, either with small black spots longitudinally arranged along each side of the back or with a black vertebral stripe and no spots. The head and nape are black with yellow markings. Tail with two black rings, one on the base and the other near the tip. The belly is red. It grows to about 30 cm long.

Occurrence:

It is only recorded in the northern part of Peninsular Malaysia and one from the Langkawi island (Lim & Mohd Sharef 1975). It is uncommon. It also occurs in Sumatra of Indonesia.

Disposition and venom:

It is strictly a terrestrial form. The specimen from Langkawi island was found in rocky places near a forest stream. Nothing is known of its habit, and also its venom.

Blue Malaysian Coral Snake (fig 28)
Malay name: Ular Pantai biru biru
Maticora bivirgata (Boie)

Description:

The Blue Malaysian Coral Snake is dark blue-black with pale bluish stripe on each side of the body. The head, tail and belly are bright red. It is the largest of the coral snakes growing to about 1.5 m long.

Occurrence:

This snake is widely distributed throughout Malaysia, in lowland and hill forests. It also occurs in Kalimantan, Sumatra and Java of Indonesia.

Disposition and venom:

It is nocturnal and a slow moving snake. A strictly ground-dwelling form and found near forest streams. Captive specimens fed on lizards and other small snakes. There was a reported case of a child bitten by this snake who died few hours after the bite. Although nothing is known about its venom, the death

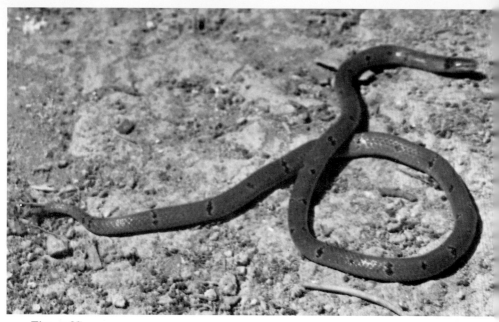

Figure 27
Callophis maculiceps.

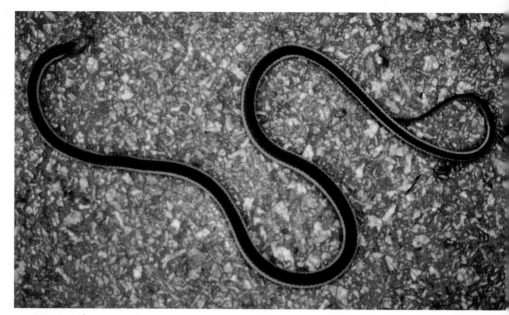

Figure 28
Maticora bivirgata.

410

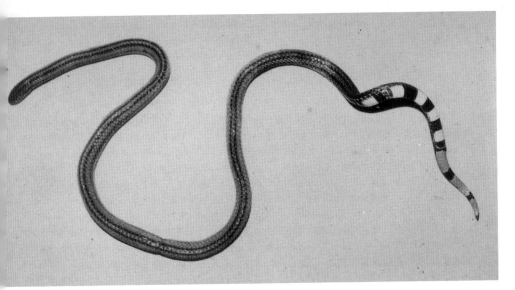

Figure 29
Maticora intestinalis.

of the child due to the bite (Harrison 1957) indicates that the venom is very potent.

Banded Coral Snake (fig 29)
Malay name: Ular Pantai belang
Maticora intestinalis (Laurenti)

Description:

The Banded Coral Snake is brown with various black, orange and white stripes on the body. The belly is banded with alternate black and white. Head brown and the tip of the tail reddish. It grows to about 30 cm long.

Occurrence:

The snake is common throughout Malaysia. It is found in a wide variety of habitats, ranging from forest to surroundings of human habitations. It also occurs in Kalimantan, Sumatra and Java of Indonesia.

Disposition and venom:

It is nocturnal. During the day when this snake is molested, it makes no attempt to escape, but will often raise its tail, displaying the bright red underside, and will writhe and tumble about turning the conspicuously barred belly uppermost, a clear case of aposematic behaviour. In a case report of a bite by this snake, the victim suffered local pain and swelling followed by giddiness and acute difficulty in breathing, and also vomiting and intestinal disturbance (Jacobson 1937).

All coral snakes are very slenderly built with very tiny mouths, probably too small to inflict an effective bite, but the few reports of snake bites by some species of this group indicate that their venom are quite potent.

Ecology of Venomous Land Snakes in Malaysia

During the period from 1948 to 1977, about 4,500 land snakes including each of the venomous species, were examined. Data on locality, habitat and food content where these snakes came from, were recorded. Some information on food habits and ecological niches of venomous snakes were reported previously by Lim (1982) and Tweedie (1983). Based on the author's personal observation, information on habitat and food habit of the land venomous snakes are presented in Tables 1 & 2.

In general, most snake species are forest dwellers. Deforestation of the primary habitats, to some extent, influenced the migration of these snakes to alternative environments. During this process, some snakes adapt well to their new habitat niches while those of the highly specialised either perished or dwindled in numbers. Agriculture development patterns by increasing monoculture practices, such as oil palm, rubber, ricefield, cocoa, orchards, etc. have been associated with parallel increments in the number of animal species which are food resources of most snake species, thus food source is another important factor in the perpetuation of snake species in their new environments.

Habitat diversification of the elapid snakes (Table 1) shows that the two cobra species have adapted well to different environments, but the Common Cobra appears to be more versatile to a wide range of habitats than that of the King Cobra. Among the three Krait species, both the Banded and the Malayan Kraits, like the Common Cobra, are found also equally adaptable to different environments, while the Red-headed Krait is shown to be habitat specific. All the Coral snake species with the exception of the Banded Coral Snake are able to conform to environmental changes.

The viperid snakes are found to be less versatile than most members of the elapid snakes (Table 1). Among the eight viper species, the Marbled or Malayan Pit Viper, is the only one that adapts well outside forest environments. The rest of the seven species are shown to be fairly habitat specific.

Snakes are very specialised feeders. Their prey is associated with the type of habitat the snakes frequent in relation to their behavioral patterns. For example, arboreal snakes tend to feed on prey which is semi-arboreal in habits, while terrestrial snakes prey usually on ground dwelling animals. Observations on the food habits of most of the venomous land snakes are presented in Table 2.

The elapid snakes are mainly terrestrial. All but the Common Cobra were found to feed on snakes, lizards and frogs. The Common Cobra was found to feed mainly on rats with frogs being occasional prey. The viperid snakes, on the other hand, are semi-arboreal with few being strictly arboreal. They appear to be more variable in their food habits. They were found to take not only warm-

TABLE 1
Distribution of Venomous Land Snakes in various habitats

	Primary forest	Secondary forest	Mangrove forest	Scrub	Fields*	Ricefield	Rubber estate	Oilpalm estate	Human+ habitat
ELAPIDAE									
Ophiophagus hannah	XX	XX	–	X	X	–	X	XX	–
Naja naja	XXX	XX	XX	XX	XX	XX	XXX	XXX	XX
Bangarus candidus	XX	X	X	X	X	X	X	X	X
Bangarus fasciatus	X	X	XXX	X	X	X	XX	X	XX
Bangarus flaviceps	X	–	–	–	–	–	–	–	–
Callophis gracilis	XX	X	–	–	–	–	–	–	–
Callophis maculiceps	X	–	–	–	–	–	–	–	–
Maticora intestinalis	XXX	XX	X	X	X	X	X	X	XX
Maticora bivirgata	XX	X	–	–	–	–	–	–	–
VIPERIDAE									
Agkistrodon rhodostoma	X	X	–	–	–	XX	XXX	–	–
Trimeresurus wagleri	XXX	XX	X	–	–	–	–	–	–
Trimeresurus popeiorum	XX	–	–	–	–	–	–	–	–
Trimeresurus sumatranus	XXX	XX	X	–	–	–	–	–	–
Trimeresurus hageni	XX	–	–	–	–	–	–	–	–
Trimeresurus puniceus	XX	–	–	–	–	–	–	–	–
Trimeresurus monticola	XX	–	–	–	–	–	–	–	–
Trimeresurus purpureomaculatus	–	–	XXX	–	–	–	–	–	–

- not observed

* Field includes lalland fields (Imperata cylindrica) and backyard gardens

+ Human habitations are places like towns, villages and farming villages

XXX very common

XX common

X rare

TABLE 2
Food habits of Venomous Land Snakes (Based on stomach contents)

| | Small mammals | | | | Reptiles | | Amphibians | | Birds | Fish |
	Ground rat	Tree mice/rat	Tree squirrel	Ground shrew	Snakes	Lizards	Ground frogs	Tree frogs		
ELAPIDAE										
Ophiophagus hannah	–	–	–	–	+	+	–	–	–	–
Naja naja	+	–	–	–	–	–	+	–	–	–
Bangarus candidus	–	–	–	–	+	+	+	–	–	–
Bangarus fasciatus	–	–	–	–	+	+	+	–	–	+
Bangarus flaviceps	–	–	–	–	+	+	–	–	–	–
Callophis gracilis	–	–	–	–	+	+	–	–	–	–
Callophis maculiceps	–	–	–	–	–	–	–	–	–	–
Maticora intestinalis	–	–	–	–	+	+	–	–	–	–
Maticora bivirgata	–	–	–	–	+	+	+	–	–	–
VIPERIDAE										
Agkistrodon rhodostoma	+	–	–	–	–	+	+	–	–	–
Trimeresurus wagleri	+	+	+	–	–	–	+	+	+	–
Trimeresurus popeiorum	+	–	–	–	–	+	+	+	–	–
Trimeresurus sumatranus	+	+	–	–	–	–	–	+	–	–
Trimeresurus hageni	+	+	–	–	–	–	–	–	–	–
Trimeresurus puniceus	+	+	–	–	–	–	–	–	+	–
Trimeresurus monticola	+	–	–	+	–	+	+	–	+	–
Trimeresurus purpureomaculatus	+	+	–	–	–	–	–	+	+	–

– not observed

+ content identified

414

blooded vertebrates, ie. rats, mice, squirrels, ground shrews and birds, but also cold-blooded vertebrates, like lizards and frogs.

Cannibalism among the elapid snakes appears to be common. This has been found in Kraits, Coral snakes and King Cobras (Lim, 1956; 1960), but has not been observed in viperid snakes.

Snake bite cases are directly associated with the environments and the degree of contact between man and snake. Among the elapid snakes, the Common Cobra and the Banded Krait are the two most dangerous species because of their close association with human surroundings. In northern Peninsular Malaysia, the non-spitting cobra *(N. naja kaouthia)* is the main cause of cobra bites, while in other parts of Malaysia, the spitting cobra *(N. naja sputatrix)* is the main cause. The bites of the King Cobra though relatively few in number, were the most lethal because of the high human toll sustained (Lim, 1982). The absence of specific reports of snake bite by other elapid snakes could be due to lack of information and probably also due to misidentification of the snake species when such bites occur, for example differentiation between the Banded and the Malayan Krait.

Among the viperid snakes, the Marbled Pit Viper is the most dangerous, causing the majority of the snake bites in northern parts of Peninsular Malaysia and again, this is due to the close association of this snake with human habitation. Among the *Trimeresurus*, *T. purpureomaculatus* is one that causes more bites than other *Trimeresurus* species, because this snake is very common in mangrove forests which are frequented by woodcutters. In the forests and plantations, *T. sumatranus* is another viper that must be considered dangerous because it is the most aggressive among the viper species, and in East Malaysia, snake bites due to this snake in plantations is quite common. Most of the other viper species are sluggish and inoffensive. Nevertheless, they are all venomous snakes, although their bites seldom kill, but if inflicted, they can cause severe injury. It is therefore important to be cautious of them. Snakes, whether venomous or not, like all other animals, vary individually in temperament, and some snakes are bound to be bolder than others.

The venom of the elapids, like the King Cobra, Common Cobra and various species of kraits are well documented except the Red-headed Krait. Nothing is known about the venom of the four species of coral snakes. Similarly, little is known of the venom of most of the viper species. With the exception of the *A. rhodostoma* venom which had been well studied, the potency of venoms of each of the remaining seven species has yet to be determined, although Tweedie (1983) stated that poisoning through bites by *T. wagleri* and *T. purpureomaculatus* was trivial in virtually all cases examined. Thus the potency of venoms of most of the viperid and some of the elapid snakes opens a field for further investigations.

Snakes bite incidence from 1960 to 1983 (Lim, 1987) have shown to be on the increase since the first report in 1958/1959 by Reid et al (1963). The yearly average snake bite cases was about 6,600 from 1980 to 1983 (Lim, 1987). Of these, 18.4% were due to venomous snake bites by land and sea snakes, and only

0.1% fatality was caused by snake bite envenomation. The results showed that among snake bite cases, only about a quarter will develop serious generalised envenomation, and although deaths, do occur, they are rare. Farmers, rubber tappers and woodcutters are the main victims of venomous land snake bites and fishermen of sea snake bites. Most bites occur in the daytime and on the foot or ankle and hands because the victim either treads on or near the snake. Male victims are in the higher risk group and the age group that is prone to snake bites falls on the most active group in the population structure (Lim, 1987). It is evident from these records, that snake bites by venomous land snakes continue to be a public hazard in Malaysia.

Summary

In Malaysia, poisonous land snakes comprise 17 species out of 105 land snake species, excluding freshwater and sea snakes. They belong to two families, the Elapidae and the Viperidae. The elapids consist of five genera represented by two cobras, three kraits and four coral snakes, and the viperids with two genera of eight species. All these snakes are brightly coloured, and a key to the identification, based on colour patterns, was constructed and followed by a detailed description of each of the 17 species.

Habitat distribution of these snakes, showed that among the elapids, the Common Cobra, King Cobra, Banded Krait and the Malayan Krait are well adaptable to different environments with the Common Cobra and the Banded Krait more versatile in their adaptability than the other two species. All the Coral snakes are rather habitat specific. All viperids, except the Marbled or Malayan Pit Viper, were found to be more habitat restricted. The latter was found to adapt itself fairly well to different habitats.

Food habits of these snakes revealed that all elapids with the exception of the Common Cobra that feeds mainly on rats, prefer other snakes and reptiles. The viperids were found to be more versatile feeders generally, and take not only warm-blooded vertebrates but also cold-blooded ones. Cannibalism among the elapid snakes were found to be common, but this has not been observed among the viperid snakes.

Venoms of some of the elapid and viperid snakes have been well established, but the potency of venoms of coral snakes and most of the vipers needs further investigation.

The prevalence of snake bite cases is influenced by the local distribution of the various species of venomous snakes, especially those that have a wider range of habitats and are commonly found near human habitations. Since the first report of snake bites in 1958/59, snake bites have been consistently on the increase in the last 2½ decades, but fortunately the fatality rate was on the decline. Despite the situation, snake bites are occupational hazards, and thus of public health importance.

References

Frith, C.B. & D.W. (1975). A case of snake bite by the shore pit viper, *Trimeresurus purpureomaculatus* (Viperidae). Nat Hist Bull Siam Soc 26:159 — 163.

Gharpurey, K.G. (1935). The snakes of India. Aryabhushan Press, Bombay. 165 pp.

Grandison, A.G.C. (1972). The Gunung Benom expedition 1967.5. Reptiles and amphibians of Gunung Benom with a description of a new species of *Macrocalamus Bull Br Mus nat Hist 23*:60 — 64.

Harrison, J.L. (1957). The bite of a Blue Malayan Coral Snake or Ular Matahari. Mal. nat. J. 11:130.

Jacobson, E. (1937). A case of snake bite *(Maticora intestinalis)*. Bull Raffles Mus. 13:77.

Lim Boo Liat (1956). The natural food of some Malayan snakes. Mal. nat. J. 10:139 —144.

Lim Boo Liat (1960). Observation on some captive snakes. Mal. nat. J. 14:181 — 187.

Lim Boo Liat (1964). Comments on some rare snakes. Fed. Mus. Journn 60 — 64.

Lim Boo Liat (1982). Poisonous snakes of Peninsular Malaysia. 2nd edition. Art Printing Works Sdn. Bhd., Kuala Lumpur 73 pp.

Lim Boo Liat (1987). Snakes of Public Health Importance. Proc of the 1st Asia-Pacific Cong on animal, plant and microbial toxins, Singapore June 24 — 27. National University of Singapore. 118 — 134.

Lim Boo Liat & Abu Bakar bin Ibrahim (1970). Bite and stings by venomous animals with special reference to snake bites in West Malaysia. Med. Journal of Malaya. 25:128 — 141.

Lim Boo Liat & Mohd Sharef bin Kararudin (1975). Notes on new locality records of some rare snakes in Peninsular Malaysia. Mal. nat J. 27:114 — 117.

Reid, H.A. & Chan, K.L. (1968). The paradox of therapeutic defrination. The Lancet. 485 — 486.

Tweedie, M.W.F. (1983). The snakes of Malaya. Singapore National Printers Pte Ltd. 3rd ed. 167 pp.

Tweedie, M.W.F. & Reid, H.A. (1956). Poisonous snakes in Malaya. Malayan Museum Popular Pamphlet Ne 11. 16 pp.

Venomous Terrestrial Snakes Of Pakistan And Snake Bite Problem

M S Khan

Herpetology Laboratory
15/6 Darul Saddar North
Rabwah 35460, Pakistan

Introduction

Pakistan is a rhomboidal strip of land stretched over an area of 803,943 km². It extends from the extreme western corner of Baluchistan, from longitude 60°52' to longitude 75°22' in the northeastern tip of Punjab; and from latitude 24° in the arid cliffs of Arabian Sea coast up to latitude 37° in the northern snowfields of Pamir.

The terrain of the country is divided into northern, northwestern highlands comprising 476, 143 km², overlooking a southeastern stretch of 327,796 km² of flat gradational surface known as the Indus Plains. The northern lofty mountains are part of the Himalayas, with moderate precipitation and mild climate. On the other hand, the northwestern hilly tracts comprise low barren hills with scanty rainfall and severe dry conditions. The southwestern part of Baluchistan is dry, desolate and a perpetual desert of rolling sand dunes. The southeastern vast plains comprise of Punjab — the upper Indus valley, cut through by five tributaries of the Indus River. It offers variable habitat conditions. Lower Indus Valley — the Sind, stretches to the sea coast. All along its east lie Cholistan and Thar deserts, while along the west, the lofty Kirthar Range of Southern Baluchistan.

Zoogeographically, Pakistan is sandwiched between Palearctic and Oriental Regions. Dominant elements of its fauna belong to these two regions, however Ethiopial elements are also present considerably, (Khan 1980). The terrain of Pakistan is subdivided into several physiographical units (Roberts, 1974; Baig, 1975) due to its complex topography, climatic conditions and vegetation, supporting entirely different species from region to region. The snake fauna of Pakistan beautifully illustrates this phenomenon. Except for widely distributed species, there are certain species which are peculiar to a region. A happy implication of this fact is that it helps in the identification of snakes of a region, especially the venomous snakes.

Checklist Of The Venomous Snakes Of Pakistan

Venomous terrestrial snakes of Pakistan belong to three families:

Elapidae	:	Cobras and Kraits
Viperidae	:	True vipers
Crotalidae	:	Pit vipers

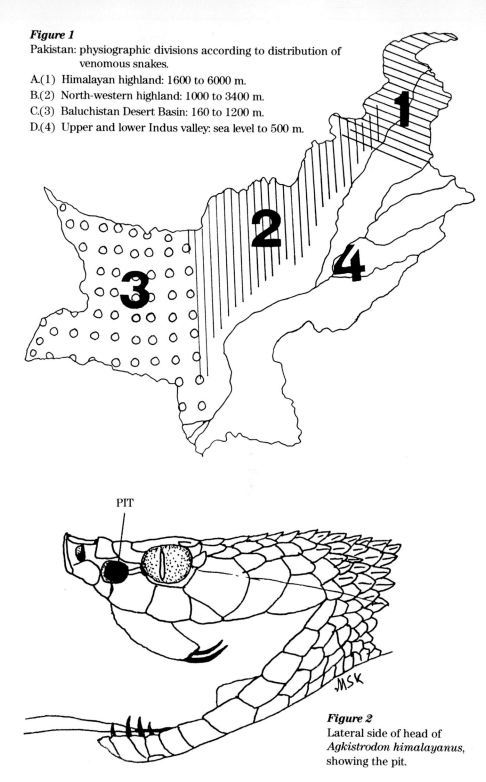

Figure 1
Pakistan: physiographic divisions according to distribution of
venomous snakes.
A.(1) Himalayan highland: 1600 to 6000 m.
B.(2) North-western highland: 1000 to 3400 m.
C.(3) Baluchistan Desert Basin: 160 to 1200 m.
D.(4) Upper and lower Indus valley: sea level to 500 m.

PIT

Figure 2
Lateral side of head of
Agkistrodon himalayanus,
showing the pit.

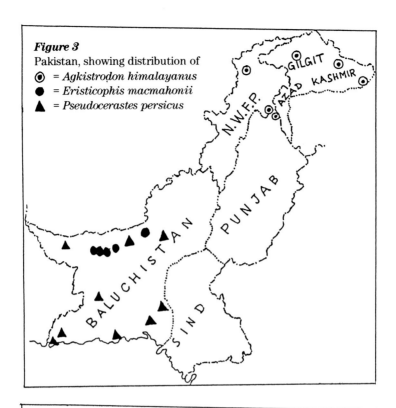

Figure 3

Pakistan, showing distribution of

⊙ = *Agkistrodon himalayanus*

● = *Eristicophis macmahonii*

▲ = *Pseudocerastes persicus*

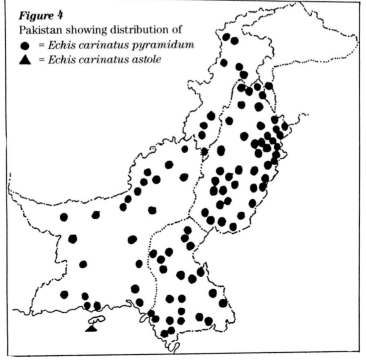

Figure 4

Pakistan showing distribution of

● = *Echis carinatus pyramidum*

▲ = *Echis carinatus astole*

While preparing this checklist, special attention is devoted to the preparation of synonymies of each recognised species to provide information in basic source material. Each species is accompanied by (1) reference to original descriptions of primary synonyms; (2) type locality; (3) distribution, world-wide and in Pakistan.

For more information, the works of considerable interest are Wall (1913); Boulenger (1890); Smith (1943); Gharpury (1962); Minton (1966); Minton et al (1968); Leviton (1967); Klemmer (1963); Deoras (1978); Harding and Welch (1980); Khan (1980, 1983); Whitaker (1982) and Golay (1985).

Family Elapidae

Bungarus caeruleus caeruleus (Schneider)

1801.   *Pseudoboa caerulea* Schneider, Hist. Amph., 2:284.
1963.   *Bungarus caeruleus caeruleus*, Klemmer, Behringwerk-Mitt., Marburg, Sonderband: 279.

Distribution :   Ceylon, Peninsular India to foothills of Himalayas, western Bengal, in Pakistan along east of Indus River, rarely extending onto the west.

Bungarus sindanus sindanus (Boulenger)

1897.   *Bungarus sindanus* Boulenger, J. Bombay Nat. Hist. Soc. 11: 73-74.
1963.   *Bungarus caeruleus sindanus*, Klemmer, Behringwerk-Mitt., Marburg, Sonderband: 279.
1985.   *Bungarus sindanus sindanus*, Khan, The Snake, 17:71-78.

Distribution :   Typical of Rajasthan, Cholistan and Thar Deserts.

Bungarus sindanus razai Khan

1913.   *Bungarus sindanus*, Pitman, J. Bombay Nat. Hist. Soc., 22:636.
1985.   *Bungarus sindanus razai* Khan, The Snake, 17:75.

Distribution :   Southern Waziristan, Dera Ismail Khan, Makerwal.

Naja naja naja (Linnaeus).

1758.   *Coluber naja* Linnaeus, Syst. Nat. 10th ed., 1:221 Type locality: India.
1943.   *Naja naja naja*, Smith, Fauna British India, 3:427 & 431.

Distribution :   Ceylon, throughout India, Bangladesh, throughout Pakistan.

Naja naja oxiana (Eichwald)

1831.   *Tomyris oxiana* Eichwald, Zool. Spec., 3:171.
       Type locality : Transcaspia.
1889.   *Naja oxiana*, Boulenger, Trans. Zool. Soc. London, 5, ser. 2:103; Pl.11, Fig.2
1907.   *Naja naja oxiana*, Stejneger, Bull. Nat. Mus. Washington, NO. 58:395.

Family Viperidae

Echis carinatus (Schneider)

1801.   *Pseudoboa carinata* Schneider, Hist. Amph., 2:285.
        Type locality: Arni, Madras, India.
1802.   *Boa horatta* Shaw, Gen. Zool., 3:359.
1803.   *Scytale bizonatus* Daudin, Hist. Nat. Rept., 5:339.
1820.   *Vipera (Echis) carinata* Merremtent. Syst. Amph. :149.
1825.   *Echis ziczac* Gray, Ann. Philos.: 205.
1837.   *Vipera echis* Schlegel, Essai Phys. Serp. 2:583.
1859.   *Vipera (Echis) superciliosa* Jan, Rev. Mag. Zool. :156.
1949.   *Echis carinatus*, Constable, Bull. Mus. Comp. Zool., Cambridge, Mass.,
        103:155.

Echis carinatus pyramidum (Geoffroy Saint-Hilaire)

1827.   *Scythale pyramidum* Geoffroy Saint-Hilaire, Descript. Egypte, Rept. :152
1949.   *Echis carinatus pyramidum*, Constable, Bull. Mus. Comp.
        Zool. Cambridge, Mass., 103:155.

Distribution :   Northern India, coastal Pakistan, Afghanistan.

Echis carinatus sochureki Stemmler

1969.   *Echis carinatus sochureki* Stemmler, Aquaterra, Bd. 6, H. 10:118-125.

Distribution :   Southern Pakistan, Afghanistan.

Echis carinatus astolae Mertens

1970.   *Echis carinatus astolae*, Mertens, Stutthg. Beit. Naturk., No. 216:3-4.

Distribution :   Island Astola, off the coast of Makran, coastal Pakistan.

Echis carinatus multisquamatus (Cherlin)

1981.   *Echis multisquamatus* Cherlin, Proc. Zool. Inst. Acad. Sciences 101:92-
        95.

Distribution   : Northwestern Baluchistan, Afghanistan.

Eristicophis macmahoni Alcock & Finn

1896.   *Eristicophis macmahoni* Alcock and Finn, Jour. Asiat.
        Soc. Bengal, 65:564.

Distribution :   Desert regions along Afghan Baluchistan border.

Vipera lebetina obtusa Dwigubskij

1832.   *Vipera obtusa* Dwigubskij, Essay Nat. Hist. Russ. Emp.:30.
        Type locality: Jelisawetpol, Transcaucasia, USSR.

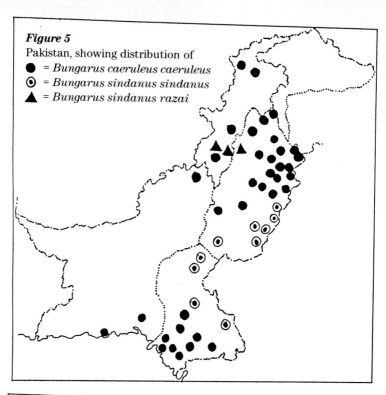

Figure 5
Pakistan, showing distribution of
● = *Bungarus caeruleus caeruleus*
◉ = *Bungarus sindanus sindanus*
▲ = *Bungarus sindanus razai*

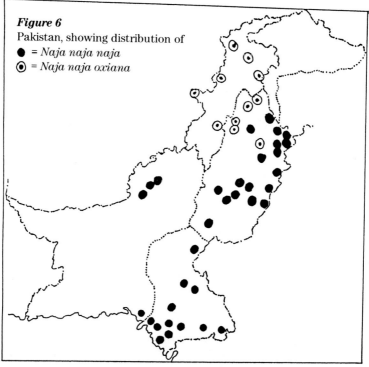

Figure 6
Pakistan, showing distribution of
● = *Naja naja naja*
◉ = *Naja naja oxiana*

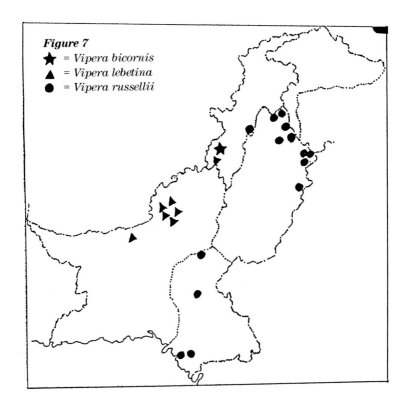

Figure 7
★ = *Vipera bicornis*
▲ = *Vipera lebetina*
● = *Vipera russellii*

1940   *Vipera lebetina obtusa*, Terentjev and Chernov, Opredel, Presmyk, Semnovod., 2nd ed. :163.

Distribution :   North and northwest highland of Pakistan, southern Afghanistan.

Vipera russelli russelli (Shaw)

1802.   *Coluber russelli* Shaw, Gen. Zool., 3:418.

Distribution :   Western Indonesia, Thailand, Taiwan, Burma, Southern Assam, Bangladesh, India, East of Indus in Pakistan.

Pseudocerastes persicus (Dumeril and Bibron)

1854.   *Cerastes persicus* Dumeril and Bibron, Erp. Gen. vii:1443.

1896.   *Pseudocerastes persicus* Boulenger, Cat. Snak. Brit. Mus. 3:501.

Distribution :   From central Asia, Afghanistan. In Pakistan it has been reported from Las Bela and Kalat.

Pseudocerastes bicornis Wall

1913.   *Pseudocerastes bicornis* Wall, Pois. Snak. Ind., :64.
         Type locality: Khajuri Kach, above Gwaleri Kolal in the Gomal pass in Waziristan.

Distribution :   Known only from its type locality.

Family Crotalidae

Agkistrodon himalayanus (Günther)

1864.   *Halys himalayanus* Günther, Rept. Brit. India: 393.
      Type locality: Garhwal, northern East Punjab, India.

Distribution :   Sikkim, Nepal, Kashmir, alpine Punjab, Chitral.

Description of Venomous Snakes of Pakistan

Differentiation of subspecies is not considered since it is of no practical importance.

Bungarus caeruleus (Figs 8 & 9)

Common name: Common krait.

Identification:

Medium sized snake with a jet black to deep blue body dorsum and a row of transverse white stripes; scales smooth, glossy; medium dorsal row of scales wider than rest; head slightly distinct from neck; eyes black small, barely visible pupil round. Average size: 70 to 80 cm.

Habitat:

This snake frequents grasslands or semidesert sandy soil. In general, it frequents suburban gardens, termite mounds, burrows of small rodents, piles of brick and rubble. *B. caeruleus* is mainly a snake of the plains but extends to an elevation of 1700 m.

Habits:

Nocturnal, becoming active quite after sunset. When alarmed, throws itself into a loose ball (Khan and Tsnim, 1986a). During day, timid and secretive.

Venom:

One of the major deadliest snakes of Pakistan. Its venom is extremely neurotoxic, including nerve paralysis, with no local signs and symptoms. Thus diagnosis of its bite is very difficult. Symptoms appear very late, resulting in death of the victim.

Distribution:

Oriental. Sri Lanka, peninsular India, to foothills, of Himalayas, Azad Kashmir, Bengal. In Pakistan, it frequents inter-riverine tracts in upper and lower Indus valley. Rarely extends along the Makran coast (Shockley, 1949), where it is extremely rare (Khan, 1980, 1983).

Naja naja (Figs 10 & 11)

Common name: Nag, Cobra.

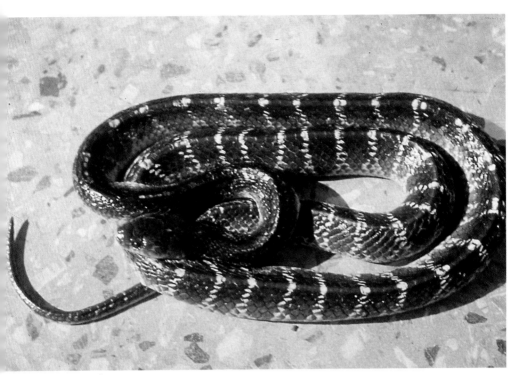

Figure 8
Bungarus caeruleus

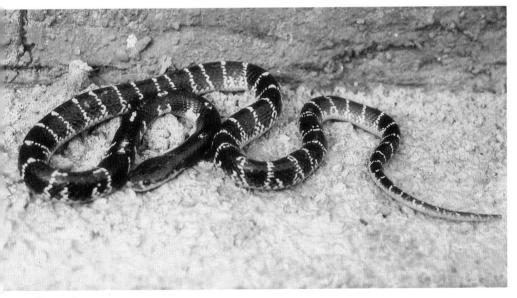

Figure 9
Bungarus caeruleus

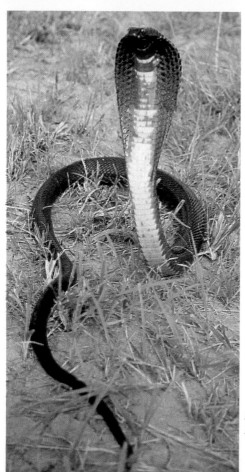

Figure 10
Naja naja naja

Figure 11
Naja naja

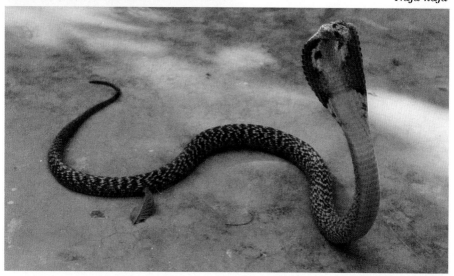

Diagnosis:

Large sized snake, with smooth scales. A hood distinguishes this snake from other snakes of the area. Third supralabial large, in contact with orbit and nasal scale; a small triangular scale between fourth and fifth supralabials — the "cuneate" often present; some of the subhood ventrals pigmented.

Body dorsum jet black, variegated to brown, a light spectacle mark on the hood dorsum may be present, and a yellow white large ocellus on its ventral side (Khan, 1984). Spectacle mark may be absent. Average length is from 1 to 2 m.

Habitat:

Naja naja frequents grassland or semidesert sandy soil. Generally frequents suburban gardens, termite mounds, burrows of small rodents, around town and villages. In sandy deserts *Naja* occurs in oases and patches of Acacia scrub. Earth dams and ruinous country are its favourite habitat.

Habit:

Nocturnal, but sometimes becoming diurnal. Cobras are shy animals and will try to avoid man, however rodents often attract them into the houses. When alarmed, anterior one-third part of body is raised above the ground, and the neck expands into a hood. It carefully surveys the surroundings, and when in danger, emits low and intermittent hisses and sways the hood slightly. However, when there is no danger, the hood is lowered and the snake escapes. When disturbed, and angry cobra strikes repeatedly, and while biting may hold on to prey or victim savagely.

Venom:

Naja venom is neurotoxic, resulting in paralysis of respiratory system and cardiac failure. Usually a less than fatal dose is injected but because of the possible fatal consequences of the bite, it must be treated promptly.

Distribution:

Oriental in distribution. In Pakistan, it is widely distributed throughout upper and lower Indus valleys. Its northwestern race *oxiana* extends into the Palearctic Region.

Echis carinatus (Fig 12 & 13)

Common name: Phoorsa, saw-scaled viper.

Diagnosis:

Body stocky, tail short and stubby; head wide and flat, squarish, covered with small keeled scales; head distinct from neck with a cross or an arrow mark at the top; six rows of lateral scales strongly oblique, each scale with cirrated keel (saw-scale); single row of scales under the tail.

Dull ground colour with a pattern of white and light brown, a lateral undulating white band on each side. Average length is from 30 to 35 cm.

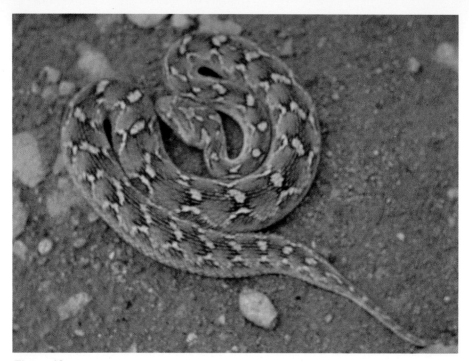

Figure 12
Echis carinatus

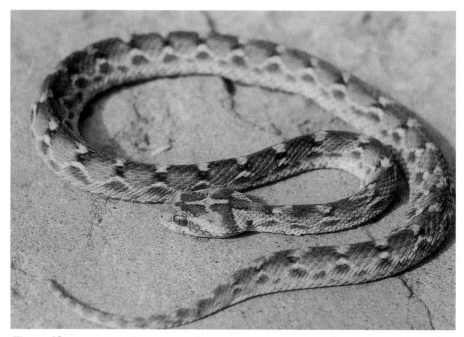

Figure 13
Echis carinatus

Habitat:

Echis carinatus occurs in a variety of habitat: rocky sandy and loose alluvial soil, with vegetation varying from sparse xerophytes to moderately dense grass and scrub. Its frequent haunts are desolate rough terrain and scrub. It avoids marshy and much humid riverine tracts and often climbs shrubs and low-lying trees up to 2 m during rainy seasons.

Habits:

Nocturnal, but in hot days becoming diurnal. *Echis carinatus* is dangerously bad tempered. When in danger, it throws itself into S-shaped loops, keeping its head raised in the centre, ready to strike. It strikes with lightning speed. At the same time its hissing and rubbing of body coils against each other produce a rustling noise. It can even move in this coiled posture at a considerable speed.

Since *Echis carinatus* dose not try to escape, it is killed in large numbers. The areas in Pakistan which once teemed with this snake are now almost devoid of it.

Venom:

Echis carinatus cause a large number of venomous bites in the area of its distribution, however the bites are rarely fatal. The venom is a strong blood coagulant, and after neutralizing body fibrin, causes bleeding due to disseminated intravascular coagulation.

Distribution:

Echis carinatus is Saharo-Sindian in distribution. In Indo-Pakistan subcontinent, it has been distinguished into several sub-species.

Eristicophis macmahoni (Fig 14).

Common name: Baluchistani leaf-nosed viper.

Diagnosis:

Body stocky, dorsoventrally flat, tail short and stubby; head short, wide, very distinct from head, covered with small keeled scales; snout flanked on either side by broad expanded "butterfly" scales with free lateral edges; body scales arranged in straight vertical transverse rows; a ridge on lateral sides of ventrals.

Dorsal ground colour khaki to tan, with a series of 20-25 lateral dark spots each surrounded partially or completely by a group of cream coloured smaller spots. Ventrum light in colour, tail base with distinct cross bands, tip yellowish.

Habitat:

Eristicophis macmahoni is a perfect sand dune dweller of the southwestern desert of Baluchistan. The snake is able to bury itself in the sand by jerky movements of its body, quite quickly and completely, except the head. It feeds on lizards.

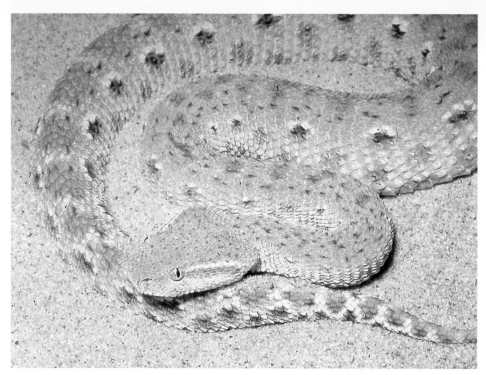

Figure 14
Eristicophis macmahoni

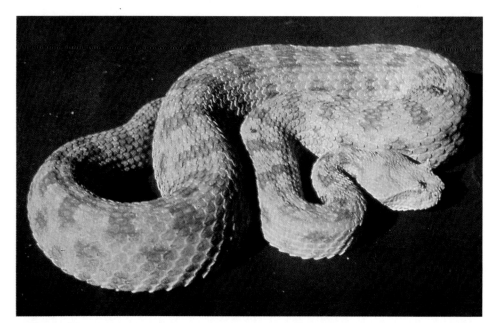

Figure 15
Pseudocerastes persicus

432

Habits:

E. *macmahoni* is nocturnal, remaining burrowed in the sand during day and becoming active during night. It is an active bad-tempered snake. When alarmed, it raises its anterior part of body in a coil, 15 to 20 cm above ground, ready to strike, and at the same time making a very loud and continuous hiss. It moves about in a rectilinear way, but when alarmed, resorts to side-winding type of movement.

Venom:

Venom of *Eristicophis macmahoni* is haemorrhagic, accompanied by much pain and local swelling, and later ulceration at the site of bite. Except reports by Shaw (1925), nothing else is known of its bite.

Distribution:

Range of distribution of *Eristicophis macmahoni* includes the desert basin of northwestern Baluchistan and extends into nearby Iran and Afghanistan. All localities are below 1200 m elevation.

Pseudocerastes persicus (Fig 15).

Common name: Persian horned viper.

Diagnosis:

A distinct erect "horn" formed by two sets of elongated scales from each orbit, head broad and flat, distinct from neck, covered with tuberculated keeled scales; keels of body scales ends in a knob; lateral scales with cirrated keels.

Dorsal ground colour pale grey or bluish grey to khaki, a medium series of transverse blotches, narrower than inter-spaces, a faint series of alternating spots on each side; a dark band from eye to angle of the jaw. Belly white. Average length is from 65 to 90 cm.

Habitat:

Pseudocerastes persicus inhabits sandy rocky hilly tracts up to an elevation of 2000 m. It lives in burrows and crevices among rocks, feeding on lizards and small mammals.

Habits:

Strictly nocturnal; side winding usual mode of locomotion. When disturbed, it hisses loudly, and throws its body into coils. However, it is placid in disposition.

Venom:

Practically nothing is known about the venom of *Pseudocerates persicus.* Sherlov et al. (1956), reported that the venom of subspecies *fieldi* found in Israel has extremely toxic venom, with little haemorrhagic or local necrotizing effects.

Distribution:

Pseudocerastes persicus extends from Azerbydzhan to the Persian Gulf and eastward to Central Afghanistan. In Pakistan, it is reported from Chagai and Kalat, in Baluchistan.

Vipera lebetina (Fig 16).

Common name: Levantine viper.

Diagnosis:

Head triangular and wide, about as high as the width, body stout, stocky, tail short and stubby. Head with small keeled scales; supraocular divided into three small scales.

Dorsum light grey or buff with minute dark punctuation giving it a dusty appearance; a series of small rectangular brown, reddish or grey blotches. Belly buff, variably clouded with grey. Tail pinkish brown. Average length is from 80 to 115 cm.

Habitat:

Vipera lebetina is a snake of dry, rocky and mountainous country with sparse to heavy vegetation and mild environments, between 1000 to 2300 m elevation.

Habits:

Nocturnal; when encountered during day, it is very sluggish and seldom responds to a stimulus. However, during night its habits are changed and it moves quickly, strikes quickly and savagely on slight provocation. It occasionally climbs low bushes.

Venom:

Bites of *Vipera lebetina* is followed by great pain and swelling at the site of bite. Later breathing becomes fast and noisy, pulse rapid. Pain felt all over the body or on the bitten part. Often the patient dies after several hours of agony.

Vipera russelli (Fig 17 & 18).

Common name: Chain viper, Daboia.

Diagnosis:

Head wide, longer than broad, covered with small scales with keels; nostril abnormally long and vertical; supraorbital scale single; body moderately long with much shorter tail.

Colour deep yellow, tan or light brown, with three rows of large oval dark black ringed blotches often narrowly edged with white, mid row of blotches often join each other to form a mid-dorsal chain; ventrum pinkish white with dark brown dots. Average length is 80 to 100 cm.

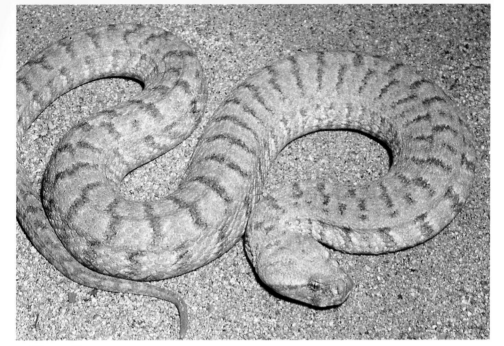

Figure 16
Vipera lebetina

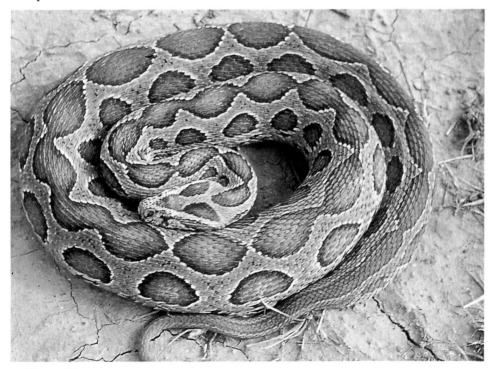

Figure 17
Vipera russelli

Habitat:

Vipera russelli frequents grassland, margins of cultivated fields, bushes and scrub along margins of marshes. It is also likely to be found in mesic rocky country. Though *Vipera russelli* is a species of the plains, it may extend to an elevation of 2300 m.

Habits:

Vipera russelli is strongly nocturnal, becoming crepuscular during cool summer days. Often climbs low trees. When disturbed, it throws itself in coils, keeping the head in the middle. When provoked, hisses loudly, squeezing and expanding the body alternately. During a strike, it hurls itself onto the body of the victim, spraying venom before biting.

Venom:

Chain viper's bite is one of the most dangerous among the Pakistani snakes. Symptoms of poisoning are difficult to distinguish from those of *Echis carinatus*. Its venom is strongly blood coagulant and causes extensive bleeding.

Agkistrodon himalayanus (Fig 19)

Common name: Himalayan pit viper.

Diagnosis:

The only Pakistani snake with a pit (loreal pit) between eye and nostril; head distinctly wide and elongated, with symmetrically arranged large scales; body scales strongly keeled; an elongated postocular extending anteriorly to separate eye from supralabials. (Fig. 2).

Dorsum brownish, mottled or variegated to form pattern of transverse bars. Ventrum white with black and red dots. Average length from 76 to 90 cm.

Habitat:

Highland snake ranging from 2100 to 4900 m in the mid and western Himalayas. It takes refuge under fallen timber, crevices in or under rocks, beneath boulders, ledges, stones and fallen leaves.

Habits:

Nocturnal; often seen close to its hiding place, to which it retreats when disturbed. It is a lazy timid snake, moving slowly from one place to another. Its food consists of millipedes, centipedes and small rodents (Khan and Tasnim, 1986b).

Venom:

Bite of *Agkistrodon himalayanus* results in intense local pain and swelling, which usually subsides within two or three days, even without treatment.

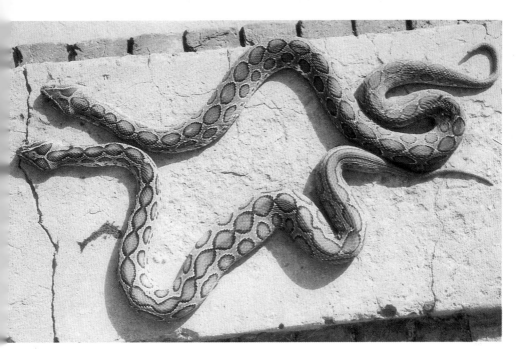

Figure 18
Vipera russelli

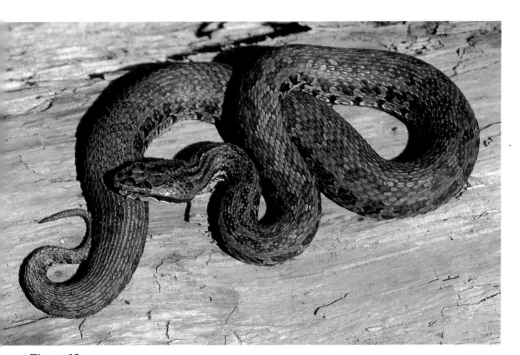

Figure 19
Agkistrodon himalayanus

437

Distribution:

A strictly West Himalayan species. *Agkistrodon himalayanus* has been reported from Chitral to Sikkim. Reports of its collection from eastern Himalayas are doubtful.

Generalized Key For Identification Of Pakistani Venomous Snakes

1. Head with small asymmetrical scales, body scales strongly keeled 2
   Head with large symmetrical scales 6
2. Single row of scales under the tail .... *Echis carinatus*
   Two rows of scales under the tail 3
3. On the upper side of eye a horn-like structure,
   on each side .... *Pseudocerastes persicus*
   No horn on the eye 4
4. Snout with abnormally enlarged scales .... *Eristicophis macmahoni*
   Snout with normal scales 5
5. Nostril crescentric, large and vertical, head
   elongated, single supraocular .... *Vipera russelli*
   Nostril more or less normal; head broad and
   flat; three supraocular .... *Vipera labetina*
6. A pit between nostril, and eye; body scales
   keeled .... *Agkistrodon himalayanus*
   No pit between nostril and eye; body scales smooth 7
7. Mid dorsal scale row of enlarged scales; body dark blue or black with
   transverse row of white narrow stripes .... *Bungarus caeruleus*
   Scales of mid-dorsal row not enlarged; body uniformly black or variegated or
   brown, without any pattern .... *Naja naja*

Snake Bite Problem In Pakistan

No snake bite data are available from any reliable source for Pakistan. Whitaker (1978) estimated 6000 to 9000 deaths in India each year due to snake bite. Figures for Pakistan should be much less, since compared to India, Pakistan has much less area; lower population. Natural jungles, which are usually the haunt of venomous snakes are lacking and there are only a few venomous species. Chances of snake-man encounter are much higher in India than in Pakistan. Northern and northwestern highland of Pakistan is thinly populated and most of the southwestern Baluchistan and southeastern Sind is desolate desert. These vast areas are rarely visited by the general public. Except for occasional bites, snakes are not a great danger compared to other animals of the area. However, most of the snake-man encounter cases are reported from Punjab and Sind, where about 95% of the country's agricultural activity takes place. Judging from occasional reports of snake bite cases appearing in newspapers, 32 deaths were reported from Punjab and 156 from Sind in 1986. If unreported cases are estimated to be thrice the above figures, the figures for

Punjab will be about 150 and for Sind about 500. Figures for N.W.F.P. and Baluchistan, naturally, are expected to be much lower.

In agricultural areas along the Eastern half of Punjab, main casualties are due to the bite of *Bungarus caeruleus, Naja naja* and *Vipera russelli.* In arid northwestern Punjab, the main offenders are *Echis carinatus* and *Naja naja; Bungarus caeruleus* becoming rare and *Vipera russelli* does not extend to this area. In the reclaimed inter-riverine tracts of Punjab, *Echis carinatus* is the main offender. The picture changes in the tableland Potwar, where the main offender is *Echis carinatus* while *Bungarus caeruleus, Naja naja* come in second catagory and *Vipera russelli* becomes rare. While in the lower Indus valley *Bungarus caeruleus, Naja naja,* and *Vipera russelli* are the main offenders, while *Echis carinatus* confines itself to more desert areas.

Bites by *Eristicophis macmahoni, Pseudocerastes persicus* , *Agkistrodon himalayanus* and *Vipera lebetina* are very rare, since their habitat is rarely trespassed by human beings.

Identification Of The Snake Involved In A Bite

Poisoning from venomous snake bite is a medical emergency. It requires immediate attention and care. Delayed or inadequate treatment may result in tragic consequences. At the same time if the bite of a non-venomous snake is not differentiated well in time from that of a venomous snake, it may lead to discomfort and deterioration of the patient's condition. For this purpose, the following observations are suggested to help the physician attending the patient to determine if the wound is inflicted by a thorn, etc., or by a snake. If it is a snake bite, was it from a venomous or non-venomous snake and was it a viper or a non-viper?

1. *Identification by fang marks*

About 57 species and subspecies of terrestrial snakes have so far been reported from Pakistan (Khan, 1982) of which 8 species (disregarding subspecies) are venomous (Khan, 1983). The chances of being bitten by a non-venomous snake is thus 75%. The matter becomes easier if the dead offending snake is brought along with the victim. It is always not possible to identify the snake from the tooth or fang marks found on the victim's body, but sometimes these marks can be very helpful.

Viperid bite : Usually results in one or two relatively large puncture wounds, 10 to 20 mm apart and of various depths, depending on the size of the snake, force of its strike and the part of victim's body. In most cases, additional tooth marks are not observable.

Elapid bite : May produce one or two relatively superficial wound marks, about 8 to 15 mm apart, depending on the size of the offending snake. Usually there are additional puncture marks along the fangs.

Note: Identification by bite marks often becomes complicated when the skin tears as a result of a struggle on the part of the victim to disengage the snake. Long and deep scratches result in a viperid bite, while an elapid bite results in superficial scratches.

2. *Identification of dead snake*

Straighten the dead snake (after making sure that it is dead) on the table: Open its mouth with the help of two forceps, and look for the fangs (large teeth) in the anterior part of the upper jaw:

If fangs are present .... the snake is venomous

If fangs are absent, all teeth are of the same size .... the snake is non-venomous

If venomous

Fangs small, not covered with a membrane .... Elapid, Cobra or Krait

Fangs large, covered with a membrane .... Viper

If the head is smashed, then look for more than two characters of the following:

Viper: 1. Body small stocky, tail very short; body scales strongly keeled;
      2. Scales under the tail in a single row;
      3. Head distinct from body with small scales;
      4. A pit between eye and nostril;
      5. Head very distinct from body;
      6. Nostril abnormally large, vertically enlarged;
      7. Reddish brown body colour.
         i) with three rows of large black brown blotches lined with white, median row of which joined to each other to form a median chain;
        ii) with a lateral row of small brown and white spots;
        iii) an undulating white band along the body latrum;
      8. Pupil of eye vertical;
      9. Supralabials separated by one to three rows of small scales from eye;
    10. Ventrals white with black brown small dots.

Elapid: 1. Body large, tail long, body scales smooth;
      2. Body jet black with transverse white stripes;
      3. Body jet black, variegated to brown, with a hood in life.
      4. Head slightly distinct from neck;
      5. Head with symmetrically arranged large shields;
      6. Some ventrals black;
      7. Supralabials in contact with orbit;
      8. Eye pupil round.

3. *Information from the victim*

If the victim is conscious, he should be interviewed. This not only reassures him, but will also divert his attention.

    a. If he describes the biting action as:
      — a sudden feeling of pin-prick .... Elapid
      — he had a struggle to dislodge the snake .... Viper
      — the snake held on, chewing the site .... *Naja*

b. Bitten while walking:
— bite above ankle .... *Naja*
— bite below ankle .... *Bungarus*, Viper
c. Bitten while watering fields at night:
— in fertile agricultural land .... Elapid
— in arid agricultural .... Viper
d. Biting preceded by:
— hissing .... Viper, *Naja*
— no hissing, sudden .... *Bungarus*
e. The snake turned its head backward to disengage itself .... Viper

4. *Identification from symptoms*

Snake poisoning depends on a number of factors:

a. age and size of victim,
b. length of time the snake holds on,
c. nature, location, depth and number of bites,
d. extent of anger, fear motivating the snake to bite,
e. amount of venom injected,
f. victim's sensitivity to venom.

Viperid bite symptoms

a. rapid onset of burning pain at the bite site,
b. swelling edema and patchy skin discoloration and ecchymosis at the area of bite,
c. extravasation of blood from bite site,
d. failure of blood to coagulate: bleeding from gums, intestinal and urinary tracts.

Cobra and krait bite symptoms

a. pain within 10 minutes at the site,
b. slow localized swelling,
c. drowsiness, weakness, excessive saliva from mouth,
d. paresis of the fascial muscle, lips, tongue and larynx,
e. pulse weak, blood pressure reduced,
f. respiration laboured,
g. petosis, blurring of vision, headache.

Krait bite

a. little or no local swelling or severe pain,
b. systemic signs are often more severe,
c. the victim is in shock,
d. marked respiratory depression and coma may rapidly develop,
e. intense abdominal pain.

5. *Geographical distribution of venomous snakes of Pakistan*

Identification of the venomous snakes becomes easy when one·is familiar with the venomous snakes of his area. For this purpose, the following key is based on the zoogeographical distribution of the snakes.

Distribution pattern of venomous snakes divides Pakistan into four biogeographic regions, each having its own fauna of venomous snakes. In the following account, each region is defined, venomous snakes listed in order of frequency of occurrence; and a key for identification is provided:(Fig 1)

	Physiographical region	Geographical limits	Venomous snakes
A.	Himalayan highland 1600 to 6000 m	Hunza, Gilgit, Swat, Dir, Chitral and Alpine Punjab	*Agkistrodon himalayanus,* *Bungarus caeruleus,* *Vipera lebetina,* *Naja naja oxiana*

Key to the venomous snakes of Himalayan highland from 1600 to 6000 m elevation

1. Head with large symmetrical shields 2
   Head with small asymmetrical scales .... *Vipera lebetina*
2. A pit between eye and nostril, body scales keeled .... *Agkistrodon himalayanus*
   No pit between the eye and nostril, body scales smooth 3
3. Median dorsal row of scales distinctly enlarged; body dorsum dark, with transverse white stripes .... *Bungarus caeruleus*
   Body dorsum, brown to variegated; a hood in life; all dorsal scales uniform .... *Naja naja oxiana*

	Physiographical region	Geographical limits	Venomous snakes
B.	North-western highland 1000 to 3400 m	Highland around Kalat, Quetta, Waziristan lower valleys of Swat, Dir, and Chitral, Kurrum Agency Peshawer area, Dera Ismael Khan, Sibi, Loralai, Zhob (Baluchistan)	*Vipera lebetina,* *Naja naja oxiana,* *Bungarus caeruleus,* *Echis carinatus,* *Pseudocerastes persicus*

Key to the venomous snakes of Northwestern highland from 1000 to 3400 m elevation

1. Head with large symmetrical shields; body scales smooth 2
   Head with small scales; body scales keeled 3
2. Mid-dorsal body scale row broader than other body scales; body dark coloured with a row of transverse white stripes .... *Bungarus caeruleus*
   All body scales similar; body brownish; a hood in life .... *Naja naja oxiana*

3. A group of scales forming a horn-like structure on each eye ....
    Pseudocerastes persicus
    No horn-like structure on eye 4
4. Scales under the tail divided .... *Vipera lebetina*
    Scales under the tail not divided .... *Echis carinatus*

C.	Baluchistan Desert Basin 160 to 1200 m	Chagai, Kharan, lower Kalat, Khuzdar, Makran, Las Bela Divisions	*Eristicophis macmahoni, Pseudocerastes persicus, Echis carinatus, Bungarus caeruleus* (only along Makran coast)

Key to the venomous snakes of Baluchistan desert basin
from 160 to 1200 m elevation

1. Head with large symmetrical shields .... *Bungarus caeruleus*
    Head with small asymmetrical scales 2
2. Single row of scales under the tail .... *Echis carinatus*
    Double row of scales under the tail 3
3. A group of scales forming horn-like elevated structure above each eye ......
    Pseudocerastes persicus
    No horn on eye, snout with abnormally large scales on sides ....
    Eristicophis macmahoni

D.	Upper and lower Indus valley, sea level to 500 m	Potwar Plateau, Salt range, Sargodha, Faisalabad, D. G. Khan, Multan, Bahawalpur, Kherpur, Larkana, Rhimyarkhan, Hyderabad, Kharachi, Divisions	*Bungarus caeruleus, Naja naja, Echis carinatus Vipera russelli*

Key to the venomous snakes of upper and lower Indus valley
from sea level to 500 m elevation

1. Head with large symmetrical shields 2
    Head with asymmetrical small scales 3
2. Mid-dorsal row of scales large and broader, body dorsum dark with white
    transverse stripes .... *Bungarus caeruleus*
    Dorsal body scales of equal size; a hood in life; dorsum brown to dark ....
    .... *Naja naja naja*
    Naja naja oxiana
3. Single row of scales under the tail .... *Echis carinatus*
    Two rows of scales under the tail .... *Vipera russelli*

Production of Antivenom Serum in Pakistan

The most reliable cure against snake bite is antivenom serum. The National Institute of Health Laboratories, Islamabad, is producing antivenom serum against the four most common venomous snakes of the country: *Naja naja, Bungarus caeruleus, Echis carinatus* and *Vipera russelli.*

The antivenom serum is made available at the District Headquarter Hospitals throughout the country. Recently, the Government has spread a network of rural centre, but due to lack of proper facilities, these centers are not supplied with the antivenom serum. When a patient is brought to a hospital, he is already in a critical condition and much precious time is lost in getting treatment of snake bite from local hakims etc. When he is referred to the District hospital, the patient often does not survive the difficulties with the transport and the distance involved.

There is a great need to equip every health centre with the antivenom serum moreover, other centres for the production of antivenom serum must be set up in other cities of the country. Publicity to this effect must be made through all media.

References

Baig, A.R. (1975). Wildlife habitats of Pakistan. Bulletin No. 5, Botany Department, Pakistan Forest Institute, Peshawar.

Boulenger, G.A. (1890). The Fauna of British India, including Ceylon and Burma. Reptilia and Batrachia. London, xvii + 541.

Cherlin, V.A. (1981). The new saw-scaled viper, *Echis multisquamatus* sp. nov. from South-western and Middle Asia. Proceedings of the Zoological Institute, Academy of Sciences USSR, 101: 92-95.

Constable, I.D. (1949). Reptiles of the Indian penisula in the Museum of Comparative Zoology, Cambridge, Mass., Bulletin Museum Comparative Zoology, 103(2): 159-160.

Deoras, P.J. (1978). Snakes of India. National Book Trust, India, New Delhi: 1-156.

Deraniyagala, P.E.P. (1951). Some new races of the snakes, *Eryx, Callophis* and *Echis.* Spoila Zeylanica, 26(2): 147-150.

Gharpurey, K.G. (1962). Snakes of India and Pakistan. Popular Prakashan, Bombay: 1-156.

Golay, P. (1985). Checklist and Keys to the terrestrial Proteroglyphs of the World. (Serpenttes: Elapidae-Hydrophiidae). Elapsoidea Foundation Culturelle, Geneva: 1-90.

Harding, K.A. & Welch, K.R.G. (1980). Venomous snakes of the World. A checklist. Pergamon Press: 1-188.

Holdridge, L.R. (1964). Life zone Ecology. Tropical Science Centre, San Jose, Costa Rica: 1-124.

Khan, M.S. & Tasnim, R. (1986a). Balling and caudal luring in young *Bungarus caeruleus.* The Snake, 18: 42-46.

Khan, M.S. & Tasnim, R. (1986b). Notes on the Himalayan pit viper, *Agkistrodon himalayanus* (Günther). Litterarura serpentium. English edition, 6(2): 46-55.

Khan, M.S. (1984). A cobra with an unusual hood pattern. The Snake, 16: 131-134.

Khan, M.S. (1983). Venomous terrestrial snakes of Pakistan. The Snake, 15: 101-105.

Khan, M.S. (1980). Affinities and Zoogeography of the Herptiles of Pakistan. Biologia, 26(1-2): 113-171.

Khan, M.S. (1982). An annotated checklist and key to the reptiles of Pakistan. Part III: Serpentes (Ophidia), Biologia, 28(2): 215-254.

Klemmer, K. (1963). Liste der rezenten Giftschlangen: Elapidae, Hydrophiidae, Viperidae and Crotalidae. Die Giftschlangen der Erde. N.G. Elwert Universitats- and Verlags-Buchhandlung Marburg: 255 — 449.

Leviton, A.E. (1967). The venomous terrestrial snakes of East Asia, India, Malaya and Indonesia. Chapter 18. Venomous animals and their venoms. Vol 1: 529-576. Academic Press Inc, New York.

Minton, S.A. Jr., Dowling, H.G. & Russell, F.E. (1968). Poisonous Snakes of the World. NAVMED P — 5099. A manual for use by U.S. Amphibious Forcus. U.S. Government Printing Office, Washington, D.C.: 1-212.

Minton, S.A. Jr. (1966). A contribution to the herpetology of West Pakistan. Bulletin American Museum Natural History, New York, 134: 27-184.

Roberts, T.J. (1977). The mammals of Pakistan. Ernestt Benn ltd. London.

Shaw, C.J. (1925). Notes on the effect of the bite of McMahon's viper (*E. McMahoni*). Journal Bombay Natural History Society, 30: 485-486.

Shockley, C.H. (1949). Herpetological notes for Ras Jiunri, Baluchistan, Herpetologica, 5: 121-123.

Shulov, A., Weissmann, A. & Ginaburg, H. (1958). Toxicity of the venoms of two sand vipers of Israel. Harefuah, Journal Medical Association of Israel, 54: 140-143.

Smith, M.A. (1943). The fauna of British India including Ceylon and Burma. Vol 3, Serpentes, xii + 583.

Stemmler, O. (1969). Die Sandrasselotter aus Pakistan: *Echis carinatus sochureki* subsp. nov. Aquaterra, 6(10): 118-125.

Wall, F. (1913). The Poisonous Terresterial Snakes of our British Indian Dominion (including Ceylon) and how to recognise them. Bombay Natural History Society, Bombay: 1-149.

Whitaker, R. (1978). Common Indian Snakes. A field guide. Macmillan Indian Limited, Delhi: 1-154.

ACKNOWLEDGMENTS:— Photographs by Dr. S.A. Minton Jr., M.S. Khan and Shekar Dattatri.

Snake Bite — A Medical And Public Health Problem In Pakistan

By Zafar ALI
Chief Biological Production Divison
N.I.H., Islamabad

Mumtaz Begum
Senior Scientific Officer
N.I.H. Islamabad

The cases of snake bites in Pakistan are abundant, as a rough estimate of nearly 40,000 cases do occur annually. It is mostly a problem of the rural areas of the country. The rural population of Pakistan is about 70%. Mostly farmers, tillers and workers, engaged in this profession are prone to snake bite, whether with poisonous or non-poisonous snakes. But bites due to poisonous snakes are about 15,000 to 18,000 annually and death occurs mostly in specifically untreated cases, according to Frayer (cited by Reid, 1967). The snake bite mortality in Pakistan is about 15 — 18 per 100,000 population. Minton Jr. (1968) reported 10,000 to 12,000 snake bite deaths in Pakistan annually. With the passage of time and increase in population death due to poisonous snake bites has increased up to 20,000 annually. These figures indicate definitely that there is an alarming situation of snake bite mortality and morbidity rate in Pakistan and as such, it is a public health hazard and a medically important issue and a threat of snake bite may create a medical emergency and a health problem in Pakistan.

Types Of Poisonous Snake In Pakistan.

Herpetologists classify venomous snakes in the following families and sub families (Manson-Bahr, 1960 Minton Jr, 1966):-

a) *Viperidae or True Vipers:*
They possess single large fang on short and otherwise toothless maxillae, permitting the fang to be erected or folded against the roof of the mouth. It includes *Vipera russelli* (Russell's Viper) and *Echis carinatus* (the saw scaled viper).

b) *Crotalidae or Pit Vipers:*
It is a sub-family of Viperidae found mostly in the New World and South-east Asia only. It is characterised by a deep pit line with sensitive heat receptors situated between the eye and the nostrils. It includes *Lacheris graminues* (Green pit viper). In Pakistan, these species are generally found in hilly regions about 5000 ft. above the sea level.

c) *Elapidae:*

They are represented by coral snakes and cobras found in all continents except Europe. These snakes have fixed fangs on the exterior ends of the maxillae; the fangs may be followed by solid teeth. It includes *Naja naja* and *Naja tripudians* and *Naja hannah.* Species of cobra are found in all parts of the country Pakistan.

d) *Colubridae:*

This family includes most of the world's snakes of about 2500 species, but the only venomous varieties in this family are some of the rear fanged reptiles seldom found outside Africa.

e) *Hydrophiidae:*

These are marine or sea snakes. They have fixed fangs on the anterior ends of the maxillae; the fangs may be followed by solid teeth. The venoms are predominantly neurotoxic and often very potent. These snakes are so unobstrusive in their habits that they rarely conflict with man. According to Minton Jr. (1966), various snake species of the Pakistan coastal waters which are commonly found include annulated sea snake *Hydrophis cyanocinctus),* yellow sea snake *(Hydrophis spiralis),* Persian Gulf sea snake *(Hydrophis lapemoides),* oriental small-headed sea snake *(Hydrophis fasciatus),* graceful small-headed sea snake *(Microcephaphis gracilis),* beaked sea snake *(Enhyrina schistosa)* and pelagic sea snake *(Pelamis platurus).*

Habits of Venomous Snakes

Ahuja and Singh (1954), Manson-Bahr (1960), Minton Jr. (1966) and Munir A.H. (1969) reported that Cobra *(Naja naja hannah* and *Naja tripudians),* Indian krait *(Bungarus candidus, Bungarus fasciatus),* Russell's viper *(Vipera russelli)* commonly called Dabois and the saw scaled viper *(Echis carinatus)* commonly called in Pakistan as Lundi or Jalebi snakes, are the common terrestrial poisonous snakes in Pakistan. These types of venomous snakes are responsible for practically all the snakes bite cases in this part of the world.

There are few other species of venomous snakes, such as the green pit viper *(Trimeresurus gramineus),* the Coral snake *(Calliophis)* and the Himalayan pit viper *(Ancistrodon),* which seldom inflict fatal bites. They are generally found in some part of province Baluchistan and in hilly parts of the country where habitants are very few.

Cobras occur in many places but are most plentiful in rather damp grassy land and around cultivated areas. They are common in villages and are occasionally found in the suburbs of urban population. Typical refuge for cobras are holes in embankments or about the bases of trees and dens of small mammals. Russell's vipers are frequently seen in grassy land, cultivated fields, salt bush scrub and the margins of marshes. They are most frequently found when low land is flooded by heavy rain or due to irrigation. *Echis carinatus* is an amazingly adaptable snake, occuring on rocky sandy and alluvial soils with vegetation, varying from sparse xerophytes to moderately dense grass and scrub. It generally avoids marsh and gallery forests. Kraits are mostly found in grassy land or semidesert areas with moderately dry alluvial soil, to some extent they are also found in marsh and suburban gardens. It seems that krait avoids very rocky or sandy terrain.

Snakes in general, and poisonous snakes in particular, are nocturnal or seminocturnal. Among human beings therefore, snake bites are more common during the night hours than the day.

Snake Venom

It is well known that considerable differences do exist in the quantity of venom collected during different times of the year. The same is true during moulting and before and after a prolonged fast. Ahuja and Singh (1954) stated that venom secretion is greater in the months of May to September than winter and spring months of the year. The incidence of snake bites is generally increased during the hotter months of the year, the peak being reached in May to August. The marked increase in summer months is due possibly to greater activities and vigour of the reptiles in hot weather. A contributory factor is that the monsoon rains which are at their maximum in July and August, flood the holes and crevices inhabited by the snakes, which are then forced to seek refuge in comparatively higher and drier areas. Also during hot weather, people used to sleep in the open on mats on the ground which increase the risk of exposure to snake bites.

Properties of Snakes Venoms

Snake venoms are pale yellow to amber coloured viscid fluid and composed of proteins, varying in composition from species to species and are mainly of two kinds. The venom of Viperidae type acts principally upon the blood vascular system while that of the Elapidae type acts upon the nervous system and brings about respiratory paralysis as reported by Brooks and Jacobes (1958) and Minton Jr. (1968). According to Ganguly and Malkana (1936), Kondo et al (1960), Anthony et al (1965), Forbes et al (1966) and Omori et al (1967) and Khan et al (1973), the viper venoms contain haemorrhagic fraction and possess proteolytic enzyme activities as well.

Chopra and Ishwariah (1931), Ganguly and Malkana (1936), Sato et al (1964), Minton Jr. (1968) and Condrea et al (1970) reported that the venom of the cobra are predominantly neurotoxic and cardiotoxic. Sarkar in 1956, cited by Manson-Bahr (1960) isolated cardiotoxin from cobra venom and concluded that the death from cobra bite is caused primarily by the failure of respiration due to paralysis of the respiratory centres. Reid (1967) reported that the venom of Krait is only neurotoxic, however, hyaluronidase as a spreading factor is present in surprisingly higher quantities in the common Indian kraits (spp. of *Bungarus*).

Ganguly and Malkana (1936) studied the chemical composition and protein fraction of Russell's viper and cobra venoms. According to them, the venom of Russell's viper contains chemical elements like carbon, hydrogen, nitrogen, sulphur and oxygen and as regards the protein fraction, this contained globulins, albumins and proteases. The cobra venom was found to contain carbon, hydrogen, nitrogen and oxygen and also phosphorus, which was not detected in Russell's viper venom. Globulins, albumins and proteases were present. The toxicity of the cobra venom was attributed mostly due to proteases, although cholinesterases found in elapid venoms, may also account for some of the toxicity.

Nakai et al (1970), studied the lethal fraction of common Indian cobra venom and showed that it possess amino acids like cystein, alanine, phenyl alanine and proline but no methionin. The molecular weight of the Russell's viper venom was established by Gralen and Swedberg (cited by Barnes and Trueta, 1941) to be over 20,000. The molecular weight of cobra venom was found to be 2,500 to 4,000 by Michel and Yung (cited by Barnes and Trueta, 1941).

Clinical Sign And Symptoms Of Snake Bites

Since snake venoms are the mixture of many toxic factors and it is still uncertain which of them are the cause of the various symptoms of poisoning displayed by the snake bite victims, Gans et al (1968) stated that the action of venom appeared to be the result of the types of various components as follows:

1) The toxins, low molecular weight polypeptides,
2) The enzymes such as proteases, phospholipases, esterases, hyaluronidases, nucleotidases and lecithinases.
3) Biologically active amines such as serotonin.

However, the clinical pattern can be divided conveniently into (a) Local and (b) Systemic poisoning (Parrish, 1961).

(a) Local Symptoms

These consist of pain, swelling, necrosis and blisters. The severity and duration of local pain are extremely variable depending upon the amount of venom injection. Ahuja and Singh (1954), Parrish (1961), Reid (1967) and Minton Jr. (1968), reported that the cobra and viper bites usually cause considerable pain and swelling, occasionally followed by necrosis. In case of cobra bites, swelling usually starts from one to three hours after the bite and reaches the maximum in 24 to 48 hours. In viper bites, it starts within a few minutes and often continues for 24 to 72 hours after bite according to the venom dose, but in all cases, at least 75% of the final swelling is reached within 12 hours of the bite. Swelling of the whole limb is common in viper bites but it is rare in cobra bites. However, in both cases, the swelling would be tender. Snake bites due to krait species are usually painless and if pain is present, it is usually of brief duration. Ahuja and Singh (1954), Monson-Bahr (1960) and Reid (1963) indicated that discoloration of skin occurred in viper and cobra bites due to extravasation of blood into subcutaneous tissues. In cobra bite, a constant feature is a dusky discoloration around the bite marks, which extend in area and deepens in colour each day. Krait poisoning is not as a rule associated with much pain, local oedema or discoloration. This is a strong contrast to the effects of Russell's viper, *Echis carinatus* and cobra species bites in which pain, swelling and discomfort are very acute.

(b) Systemic Symptoms

Dubois and Geiling (1959), Manson-Bahr (1960) and Dreishbach (1961), stated that the physiological action and systemic symptoms produced by snake venoms could be classified into two groups: (i) Elapidae and (ii) Viperidae.

(i) *Elapidae Systemic Symptoms*

The venoms of elapids that include cobra and krait are predominantly neurotoxic and often very potent. Manson-Bahr (1960) and Reid (1967) indicated that the earliest symptoms were of feeling of drowsiness or intoxication which started from 15 minutes to 5 hours after cobra bite depending upon the amount of venom injected by snake. Generally an hour after the bite, the patient becomes dull, apathetic and is unable to stand having nausea and vomiting, with profuse salivation and paralysis of the tongue and larynx. Soon the respiratory centres become involved, and respiration ceases entirely. The patient remains conscious until respiratory failure is advanced. Ahuja and Singh (1954) reported that in severe poisoning, the patient was unable to speak, cough, swallow, protrude his tongue or move the lower jaw. In severe poisoning, the patient could not turn his head or turn to the side. Complete limb paralysis never occurred and even shortly before death, the victim could move some part of his limb. Severe abdominal pain was observed in krait bite, which was confined to epigastrium but often was generalized. Dubois and Geiling (1959) and Dreisbach (1961) stated that the neurotoxin of cobra venom produced both convulsions and paralysis whereas krait venom could only cause muscular paralysis. In severe cobra poisoning, cardiovascular depression as shown by sweating, cold extremities and hypotension could be more prominent than neurotoxic effect. However, it was doubtful whether these cardiovascular changes were from direct venom effect or secondary to carbon dioxide retention and acidosis from respiratory failure. According to Reid (1967), primary cardiovascular depression could not be noticed in krait poisoning. Other effects of elapid poisoning were fever and urticaria in laboratory personnel working with snake venoms, presumably due to venom allergy (Mendes et al 1960).

(ii) *Viperidae Systemic Symptoms*

The venoms of viperidae that include Russell's viper *Echis carinatus* and pit vipers are predominantly haematoxic and cytolytic. Forbes et al (1966) and Omori et al (1967) indicated that haemorrhage was the outstanding symptom of systemic viper poisoning mainly by damage to vascular endothelium by venom haemorrhagic constituent. Clotting defect was most common in these cases and the defect persisted for many days after the haemorrhage spontaneously ceased if specific antivenin was not given.

Dubois and Geiling (1959) and Dreisbach (1961) indicated that haemotoxic effects of viperidae venoms were mainly due to enzymatic destruction of cell walls and tissues. They contained high percentage of proteolytic enzymes which caused destruction of endothelium of blood vessels, haemolysis of RBCs and other cells. The cytolytic venoms could cause wide-spread haemorrhages, haemoptysis, haematuria and as a result of necrosis of renal tubules also extensive haemorrhages at the site of injection. The resulting haemorrhages produced functional impairment throughout the body. Manson-Bahr (1960) indicated no paralysis of muscles in case of viperidae poisoning but the viperine toxin produced vasomotor paralysis.

Points of Identification of Venomous and Non-Venomous Snakes (A General Guide For Medical Persons):

It has been observed that there is a general desire by those who are not well acquainted with the snakes to identify between venomous and non-venomous varieties of the snakes. To meet this requirement, various criteria have been proposed by different authors but none of the proposed criteria, however, have provided to be satisfactory. Even cursory examination is not always sufficient to decide the factor, because in some cases a striking resemblance between snakes of totally different affinities, by which even the most experienced people and the specialists may at first be misled and deceived. In short, it is beyond doubt that it is only the examination of dentition which can afford to supply the actual positive information as to its being venomous or non-venomous nature of an unidentified or unknown snake.

The venom gland of a snake can always be traced on either side above the upper jaw, below and behind the eyes. In some elapid forms, the venom glands even extend far back along each side of the body. These glands communicate by a duct with the fangs, which are enlarged, channelled or 'perforated' teeth. The difference between channelled and perforated fangs is but of degree. The term 'perforated' generally used in such cases is anatomically incorrect.

In venomous snakes, venom fangs in varying sizes are always present and directly connected through a duct to venom gland. These fangs are either single type or fixed type on upper maxillae. Other points of identification are the arrangement of scales and counting.

In order to distinguish a venomous snake from a non-venomous snake, all medical officers should be able to tell whether a snake is venomous or not. The size, colour and marks on the body of a snake are not sufficient to identify it. The general method, employed in distinguishing a venomous snake from a harmless, non-venomous is as follows:

(i) *Examination of belly scales:*
   First turn the snake over belly upwards:
   a) If the belly scales are small like those on the back or moderately large, but do not extend the breadth of the belly, the snake is not poisonous.
   b) If the body scales are large and cover the entire breadth, the snake may be harmless or venomous.
   To decide this, look at the top of the head as follows:
   — If the scales on the head are small, the snake is venomous and may be one of the vipers.

— If the scales on the head are large, it may be harmless or may be poisonous.

(ii) *Examination at the side of the face:*
   a) If there is a conspicuous opening or 'pit' between the eye and the nostril, it is poisonous and is one of the pit vipers.
   b) If the third labial touches the eye and nasal shields, it is venomous, may be a Cobra, king cobra or a coral snake.
   c) If a snake has large shields on the top of the head, but has no 'pit' and the third labial does not touch the nose and eye, look for the following points:-
      i) Central row of scales on back will be enlarged.
      ii) Under surface of mouth with only four infralabials, the fourth one will be the largest. Be careful not to count the central scale, because it is cranial.

If characters (i) and (ii) are present, it is a venomous snake and is one of the kraits, and often has bands or half rings across the back.

It is to be noted that if a snake has large scales on the top of its head but does not possess the points described as above, the snake will be harmless or non-venomous.

Recognition of sea snakes is comparatively easy by their valved nostrils and vertically flattened tails. They are all poisonous with the exception of a single species found in creeks and estuaries, which can be easily recognised as being the only species with a flat tail, which has its head covered with timely scales instead of large shields. The sea snakes, although possessing very potent venom, have a narrow gape, and rarely bite effectively.

Treatment of Snake Bite (as practised in Pakistan)

In the treatment of snake bites, the type of venom that could be injected by the snake, along with the signs and symptoms which are likely to be produced in the victim should be noted.

First Aid Treatment

First aid in case of a snake bite consist of the following:

a. Wipe off the excess venom lying on the skin.
b. The site of the bite should be washed thoroughly, preferably in a stream of running water.
*c. The wound should be sucked with a suction cup or with the mouth provided one is sure that there is no abrasion in the buccal cavity including lips or gums, etc.
d. In the case of bites by very dangerous snakes, the wound should be incised to its full depth to promote bleeding and suction should be applied afterwards. (N.B. This measure is of doubtful nature in the case of bites like that of Elapid

---

*Controversial

453

snakes, because in these cases, venom is absorbed very quickly and in the case of snakes which are not very poisonous, incision may do more damage than the actual bite. It is not recommended at all in these cases).

e. A tourniquet should be applied about two to four inches above the site of bite on a limb between site and the heart. This step is necessary to localize the effect of venom. The tourniquet should be tight enough to block the superficial venous and lymphatic return. The idea of a tourniquet is not to block the arterial flow of the blood. The tourniquet should be released for about one and a half minutes after every ten minutes.

f. Exercise should be avoided altogether. Patient should be put to bed. Bitten limb should be immobilized by splinting.

g. Treatment for shock or respiratory paralysis should be given at once if considered necessary.

h. Application of potassium permanganate to the wound is not recommend at all.

i. Medical aid should be obtained as early as possible.

Specific Treatment

Prognosis is considered to be very good in cases where a specific antivenin of good manufacture is made available and is injected when early signs of systemic poisoning become clinically evident. Haemorrhagic signs indicate a viper venom. Neurotoxic signs combined with local swelling indicate krait venom. Muscular weakness and myoglobinurea indicate sea snake venom (Reid, 1968).

Only the specific antivenin is recommended when signs of systemic poisoning are clinically evident. It should always be borne in mind that a routine practice to inject an antivenin in all cases of suspected snake bites may prove dangerous.

Snake bite or snake venom poisoning is always considered to be a medical emergency which requires immediate attention by the physician. A delay in instituting medical treatment may lead to tragic consequences. In most cases, first aid measure will already have been instituted. Now it will be the duty of attending physician to evaluate these measures before determining the course of subsequent treatment. In cases where a patient arrives after about an hour or more of the bite and no first aid measure had been initiated, the physician should put him to bed, immobilize the affected part, clean the wound but should never try to incise or excise the wound as this will be of no value after such a delay.

A routine history should be taken and a physician examination should be done at once without loss of time. The identity of the offending snake, its size, the time of bite and the details of all first aid measures employed should be clearly recorded. Inquiry should be made concerning previous snake bite, allergies and whether or not patient has previously been exposed to horse serum.

Patient's blood should be drawn for typing, cross-matching, blood clotting, complete blood count and haematocrit values determination. Urine analysis is also essential. Determination of the sedimentation rate, prothrombin time, carbon dioxide combining power, urea nitrogen, sodium, potassium are also advised. In severe poisonings, an electrocardiogram and a blood platelet count should be done. Serum bilirubin, red cell fragility tests and renal function test are also advised. Studies of the haematocrit, complete blood count and haemoglobin concentration should be carried out several times a day. In viper venom poisoning, it is especially important to perform urinalysis with particular attention being given to the presence or absence of red cells.

In all patients, pulse, blood pressure and respiration should be recorded regularly. Anti-shock therapy, tracheostomy set and positive pressure breathing apparatus should always be kept in order and ready at hand for operation.

Continued close observation by the physician is essential because the course of prognoses is highly unpredictable and a patient showing steady recovery may take a turn for the worse.

The following measures may be adopted for treatment of snakes bite victim:

1. Early administration of poly antivenin intravenously. A few minutes may mean the difference between life and death. After assuring the type of snake involved, specific monovalent antivenin in sufficiently large quantity to start with, should be given instead of repeating the small doses which may cause anaphylactic reactions sometimes even in cases where patients have been tested for allergic reactions, that is, negative skin or ophthalmic test.

2. Parenteral fluid should always be given following a severe envenomation. It may be necessary to add vasopressor drug to the solution. Avoid using corticosteroids, particularly if antivenin has or is being administered.

3. The nature of injury may predispose to infection and pathogenic bacteria may get entrance into wound, therefore a broad spectrum antibiotic should always be given if the reaction to envenomation seem severe.

4. The prophylactic use of tetanus may be considered if necessary.

5. Changes in electrolyte and fluid balance should be treated immediately as they are most likely to occur due to acute changes associated with the tissue damage produced by the venom, loss of blood and intracellular fluid which may occur.

6. Analgesic and sedative (Aspirin, codeine, morphine and phenobarbital) may be considered if near shock conditions and respiratory deficit leading to failure is not a problem. Local "Block" with procaine and topically applied lotions or ointments are rarely effective.

7. At the very first sign of respiratory distress, oxygen should be given and artificial respiration should be resorted to. A tracheostomy may be indicated particularly if trismus, laryngeal spasm and excessive salivation are present. The drugs used for respiratory centre stimulant have proved to be of no value.

8. In case renal shut down occurs or its signs do appear, routine, emergency measures should be taken. In such cases, the possibility of shock, fluid restriction, electrolytic balance diet administration of digitalis must be considered. The site of the wound should be cleaned, covered with sterilized

dressing and kept dry. Fasciotomy is recommended only when circulation is seriously threatened.

9. Try to avoid the use of antihistamines, ammonia on the wound, or even corticosteroids and cryotherapy as these measures are either of doubtful value or contraindicated.

10. Atropine can be used as a parasympatholytic drug and EDTA (Etylenediaminetertraacetic acid) has been suggested as an agent for combating the tissue effect produced by certain viper venom enzymes.

To administer Antivenin (Anti Snake Venom) after proven snake bite cases, polyvalent and specific monovalent anti snake serum is prepared against four kinds of snakes, that is, Cobra, Russell's viper, *Echis carinatus* and Krait, at the National Institute of Health, Islamabad, Pakistan. The production is carried out as per recommended methods of WHO and as per modified method introduced by Albert Hansen for the preparation of purified anti-toxins in 1948.

The annual production is from 2,500,000 mls to 3,000,000 mls and the final product is 250,000 doses consisting of 10 ml per single dose bottles, and this amount practically meets the demand of the country. The Government of Pakistan do not import a single dose of anti-snake serum from any other country. The inprocess control and final quality control of the product is carried out at the National Institute of Health and it is also a practice to get our samples tested at WHO Collaborating Centres for the control of Antivenom, Liverpool School of Tropical Medicine, Birmingham, UK and Razi Institute, Teheran, Iran. The product prepared at N.I.H. Islamabad, meets all the minimum requirements of potency and it is completely non-toxic and non-pyrogenic. It is prepared in two forms (1) liquid and (2) freeze dried. An ampule of diluent containing 10 ml non-pyrogenic triple distilled water prepared by NIH is being supplied with freeze dried antivenom serum.

An instruction leaflet for proper use of polyvalent and monovalent anti-snake serum is being supplied with each and every vial of antivenin. The leaflet is a guideline for judicial use of antivenom serum for a snake bite victim by medical doctors or qualified attendants. The contents of the leaflet for use of antivenom serum, (liquid and freeze dried), prepared at NIH, Islamabad, are seperately be given which are as follows:

Instructions For The Use Of Concentrated Anti-Snake Venom Serum (Freeze Dried) — (Having Shelf Life For Five Years)

I. The Antivenin is a purified concentrate from the serum of horses immunized against the venoms of Cobra, Russell's Viper, Echis Carinatus and Krait. Each bottle contains 10 ml. of the Polyvalent antivenin.

II. In the case of Cobra, R. Viper, Echis and Krait bite, the serum should be injected intravenously or subcutaneously. It is much more effective when given intravenously.

III. Treatment of Cobra and Krait bite:—

(a) In the case of bites on the limbs apply a tourniquet in order to prevent and control the flow of poisoned blood and lymph from the area of the bite. In the case of the leg apply the tourniquet above the knee and in the

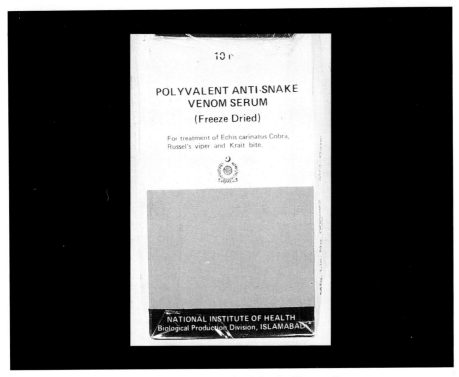

Photograph of Polyvalent Anti Snake Venom Serum,
prepared at N.I.H. Islamabad.

case of the arm above the elbow. Do not keep the tourniquet longer than
30 minutes at a time.

(b) Make a crucial incision at least ¼ inch deep over the fang wounds about
one inch long and encourage bleeding to wash out the poison. Syringe out
the wound with a three percent solution of potassium permaganate:
apply a wet antiseptic dressing.

(c) Inject intravenously at least 50 ml. concentrated serum, initially.
Injection may be repeated depending on the condition and response of
the patient.

When the biting snake is a large one or the symptoms continue, the doses
may be increased and repeated.

If the case is seen late and when symptoms have developed, intravenous
injection should always be employed.

(d) Additional methods of treatment which may be used are the
administration of hot coffee, and the injection of 1 ml. of 1 in 1:1000
solution of adrenalin or any suitable antihistaminic substance.

IV. Treatment of Russell's Viper and Echis carinatus bite:

(a) The same procedure of the application of a tourniquet and incision and
local treatment should be followed.

457

(b) The serum is equally potent against Russell's viper, Cobra, Krait and Echis carinatus Venoms. Two to four bottles intravenously or subcutaneously will be sufficient unless a large dose of the venom has been injected, by the snake.

As the venom is liable to partly fix locally at the site of the bite, one quarter of the antivenin dose should be injected into the area where the fang wounds are seen.

(c) The injection of adrenalin 1 ml. of 1:1000 or a solution of ephedrine of ¾ grain tablet in 1 ml. of water is valuable supportive therapy.

V. Injection of serum:-

The serum is sterile and preserved with an antiseptic. Reconstitute with given diluent. The syringe and needle used for injection should be sterilized before use. It is essential that the injection should be given at the earliest possible moment. Subcutaneous injection should be given under the loose skin of abdomen or thigh. Intravenous injection should only be administered by a physician. The serum should be injected slowly. Due precautions should be taken to test for any serum reaction.

VI. The serum should be stored at a refrigerator temperature i.e. 2 — 4°C and in a dark place and should not be exposed to light.

Persons who make use of the serum should communicate the results to:

National Institute of Health
(Biological Production Division)
Islamabad (Pakistan)

Instructions For The Use Of Concentrated Anti-Venom Serum (Liquid) (Having Shelf Life of two years.)

I. The Antivenin is a concentrate from the serum of horses immunized against the venoms of Cobra, Russel's Viper, Echis carinatus and Krait. Each bottle contains 10 ml. of the Polyvalent antivenin.

II. In the case of Cobra, R. Viper, Echis and Krait bite the serum should be injected intravenously or subcutaneously. It is much more effective when given intravenously.

III. Treatment of Cobra and Krait bite:-

(a) In the case of bites on the limbs, apply a tourniquet in order to prevent and control the flow of poisoned blood and lymph from the area of the bite. In the case of the leg apply the tourniquet above the knee and in the case of the arm above the elbow. Do not keep the tourniquet longer than 30 minutes at a time.

(b) Make a crucial incision at least ¼ inch deep over the fang wounds about one inch long and encourage bleeding to wash out the poison. Syringe out the wound with a three percent solution of potassium permanganate: apply a wet antiseptic dressing.

(c) Inject intravenously at least 50 ml. concentrated serum, initially. Injection may be repeated depending upon the condition and response of the patient.

When the biting snake is a large one or the symptoms continue the doses may be increased and repeated.

If the case is seen late and when symptoms have developed, intravenous injection should always be employed.

(d) Additional methods of treatment which may be used are the administration of hot coffee, and the injection of 1 ml. of 1 in 1: 1000 solution of adrenalin or any suitable antihistaminic substance:-

IV. Treatment of Russel's Viper and Echis carinatus bite:-

(a) The same procedure of the application of a tourniquet and incision and local treatment should be followed.

(b) The serum is equally potent against Russel's Viper, Cobra, Krait and Echis carinatus Venoms. Two to four bottles intravenously or subcutaneously will be sufficient unless a large dose of the venom has been injected, by the snake.

As the venom is liable to partly fix locally at the site of the bite, one quarter of the antivenin dose should be injected into the area where the fang wounds are seen.

(c) The injection of adrenalin 1 ml. of 1: 1000 or a solution of ephedrine of ¾ grain tablet in 1 ml. of water is valuable supportive therapy.

V. Injection of serum:-

The serum is sterile and preserved with an antiseptic. The syringe and needle used for injection should be sterilized before use. It is essential that the injection should be given at the earliest possible moment. Subcutenous injection should be given under the loose skin of abdoment or thigh. Intravenous injection should only be administered by a physician. The concentrated serum should be injected very slowly. Due precautions should be taken to test for any serum reaction.

VI. The serum should be stored at a refrigeration temperature *i.e.* 2-4C and in a dark place and should not be exposed to light. The date of expiry is marked on each bottle and when approaching the expiry date the dose should be increased.

Persons who make use of the serum should communicate the results to

The Chief,

Biological Production Division,
National Health Laboratories,
(ISLAMABAD) PAKISTAN.

References

1. Ahuja, M.L. & Singh, G. (1954). Snake bite in India. Ind. Jr. Med. Res. 42: 661-0686.
2. Anthony, T., Gordon, P., James & Chua, A. (1965). Some biochemical evidence in support of the classification of venom and snakes. Toxicon, 3: 5-8.
3. Barness, J.M. & Trueta, J. (1941). Absorption of Bacteria, Toxins and snakes' Venoms from the tissues. Lancet, 1:623-626.
4. Brookes, V.J. & Jacobes, M.B. (1958). Poisonous snakes, pp 197-200. In V.J. Brookes and M.B. Jacobes. Poisons, D; Van Nortrand company. Princeton, New Jersey.
5. Chopra, R.N. & Ishwariah, V. (1931). An experimental investigation into the action of the venom of the Indian Cobra, Ind. Med. Jr. Res., 18: 1113-1125
6. Condrea, H., Barzilay, M. Mayer, J. (1970). Role of Cobra venom direct lytic factor and Ca in promoting the activity of snake venom. Phospholipase. A. Biochem. Biophys. Acta, 210: 65-73.
7. Dreisbach, R. H. (1961). Reptiles — Diagnosis and treatment pp 327-330. In R.H. Dreisbach, hand book of poisoning, 3rd. ed. Lange Medical Publications, California.
8. Dubois, K.P. & Geiling, E.M.K. (1959). Food poisoning; Plant and Animal poisons. pp 245-6. In K.P. Dubois and E.M.K. Geiling. Text book of Toxicology, Oxford University Press, New York.
9. Forbes, C.D., Turpie, A.G.G., McNicol, G.P. & Douglas, A.S. (1966). Studies on East African snakes; Mode of action of *Echis carinatus'* venom, Scot. Med. J. 11: 168-175.
10. Ganguly, S.N. & Malkana, M.T. (1936). Studies on Indian snakes' venom, Part II, Cobra venom, its chemical composition, protein fractions and their physiological action; Ind. J. Med. Res. 24: 281-286.
11. Ganguly, S.N. & Malkana, M.T. (1936). Studies on Indian snakes' venom, Part I, Daboia vanom, its chemical composition, protein fractions and their physiological action; Ind. J. Med. Res. 23: 997-1006.
12. Gans, C. & Elliott, W.B. (1968). Snake venoms. Production, Injection and Action. Advances Oral Biol. 3: 54-8.
13. Khan, Z.H., Jan, Z.A. & Mukhtar, A. (1973). Fractionation of Russell's viper venom by chromatography on C.M. Cellulose with special reference to biological activities. A preliminary report, Jap. J. Med. Sc. & Biol. 26(1): 39-43.
14. Kondo, H., Kondo, S., Ikezewa, H., Murata, R. & Ohsaka, A. (1960). Studies on the quantitative method for determination of haemorrhagic activity of Habu snake venom, Jap. J. Med. Sc. & Biol. 13: 43-51.
15. Manson-Bahr, P.H. (1960). Animal poisons. pp 817-25. Manson's Tropical Diseases. 15th ed. Cassel and Company, London.
16. Mendes, E., Cintra & Corres, A. (1960). Allergy to snake venom. J. Allergy, 31: 68-73.
17. Minton, S.A. Jr. (1966). A contribution to the herpetology of West Pakistan. Bulletin American Museum Natural History, New York, Vol. 134: 27-184, Article 2.
18. Minton, S.A. Jr. (1968). Snake bite, pp 420-426. In Cecil Locbis Text Book of Medicine, 12 ed. edited by Beeson, P.B. & McDermott, W.W.B. Saunders Company, Philadelphia.
19. Minton, S.A. Jr. (1968). Paraspecific protection by elapid and sea snake antivenin. Toxicon 5: 47-55.
20. Muneer, A.H. (1969). Survey of the species of snakes found in Pakistan. A.F. Med J. xix(1): 1-19.
21. Nakai, K., Nakai, C., Saskai, T., Kakiuchi, K. & Hayaschi, K. (1970). Purification and some properties of Toxin A. From the venom of Indian Cobra. Wetersissenschagten, 57: 382-88.

22. Omori—Satoh, T., Ohsaka, A. Kondo, H. (1967). A simple and rapid method for separating two Haemorrhagic principles in the venom of *Trimeresurus flavoviridis*. Toxicon 5: 17-24.

23. Parrish, H.M. (1961). Snake venom poisoning. Medical Times, 89: 595-602.

24. Reid, H.A. (1967). Symptomatology, Pathology and Treatment of Land Snake bite in India and South East Asia, pp 611-642. In H.A. Reid, Venomous Animals and their venoms. Vol 1, Academic Press, New York.

25. Reid, H.A., Theam, P.C., Chan, K.E. & Baharom, A.R. (1963). Clinical effects by bites by Malayan viper *(Ancistrodon rhoclostoma)*. Lancet, 1: 617-621.

26. Sato, I., Rayan, K.W. & Mitsuhashi, S. (1964). Studies on Habu Snake venoms. VI Cyto-toxic effects of Habu *(Trimeresurus Flavoviridis hallowell)* and cobra *(Naja naja)* venoms on the cell in vitro. Jap. J. Exp. Med. 34: 119-124.

Venomous Snakes of Medical Importance in the Philippines

M. Toriba

The snakes of the Philippines were described by Taylor (1922) and later by Leviton (1961 etc.) in detail. Therefore the account on the classification and distribution of the snakes in this article is a summary of their works.

The snake fauna of Philippines is related to Western Indonesia and Malaysia, but it lacks viperine snakes and the genera, *Bungarus* and *Agkistrodon* (Auct.). Leviton (1963) recorded 39 islands as being inhabited by snakes, of which 18 have venomous ones. Out of more than 60 species of snakes, seven are known to be venomous, of which three are *Trimeresurus* and four are elapid snakes. Opisthogliphous snakes are not included here. The distribution of the venomous snakes are summarized in Table 1, in which islands are arranged corresponding to the subdivision by Leviton (1963). *Calliophis c. calligaster* was listed in the snake fauna of Samar Island by Leviton (1963). It was, however, omitted from that island in his later work (Leviton, 1964a).

Crotalinae

Three species of the genus *Trimeresurus* are recognized, of which two are endemic to the Philippines. *T. flavomaculatus* (Gray) is distributed in most of the larger islands except Palawan and Central Visayan group, whereas *T. schultzei* Griffin is restricted to Palawan group. These two species resemble each other in appearance, although they are different in some morphological features such as the hemipenes and are considered not to be closely related.

T. flavomaculatus is divided into three subspecies, of which two are seen in only Batan and Polillo respectively, and distinguished from nominate subspecies by coloration. The subspecies in Batan, *T. f. mcgregori* Taylor, is remarkable in lacking all pigmentation except xanthophores. *T. f. halieus* Griffin from Polillo has coloration similar to nominate subspecies except in lacking green or yellowish green series of spots or a stripe along the outer scale row. General coloration of *T. flavomaculatus* is green to brownish with a series of irregular dark blotches or crossbars on dorsal body. It lives in damp areas in some islands and feeds on frogs, geckos, fishes and probably mammals. It is oviparous.

T. wagleri (H. Boie) is sometimes placed in the genus *Tropidolaemus* Wagler. It inhabits throughout the Philippines and westward to Sumatra and the Malay Peninsula. This arboreal pit viper is docile and has conspicuous coloration which is very variable in the Philippines. Ground colour is greenish on which white to yellowish or brownish narrow crossbars are present with

TABLE 1
The distributions of venomous snakes
in each island of the Philippines

Species	T.f.	T.s.	T.w.	N.n.	O.h.	C.c.	M.i.
Batan	m						
Camiguin	f						
Luzon	f		w	p	h	c	p
Polillo	h					m	
Mindoro	f			p	h	c	
Panay						g	
Negros	f		w		h	g	
Cebu						g	
Samar			w	s			p
Leyte	f		w	s			
Bohol	f			s			
Mindanao	f		w	s	h		p
Basilan			w				
Jolo	f		w		h		s
Busuanga							b
Culion							b
Palawan		s	w	m	h		b
Balabac		s	w		h		b

Presence of a snake is shown by a letter which is the abbreviation of specific or subspecific name.
Abbreviations are as follows:

T.f.	=	*Trimeresurus flavomaculatus*		(under N. n.)	
T.s.	=	*Trimeresurus schultzei*	p.	=	*N. n. philippinensis*
T.w.	=	*Trimeresurus wagleri*	s.	=	*N. n. samarensis*
N.n.	=	*Naja naja*	m.	=	*N. n. miolepis*
O.h.	=	*Ophiophagus hannah*	(under O. h.)		
C.c.	=	*Calliophis calligaster*	h.	=	*O. hannah*
M.i.	=	*Maticora intestinalis*	(under C. c.)		
(under T.f.)			c.	=	*C. c. calligaster*
f.	=	*T. f. flavomaculatus*	m.	=	*C. c. mcclungi*
m.	=	*T. f. mcgregori*	g.	=	*C. c. gemianulis*
h.	=	*T. f. halieus*	(under M. i.)		
(under T.s.)			p.	=	*M. i. philippina*
s.	=	*T. schultzei*	s.	=	*M. i. suluensis*
(under T. w.)			b.	=	*M. i. bilineata*
w.	=	*T. wagleri*			

black borders. The most varied patterns are seen in Mindanao. This viper is common in lowland jungles. It feeds on reptiles or mammals.

Elapidae

Out of four species, only *Calliophis calligaster* is endemic to the Philippines. Others have a wider range, especially *Naja naja* which extends to Central Asia. Although intraspecific variation of *Naja naja* shows some complexity, three subspecies in Philippines are clearly defined. *N. n. philippinensis* Taylor, which possesses highly toxic venom, inhabits Luzon and Mindoro. Its coloration is light brown to olive brown without any distinctive cross bands. It exceeds 1 m in length. It is common in Luzon and probably the most important snake in Philippines. Frogs and snakes are known as its diet. *N. n. samarensis* Peters, which inhabits eastern Visayan islands and Mindanao, is dark brown to black in colour with a trace of a light lateral line. Interstitial skin is yellowish. A broad black crossbar present on the posterior throat. Mammals are recorded as its food in addition to frogs and snakes. *N. n. miolepis* (Boulenger) occurs in Palawan Archipelago and Borneo. Its dorsal colour resembles that of *N. n. samarensis* but it lacks the dark band on the throat. *Naja naja* is absent in western Visayan islands.

Ophiophagus hannah (Cantor) is known as the largest venomous snake in the world. It is distributed throughout the Philippines except Visayan group in which only Negros island is inhabited. It extends westward to India. Coloration is light to dark olive brown with many whitish transverse bands on interstitial skin of the dorsal body. Young individuals have darker and more vivid coloration. Taylor (1922) mentioned a specimen from Balabac, which was 4.25 m in length. On its ecology in the Philippines little is known, but it probably feeds on snakes.

Genera *Calliophis* and *Maticora* are differentiated by the shape, size and location of venom glands. The venom gland of the latter is markedly elongate and extends to the body cavity in contrast to the normal gland in the former. Appearance is similar in these genera, but in colour pattern *Calliophis* is banded and *Maticora* is striped in the Philippines.

As shown in the table, ***Calliophis calligaster*** (Wiegmann) is represented by three subspecies. They are differentiated by coloration and ventral count. On dorsum, black rings and reddish bands are arranged alternately and separated by narrow white annuli from each other. In *C. c. gemianulis* (Peters), these black rings are divided by narrow white annuli. *C. c. calligaster* has higher number of ventrals than the other two subspecies and in this respect *C. c. mcclungi* (Taylor) is distinguished from nominate subspecies. Reddish part of the body becomes blackish in the adults. They are secretive snakes and some burrowing snakes were recorded as its diet.

In ***Maticora intestinalis*** (Laurenti), three subspecies are known from the Philippines. They are distinguished by coloration. In the Philippine forms, basically a light mid-dorsal stripe and a light brown dorso-lateral stripe are present on the dorsal body and black and light crossbars are arranged alternately on venter. *M. i. bilineata* (Peters), which inhabits Palawan

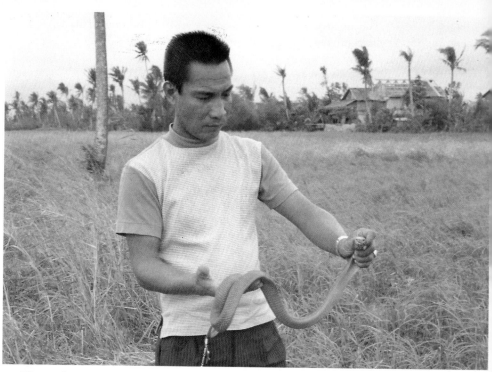

Figure 1
Naja naja philippinensis at Luzon. Courtesy of Dr. Yoshiharu Kawamura.

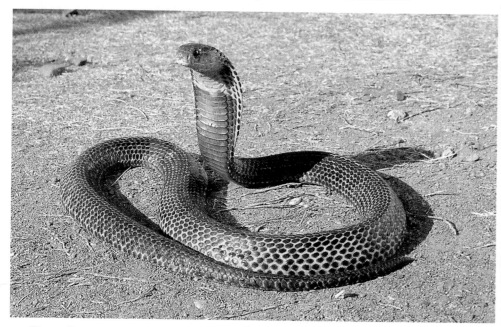

Figure 2.
Naja naja samarensis from Mindanao.

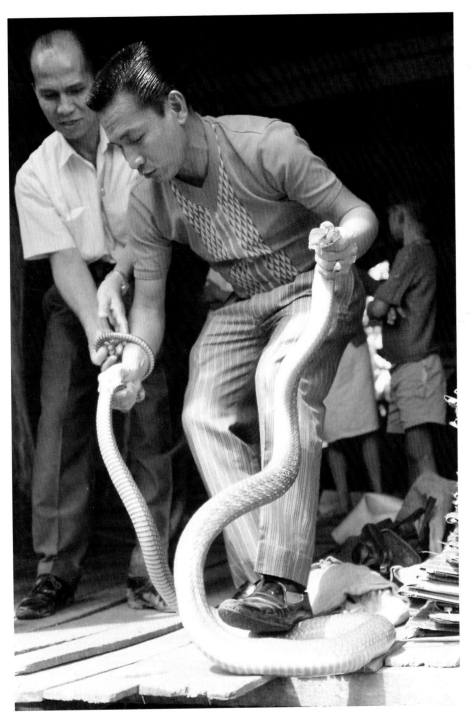

Figure 3.
Ophiophagus hannah at Luzon. Courtesy of Dr. Yoshiharu Kawamura.

Archipelago, has the condition where the black crossbars on venter do not contact with black marking on the side. Dorso-lateral stripe is narrow and a distinct white line is present on the side. Two other subspecies, *M. i. suluensis* (Steindachner) and *M. i. philippina* (Gunther), are distinguished by cranial coloration and light ventral bands. In the former, prefrontals are lighter (it may be red in life) than the other part of head and light crossbars on venter do not extend onto side of body above the first scale row. Little is known about its habits.

Snake bite cases and their treatment.

There were very few reports on snake bite cases in the Philippines. Reyes and Lamanna (1955) reported older records before 1940, in which 183 annual deaths due mainly to cobra, were recorded. Recent study was made by Sawai et al. (1971) who investigated the statistics of snake bites cases during 1965-1969 and 304 clinical records in 1969 from 15 hospitals. Two thirds of the bites occurred at rainy season from July through December, although bites were recorded throughout the year. Majority of the bites occurred on males. Among ages, the bites on teens were most frequent. Majority of the bites occurred while working in fields. Lower legs especially feet were most frequently bitten. Among 304 cases with clinical records, the species responsible for the bites could not be identified in 231 cases; cobra bites 35, king cobra 1, sea snakes 2 and remaining 35 were non-venomous snakes. Therefore the cobra is the most important snake regarding snake bite cases in Philippines. Sawai et al. (1971) also quoted statistics of snake bite deaths in 1968 from Disease Intelligence Center of the government of the Philippines. In that year 294 deaths were recorded in the country, of which 237 occurred at Luzon and 36 in Mindanao.

Among 24 cases of cobra bites examined by Sawai et al. (1971), 12 cases showed definite swelling and 11 indicated paralytic symptoms as drowsiness, ptosis of eyelids, unconsciousness, dizziness, drooling of saliva, vomiting, dyspnoea and blurred vision. All the fatal cases had some of the paralytic symptoms and the average time from the bite to death was about three and a half hours. Most of the patients bitten by the cobra received monovalent antivenin produced by National Serum Vaccine Laboratories of the Philippines. Because effectiveness of such an antivenin depends on the time interval between bite to the administration since the neurotoxin of the Philippine cobra affects the patients very quickly, Watt et al. (1986) considered that anticholinesterases may be effective in the paralysis caused by snake neurotoxin and tried edrophonium in the patients bitten by *Naja n. philippinensis*. Based on the positive results, they recommended a test of edrophonium in the patients with signs of neurotoxic envenoming by snakes.

The LD_{50} of *N. n. philippinensis* is 3.3 μg per mice i.v. injection and 3.6 μg in s.c. injection (Christensen, 1966), while that of *O. hannah* is 1.6 mg/kg in i.v. and i.p. injection on mice (Kocholaty et al., 1971). The neurotoxin of *N. n. philippinensis* was purified by Hauert et al. (1974) and two toxins of *O. hannah* were purified by Joubert (1973). The amino acid sequences of these toxins were also determined. On the other hand, the venom of *T. wagleri* was examined by Minton (1968) using the snakes from Malaya.

References

Christensen, P.A. (1966) Venom and antivenom potency estimation. Memorias do Instituto Butantan, 33: 305-326.

Hauert, J., Maire, M., Sussman, A. and Bargetzi, J.P. (1974) The major lethal neurotoxin of the venom of *Naja naja philippinensis*. Purification, physical and chemical properties, partial amino acid sequence. International Journal of Peptide and Protein Research, 6: 201-222.

Joubert, F.J. (1973) Snake venom toxins. The amino acid sequences of two toxins from *Ophiophagus hannah* (King cobra) venom. Biochimicaet Biophysica Acta, 379: 345-359.

Kocholaty, W.F., Ledford, E.B., Daly, J.G. and Billings, T.A. (1971) Toxicity and some enzymatic properties and activities in the venoms of Crotalidae, Elapidae and Viperidae. Toxicon, 9: 131-138.

Leviton, A.E. (1961) Keys to the dangerously venomous terrestrial snakes of the Philippine Islands. Silliman Journal, 8: 98-106.

Leviton, A.E. (1963) Remarks on the zoogeography of Philippine terrestrial snakes. Proceedings of the California Academy of Sciences, 4th series, 31: 369-416.

Leviton, A.E. (1964a) Contributions to a review of Philippine snakes, III. The genera *Maticora* and *Calliophis*. Philippine Journal of Science, 92: 523-550.

Leviton, A.E. (1964b) Contributions to a review of Philippine snakes. V. The snakes of the genus *Trimeresurus*. Philippine Journal of Science, 93: 251-276.

Leviton, A.E. (1965) Contributions to a review of Philippine snakes. VII. The snakes of the genera *Naja* and *Ophiophagus*. Philippine Journal of Science, 93: 531-550.

Minton, S.A., Jr. (1968) Preliminary observations on the venom of Wagler's pit viper *(Trimeresurus wagleri)*. Toxicon, 6: 93-97.

Reyes, A.O. and Lamanna, C. (1955) Snakebites mortality in the Philippines. Philippine Journal of Science, 84: 189-194.

Sawai, Y., Koba, K., Okonogi, T., Mishima, S., Kawamura, Y., Chinzei, H., Ibrahim, A.B.B., Devaraj, T., Phong-Aksara, S., Puranananda, C., Salafranca, E.S., Sunpaico, J.S., Tseng, C.S., Taylor, J.F., Wu, C.S. and Kuo, T.P. (1971) An epidemiological study of snakebites in the Southeast Asia. The Snake, 3: 97-128. (in Japanese with English summary).

Taylor, E.H. (1922) The snakes of the Philippine Islands. Bureau of Sciences, Manila.

Watt, G., Theakston, R.D.G., Hayes, C.G., Yambao, M.L., Sangalang, R., Ranoa, C.P., Alquizalas, E. and Warrell, D.A. (1986) Positive response to edrophonium in patients with neurotoxic envenoming by cobras *(Naja naja Philippinensis)*: A placebo-controlled study. New England Journal of Medicine, 315: 1444-1448.

Venomous Snakes of Medical Importance in Taiwan

Bungarus multicinctus

Contour of head — broad oval; dorsal shields — large, smooth and glossy; fangs — short, rigid, located in upper jaw between eye and nose.

Upper body — barred with distinct black and white bands, 34 to 45 broad black bands on body, and tail — 8 to 15 black bands, the last band is at the end of tail; a row of hexagonal scales (about 3/2 to 2 the size of body scales) along vertebral line, from head to anterior tail.

Ventral scales — large, smooth and glossy, 205 to 216; subcaudals — 44 to 48; scale counts — 15-15-15.

Distribution:

B. multicinctus is very common on Taiwan. It apparently occurs in all areas of the island at lower altitudes, perhaps below 2000 feet. Except in Taiwan this species occurs on Hainan and is widely distributed in the provinces of southeastern China.

Naja naja

Body — may be considerably flattened when angry or "hooded"; fangs — rigid, short to medium length located anterior to middle of upper jaw.

Upper body and tail — light grey tan to dark grey black; in the expanded part of neck is a spectacle like design when it is angry or hooded, except this and irregularly spaced, ill-defined vertical lines on body, this usually uniform in color.

Ventral scales — large, smooth glossy, some may have light grey posterior border, 165 to 175; subcaudals — 43 to 48 pairs; scale counts — 21-21-15.

Distribution

Records are incomplete but indications are that this snake may be found anywhere on the island at low altitudes. The Taiwan cobra apparently is more common in the west central and southern parts of Taiwan. The same species occurs commonly on Hainan and in a number of the Southeastern provinces of mainland China.

Agkistrodon actus

Dorsal contour of head — broad triangle; nose — rapidly tapered to knobbed tip, i.e. prominent turned up snout; upper head — uniform rich dark

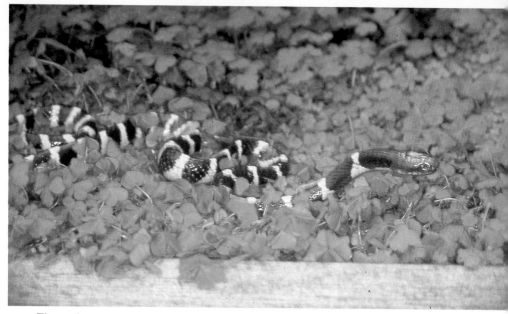

Figure 1.
Bungarus multicinctus Blyth

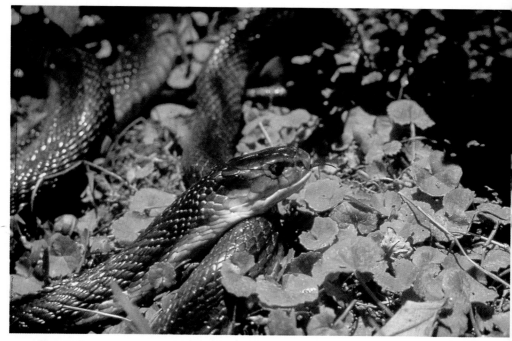

Figure 2.
Naja naja atra (Cantor)

brown to chocolate brown, prominent dark brown oblique stripe extending from eye posterior to and beyond corner of mouth; prominent pit midway between eye and nostril; dorsal shields — large, broad, dull, tuberculated surface; smaller scutes on back of head strongly keeled; tongue — black; fangs — large, retractable, located in fleshy sheath in anterior part of upper jaw.

There are 19 to 22 dark triangular designs on side of body, apex of each directed dorsally, usually uniting at vertebral line with similar design from opposite side, base of triangular designs usually on second or fourth row of scales; upper tail — five or six dark designs, which form broadly fused triangles, bands over top, posterior third of tail dark brown to black; body scales — from parietls to tip of tail, rough in appearance and touch, strongly keeled, dull.

Ventral body — white to light cream, irregular areas of designs involving (one or several ventrals) of black from neck to mid-tail; ventral scales — alrge, smooth gloosy, 160 to 166; subcaudals — 51 to 56 pairs; scale counts — 21-21-17.

Distribution

Records and literature indicate that it occurs in central mainland China and Viet Nam.

Trimeresurus stejnegri

Dorsal contour of head — broad, roughly triangular; prominent pit (pit viper), three to five times size of nostril between eye and nostril; eye — distinctly rusty brown or brick red, flecked with cream; iris — vertically elliptical, black with narrow margin of cream or light orange; dorsal shields — no true shields, head covered with small scales; upper head — frequently with white or light cream line extending from lower edge of eye posteriorly over corner of mouth and onto sides of neck (live variable, a sexual characteristic, usually more prominent in male), in males white line may be bordered with brick red or rust; fang — long, moveable, in fleshy sheath in anterior part of upper jaw.

Upper body — uniform dark green of chartreuse, white or cream line or a combination of this and brick red line, (involving first and second scale rows) above latero-ventral junction; white line only in females; in males with both white and red line; upper tail — variable, may be same green as rest of upper body, but usually tinged with dull diffuse rusty red; body scales — rough, with well-developed keels, dull in appearance.

Ventral body — uniform bright green lighter than dorsal body; underside of tail — subcaudals clearly differentiated by narrow white margins, distal quarter to third of tail tinged with dull, diffuse rusty red; ventral scales — large, smooth, gloosy, 156 to 172; subcaudals — 63 to 72 pairs; scale counts — 21-21-15.

Distribution

T. stejnegri is found throughout Taiwan. It occurs more commonly at the lower altitudes of wooded, shrub and mountainous areas. The same or a closely related species of *Trimeresurus* occurs on the island of Hainan and in the eastern provinces of mainland China.

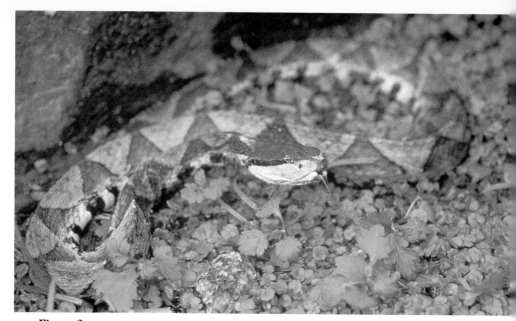

Figure 3.
Agkistrodon actus

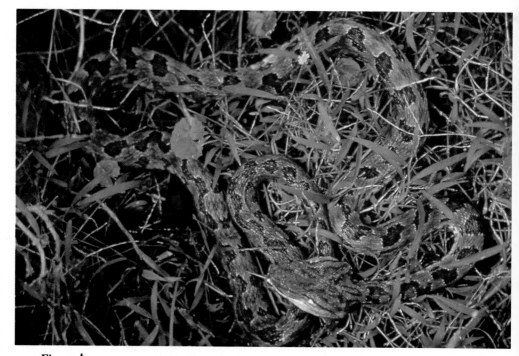

Figure 4.
Trimeresurus mucrosquamatus (Cantor)

Trimeresurus mucrosquamatus

Dorsal contour of head — broad, distinctly triangular; large triangular pit between nostril and eye; eye — light brown to tan dappled with cream which blends well with colour of head; iris — vertically elongate oval or elliptical, black surrounded by well-defined band of yellow; dorsal shields — no true shields, head covered with small scales; prominent dark band extends from eye to corner of mouth; a second pair of longitudinal designs extends from nostril over eye and posteriorly, parallel with band back of eye; tongue — dark grey to black, stem lighter than branches; fangs — large (1/4 to 5/8 in.), moveable, in sheath in anterior part of upper jaw.

Upper body — light brown to brown with many designs of chocolate to brown black; 40 to 60 dark areas or designs meet at, or cross, the vertebral line; 15 to 20 designs on tail; other dark designs involving three to six scale rows and separated by three to six rows of scales from longitudinal broken line on each side of body; body and tail scales — dull, rough to touch, heavily keeled.

Ventral scales — large, smooth, glossy, 205 to 214; subcaudals — 80 to 94 pairs; scale counts — usually 29-27-21 but variable.

Distribution

T. mucrosquamatus is very common and widely distributed in Taiwan. It also occurs in the provinces of southeast China.

Vipera russelli

Dorsal contour of head — triangular; iris — vertically elliptical black with conspicuous grey to yellow border; angular ridge from upper eye to nostril; upper head — three large prominent designs on head; dorsal scutes — most scales equal in size, heavily keeled, rough; tongue — dark grey to black, outer branches grey; fangs — large (3/8 to 5/8 in.) hinged from upper jaw.

Upper body and tail — brown to grey brown or chocolate, entire upper body with blotches or designs of variable size, shape & distribution; 23 to 28 (depending on fusion) prominent designs, usually with narrow grey to light brown borders along dorsal part of body; a second series of similar blotches on side of body, these tend to alternate with dorsal designs; one longitudinal line of small designs of variable size & shape occur above and one below the lateral line of medium size blotches; body & tail scales — heavily keeled, rough, dull.

Ventral body — one to five semicircular designs of ventrals, base of design on posterior edge of scale, these erratic in distribution but frequently arranged in checker-board fashion; ventral scales — very large, smooth, glossy, 158 to 168; subcaudals — 40 to 46 pairs, scale counts — (variable), 29(30)-27(29)-21.

Distribution

This snake, a true viper, has been collected in the southern third and on the eastern side of the central mountain range in Taiwan. Geographical races of *Vipera russelli* range from Ceylon northwards through India and to the western Himalayas. It has been taken also in Kwang-tung Province of mainland

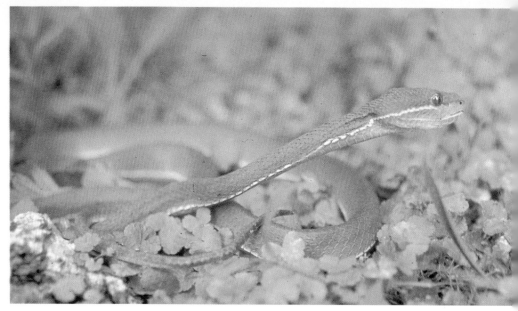

Figure 5.
Trimeresurus gramineus stejnegeri (Schmidt)

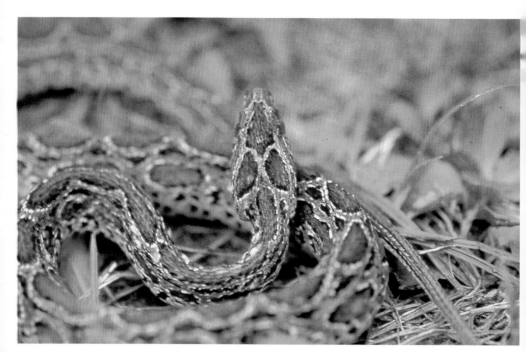

Figure 6.
Vipera russellii formosensis (Maki)

476

China. Apparently those common to mainland Asia attain a larger size than the Taiwan form.

Acknowledgement: This chapter was abstracted by Mr. Jun-Tsong Lin and the photographs also supplied by him.

Venomous Snakes, Their Bites And Treatment in Sri Lanka

Anslem de Silva

Dept of Community Medicine, Faculty of Medicine
Peradeniya, Sri Lanka

Introduction

Sri Lanka is a tropical island lying in the monsoon region of South East Asia. The climate and vegetation vary from semi arid deserts to evergreen tropical rain forests and cool mountain forests. Topographically a major portion of Sri Lanka is plains with central mountain regions.

A diverse assemblage of snakes occupy many ecological niches of the island. The snakes of Sri Lanka include some of the most primitive snakes. (Family Aniliidae, Typhlopidae and Uropeltidae) as well as recent ones and are considered to be one the best snake faunas of the world (de Silva 1982, 1986b). Furthermore it includes all the known families of venomous or medically important snakes such as the kraits and cobra (Family Elapidae), sea snakes (Family Hydrophiidae), Russell's viper, saw-scaled viper, Hump-nosed vipers and Green pit viper (Family Viperidae). Although there are eleven species of ophisthoglyphous snakes of Family Colubridae, they have, up to date, not caused any serious bites. The common krait *(Bungarus caeruleus)*, Cobra *(Naja naja naja)* and Russell's viper *(Vipera russelli pulchella)* are commonly found near human habitations and account for approximately 97% of deaths due to snake bite envenomation in Sri Lanka (de Silva and Ranasinghe 1983). Further, the available data (de Silva 1981, 1987b; Sawai et al 1983) suggest that the victims of the common krait *(Bungarus caeruleus)* run a greater risk of death than from any other snakes in Sri Lanka. As regards to snake bite and traditional management, there is evidence to suggest that these two had been in existence in Sri Lanka from pre Christian times (de Silva 1981, 1987; de Silva et al 1983; de Silva & Uragoda 1983). At present there is a high incidence of snake bite in the country, with one of the highest death rates (average for 1975 to 1979 = 5.3/100,000 population) recorded in the world. Most of these deaths occurred without receiving antivenom serum (AVS).

In the field of management of snake bite envenomation, there are at present two major systems in Sri Lanka. The ancient traditional system (Ayurveda) is a well established part of Sri Lankan culture and the most widely sought form of treatment (de Silva & Uragoda 1983). The other is the Allopathic or Western system. Initially, the majority of people were unaware of the availability of antivenom serum or had faith in the Allopathic system. However, there is now evidence that more people are aware of antivenom serum and steadily accepting Allopathy (de Silva & Ranasinghe 1983).

A knowledge of the island's topography, climate, vegetation and biology of medically important snakes, epidemiological aspects of snake bite, treatment and demographic trends are important in designing a national strategy for the prevention, control, treatment of snake bite and conservation of snakes. These aspects pertaining to Sri Lanka are dealt in this chapter.

Location

Sri Lanka (formerly Ceylon) is a tropical island situated in the Indian ocean at the southern tip of the peninsula of India between latitudes 5° 55' – 9° 51' N and longitudes 79° 41' – 81° 54' E.

Physiography

The island is 65,584 km^2 in area of which 64,742 km^2 is land and the rest, inland waters. The island is 435 km long and the widest breadth 225 km. The coast around Sri Lanka is a plain, where it is narrowest in the southwest but broadens and is flatter in most other parts. The central part of the island is mountainous and forms the 'Central Highlands' with the highest elevation of 2,525 m.

Geologically and physically, Sri Lanka is the southern continuation of India, separated by the narrow strip of shallow sea, the Palk Strait and the Gulf of Mannar during the Miocene (Peiris 1976). Moore (1960) even considers temporary land connections between Sri Lanka and India four times during the Pleistocene period coinciding with each glacial period and separation from each other during inter-glacial periods. These land connections have favoured the spread of fauna from mainland India to Sri Lanka and even reinvasion. Hence a majority of Sri Lanka's snake fauna has affinities with that of South India.

Some recent studies of snakes (Deraniyagala 1955, de Silva 1983g 1987a, de Silva and Toriba 1984, de Silva 1980, Gans & Fetcho 1982) show that their distribution is mainly influenced by the climate, rainfall, altitude, vegetation, soil and the availability of food. It is important to have a fair knowledge of these aspects to understand the distribution of snakes, as it reflects on snake bite, helps in stocking specific AVS and prevention of snake bite.

Climate

Sri Lanka is a tropical island. Its maritime influences make it free from thermal extremes. The country receives its rainfall during two seasons, (a) the southwest monsoon from late May to late September felt in the south, west and the central hills and (b) the northwest monsoon from December to February bringing rain to the lowlands in north, north central, northeast and southeast, and central hills facing the north and east. In addition to these two monsoons, inter-monsoonal rains occur in many parts of the island during March to April and October to November.

However, the inter-monsoonal rains occur much more over the central hill country and the southern and western lowlands than over the northern and eastern lowlands. Hence the southwest quadrant of the island receives heavy, seasonally well distributed, reliable rainfall throughout the year. But the rainfall in the rest of the island is relatively low, less reliable and restricted to a shorter period.

Owing to this pattern in rainfall, two distinct zones, the wet zone and the dry zone are demarcated. Further the border areas in between these two zones form a recognizable distinct 'intermediate zone' (Fig 1). This zone consists of mixed features in the flora and fauna seen in both the dry and wet zones. Of Sri Lanka's total land area, 65% constitute the dry zone. The wet and intermediate zones consist of 23 and 12 percent respectively (Peiris 1976). Some recent studies (Crusz 1984, de Silva 1987a, de Silva 1980, Gans & Fetcho 1982) indicate that the distribution of many species of snakes are influenced by these climatic zones eg. *Bungarus ceylonicus* is mainly confined to the wet and intermediate zones (de Silva 1987a); *Echis carinatus* is confined to the arid coastal areas of the dry zone.

Soil and Vegetation

According to some soil studies (Moorman and Panabokke 1961, Wijesinghe (1981), Gaussen, Legris, Viart and Labroue 1964, Peiris 1976), the soil of Sri Lanka is grouped under 8 - 18 major soil groups. Of these, red yellow podzolic soils and latosolic soils are the dominant groups in the wet zone with 82% of this zone consisting of red yellow podzolic soils (Peiris 1976). The predominant soil groups in the dry zone are reddish brown earths, while the intermediate zone consists of features seen in both dry and wet zones.

The vegetation is grouped under seven vegetational zones (Gaussen et al 196). Recent studies of the distribution of fauna of Sri Lanka is based on these seven vegetational zones (fig 2), (Crusz 1984, Eisenberg & Mckay 1970, de Silva 1981) eg. *Bungarus ceylonicus* is confined to the rain forests and grassland zone.

Elevation

According to height and slope characteristics the island is divided into three peneplains or erosion levels (Vitanage 1972) (fig 3).

1. The coastal lowlands with elevations from the sea level to 270 m. There are isolated inselbergs.
2. Uplands with elevation from 270 - 1,060 m.
3. Highlands with a series of well defined high plains and plateaus, rimmed with mountain peak and ridges. Elevation from 1,060 to 2,420 m from above mean sea level.

Snakes of Sri Lanka

It is clear that some taxa presently found in Sri Lanka are from the stock that had undergone a process of evolution in isolation for a few million years. The climate, relief, vegetation and geology of Sri Lanka have contributed to this evolution. Hence, many have evolved into endemic species, subspecies, a few genera or even a few showing morphological variations, from the respective

481

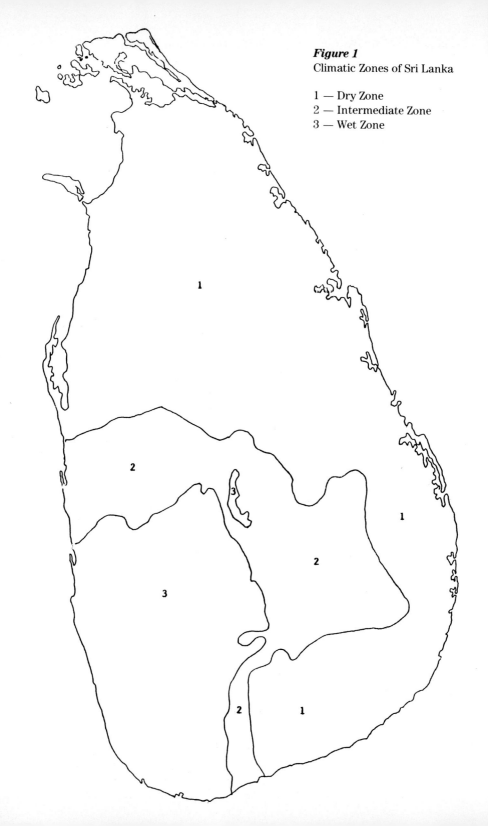

Figure 1
Climatic Zones of Sri Lanka

1 — Dry Zone
2 — Intermediate Zone
3 — Wet Zone

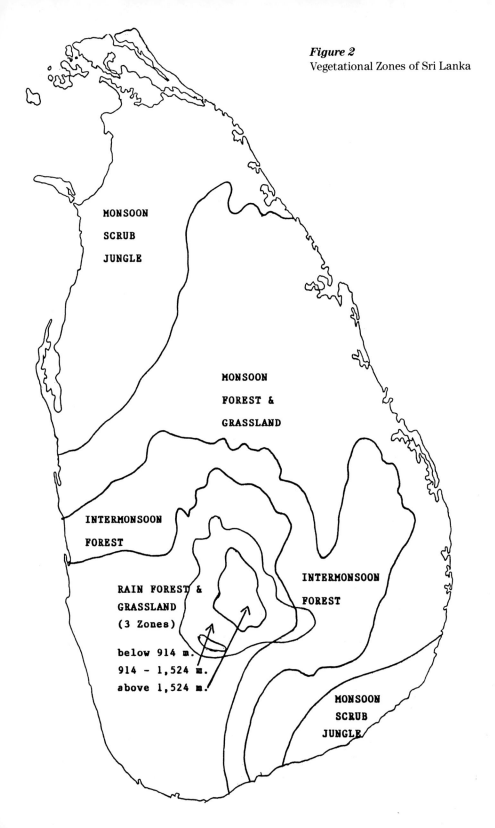

Figure 2
Vegetational Zones of Sri Lanka

MONSOON
SCRUB
JUNGLE

MONSOON
FOREST &
GRASSLAND

INTERMONSOON
FOREST

RAIN FOREST &
GRASSLAND
(3 Zones)

below 914 m.
914 - 1,524 m.
above 1,524 m.

INTERMONSOON
FOREST

MONSOON
SCRUB
JUNGLE

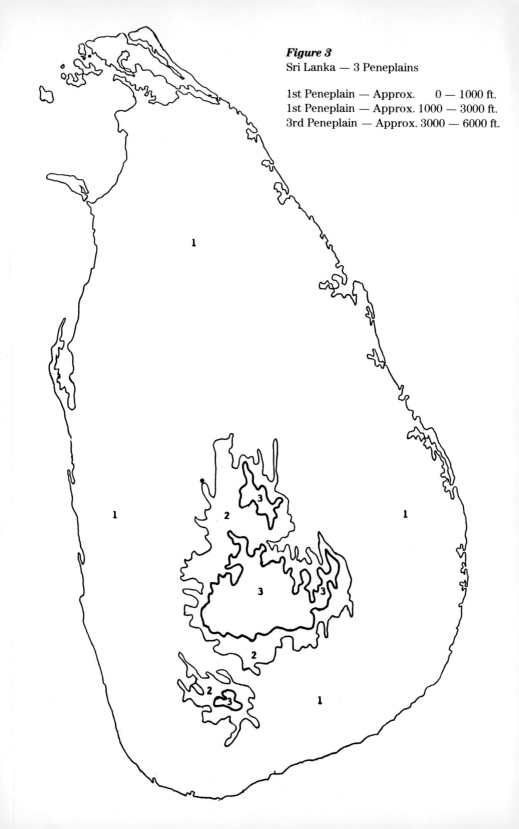

Figure 3
Sri Lanka — 3 Peneplains

1st Peneplain — Approx.   0 — 1000 ft.
1st Peneplain — Approx. 1000 — 3000 ft.
3rd Peneplain — Approx. 3000 — 6000 ft.

Figure 4
Provinces of Sri Lanka

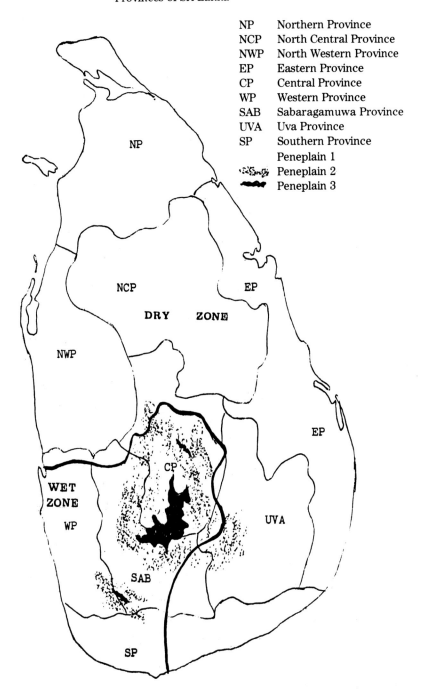

NP	Northern Province
NCP	North Central Province
NWP	North Western Province
EP	Eastern Province
CP	Central Province
WP	Western Province
SAB	Sabaragamuwa Province
UVA	Uva Province
SP	Southern Province
	Peneplain 1
	Peneplain 2
	Peneplain 3

Indian and Indo-Malayan forms with whom they have close affinities (see Deraniyagala 1955, de Silva, P.H.D.H. 1980). Deraniyagala (1955) considers some forms in Sri Lanka to be closer to the original stock than the Indian ones. In fact, some studies on reptiles and amphibians have indicated that Sri Lanka has a much higher number of relict forms than continental south India (Senanayake, Soule & Senner 1977). Moreover, within Sri Lanka, many species are highly polymorphic in their colouration, typical examples of which are the striking colour variations seen in *Ahaetulla nasuta*, *Bioga forsteni*, *Hypnale hypnale* (which exist as three species) *Naja naja naja* and *Pelamis platurus*. Hence the venomous snakes of Sri Lanka forms an important group in the Asia-Pacific region, not only taxonomically but also for the high incidence of snake bite and for some clinical symptoms produced.

Recent literature records the number of species and subspecies of snakes in Sri Lanka at 92 (de Silva 1980, de Silva 1980a) and 93 (de Silva 1982). This was assuming that some of the species and subspecies erected by Deraniyagala (1945, 1951, 1954, 1945 and 1975) and Taylor (1947 and 1950) were considered as valid formerly. However, some recent observations (de Silva 1986, 1986b, Mahendra 1984, and Gans and Toriba personal communication 1986 and 1987) show some doubt on the validity of some of these species. Considering this, de Silva (1986b) ascertained 87 species. However, the exact number has not been determined. This doubt also stands in respect of the number of species of our venomous water snakes (sea and river).

The venomous snakes of Sri Lanka are well documented, from early Christian periods in traditional literature in Eastern languages (Pali, Sinhala, Sanskrit and Tamil) and in European languages from the 17th century to present times, appearing either in a page or two or as a chapter in a book dealing with Sri Lanka or in papers dealing exclusively with snakes. Some data from these early literature are incorporated in the present work.

The criteria used to categorise venomous snakes here are snakes which possess venom apparatus (either with venom gland or Durvernoy's gland) which could cause from mild local reactions to systemic envenomation that may culminate in death. According to this criteria the venomous snakes of Sri Lanka could be placed into the three groups:

1. Highly venomous snakes where a significant proportion of bites, produce systemic envenomation and posssibly culminating in death (eg. sea snakes, kraits, cobra, Russell's viper and saw-scaled viper).
2. Moderately venomous snakes where there are occasional reports of systemic envenomation and death (eg. hump nosed vipers) or severe local reactions (eg. hump nosed vipers and green pit viper).
3. Mildly venomous snakes where there are no reported deaths, systemic, or severe local reactions but where the venom gland or Durvernoy's gland, and fangs which are canalised or grooved are present with accounts of mild local envenomation reports by some species (eg. cat snakes, and green vine snakes).

Taxonomically the venomous snakes (excluding Hydrophiidae) of Sri Lanka belongs to the families, genera and species as shown in Table 1. There are

TABLE 1
Distribution of venomous snakes * of Sri Lanka

Family	Genus	Species
Colubridae	*Cerberus*	*C. rhynchops rhynchops*
	Gerarda	*G. prevostiana*
	Chrysopelea	*C. ornata ornata*
		C. taprobanica
	Boiga	*B. trigonata trigonata*
		B. ceylonensis
		B. barnesi
		B. forsteni
	Balanophis	*B. ceylonensis*
	Ahaetulla	*A. nasuta*
		A. pulverulenta
Elapidae	*Calliophis*	*C. melanurus*
	Bungarus	*B. caeruleus*
		B. ceylonicus
	Naja	*N. naja naja*
Viperidae	*Echis*	*E. carinatus*
	Vipera	*V. russelli*
	Hypnale	*H. hypnale*
		H. nepa
		H. walli
	Trimeresurus	*T. trigonocephalus*

*Except Family Hydrophiidae.

21 species and subspecies of snakes which possess venom apparatus. However, some snakes are rare, (eg. *Balanophis ceylonensis, Hypnale walli, Hypnale nepa* and *Boiga barnesi)* and confined mainly to the rain forests, and forests and hence rarely encountered by humans. On the other hand, *Calliophis melanurus* though widely distributed is rarely encountered due to its secretive nature. A few, *Gerarda provostina* and *Hydrophis biterbiculatus* are known only from single records of specimens.

However, the venomous snakes responsible for high incidence of snake bite morbidity and mortality in Sri Lanka like the cobra, kraits and Russell's viper are relatively common, widely distributed on the island and often encountered in human, habitations (house, compound, plantations and farmland). Thus the people who are living mainly in rural areas become the most vulnerable group for snake bite. The majority (79%) of people in Sri Lanka live in rural areas (Census 1981). Consequently Sri Lanka records one of the highest death rates due to snake bite envenomation in the region and perhaps in the whole world. Recent studies (de Silva 1976a, 1980, 1981; de Silva & Ranasinghe 1983; de Silva, Jayatilleke & Ranasinghe 1983, de Silva 1987, Sawai et al 1983), indicate snake bite in Sri Lanka to be a serious medical and public health problem. Ecological studies of these snakes which cause high snake bite morbidity and mortality show the preponderance of these snakes near human habitations due to availability of food and water, ecological niches and absence of most of their natural predators.

Following is an account of the venomous land snakes of Sri Lanka. An attempt is made to record all the known taxa which possess venom apparatus (Venom or Duvernoy's gland) and the latest accepted nomenclature changes available at the time of writing are given. Each taxa is briefly described as follows: historical aspects, identification, morphology, ecology, action of venom, clinical features with an authentic case report where the offending snake is known.

Family Colubridae

The family colubridae comprises the largest group of ophidian species in the world. The majority of species in Sri Lanka belongs to this family. They live in various ecological niches, ranging from sub fossorial, arboreal and aquatic. The majority are terrestrial. However, a terrestrial snake may be found on a high tree or in water.

Their feeding habits also show a marked diversity. The fossorial species feed on earthworms and insect larvae, the terrestrial and arboreal forms feed on a wide array of animals (frogs, toads, small mammals, birds, lizards, snakes and eggs) whilst the aquatic ones feed on frogs, fish and other aquatic animals.

The gland which produces venom in colubrid snakes is known as Duvernoy's gland and not all colubrid snakes have this (Taub 1966, 1967). The Duvernoy's gland is a tubuloacinous gland composed of predominantly serous cells. The secretions enter the oral cavity via a single duct which generally opens in the oral mucosa near the posterior maxillary teeth (Taub 1967). The colubrid snakes described in this paper are the ophisthoglyphous or rear-fanged snakes. These fangs are grooved which helps to carry the venom during bite. However, Stejenger's (1893) observations show that the presence of grooved rear-fangs is not a necessity for the introduction of the secretion of Duvernoy's gland into the prey.

Although most of these snakes that are described under this family have not caused any serious medical problems, a few brief reports of mild local envenomations due to some species have been published (de Silva 1976, de Silva & Aloysius 1983). Reports of envenomation due to the so called non-venomous colubrid snakes continue to appear (da Silva & Buononato 1983/1984, de Silva & Aloysius 1983, Mamonov 1977, Mather et al 1978, Maretic & Russell 1979, Minton 1978, Ogawa & Sawai 1986). In recent times, the bites of the rear fanged *Rhabdophis tigrinus* and *R. subminiatus* have been reported to cause systemic poisoning (Mather et al 1978) or even death (Ogawa & Sawai 1986). This snake was earlier considered to be not dangerous.

Ophisthoglyphous Colubrid Snakes Of Sri Lanka

Family Colubridae

Sub family Homalopsinae

Genus: *Cerberus* Cuvier, 1829

C. rhynchops rhynchops (Schneider) 1799

English name — Dog-faced water snake

Local (Sinhala name) — *Kunudiya kaluwa*, (Tamil name) — *Appu Ar pambu*

Historical aspects:

Patrick Russell mentioned it in his classic work 'An account of Indian Serpents' in 1796.

Distinctive morphological features:

Dog-faced water snake is a medium sized (av. 600 mm) stout bodied, dull-coloured snake with a small, pear shaped head. Nostrils are situated more dorsally and are narrow slit-like. Scales on the body are rough (keeled). Tail is short and slightly compressed. It grows to about 1,200 mm in length.

Colour:

The common dorsal colour is greyish or dark chocolate brown with indistinct irregular dark cross bars. Ventrally, light yellow or creamy white with distinct black markings (fig 5). A conspicuous black stripe from the snout runs through the eye to the neck. When out of water its body dries up and gives a dull dry appearance.

Identification:

1. The distinctive bodily features described above.
2. Its coloration.
3. The ventrals are not wide (does not extend the whole ventral width like in most colubrid, elapid and viperid snakes).

Habits:

It is an aquatic snake preferring brackish water and is an excellent swimmer. It is active during day as well as night. Wall (1921) and de Silva (1980) consider it to be a diurnal snake while Whitaker (1978) considers it to be mainly nocturnal. When compared to other water snakes like *Xenochrophis piscator* which usually bites readily and savagely, *rhynchops* is an inoffensive and a quiet snake. It gives birth to about 10 young.

Food:

If feeds voraciously on fish. Wall (1921) records caudal luring of fish by *Cerberus rhynchops* at times.

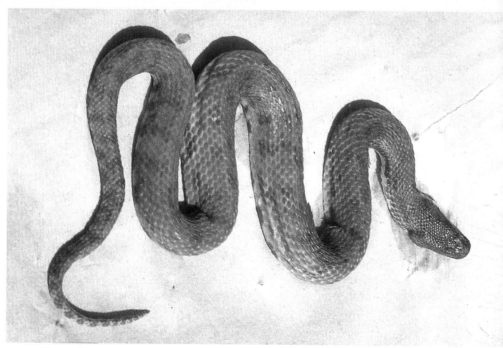

Figure 5
Cerberus rhynchops rhynchops (Photo — A. de Silva)

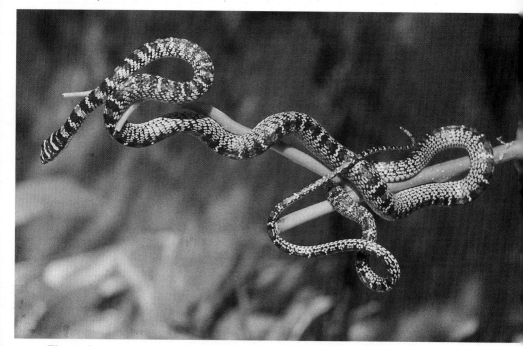

Figure 6
Chrysopelea ornata ornata (Photo — A. de Silva)

Habitat and Distribution:

It is found in crab holes, under rocks, logs and in muddy areas in lagoons, streams, creeks, rivers estuaries and mangrove swamps in the coastal areas of Sri Lanka. Taylor (1950) records capturing one specimen in a salt water lagoon at north of Trincomalee. I have observed them around Negombo (W) lagoon. It could be considered as a common snake.

Defense and Action of Venom:

On provocation it hisses, (Wall 1921), bites and produces an offensive odour and is sometimes accompanied by discharging of cloacal contents. *C. rhynchops* is an ophisthoglyphous snake and the maxillary teeth are followed by a pair of grooved fangs. However, traditional physicians believe that this snake can cause envenomation which may require treatment. According to the traditional system, the bite would give rise to symptoms such as pain, swelling and burning sensations at the site of the bite (D.G. Vijepala, personal communication 1983).

Genus: *Gerarda*, Gray, 1849

Gerarda prevostiana (Eydoux and Gervais), 1832-1837

English name — Gerard's water snake

Local (Sinhala name) — *Diyawarna (G. prevostiana* superficially resemble *Atretium schistosum* (Daudin), the Olivaceous keelback — a common water snake in Sri Lanka which is also known as *Diyawarna)*

Historical aspects:

First referred to by Eydoux & Gervais in 1837. Haly (1886) records one specimen captured in Kelani river, Colombo, by one Mr. H.F. Fernando. Wall (1921) considers that specimen no. 99 in Colombo Museum to be this. Gyi (1970) records one specimen from Sri Lanka without referring to any specific locality at the Field Museum of Natural History, U.S.A. (No. 121532). De Silva (1982) included it in his list of rare snakes of Sri Lanka. The following account of *prevostiana* are from Wall (1921) and Gyi (1970).

Distinctive morphological features:

A small snake (av. 600 mm), head as broad as the body. Nostrils slit-like, valvular and on dorsal side. Body moderately long with smooth scales. Tail short.

Colour:

The dorsal ground colour of the body is uniform dark olive green or grey. The ventral aspect of the body is grey or buff, except the throat and neck which is yellow or white. On the lateral sides of the body there is a white or yellow line.

Identification

1. Its morphology and coloration.

2.   The costals in 17 rows at midbody which reduces to 15 to 13 anterior to the vent.

Habits:

It is an aquatic snake, which sometimes comes to the land. According to Wall (1921) it is a lethargic snake on land, and does not attempt to bite. Being an aquatic snake it feeds on fish. Observations on its reproductive habits are not available.

Habitat and Distribution:

Habitat not known. It is known to inhabit coasts and estuaries and rivers. Haly (1886) records one from Kelani river.

Defense and Action of Venom:

The maxillary teeth are followed by a pair of enlarged, grooved teeth (Gyi 1970). Nothing is known on the action of its venom and there are no records of its bites.

Status:

Very rare snake, known only from two specimens,

Family — Colubridae
Sub family — Boiginae

Genus: *Chrysopelea* Boie, 1826.

There are two species *(ornata* and *taprobanica)* representing this genus.

Chrysopelea ornata ornata (Shaw), 1802

English name — The ornate snake, Gold and black snake, flying snake.
Local (Sinhala name) — *Malsara, Polmal karawela,* (Tamil name) — *Parrakum pambu.*

Historical aspects:

The first reference to this snake was by Seba in 1734. Ferguson (1877) was one of the first few to provide a brief account of the Sri Lankan form. Deraniyagala (1945) showed that there is slight difference in scales and colour from the Indian form and named it *C. ornata lankave* and subsequently re-named it *C. ornata sinhaleya* (Deraniyagala 1955) without providing reasons for this change. The validity of this subspecies has been doubted by Constable (1949). Mertens (1965) considered the form found in India and Sri Lanka to be of one subspecies, *C. ornata ornata.*

Distinctive morphological features:

It is a slender, medium/small snake. Average length about 600 mm and can grow to 1,200 mm. Head fairly flat and oval shaped, neck distinct. Tail cylindrical, slender and long, being about 1/4 its total body length. Ventral scales have lateral folds which are used in climbing.

Colour:

Head black with yellow cross-bars. Dorsal aspect of the body pale greenish-yellow with more or less distinct black cross bands. These are distinct along vertebral line and fades laterally. There is a series of red/orange flower-like spots along the spine separated by two black cross-bars. Ventral side is dull green. Due to its attractive coloration, it is considered as one of the most beautiful snakes of Sri Lanka (fig. 6).

Identification:

1. General body features and striking colour pattern.
2. The lateral folds or keels of the ventral scales.

Habits:

It is a diurnal snake, arboreal in habits. However, it may be often encountered on the ground. It is an active, fast moving snake. It has the curious habit of leaping from branch to branch, sometimes even 'gliding' down by extending the ribs and slightly arching the body. Of their temperament, most specimens observed were extremely nervous and bite savagely at the slightest provocation while a few were docile and able to be handled freely without being bitten. *Chrysopelea ornata ornata* is oviparous. The female lays about 6 — 12 eggs.

Food:

The ornate snake prefers to feed on Gekkonidae. It was often observed that it swallowed its prey alive. It also feeds on frogs, other lizards, birds and mice.

Habitat and Distribution:

It is found on small shrubs, trees and coconut palm, and mainly confined to forest patches and seldom near human habitations. Abercromby (1913) recorded it from Polgahawela (NW). According to Wall (1921) and Deraniyagala (1955), *ornata* is recorded from Veyangoda, Gampaha, Matugama (all W); Punagala (below 1,000 ft.), Wewalwatta (Ratnapura district), Balangoda, Pelmadulla (all Sab.), Kantalai (E). I have observed it in Gammana (Agalawatte) (W), Kataragama, Galle, Akuressa, Deniyaya (all S) and Kurunegala (NW). Gamini de Silva (personal communication 1983) records it from Labugama (Sab.) and from Randenigala (NC) (S.M.X. Corea, personal communication, 1987). These data suggest that it is yet confined to the first peneplain of the wet and dry zones (figs 1 and 3).

Defense and Action of Venom:

The last three or four maxillary teeth are enlarged and grooved (de Silva 1980). The author and six colleagues were bitten savagely by this snake, but there was not even a local reaction in all these cases.

Status:

This is an uncommon snake — Many in Sri Lanka and in India (Whitaker 1978) consider it to be a highly venomous snake.

Genus: *Chrysopelea* Boie, 1826

Chrysopelea taprobanica Smith 1943
English name — Sri Lanka flying snake
Local (Sinhala name) — *Dangaradanda*

Historical aspects:

Malcolm A. Smith (1943) first described this species and regarded it as peculiar to Sri Lanka. However, Constable (1949) had described one received from R. H. Beddome (Museum of Comparative Zoology .S.A. 47881) from a locality "near Madras". Taylor (1950), Deraniyagala (1955) and de Silva (1980) consider *taprobanica* to be endemic in Sri Lanka. But Mahendra (1984) following Constable (1949) included India for its range.

However, the locality referred to by R.H. Beddome needs confirmation as Beddome had collected many snakes from Sri Lanka during the latter part of 19th Century. Also, *C. taprobanica* was not reported or collected by other herpetologists from South India.

Distinctive morphological features:

Its morphological features are similar to *C. ornata ornata* and grows to about 900 mm in length.

Colour:

Dorsally, from neck to tail, is a series of wavy or zig zag black bands on the greyish brown or greenish brown background colour. Head coloration is similar to *ornata*.

Identification:
1. Its body features and colour pattern.
2. It could be distinguished from *ornata* by having an individual scale preceding the anal scale.

Habits:

Its habits are similar to *ornata*. However no observations or records were made on its reproductive habits.

Food:

Similar to *ornata*.

Habitat and Distribution:

Its habitat is similar to *ornata*. However its distribution show that it is found only in the dry zone. Smith (1943) records Kantalai (E) and Kurunegala (NW), Taylor (1950) 19 km north of Trincomalee (E). Deraniyagala (1955) adds Sigiriya (C) and Jaffna peninsula (N). De Silva (1969), Wilpattu (NW), Gamini de Silva (personal communication 1983) Yala (S) and Polonnaruwa (NC).

Defense and Action of Venom:

Ophisthoglyphous snake, nothing is known of the effects of the venom nor has any work been done.

Status:

Available evidence suggests it to be an uncommon snake.

Genus: *Boiga* Fitzinger, 1826

English name — Cat snake
Sinhala name — *Mapila*
Tamil name — *Poonai pambu* or *Wollai Pambu* (Whitaker 1978)

Snakes of this genus found in Sri Lanka have some distinct common features. The head is subovate and markedly depressed. Eyes are large and pronounced and the pupils are vertical, like that of a cat from which it received its common English name. Their distinctly constricted necks give them a viperine appearance. The body is long, slender and fairly compressed laterally. Tail is long and cylindrical. They are ophisthoglyphous snakes having posterior fangs. Many in Sri Lanka consider these snakes to be highly venomous which is probably due to their viperine appearance, and wrong identification. However it is of interest to note that the traditional physicians for many centuries had prescribed many herbal medicines for envenomation by *Boiga* species.

The following four species are found in Sri Lanka.

Boiga trigonata (Schneider) 1802
English name — The Gamma snake, common cat snake
Local (Sinhala name) — *Ran mapila*, (Tamil name) — *Chingihahu*

Historical aspects:

Russell illustrated it in 1976 and Schneider named it in 1802. Ferguson (1877) provided a brief note of this snake. The presence of two colour variations in the range (India and Sri Lanka) was recorded by Wall (1921) and Smith (1943). On the basis of these colour patterns, Mahendra (1984) regarded them as two subspecies. The form in Sri Lanka and India is *B. trigonata trigonata* (Schneider).

General morphological features:

As described under the genus. Its average length is 75 cm and reaches a maximum of 1 m.

Colour:

The dorsal colour in some are light yellowish brown to greyish brown. The head has a distinct "Y" mark. There is a vertebral series of creamy white or pale yellowish brown markings which are brownish-black edged (fig 7). These branch laterally. Ventral aspect is creamy white and has a black or brown row of spots on the outer margins. It was observed in nearly 50 specimens from different parts of the country that these markings were fairly constant.

Identification:

1. The morphological features and coloration.
2. Scale rows 21 up to mid-body.

Habits:

It is a nocturnal, arboreal snake. However it could be occasionally observed moving on the ground and at the base of mana grass *(Cymbopogon nardus* (L). When compared to *Boiga ceylonensis* and *Boiga barnesi* it is fairly temperamental and tries to attack. It is oviparous and the female lays an average of 7 eggs.

Food:

It mainly feeds on geckos and calotes lizards.

Habitat and Distribution:

During the day, they often sleep in tree holes, thatched roof, in between heaps of stones, bricks, stacks of wood and also at the base of mana grass (the dead grass at the base camouflages well with *trigonata* and is also fairly cool). As regards its distribution, the available records suggest that it is found in all the climatic zones and ascends up the second peneplain. Wall (1921) records it from Haldumulla (U), Taylor (1953) records it from Namunukula (U) 3,000 —4,500 ft altitude, Deraniyagala (1955) adds Jaffna. The author observed them at Matara, Tissa (S); Horana (W), Gampola, Peradeniya and Kandy (All C).

Defense and action of venom:

In the attack posture, *B. trigonata* raises its forebody which is formed into loops and lashes out, simultaneously often vibrating its tail. Ophisthoglyphous snake. The last two maxillary teeth are enlarged and grooved. There are no reports of its bite in Sri Lanka.

Status:

A common snake, but many people kill it.

Boiga ceylonensis (Gunther) 1858
English name — Sri Lanka cat snake, Gunther's cat snake
Local (Sinhala name) — *Nidi mapila*, (Tamil name) —

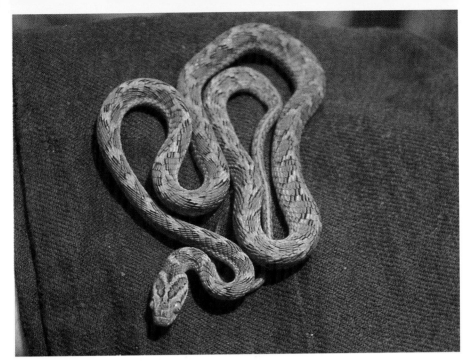

Figure 7
Boiga trigonata trigonata (Photo — A de Silva)

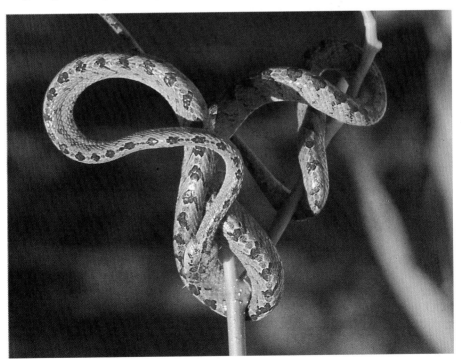

Figure 8
Boiga ceylonensis (Photo — A de Silva)

Historical aspects:

Gunther described this snake in 1858 from a Sri Lankan specimen. Deraniyagala (1955) considered the species which occurs in Sri Lanka and India to be two subspecies and the form in Sri Lanka to be the "forma typica".

General morphological features.

As described under the genus: The average length of *B. ceylonensis* is about 75 cm and may grow up to 1.35 m.

Colour:

The dorsal colour varies between light reddish brown to dark reddish brown. There is a series of dark brown or brownish black vertebral blotches which may extend on to the lateral sides (fig 8). These in some, gives a striped appearance. The head is brown with a dark or light brown lung shaped mark on it and a postocular stripe. The ventral aspect is pale reddish brown with a mixture of grey or yellow and speckled or spotted with brown. In some, from the neck to mid-body is yellow.

Identification:

Identified by the morphological features and its colour.

Habits:

The habits of *Boiga ceylonensis* is similar to *B. trigonata*. However, in temperament they appear milder. Occasionally they have been observed to bite without much provocation.

Food:

It feeds on geckos, *Calotes* and *Mabuya* species.

Habitat and distribution:

Habitat of *B. ceylonensis* is similar to *B. trigonata*. Regarding its distribution, Wall (1921) records Sigiriya, Kandy, Peradeniya, Nanu Oya (all C), Badulla (U), Moneragala and Horana (W). Deraniyagala (1955) adds Namunukula (U), de Silva (1969) records Kalutara. Horana (W), Ratnapura and Kahawatta (Sab.); Passara, Bandarawela, Haputale (all U); Kotmale, Gammaduwa (C). Author observed it to be quite common in Gampola, Weligalla, Kegalle, Gallakelle Estate (Mademahanuwara) (all C), Polonnaruwa (NC), Kahawatta (Sab.), Kosgama (W). Gamini de Silva (personal communciation 1983) adds Labugama — Kalatuwawa (Sab.), Udawalawa (S), Anuradhapura (NC). Abercromby (1913) records Matale and Bogawanthalawa (C), Anuradhapura (NC), Polgahawela, Horana and Kalutara (W). These data suggests that it is common in the three peneplains and the three climatic zones.

Defense and action of venom:

It is an ophisthoglyphous snake. Deraniyagala (1955) describes a case of a chicken weighing 12 ozs dying 47 minutes after being bitten by this snake. A post mortem of the chicken showed abundant blood clots in the peritoneal cavity and the atria of the heart was congested. I was bitten on several occasions while handling this species and on only a few occasions was there a slight swelling at the site of bite, which usually subsided in an hour (de Silva and Aloysius 1983).

Status:

B. ceylonensis is a common snake and at present it is getting overkilled (de Silva 1984).

Boiga barnesi (Gunther) 1869
English name — Barnes' cat snake
Local (Sinhala name) — *Panduru mapila*

Historical aspects:

This snake was first described by Gunther in 1869 from a collection made by R.H. Barnes. Subsequently, Willey (1903) recorded two specimens from the Colombo Museum collection.

Distinctive morphological features:

As recorded under the genus. However, the available records and specimens observed show that *barnesi* is the smallest of the genus *Boiga* in Sri Lanka and grows to about 90 cm in length.

Colour:

The dorsal colour of the body is a mixture of purple and brown. There is a series of brown blotches, not as distinct as in *B. ceylonensis*. Ventrally it is greyish white with dark mottling.

Identification:
1. Morphological features and the coloration.
2. Presence of 2 — 3 preoculars.

Habits:

Similar to other species of the genus, except that it has not been recorded inside human dwellings, whereas the other species of *Boiga* usually are. Also nothing is known of its breeding habits except for the record of observing two eggs in a preserved museum specimen (de Silva 1969).

Food:

Similar to *ceylonensis*.

Habitat and distribution:

This snake is mainly confined to forests where it lies during the day in tree holes, shrubs, crevices etc. Regarding its distribution, Deraniyagala (1955) records Haputale (U), Balangoda (Sab.), Talagasmankada (S), Gammaduwa, Matale and Kandy (all C). Author observed this species from Udawattakelle, Kandy. It is mainly confined to the wet zone.

Defense and action of venom:

Nothing is known yet.

Status:

Uncommon and seldom met. Endemic to Sri Lanka.

Boiga forsteni (Dumeril, Bibron and Dumeril) 1854
English name — Forsten's cat snake
Local (Sinhala name) — *Naga mapila*

Historical aspects:

It was first brought to scientific notice by Dumeril and Bibron in 1854.

Distinctive morphological features:

Its general features conform to the characteristics of the genus, except that this is the largest among the cat snakes in Sri Lanka, growing up to an average of 1.2 m. De Silva (1969) records a female in the Colombo Museum collection measuring 1.73 m long. The largest in my collection measured 1.8 m (de Silva 1976). Deraniyagala (1955) records a specimen 2 m long.

Colour:

In coloration this snake is highly polymorphic. Four colour variations have been observed. Of these the most striking colours are: in one, the dorsal colour is grey with black and white markings giving a checkered appearance (fig 9). Ventral colour is white often with black mottling. In the other variety the dorsal colour is uniform red or crimson brown (fig 10). This is known as the *"Le mapila"* (Blood cat snake) locally and many people fear that it sucks the blood of sleeping humans.

Identification:

Identified by its bodily features and colour.

Habits:

Similar to *B. trigonata*, in captivity they become very 'tame'.

Food:

It feeds on calotes, lizards, birds, chicken, poultry eggs and small mammals.

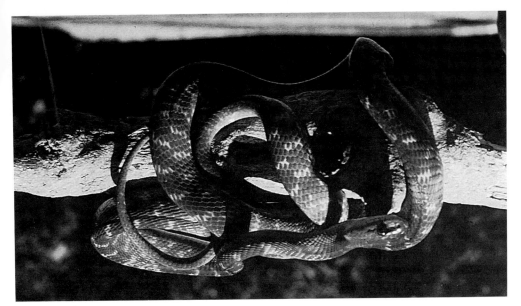

Figure 9
Boiga forsteni (black colour) (Photo — A de Silva)

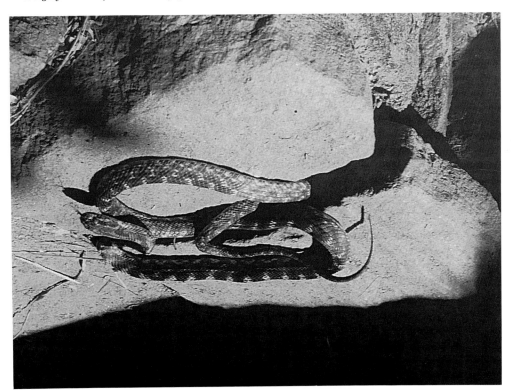

Figure 10
Boiga forsteni (reddish brown colour) (Photo — A de Silva)

Habitat and distribution:

They usually live in holes in large trees. It was observed that they usually frequent the same hole for months. Also, it was observed many times that they come to roofs of houses.

Regarding its distribution, Abercromby (1913) records Anuradhapura (NC), Wall (1921) Henaratagoda (W), Galatura (below 150 m), Massena Estate Balangoda (1,000 m) (Sab.) Taylor (1950) 12 miles north of Trincomalee, Deraniyagala (1935) records, Dodampe (near Ratnapura) and Hatagala (Dehiovita) (Sab.), Matugama (W), Vatapola (NC), Colombo Museum collection are from; Kalutara (W), Madampe, (NW), Kahawatta (Sab.), Anuradhapura (NC), Kudremalai, Mullaittivu (N) (de Silva 1969). Pearless (1909) records it from Badulla (U) (680 mm).

I have observed it in Serukelle (NW), Anuradhapura, Polonnaruwa, Galnewa and Talawa (all NC), Naula (C), Labugama (Sab.), Telijjawila (S), Horana (W). The available locality suggests that *Boiga forsteni* is widely distributed in the first and second peneplains of the three climatic zones.

Defense and action of venom:

When cornered or irritated, it threatens by hissing fiercely and at the same time raising its forebody and looping into a figure of eight. Nicholls (1929) recorded that he could not extract sufficient venom from a large Forstenis' cat snake to kill a guinea pig. I was once bitten by a large *B. forsteni* and although no local effects were observed there was giddiness which lasted for about 10 minutes (de Silva & Aloysius 1983).

Status:

This is an uncommon snake compared to *B. ceylonensis* or *B. trigonata*. However, at present it is losing much of its habitation due to clearing of forests for vast agriculture programmes in the country. Occasional specimens entering human dwellings in the night are often killed. Many people in Sri Lanka attribute deaths caused by *Bungarus* envenomation to *Boiga forsteni*.

Genus — *Balanophis* Smith 1938

The generic name *Balanophis* was instituted by Malcolm Smith in 1938. However Malnate (1960) and Malnate & Minton (1965) considered *Balanophis ceylonensis* congeneric with *Rabdophis*. However, this allocation is now doubted by many (Underwood, Toriba, personal communication, 1985) due to difference in some characters. Hence in this report, Smith's generic name *Balanophis* is used. This genus is represented by a single species *ceylonensis* which is found only in Sri Lanka.

Balanophis ceylonensis (Gunther) 1858
English name — Sri Lanka keelback, Blossom krait
Local (Sinhala name) — *Nihaluwa, mal karawala*

Historical aspects:

This snake was first brought to scientific notice by Gunther in 1858. However, only a little is known about its ecology.

General morphological features:

It is a small snake of average length 30 cm. Smith (1943) records a male 50 cm and female 46 cm long. Body is moderately elongate and cylindrical. The dorsal surface appears rough due to the keeled scales. Head is small with large eyes and a fairly evident neck. Tail is moderate. Superficially, it closely resembles the body features and coloration of a very common snake in Sri Lanka, the buff striped keelback *Amphiesma stolata*.

Colour:

Dorsal ground colour is greyish blue. Head is dull orange or brownish. Body has a series of indistinct black cross bars with a light orange or brown spot (fig 11). The ventral surface is light bluish grey.

Identification:

Its colour and bodily features.

Habits:

It is a slow moving, inoffensive, terrestrial snake, which lives most part of the day under decaying vegetation. When excited it expands and flattens its body exhibiting scarlet interstitial skin. It is an oviparous snake. Abercromby (1913) and Deraniyagala (1955) recorded brief descriptions of eggs and young.

Food:

Deraniyagala (1955) recorded hatchlings feeding on grasshoppers and de Silva (1969) recorded finding a partially digested frog in the gut of a preserved specimen.

Habitat and distribution:

B. ceylonensis is mainly confined to forests and rain forests and is found lying within decaying wet vegetation. Its colour harmonises well with the fallen leaves. Following are some localities where this snake has been collected or seen. Haly (1886) Udugama (S), Wall (1921) Peradeniya (C), Punagala Estate (Yatiyantota) (Sab.), Lennock Estate (Uva) (915 — 1,220 m) Balangoda (Sab.), Deraniyagala (1955) records Deniyaya (S), Varigama mountains (Pelmadulla) (Sab.) Yatiyantota (Sab.), Kegalle (Sab.), Bandarawela (Uva) and from Uva patnas, de Silva (1969) adds Kuruvita (Sab.). I have observed them at Labugama and Sinharajha forests. This data suggests that *Balanophis* is confined to the wet zone forests and rain forests from about 150 — 1,525 m above sea level.

Defense and action of venom:

Maxillary teeth followed by two enlarged, curved, grooved fangs (Smith

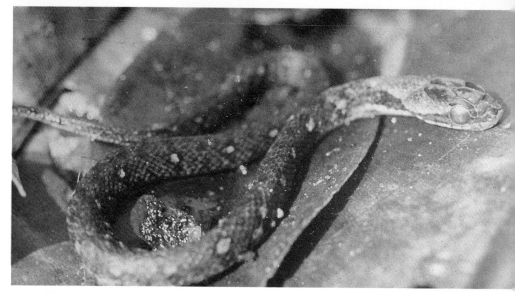

Figure 11
Balanophis ceylonensis (Photo — S. Kotagama)

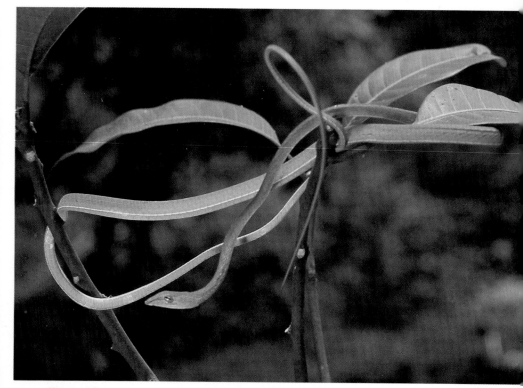

Figure 12
Ahaetulla nasuta (Photo — A de Silva)

1943). I (de Silva and Aloysius 1983) have observed a person who kept this snake as a pet, being bitten on his hand. There was pain, swelling and redness of the hand and a complaint of headache which subsided within two days. Furthermore, people living near Sinharajha rain forest fear this snake as much as they fear a viper (P.B. Karunaratne, personal communication 1986).

Status:

It is an uncommon, secretive snake, mainly confined to rain forests. It has lost much of its habitat.

Genus: *Ahaetulla* Link 1807

There are two species of snakes (*nasuta* and *pulverulenta*) belonging to this genus in Sri Lanka.

Ahaetulla nasuta (Lacepede) 1789

English name — Green vine snake, green whip snake, eye pecker.

Local (Sinhala name) — *Ahaetulla*, (Tamil name) — *Kan kuthi pambu, pachchai pambu.*

Historical aspects:

Lacepede made a brief description of it in 1789. The Portuguese historian, Ribeiro, mentioned in his book about history of Sri Lanka in 1685, the tendency of this snake to dart at the victim's eyes.

General morphological features:

It has a long, slender and markedly compressed body. The average length is 90 cm. Specimens over 1.5 m are not uncommon and the largest I had measured was 1.675 m. Largest in Colombo Museum is 1.68 m (de Silva 1969). Wall (1921) records one 1.944 m long. The head is fairly depressed and acutely pointed with a rostral appendage. Tail is cylindrical and long.

Colour:

The head, dorsal side of the body and whole tail of the commonly seen and well distributed colour variety is grass green (fig. 12), and the ventral aspect is light green or yellowish greeen with two white lines on either side. The dorsal scales are dull and hence not shiny. There are occasional colour variations. Wall (1921) and Deraniyagala (1955) record four such colorations. However, the most unusual coloration for a "Green" vine snake is rose pink dorsally with pinkish buff ventrally.

Identification:

The striking bodily features and the coloration.

Habits:

Ahaetulla nasuta is a diurnal and an arboreal snake, but may descend to the ground like other arboreal snakes. It moves fast in its arboreal habitats. I have further observed many times how it entangles itself with its long prehensile tail onto branches of trees, or when captured entangles the hand. The vine snake produces about 5 — 12 live young ones.

Food:

Feeds on calotes and gecko lizards, birds, frogs, mice and occasionally, other snakes. Whitaker (1978) observes the Sri Lanka form catching and feeding on fish.

Habitat and distribution:

It is found in low bushes, shrubs, and trees, especially near streams and in forests. It is equally commonly found on hedges near human habitations. *Ahaetulla nasuta* is well distributed in the island, in the three climatic zones and the three peneplains.

Defense and action of venom:

When cornered or provoked it rears its head and forebody, curves and dilates thus exposing the black and white pattern of the skin (fig 13). Often simultaneously it opens its mouth wide, presenting a menacing appearance. It has the tendency of attacking the face, perhaps attracted by the eyes, which has earned it the ancient Sinhala name 'Ahaetulla' (= 'eye picker'), a feature observed by many ophiologists. *A. nasuta* is an ophisthoglyphous snake, with grooved fangs. Although it is fairly common snake encountered by people, very seldom are people bitten by it. As regards its venom, Alcok and Rogers (as quoted by Wall (1921) observes close resemblance of its venom to that of the cobra. I have observed about seven people bitten by *nasuta* (including the author) and noted no reaction, local or systemic except in three people where there was slight pain and swelling at the site of bite, which subsided in a few hours. Wall (1921) observed a sampwallah in Bangalore bitten on the hand which resulted in swelling up to the forearm and causing numbness (without systemic poisoning) which subsided in two days. For Sri Lanka, Abercromby (1910) record his servant suffering for a couple of days from local pain and swelling. Further, this particular snake has bitten a wild kitten which died of great pain. Symptoms recorded are giddiness, followed by spasms and insensibility.

Status:

A common snake. However, recent observations show that many are being killed.

Ahaetulla pulverulenta (Dumeril, *Bibron & Dumeril*) 1854.
English name — Brown speckled whip snake
Local (Sinhala name) — *Henakandaya*, (Tamil name) — *Komberimookan*

Historical aspects:

First described by Dumeril, Bibron & Dumeril in 1854. In fact the

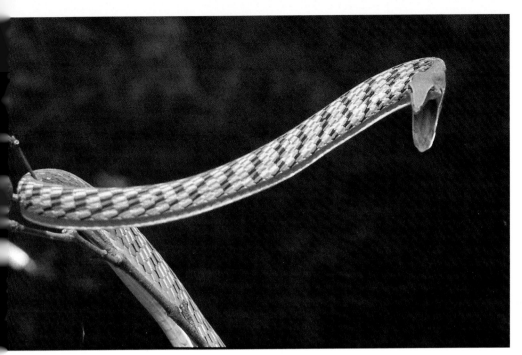

Figure 13
Ahaetulla nasuta (Threat posture) (Photo — A de Silva)

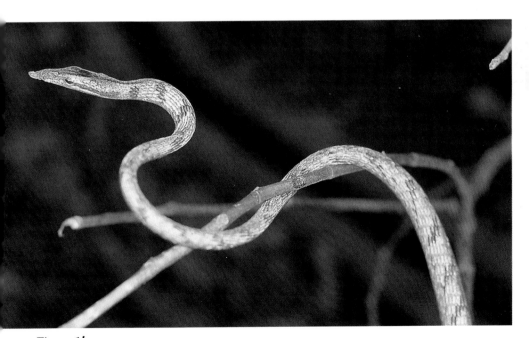

Figure 14
Ahaetulla pulverulenta (Photo — A de Silva)

Portuguese historian, J. Rubeiro, briefly mentioned this snake in 1685. Deraniyagala (1955) considered the Sri Lankan taxon to be a subspecies considering Smith's (1943) observations of differences in the ventral and sub caudal counts. However de Silva (1969) showed that the available evidence does not justify this.

General morphological features:

Similar to *A. nasuta* except that it is slightly smaller than the former, the average length being 90 cm. De Silva (1969) recorded a specimen 1.522 m long. Also *pulverulenta* has a prominent rostral appendage with small scales.

Colour:

General body colour is light brown or a mixture of light brown and grey. There are dark brown uneven markings, on the body and on the head (fig 14). Ventral aspect is reddish brown.

Identification:

Morphological features, specially the rostral appendage with small scales and its colour.

Habits:

Similar to *A. nasuta*.

Food:

Geckos, lizards and frogs.

Habitat and distribution:

It is found on low shrub and trees in forested areas. Abercromby (1910) records thatched roofs. As regards its distribution, Kandy (C), Matale (C), Anuradhapura (NC), Kurunegala (NW), Ratnapura (Sab.), Balangoda (Sab.), Horana (W),Wadduwa (W) are recorded by Abercromby (1913). Wall (1921) adds Weuda (NW), Galle (S), Veyangoda (W), Kalupahana (Sab.), Haladamulla (Uva), Peradeniya (C), Rasagala (Balangoda) and Punagala (Yatiyantota) (Sab.). Deraniyagala (1955) adds Eluvankulam, Colombo Museum collection localities as recorded by de Silva (1969) are Matugama (W), Ratnapura (Sab.), Bellanbandipalassa, Kitulgala (Sab.), Mousakanda, Taylor (1950) adds 19 km north of Trincomalee. According to these collection localities, it is evident that *pulverulenta* is mainly confined to the first and second peneplains and the three climatic zones of Sri Lanka.

Defense and action of venom:

Threat posture is similar to *A. nasuta*. It is an ophisthoglyphous snake with grooved fangs. Nothing is observed or recorded of is venom or bites. Except for a rather curious ancient record by Rubeiro (1685) in which the victim lived for some years without being cured of his symptoms. Further, it is popularly believed to be so venomous that the victim is supposed to be paralysed and wither away as if he had been struck by lighting. Hence the local name *Henakandaya* (= Thunderbolt snake).

Status:

It is not as common as the other members of the genus.

Family Elapidae

This is medically the most important group (except one species) of snakes in Sri Lanka. Their fangs are situated anteriorly in each maxilla (proteroglyphous). Hence their bites are more effective than the ophisthoglyphous snakes. Their venom is highly toxic, being mainly neurotoxic. Snakes of Family Elapidae, *Naja naja* and the two species of *Bungarus* accounts for 51 - 55 percent of deaths due to snake bite envenomation in Sri Lanka (de Silva 1976a and 1987a). Furthermore the majority of these bites took place in or near human dwellings. This was specially evident in krait bites. In a study of a total of 86 krait bites, all occurred inside residences (de Silva 1986a). The family is represented in Sri Lanka by three genera with four species (Table 1). They range from the small slender, 30 cm long *Calliophis melanurus* to the thick-bodied 1.8 m long *Naja naja naja*.

With regards to the distribution, all elapids are well distributed compared to some species of the family Viperidae.

Genus: *Bungarus* Daudin, 1803

In Sri Lanka there are two species of snakes of the genus *Bungarus;* *caeruleus* and *ceylonicus*.

Bungarus caeruleus (Schneider) 1801

English name — Common krait
Local (Sinhala name) — *Thel karawela, Magamaruwa* (in the dry zone it is erroneously called *Mapila* and *Habara*). (Tamil name) — *Yettadi viriyan, Karuvelan pambu*

Historical aspects:

The ancient traditional literature on the treatment of snake bite in Sri Lanka includes herbal remedies for krait bite envenomation (Rev. Principal, Mayurapada Pirivena (1272 — 1284 AC *"Pra Yoga Ratnavaliya"*) (Gnanawimala 1943). Knox (1681) too, provides a brief note on the kraits. In scientific literature Seba illustrated it in 1735.

General morphological features:

B. caeruleus is a medium sized snake growing to an average of 75 — 90 cm to a maximum of 1.5 m. Head is subovate, eyes are small and nostrils large. Neck fairly distinct. Body is long and cylindrical.

Colour:

The dorsal colour of the body and head varies from dark steel blue-black and seldom with a slight trace of brown. From neck to tail there is a series of thin white cross bands usually arranged in pairs (fig 15). These tend to reduce to vertebral white spots or may disappear completely with age (fig 16). The belly is lustrous white. The scales on the body are highly glossy.

Identification:
1. Its morphological features and colour.
2. Hexagonal enlarged vertebrals (fig 17).

Habits:

B. caeruleus is a terrestrial snake, and nocturnal in habits. It is rarely seen by day. Only on two of nearly 100 observations was the snake seen during day time. Of its temperament, most observers (Wall 1921, Deraniyagala 1955, de Silva 1976, de Silva 1980) state that it is of "inoffensive disposition" or "least aggressive". The observations made on many live snakes during "day time" confirmed these statements (except very few instances). However, its behavioral pattern completely changes from dusk. Being cryptozoic it becomes active at dusk (from 6 to 8 pm) and in the night, most are vicious and bite without provocation. A recent study (de Silva 1987b) confirmed this. In fact, Ponnambalam (1939) records one fatal instance where *B. caeruleus* had attack without any provocation. A similar behavioral pattern has been observed by Khan & Tasnim (1986) for Parkistani specimens. The female lays 5 to 10 eggs and stays with them.

Food:

They feed mainly on other snakes and young rodents. During dry season, they become extremely 'fond' of water.

Habitat and distribution:

During the day they stay in termite mounds, rodent holes, among the debris of wood, stones and in coconut estates underneath heaps of coconut husks and leaves. In the dry zones it was observed a few times, in the crevices and holes of wattle and daub houses (huts).

As regards its distribution, the following are some localities found in the literature. Wall (1921) records Jaffna (N), Polgahawela and Veyangoda (W). Ponnambalam (1939) Ottaimavadi (E), Taylor (1950) adds Negombo (W), Deraniyagala (1955) Colombo, de Silva (1980) Polonnaruwa (NC). I have observed it at Madurankuli, Puttalam, Tabbowa, Chilaw, Bandarakoswatte, Serukele (all NW). Many parts of Anuradhapura, Galnewa, Maha Illuppallama, and Polonnaruwa districts, Bakamuna, Dammina (Piburattwa) (all NC), Gamini de Silva (personal communication 1983) Wilachchiya, Polonnaruwa (NC), Kataragama (S). These locality data suggest that *caeruleus* is confined mainly to the dry zone (mainly North, North west, North central and North eastern up to South), Intermediate zone (there are no records of it from the

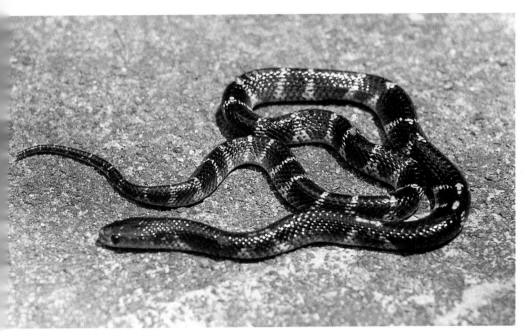

Figure 15
Bungarus caeruleus (Photo — A de Silva)

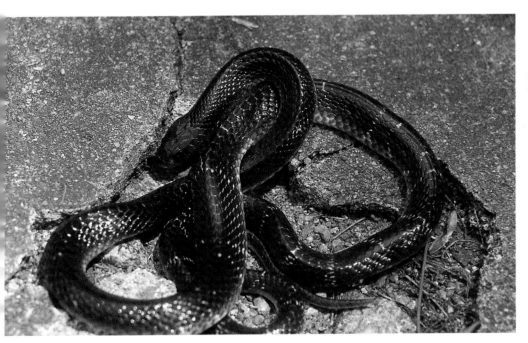

Figure 16
Bungarus caeruleus (adult with reduced white bands) (Photo — A de Silva)

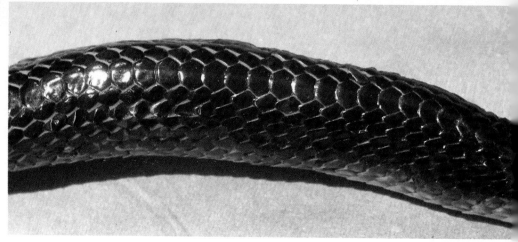

Figure 17
Enlarged vertebrals (Photo — A de Silva)

hilly areas and the Southern portion of this zone). Two localities recorded by Wall (1921) Polgahawela (NW), and Veyangoda (W) are within the wet zone, however they are situated close to the boundary (fig 18).

Defense and action of venom:

Bungarus caeruleus will not exhibit any conspicuous threat posture like most other snakes except its rather sudden nervous darts, with its body slightly inflated and flattened. As defense, 'balling' was often exhibited during the day.

Bungarus caeruleus is a proteroglyphous snake. Their fangs are small when compared with that of *Vipera russelli* or *Trimeresurus trigonocephalus*.

Bungarus caeruleus bites are common in Sri Lanka. One of the earliest case reports of *B. caeruleus* bites from Sri Lanka is by Pereira (1875). But it is reported under the name Mapila (a Sinhala name for *Boiga* erroneously used for kraits). The symptoms recorded are typical of krait poisoning. Ponnambalam (1939) reports a fatal bite in which the offending snake.(*B. caeruleus* 2' 8½" long) had been immediately killed and sent for identification. The victim had the following symptoms: Burning pain in the bitten part 30 mins after bite, dizziness, pain all over body, slight swelling around bite, difficulty in breathing, drooping of head, ptosis, slurred speech, loss of taste, severe abdominal pain.

Fernando and Dias (1982) in their case report records the following clinical features and the course of management. The victim was admitted to the hospital 15½ hours after the bite. Initially he had been treated by a traditional snake bite physician. On admission the patient was drowsy. He also had bilateral ptosis, complete ophthalmoplegia, slurred speech, bilateral coarse crepitations in the lungs, and the tenderness of the abdomen. He was managed with antisnake venom (AVS) and ventilation which are considered most important in krait bite management.

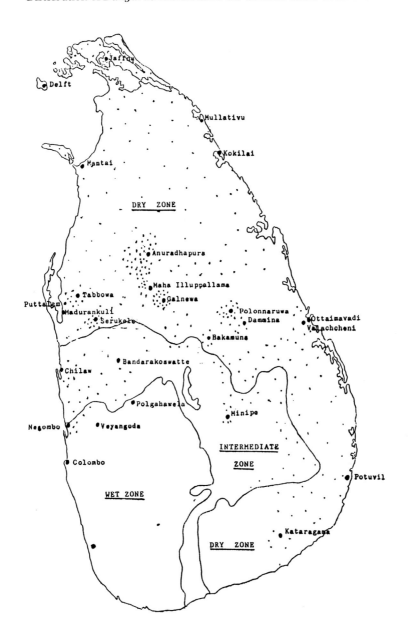

Key

•   Localities in the literature and sites collected

⋰⋱   Commonly found

∴   Probable extended distribution

In a study (de Silva 1987b) of 27 fatal cases of *B. caeruleus* bites where the offending snakes were killed and some sent for identification, the following were observed. Bites occurred while sleeping on the ground in the night. Lack of pain for some time. Negligible swelling in a few, abdominal tenderness, salivation, respiratory distress, slurring of speech and ptosis. Wall (1921) records that 'violent' abdominal pain is peculiar to krait envenomation.

Status:

Many early authors considered it as a rare snake. Recent field observations, however showed that it is a fairly common snake in the dry zone. However, due to vast agricultural programmes in the dry zone (Mahaweli River Development Project) most of their natural habitats are getting destroyed and in the process, many get killed.

Bungarus ceylonicus Gunther 1864
English name — Sri Lanka krait
Local (Sinhala name) — *Mudu karawala*, (Tamil name) — *Kundan karawila*

Historical aspects:

A brief taxonomical account of it was given by A. Gunther in 1864. Deraniyagala (1955) considered *B. ceylonicus* to occur as two subspecies. *B. c. ceylonicus* and *B. c. karawala* on the retention of white cross bars and that the latter to be of smaller size and is found above 760 m. However, recent observations and studies (de Silva 1987a, de Silva & Pereira 1987) show that these criteria are insufficient for this separation.

General morphological features:

Its general features are similar to those of *B. caeruleus* except that it is smaller in size. Average length is about 70 cm to usual maximum length of 90 cm. However specimen over 1 m in length are on record, including two unusual records of 1.153 m (de Silva 1979) and 1.346 m long (de Silva and Pereira 1987).

Colour:

Dorsal colour is shiny steel blue black with distinct white bands (fig 19). This colour pattern extends to the ventral side of the body, but they are pale and diffused and are not distinct as on the dorsal side. With age the white dorsal bands reduce to white vertebral spots. These spots gradually disappear causing the dorsal aspect of the body to appear completely black. Their scales are smooth and shiny.

Identification:

1. Morphological features and colour.
2. Fifteen scale rows along the whole body length and enlarged vertebrals.

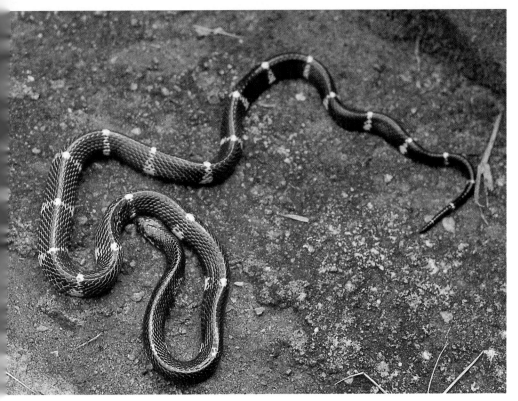

Figure 19
Bungarus ceylonicus (Photo — A de Silva)

3. It could be distinguished from *B. caeruleus* by the white broad bands and
    black bands on the ventral surface.

Habits:

Bungarus ceylonicus is a terrestrial snake with nocturnal habits. During
the day they stay in their favorite niches. The female lays eggs and gravid
specimen in the author's collection contained six eggs (de Silva 1987a).

Food:

It feeds on other snakes specially earth snakes (Uropeltids and Aspidura
species), skinks, geckos and occasionally small mammals (Wall 1921, 1923 and
1924, de Silva 1979 and 1987a).

Habitat and distribution:

The Sri Lanka krait prefers a cool moist habitat. During the day they
conceal themselves under perishing vegetation, in forest and cultivated land, in
termite mounds, under stones, in burrows in embankments and crevices.
Regarding its distribution, the following are some localities recorded.

Abercromby (1913) Colombo and about(w), Kandy, Rangala, Dimublla and Hanguranketa (all C), Badulla (U), Balangoda (Sab.). Wall (1921) adds, Peradeniya (C), Kalupahana, Haladamulla and Punagala (Yatiyantota) (all Sab.) and Matugama (W). Deraniyagala (1955) adds Ratnapura (Sab.), Welimada (C), Guruthalawa (C), Bandarawela and Namunukula (U). Fernando (1977) Horton plains (C) (2,358 m). The author has observed them in Welikanda, Hatugoda, Sinhapitiya, Mahara, Tambiligala, Udaovita (all in Gampola 490 m), Peradeniya University grounds and Mahakanda, Palledeltota, Pussellawa, Pupuressa, Hakgala (1,700 m), Muruthalawa, Medamahanuwara (all in C), Kahawate (Sab.), Opatha and Kanneliya forest (S). These data show that *Bungarus ceylonicus* is found from about mean sea level up to 2,358 m or in the three peneplains of the wet and intermediate climatic zones. (Fig 20).

Defense and action of venom:

When provoked their bodies are thrown into loose coils, the head is usually hidden beneath the coils and the tongue is frequently put out. On touching their bodies, they show signs of irritability with convulsive jerkings of the body. Like *B. caeruleus*, no particular threat posture was observed, except slight flattening of the body. *B. ceylonicus* is milder in temperament when compared to *B. caeruleus*. Out of 35 specimens observed, only one, a juvenile, was observed to bite a stick. Recently when a battery operated stunning rod (Hayashi and Tanaka 1982) for immobilizing, was tested on a large (90 cm) *B. ceylonicus*, it bit a piece of cloth savagely.

A few cases of *B. ceylonicus* bites (where the offending snake had been captured and identified) are recorded. One of the first cases on record is by Green (1908). Symptoms recorded are, 1½ hours after the bite the victim was drowsy and was worse 6 hours after the bite. At this stage he had been given a little 'Whiskey' after which he had vomited (yellow colour). Ten hours after the bite, the man was 'feverish' and 'insensible' and died 12 hours after the bite. I (de Silva 1979) have observed a case of mild envenomation where a young girl was bitten by a *Bungarus ceylonicus* (the offending snake *B. ceylonicus* was captured alive and brought with the patient and identified). There was no pain or swelling. She was only feeling drowsy from which she recovered.

Status:

Bungarus ceylonicus is not an uncommon snake in certain localities like Matugama (altitude 15 m) and Gampola (altitude 490 m). However, at present it is losing most of its habitat.

Genus: *Calliophis* Gray 1834

***Calliophis melanurus* (Shaw) 1802**
English name — Sri Lanka coral snake, slender coral snake
Local (Sinhala name) — *Depath Kaluwa*

Historical aspects:

A brief account of a specimen from Sri Lanka was first given by Haly in

Figure 20
Distribution of *Bungarus ceylonicus* in the Climatic Zones of Sri Lanka

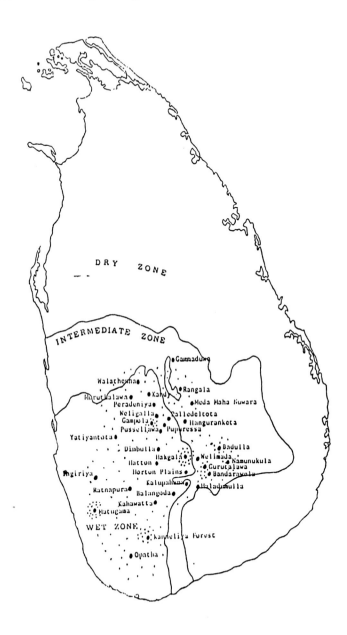

Key

•   Localities in the literature and sites collected

   Commonly found

∴   Probable extended distribution

1886. In 1951, Deraniyagala considered it as an endemic subspecies, and named it *Calliophis melanurus sinhaleyus*. However, this requires further study.

General morphological features:

These are generally small (average length 20 cm and maximum about 37.5 cm) slender, cylindrical snakes. The snake has a rounded snout with an indistinct neck and resembles a thin pencil. From head to the tail, the body is of similar girth with a short tail.

Colour:

Dorsally the body is light brown, with a darker brown spot on each scale. The head and neck is black above with yellow spots on the occiput. Tail has two distinct black rings (fig 21). Ventral aspect of the body brownish yellow, and near the vent, a distinct red or scarlet patch (fig 22). Tail is blue and gray. Scales on body are smooth.

Identification:

1. Morphological features and colour
2. Costal scales on the body in 13 rows

Habits:

It is a terrestrial snake, which hides during the day. Wall (1921) and de Silva (1980) consider it to be a diurnal snake but more nocturnal in activities. Whitaker (1978) has observed the Indian specimens to be nocturnal and occasionally active in early morning. Specimens when freely handled did not attempt to bite. They burrow into loose sand. Regarding their reproductive habits nothing was observed nor recorded in the literature. However, an Indian species is recorded to lay eggs (Whitaker 1978).

Food:

It was observed to be ophiophagus and feeds on other small nonvenomous snakes and once cannibalism was also observed.

Habitat and distribution:

In the dry zone they are confined to the scrub jungles and monsoon forests including near human habitations. During the day they lie under decaying vegetation, underneath logs, under rubble and also burrow in loose sand. As regards their distribution the following are recorded in the literature. Haly (1886) Tissamaharama (S), Willey (1903) Hopewell estate (Balangoda) (Sab.), dock yard (Trincomalee), near Kantalai tank (E), Abercromby (1913) adds Matale (C). Taylor (1950) Clodagh estate (Rattota) (C), Deraniyagala (1949) Pallewela (W), (1951) Anuradhapura, Okanda, Manampitiya, Mihintale, Horivila, Lahugala (all NC), Nalugas Aru and Balangoda (Sab.), Deraniyagala (1955) adds Wilpattuwa (NW). Gamini de Silva (personal communication

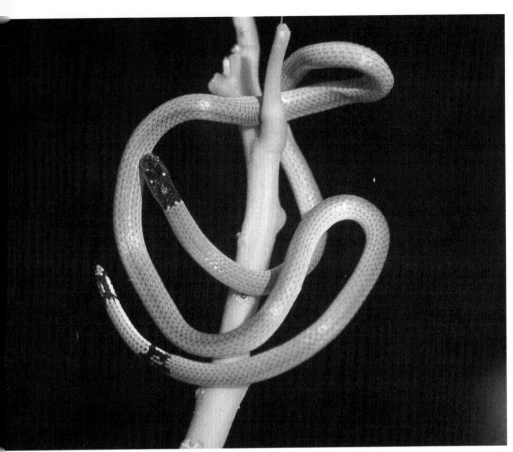

Figure 21
Calliophis melanurus (Photo — A de Silva)

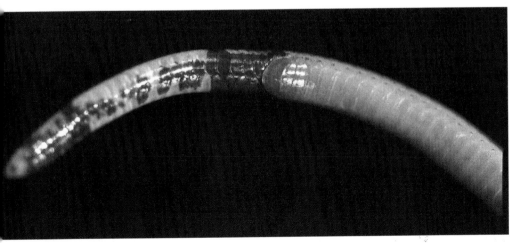

Figure 22
Calliophis melanurus (Red patch near vent) (Photo — A de Silva)

1983) Polonnaruwa, Puttalam. I have observed it from Chilaw and Serukele (NW), Galenbindunuwewa (NC) and Matale (C). Cyril Wijesundara (personal communication 1987) Lunawa (Ambalantota) (S). These localities suggests that Sri Lanka coral snake is mainly confined to the first peneplain in the dry zone. However, records of it from Matale and Balangoda show that it is found in the intermediate and wet zones up to the second peneplain. (Fig 23).

Threat posture and action of venom:

Observations made on seven live specimens did not show any attacking postures except the common defensive or threat posture of curling its tail, exhibiting the bright scarlet patch. *C. melanurus* is proteroglyphous. The effects of its venom are unknown. It has not been known to cause any problem for human beings in Sri Lanka to date. According to Sir Joseph Fayrer (1872) (as quoted by Willey 1903) the venom is virulent, and fowls, bitten by some species of *Calliophis* died within 1 to 3 hours.

Status:

Most works pertaining to Sri Lanka ophiology states it is a rare snake. However recent field observations show that in certain areas of the dry zone it is not uncommon.

Genus: *Naja* Laurenti 1768

In Sri Lanka the genus *Naja* is represented by one subspecies, *Naja naja naja* (Linne)

Naja naja naja (Linne) 1758

English name — Cobra
Local (Sinhala name) — *Naya, Nagaya* (Tamil name) — *Nalla pambu, Naga pambu*

Historical aspects:

The cobra is the most well known snake in Sri Lanka from pre Christian times. Age-old customs and tradition regard it as a deity, a guardian, an evil or a reincarnation of a departed family member. It is the most widely used reptile motif in art and sculpture in Sri Lanka (de Silva, 1973 and 1986). Furthermore, elementary biological notes on it were recorded even many centuries before Linnaeus described *Naja* in 1758. Many early authors such as Ribeiro (1685), Knox (1681) gave brief accounts of the cobra. Deraniyagala (1945) considered it to be an endemic subspecies.

General morphological features:

Cobra is the largest elapid snake in the country. Its average length is 1.2 m and specimens over 1.65 m are not uncommon. The record size in the author's collection was a female 1.85 m long. Its head is depressed and broad behind, neck and forebody is remarkably dilatable which forms the characteristic hood. Body is fairly thick. Tail is cylindrical slightly tapering and short.

Figure 23
Distribution of *Calliophis melanurus* in the Climatic Zones of Sri Lanka

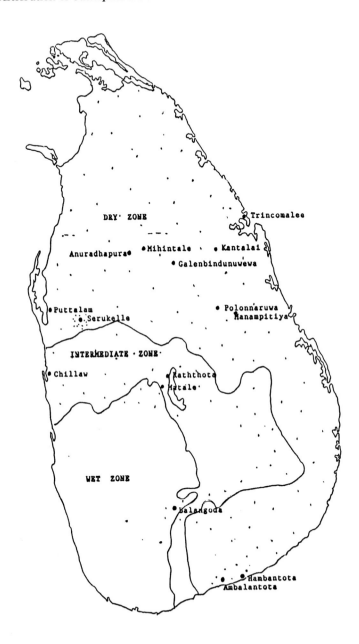

Key
- •   Localities in the literature and sites collected
- ⁑   Commonly found
- ∴   Probable extended distribution

Colour:

Its general body colour varies from light reddish brown to black. There are fine white single or double cross bands. In the young the ventral side is creamy white with black or brown bands distinct in the anterior half. These tend to diffuse with age. In adult black coloured cobra, the ventral surface is grey and in others, creamy white. Several albinos have also been recorded. Deraniyagala (1955) mentions that the specimens found in North (Jaffna) are usually yellowish. In the Sri Lankan cobra, the dorsal aspect of the hood has the characteristic "Spectacle" "Binocellate" or "Mask" markings (fig 24). But observations made on nearly 500 cobras from different parts of the country show that the markings on the dorsal aspect of the hood are variable. However it was observed that the two black spots on the ventral aspect of the hood is a constant characteristic feature (fig 25).

Identification:

1. The well developed hood with markings on the dorsal and ventral aspects of it.
2. Its bodily features and colour.

Habits:

Naja naja is a terrestrial and diurnal snake. However observations made on captive specimens (including a few day-old hatchlings) showed that they were active during the night too.

Cobras have a habit of living close to human habitations and it was also observed many times in the busiest places too. They are good in climbing and swimming and have been observed climbing on tall trees preying on birds and squirrels on several occasions. Further it was observed that larger cobras usually bask in the sun in the afternoons. The female lay 10 — 30 eggs and incubates them. Artificially incubated eggs took 58 — 90 days to hatch.

Food:

It feeds on a wide variety of animals such as frogs, toads, many species of small mammals, birds and bird eggs (especially poultry eggs), lizards. Like kraits it is also ophiophagus in habit. Cannibalism too has been observed.

Habitat and distribution:

Naja is very common and widely distributed in the island. They are often met on cultivated land (paddy and coconut) where they hide in rat holes or termite mounds (these sites are often used for laying eggs). It has been recorded from all the peneplains (except in the highest altitudes), vegetational and climatic zones.

Defense and action of venom:

Of the Sri Lankan snakes, the cobra exhibits one of the most impressive warning mechanism or threat posture. In this posture it raises the forebody

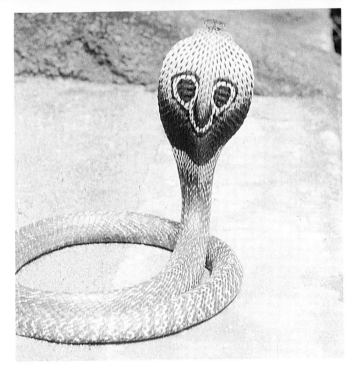

Figure 24
Naja naja naja (Dorsal aspect of hood) (Photo — A. de Silva

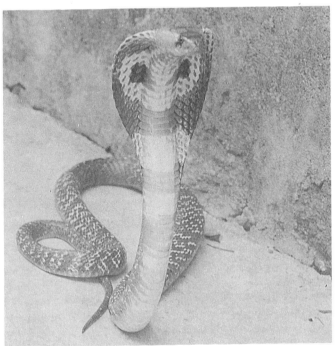

Figure 25
Naja naja naja (Ventral aspect of hood) (Photo — A de Silva)

about 1/3 to 1/4 of its body length (it was observed that the cobra usually raises its forebody more than this when confronted by a mongoose), erects or spreads its neck ribs and distends the hood thus showing the two large eyes like black spots on the ventral aspect and its well known "spectacle" or "mask" markings which too also appear like eyes. At this stage it often hisses and may open its mouth and attack.

Naja is a proteroglyphous snake. The maxillae have the fangs anteriorly. Though it is a common snake in Sri Lanka accounting for a large number of deaths (34%, de Silva 1976a), there is a paucity of literature on clinical features where the identity is definitely established as *Naja naja naja*.

Bobeau (1912) records pain and numbness of the bitten limb. Deraniyagala (1955) records immediate burning sensation of the site of bite, swelling and turned into pitch dark the following day, ptosis, bloodshot eyes (opthalmoplegia and oliguria). The victim (the person in charge of live snakes of the Colombo National Museum) resorted to traditional medicine. However, subsequently two fingers had to be amputated as they became infected and gangrenous.

Thanabalasundrum and Vidyasegara (1969) record vomiting of blood, bleeding par rectum, dark urine, bilateral ptosis, palatal and pharyngeal paralysis.. Sawai et al (1983) in a study of fatal cases records dysphonia, respiratory paralysis, ptosis, unconsciousness, local pains and swelling. However, in these two studies the offending cobra was not seen by the authors.

The following signs and symptoms were observed from the author's personal experience.

1. Immediate burning pain which spread up the limb.
2. Maximum swelling reached around 24 hours after bite.
3. Dark discoloration around site of bite and tenderness.
4. In five cases necrosis was observed (fig 26).
5. In one case, a colleague vomitted blood about 30 minutes after the bite.
6. No other systemic effects were observed.

Only in two instances did the victims receive antivenom serum.

Family Viperidae Laurenti, 1768

Family Viperidae is represented in Sri Lanka by snakes belonging to the major sub families — Viperinae and Crotalinae. There are six species of snakes belonging to four genera, compared to four species in the family Elapidae.

Of the vipers, four species are small (average being 30 cm) of which the smallest being *Echis carinatus* (Saw scaled viper or carpet viper) grows to an average of 20 cm. The other two species are relatively larger with *Vipera russelli* representing the largest among them, growing to an average length of 90 cm.

However, at present there is no specific antivenom against the crotalid snakes. Some hospitals in Sri Lanka use the Haffkine Polyvalent serum which does not include antibodies against *hypnale*. Some doctors consider it effective in *H. hypnale* envenomation. However, work is in progress on this aspect.

Snakes of family Viperidae and Elapidae are the medically most important snake as they are responsible for almost all the deaths due to snake bite envenomation of the island.

Epidemiological studies (de Silva 1976a, 1981; de Silva & Ranasinghe 1983; de Silva, Jayatilleke & Ranasinghe 1983, Sawai et al 1983) and clinical studies (Karunaratne 1970, Visuvaratnam, Vinayagamoorthy & Balakrishna 1970, Yoganathan 1973, Peruminar 1975, Jayarajah & Gopalakrishnakone 1981, Jayarajah 1984, Jahubar, Subramaniam & James 1984, Sreeharan & Ganeshamoorthy 1984) show a high incidence of viperine bites. This may be due to the following reasons:

1. Abundance of vipers in plantations.
2. Their procryptic coloration escapes detection, hence humans usually tread on them.
3. Widely distributed.
4. Their biting system (including large fangs) are more effective than cobra.
5. Their habit of coming to roads and paths at dusk.
6. Prolific breeders — their habit of giving birth to live young may be an advantage over egg laying.

Following are the six species of viperine snakes found in Sri Lanka.

Sub family — Viperinae
Genus: *Echis* Merrem, 1820

Represented in Sri Lanka by one species.

Echis carinatus, Schneider, 1801

English name — The saw-scaled viper, or Phoorsa
Local (Sinhala name) — *Vali polonga*, (Tamil name) — *Surutai pambu*

Historical aspects:

Russell had first illustrated it in 1796. Ferguson (1877) was the first to refer it from Sri Lanka. Deraniyagala (1951) considered it to be an endemic subspecies and named it *Echis carinatus sinhaleyas* initially and subsequently (Deraniyagala 1955), *E. c. sinhaleya*.

General morphological features:

It is a small snake. Average length about 20 cm and maximum 30 cm. Head is subovoid and snout is short, eyes are large — body is stout and tail short. Scales on body rough (strongly keeled) and the scales on the costals are serrated.

Colour:

The scales are dull. The dorsal surface of the body is a mixture of light brown, red and yellow, sometimes darker brown. There are dark brown blotches, encircled by a white border. Head bears the characteristic white cross or spear-like mark (fig 27). Belly is often white, sometimes with brown mottling.

Identification:

1. The white cross-like mark on the head (sometimes referred to as bird-foot mark).
2. Its bodily features, and strongly keeled costal scales.

Habits:

E. carinatus is mainly nocturnal in habit, though they may come out to bask in the sun, or immediately after rain come to open places during the day. They are active and highly irritable and may attack and bite at the slightest disturbance. Wall (1921) considered it to be the 'most vicious snake'. Semiarboreal tendencies too were observed, as during the day many were observed among branches, of small shrubs. Further it was observed that in areas where it is common it may be found in large numbers. The female gives birth to about five live young ones.

Habitat and distribution:

It is confined to the arid coastal plains of North, North West and East. Its favorite habitats are under cover of small thorny plants, leaf litter, under rocks inside crevices, in small scrub jungles in open dry tracts. Deraniyagala (1955) includes Iranative (an island north of Sri Lanka). Fernando (1962) records it for the first time from Yala (South East) Sri Lanka. (Fig 28)

Defense and action of venom:

During the threat posture, the *Echis carinatus* forms its body into a series of "S" shaped loops or coils, these coils are kept in motion and as they rub against each other, a hissing sound is produced due to the serrated costal scales. It is always ready to attack, which it does with lightning speed.

Their fangs are canaliculate, and are comparatively large for a small snake. Its venom is considered extremely toxic and according to Warrel (1983), *Echis carinatus* bites and kill more people than any other species of snake. However, in Sri Lanka, perhaps due to its limited area of distribution, bites due to *Echis carinatus* is not very common. Deraniyagala (1955) even considers the form in Sri Lanka to be not fatal to man.

As regards its bite, Deraniyagala (1955 and 1960) records two cases and Stemmler (1965) records one. Deraniyagala (1955) reported the following local symptoms.

1. Bitten on foot, immediately felt something akin to an electric current running from the site of bite up to neck.
2. Ten minutes later felt stinging pain at site of bite.
3. Thirty minutes later foot commenced to swell.
4. Three hours later had stabbing pain on top of head and burning sensation of eyes.

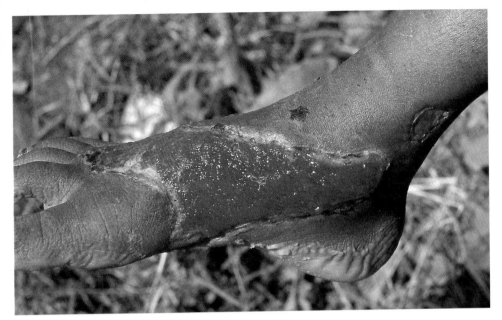

Figure 26
Necrosis due to cobra envenomation (Photo — A de Silva)

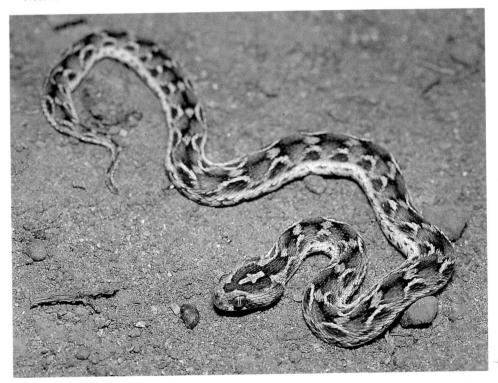

Figure 27
Echis carinatus (Photo — M. Toriba)

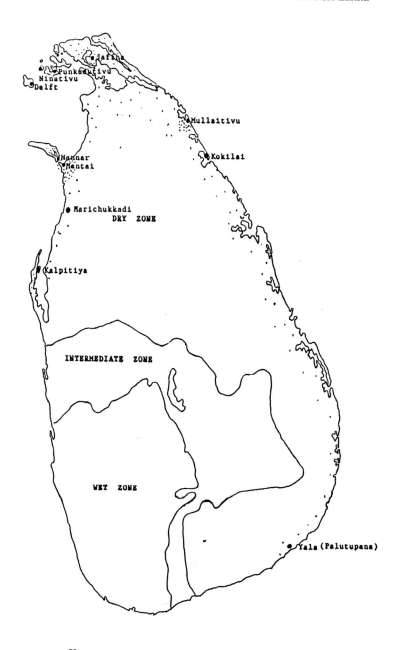

Key

●   Localities in the literature and sites collected

⠿   Commonly found

∴   Probable extended distribution

5. About 48 hours after bite swelling of foot intense, with severe stinging pain at site of bite. Following traditional treatment, for four days swelling and pain had completely subsided.

As regards Stemmler's case (1965), there was only slight pain and swelling which subsided within two days. But blisters formed near site of bite about five minutes after bite took nearly six days to heal. However, work of Gopalakrishnakone (Gopalakrishnakone 1981, Gopalakrishnakone, Reid & Theakston 1981) on experimental animals (rats) showed disseminated intravascular coagulation, fibrin clots in the lung arterioles, fibrin in kidney glomeruli, haemorrhages in the cortical and medullary region.

Status:

Taylor (1950) considered it to be a relatively recent introduction. Its habitats are not greatly disturbed.

Genus: *Vipera* Laurenti, 1768.

This genus is represented in Sri Lanka by one species.

Vipera russelli (Shaw) 1797
English name — Tic-Polonga, Russell's viper, Daboia
Local (Sinhala name) — *Thith Polonga*, (Tamil name) — *Kannadi viriyan*

Historical aspects:

Although *Vipera russelli* was first described by Russell in 1796, literature on traditional treatment for snake bite, records medicines (herbal in origin) for various systemic poisoning effects due to its venom many centuries before 1796. Knox (1681) too provides a brief account of it. Davy (1821 and 1839) illustrates it and records a few elementary experiments on its venom. Deraniyagala (1945) considered that the *Vipera russelli russelli* found in Sri Lanka to be a distinct endemic subspecies and named *V. russelli pulchella* (Gray). Obst (1983) subdivides the genus *Vipera* into three morphologically and zoogeographically defined groups, and considers the name *Daboia* Gray, 1842 as the generic name for 'Oriental vipers' which includes *Vipera russelli*. Some other herpetologists too consider that Gray's old genus *Daboia* should be resurrected for *russelli*.

General morphological features:

Russell's viper is a heavy medium sized snake. It's average length is about 90 cm and could grow up to 1.5 m. Its head is large and triangular, with a distinct neck, body stout, robust and cylindrical. Tail is short, stout and tapering. Body surface is rough due to strongly keeled scales.

Colour:

The general ground colour of the body is a mixture of dull red and brown, or yellow and brown. On the head is a 'V' shaped mark. The apex pointing towards the snout. On the dorsal aspect of the body there are three rows of large oval or elliptical dark spots, two on the sides along the body. The row of spots along the vertebrae is distinct and sométimes chain (necklace) like (fig 29). Inside the spots is dark reddish brown. The ventral aspect is off white and speckled.

Identification:

1. Colour and bodily features.
2. Distinct chain like spots along the mid dorsal aspect and 'V' shape mark on the head.
3. Nostrils are large.

Habits:

Russell's viper is a fairly sluggish snake, nocturnal in habits. Though sluggish, it was observed many times in the wild that they escape and move very fast. When compared to other species of the family Viperidae, Russell's viper is a prolific breeder giving birth to 5 — 65 live young ones. When compared to kraits and cobras, Russell's vipers seldom enter houses. In the dry zones after rain, they usually come to mecadamised roads or gravel roads in the night.

Food:

Its main stay is rats, though occasionally it may feed on birds and lizards. It could live without food for few months.

Habitat and distribution:

Russell's vipers are found in scrub jungles and grasslands bordering plantations. Its colour and markings harmonises well with the dried vegetation where it often lies during the day. It is found in the three climatic zones and the three peneplains. Highest altitude on record is that of Fletcher (1908) from Diyatalawa at 1,200 m above sea level and Wall (1921) from Hakgala, 1,700 m.

Defense and action of venom:

When cornered it assumes a defensive posture by throwing its body into 'S' shaped loops and arches its neck and hisses fiercely and powerfully. No other snake in Sri Lanka emits such a loud sound. As Wall (1921) states "the hiss once heard is not easily forgotten". When striking it hurls itself with speed and bites with determination.

Vipera russelli is a solenoglyphous snake, and the maxilla bears only large canaliculate movable fangs.

Clinical features following envenomation due to *Vipera russelli pulchella* is fairly well documented (Ameratunge 1972, Deraniyagala 1955, Kumaranayake 1971, Jayarajah 1984, Munasinghe & Kulasinghe 1965, Nimalasuriya 1971, Perumainar 1978, Sawai et al 1983, Spaar 1910, Thanabalasundrum & Vidyasagara 1969, Visuvaratnam Vinayagamoorthy & Balakrishnan 1970 Warrell 1986). Pain and swelling are some of the marked symptoms, the

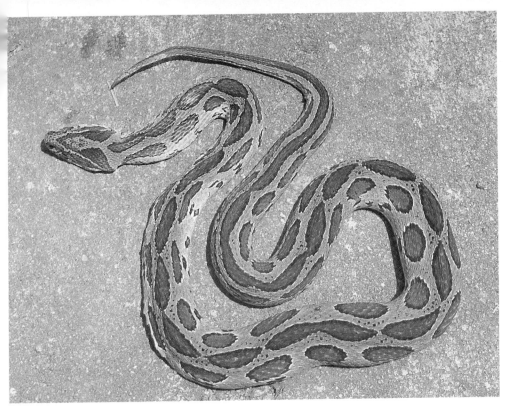

Figure 29
Vipera russelli pulchella (Photo — A de Silva)

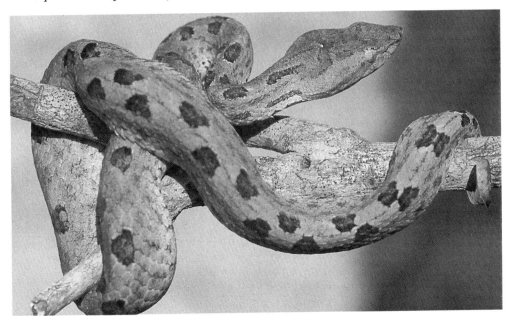

Figure 30
Hypnale hypnale (Photo — A de Silva)

systemic effects due to neuromyotoxicity (ptosis, external opthalmoplegia, paralysis, of the muscles of deglutition and respiration, inability to open mouth and protrude the tongue). Intravascular haemolysis, renal failure and myoglobinuria.

Case history:

A young girl (17 years) was bitten on the left foot by a large *V. russelli*. This snake was killed. Victim had pain and swelling. Within one hour after she had ptosis, and was unable to open the mouth 6 hours after the bites. She had bleeding from nose, mouth and ears, and died 17 hours after bite (personal observation).

Sub family: Crotalinae
Genus: *Hypnale* Fitzinger, 1843

The following three species are recorded from Sri Lanka. All are more or less similar in general appearance.

Hypnale hypnale (Merrem) 1820

English name — Merrem's Hump-nosed viper
Local (Sinhala name) — *Polon thelissa, Kuna katuwa,* (Tamil name) — *Viriyan pambu, kopi viriyan*

Historical aspects:

This snake was first described by Seba in 1734. But traditional literature recorded many prescriptions for various symptoms caused by *Hypnale* envenomation many centuries before Seba. Davy (1821) illustrated it in his book on Sri Lanka and also recorded a few elementary experiments with its venom. Gloyd (1977) considered that the species found in South India and Sri Lanka, hitherto placed in the genus *Agkistrodon* are distinct from all others, thus warranting revival of the generic name *Hypnale* (Fitzinger, 1843) for these snakes.

General morphological features:

Hypnale hypnale is a small and stout snake. Its average length is 37.5cm (n= 28) and maximum 56.5 cm. Its head is flat and triangular with a distinct neck. Its snout ends in a wedge or hump-like prominence. Body is short, stout and cylindrical. Tail is short and tapering.

Colour:

This snake is highly variable in colour. It ranges from light yellow with a mixture of brown to black and grey ones. However, the most common and widely distributed one had its dorsal aspect of the body, a mixture of light brown, yellow and a trace of red. There is a series of dark brown oval, or triangular spots on either side of the spine along the body (fig 30). The ventral aspect is light yellowish brown or greyish and with mottling. The posterior end of the tail is usually creamy white. This is lighter in the young.

Identification:
1. Flat triangular shaped head, with its wedged shape snout (fig 31), the head has large scales and other bodily features.
2. Presence of a pit "Loreal pit" between the eye and nostril.

Habits:
Hypnale hypnale is a terrestrial snake, nocturnal in habits. However, their semi arboreal habits too are on record (Wall 1921, Smith 1943, de Silva & Toriba 1984). When they are on the ground, they have a curious habit of keeping their heads raised and pointing at an angle of about 45° (Fig. 31 & 33). The females produce live young and the brood ranges from 3 — 18 (de Silva & Toriba 1984). The tail is creamy white in the young and is known to be used in luring prey animals (Henry 1925).

Food:
It feeds on frogs, geckos, calotes, skinks and mice. Also known to feed on reptile eggs (Wall 1905).

Habitat and distribution:
It is found in plantations of rubber, coconut, coffee, tea, cocoa, banana and others, in forests and grasslands. During the day they lay at the base of small shrubs and grass, or may be found under logs or leaf litter. It is widely distributed and is found in all the three climatic zones, and in the three peneplains up to about 1,250 m above sea level. (Fig 32).

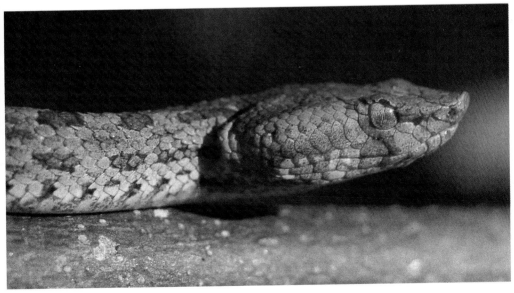

Figure 31
H. hypnale (Head lateral view) (Photo — A de Silva)

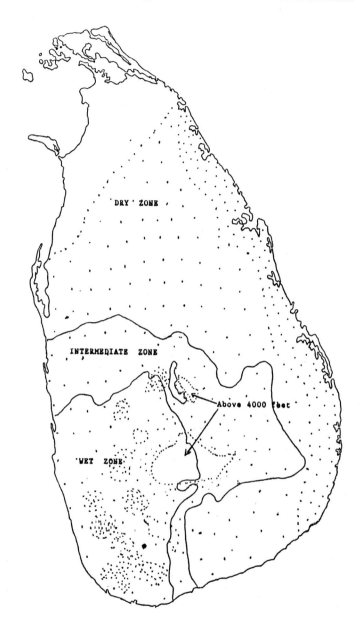

Key

∴ Probable extended distribution
(Individual localities not indicated as commonly found in the extended distribution)
⠒⠒⠒ Commonly found

Defense and action of venom:

These snakes are active and fierce and strike without hesitation. In its defensive posture, it forms its body into loops, with the head and forebody slightly raised and retracted. It flattens itself to the ground, and sometimes vibrates its tail. At this stage it strikes rapidly.

Hypnale is an solenoglyphous snake and the maxilla contains large canaliculate fangs. Bites by *H. hypnale* are common in Sri Lanka, however fatalities are extremely rare. Varagunam & Panabokke (1970) and Perumainar (1975) recorded two cases of fatal bites, where the victims had extensive kidney damage (bilateral cortical necrosis).

There are many cases of *H. hypnale* envenomation on record (Abercromby 1911, Biddell 1951, de Silva & Aloysius 1983, Green 1910, Pearless 1909, Pereira 1875). In most of these instances the victims had only pain and swelling which subsided within a few days. Deraniyagala (1955) recorded a case where the victim had pain, local swelling, burning sensation in stomach and eyes. The patient had been slightly delirious, and had been unconscious for nearly five days, but recovered completely after a month.

Perumainar (1975) records more severe systemic effects, like cardiovascular, neurological, haematological, and renal manifestations in addition to the local symptoms. These cases suggest that if a large dose of *hypnale* venom is injected during a bite it may prove fatal.

Status:

Though *H. hypnale* is a common snake, it is loosing some its natural habitats and many get killed in plantations.

Hypnale nepa (Laurenti) 1768

English name — Montain hump nosed viper, Millards hump nosed viper.
Local (Sinhala name) — *Mukalan thelissa, Geta polonga, Kunakatuwa,*
(Tamil name) — *Viriyan pambu*

Historical aspects:

It was first described by Laurenti in 1768, but the type locality given as Madagascar was an error. However many centuries before this the traditional physicians and literature on management prescribed many medicaments for both species, thus suggesting that the early snake bite physicians of Sri Lanka had observed their difference.

General morphological features:

Morphologically *H. nepa* closely resembles *H. hypnale* except for the distinguishing wart-like cluster of small scales at the tip of its snout (fig 33). Further the *nepa* is slightly shorter in length than *hypnale*. The general ground colour and pattern is similar to *H. hypnale* (fig 30).

Identification:

Similar identifying characters like *H. hypnale*. It could be distinguished

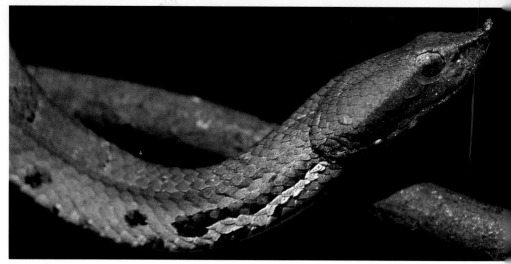

Figure 33
Hypnale nepa (Head lateral view) (Photo — A de Silva)

from *H. hypnale* by the presence of the wart like cluster of small scales at the tip of its snout (Fig. 33) and the presence of hemipenial spines.

Habits:

Similar to the former. Its reproductive habits are under study.

Food:

Similar to *H. hypnale.*

Habitat and distribution:

Hypnale nepa is mainly confined to rain forests and other forests where during the day they lie under leaf litter, logs, stones and at the base of grass, weeds and cardamoms. Observations and available records are within the three peneplains of the wet zone. (Fig 34)

Defense and action of venom:

Defensive behaviour is similar to *H. hypnale,* but are mild in temperament. A recent study (de silva 1989) of four cases of *H. nepa* bite showed that all the victims had only pain and swelling which subsided within 3-5 days. All resorted to traditional treatment.

Status:

Many get killed and lose habitats during clearing of montain forests for cultivation.

Figure 34
Distribution of *Hypnale nepa* and H. walli in the Climatic Zones of Sri Lanka

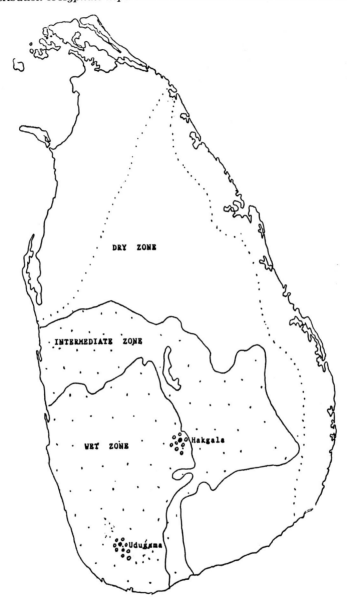

Key

∴ Probable extended distribution
  (Individual localities not indicated as commonly found in the extended distribution)
∷∷ Commonly found
○ Hypnale walli

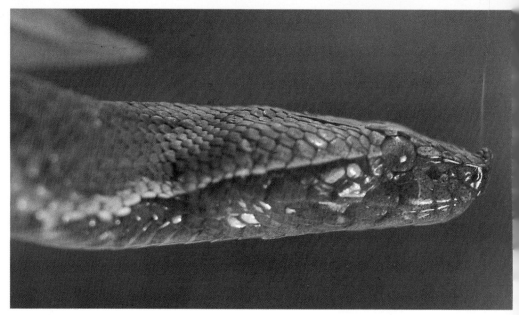

Figure 35
Hypnale walli (?) (Head lateral view) (Photo — A de Silva)

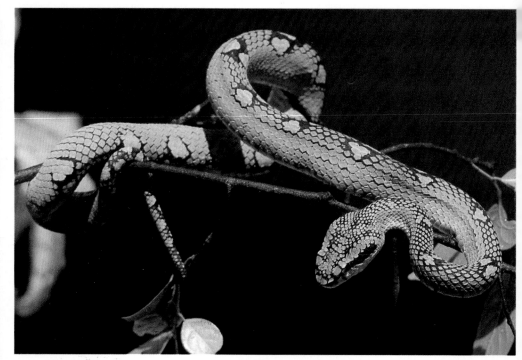

Figure 36
Trimeresurus trigonocephalus (Photo — A de Silva)

Hypnale walli Gloyd 1977

English name — Gloyd's hump nosed viper

Local (Sinhala name) — *Kuda mukalan thelissa, geta polonga*

History:

Howard K. Gloyd described this snake in 1977, but its marked similarity to *H. nepa* requires further study in order to confirm whether it is a valid species or not.

General morphological features:

Similar to *H. nepa*, but relatively small, stout-bodied and short-tailed (Gloyd 1977).

Colour:

Similar to other species of the genus (fig 35).

Identification:

1. Morphological features and colour.
2. It is separable from *hypnale* and *nepa* by the fewer ventrals and subcaudals.

Habits:

Similar to *nepa*. Its reproductive habits are being investigated.

Food:

Similar to *hypnale*.

Habitat and distribution:

They are found in rain forests under leaf litter, logs on the base of small weeds. At Hakgala (U); (1,700 m). They were observed at the base of grass *Chrysopagon zeylanica* and *Eupatorium reparium*. The holotype of Gloyd (1977) had been from Kanneliya forest, Udagama (S) paratypes from Hakgala (U). It has been collected from Sinharaja primary rain forest too. This distribution data suggests that it is found in all the peneplains but mainly confined to rain forests with high rainfall.(Fig 34)

Defense and action of venom:

Defensive postures are similar to *H. hypnale*. However, it was observed that they were not as temperamental as *H. hypnale*.

Status:

Similar to *H. nepa*.

Genus: *Trimeresurus* Lacepede 1804.

Only one species is found in Sri Lanka.

Trimeresurus trigonocephalus (Sonnini and Latreille) 1801
English name — Green pit viper
Local (Sinhala name) — *Pala polonga*, (Tamil name) — *Pachi viriyan*

Historical aspects:

Sonnini and Latreille described this snake in 1801. But there is evidence that the ancient snake bite physicians of Sri Lanka knew about the moderate nature of its venom (de Silva 1983).

General morphological features:

The green pit viper is a medium sized snake, growing to an average of 75 cm and a maximum of 1.3 m. Its head is large, broad and triangular. Neck distinct. Body robust, cylindrical and the tail short and prehensile.

Colour:

Dorsally the body is green, (seldom yellowish-green or turquoise-blue), mottled and variegated with black markings from head to tail (fig 36). A black stripe runs from the eye to the angle of the jaw on each side. However, in about 4%, the variegated black markings are absent, except for the postocular black stripe (de Silva 1982a). The belly is light green with a light touch of yellow. Posterior end of the tail is black.

Identification:
1. Bodily features and colour.
2. Presence of a large loreal pit between the nostril and eye.

Habits:

T. trigonocephalus is an arboreal snake, nocturnal in habit, but often descends, to the ground in search of food and water. Adults are sluggish. Though cobras and kraits are frequently found in and around human dwellings, green pit vipers are rarely seen closer to human habitats. The female produces about 5 — 26 young (de Silva 1983).

Food:

The food of *trigonocephalus* consists of frogs, geckos, rats, mice and birds.

Habitats and distribution:

The green pit viper may be found on tall trees or low shrubs and bushes in forests and rain forests, on reeds *(Ochlandra stridula* Thw) near streams. It may be found in plantations like cardamoms, cocoa, coffee and tea, and is widely distributed in the country. Found in all the peneplains (from sea level to about 1,825 m) and the climatic zones. However, field observations and available records show that it is common in the wet zone from 153 — 1,075 m altitude (de Silva 1983). (fig 37)

Figure 37
Distribution of *T. trigonocephalus* in the Vegetational Zones of Sri Lanka

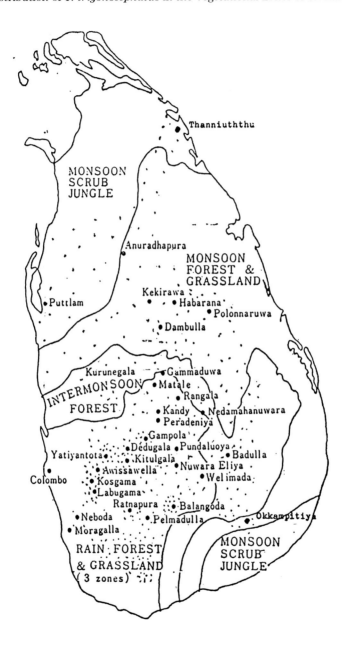

Key
- ● Localities in the literature and sites collected
- ⫶⫶⫶ Commonly found
- ∴ Probable extended distribution

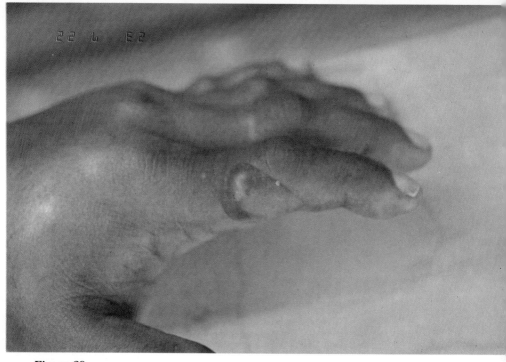

Figure 38
Blister and swelling due to *T. trigonocephalus* envenomation (Photo — M. Toriba)

Defense and action of venom:

T. trigonocephalus is an solenoglyphous snake. Its fangs are large. Though a sluggish snake, it may strike with great speed. In its defensive posture, it raises and retracts its forebody and lashes out. When disturbed, it sometimes vibrates its tail. Hissing is extremely rare. Of nearly 100 specimens observed, only one hissed (de Silva & Aloysius 1983).

Of its bite, Wall (1921), Deraniyagala (1955) and Goonaratne (1968) recorded local symptoms (pain and swelling) within subsided within a few days. Ptosis also has been observed (de Silva 1983). A detailed case report of green pit viper poisoning is available (Fig. 38) (de Silva 1983). These suggests that there are no authentic records of death or severe systemic envenomation due to *T. trigonocephalus*. However, subcutaneous administration of venom to experiment animals have produced acute tubular necrosis (Gopalakrishnakone 1975).

Status:

T. trigonocephalus is not an uncommon snake. However, recent observations show that many get killed and lose their habitats due to vast clearing of forests.

Medically Important Snakes Of Sri Lanka (Summary)

(refer text for colour, morphological features and distribution)

1. Kraits (*Bungarus caeruleus* and *ceylonicus*). Scales along the vertebra (vertebrals) are enlarged (Fig. 17). Fourth scale of the lower lip is the largest.
2. Cobra *(Naja naja naja)*. Distinct hood with markings on dorsal (Fig. 24) and ventral (Fig. 25) aspects.
3. Sea snakes (Hydrophiidae). Belly scales reduced. Tail flat and rudder like.
4. Saw scaled viper *(Echis carinatus)* small snake, with a distinct cross mark on the head (Fig. 27).
5. Russell's viper *(Vipera russelli)* head triangular shaped with a distinct 'V' shape mark. Three rows of large spots along the dorsal aspect of the body. Central row distinct. (Fig. 29).
6. Hump nosed viper *(Hypnale* species). Moderately venomous. Flat triangular shaped head (Fig. 30). Snout ends in a hump and a pit between eye and nostril (Fig. 31, 33 & 35).
7. Green pit viper (*Trimeresurus trigonocephalus)* Head broad and triangular. A pit between eye and nostril (Fig. 36).

Research Work On Venoms In Sri Lanka

According to traditional literature, all venomous snakes have four fangs. In addition, traditional literature records the belief that venomous snakes commence producing venom only after the hatchlings are exposed to sun. Furthermore, the potency of the venom was believed to vary according to the place and the day. These observations though of no scientific value in modern context, point to the fact that several centuries before the modern ophiologists, the ancient traditional snake bite healers of Sri Lanka have observed them.

Davy (1821 and 1839) conducted some elementary experiments with the venoms of Sri Lankan snakes *(Naja naja, Vipera russelli* and *Hypnale* species). This could be stated as the first scientific step taken on this aspect in Sri Lanka.

Nearly a century later, Bobeau (1912 and 1913) worked on the venoms and venom glands of snakes of Sri Lanka. Deraniyagala (1955) conducted a few elementary animal experiments to demonstrate the envenoming by *Boiga ceylonensis* and *Bungarus ceylonicus*. Somanader (1957) recorded brief observations of the venom of *H. hypnale* and *H. nepa*, Mangili (1959) included venoms of snakes of Sri Lanka *(Naja naja* and *Hypnale nepa)* in a brief study on the action of snake venoms on blood and Ponnambalam (1960) of *Naja, V. russelli* and *Bungarus* species.

Modern research on the structure of the venom gland and the action of venoms were conducted by Perumainar (1973, 1975 and 1975) and more extensively by Gopalakrishnakone (Gopalakrishnakone & Jayatilaka 1974, 1975, 1975a Gopalakrishnakone 1981, Gopalakrishnakone et al 1981 and; Jayatilaka, Gopalakrishnakone & Alcorn, 1981). Since this encouraging work, hardly any research has been conducted on the venom gland, venoms and its action of snakes of Sri Lanka. Many species (most of family Colubridae, especially *Boiga* species and *Balanophis ceylonensis*, of the Elapidae,

Calliophis melanurus and *Bungarus ceylonicus*, sea snakes mainly confined to Sri Lankan coastal water and Viperid snakes) remain to be studied. Further, the clinical features manifested due to envenomation by some Sri Lankan snakes are fairly distinct from what has been reported from other countries in the region (Karunaratne & Panabokke (1972), Warrell (1986).

Pattern of snake bite in Sri Lanka: A review

It is evident that all the venomous land snakes which inhabit Sri Lanka at present would have been on the island before it 'separated' from mainland India. Thus it could be assumed that the early inhabitants of the island would have been bitten by snakes occasionally. This is substantiated by having well organised traditional system of management of snake bite, few centuries before the Christian era. This suggests that the tradition has been evolving since that time.

Though some of the colubrid snakes discussed in this paper too are frequently found in houses, they have caused no serious medical problems, except for mild local reactions in some cases. Nevertheless reports of envenoming due to presumably nonvenomous colubrid snakes continue to appear in recent times (Burger 1974, de Silva 1976, de Silva & Aloysius 1983, Manonova 1977, Maretic & Russell 1979, Mather Mayne & McMonagle 1978, Kono & Sawai 1975).

It is also interesting to note that the traditional snake bite physicians of Sri Lanka who practice an ancient art which goes back to more than 2,000 years, regarded most of the colubrid snakes described in this paper, as venomous and prescribed medicines for their bites. It is evident from these that the ancient Lankan physicians were familiar with the local and systemic effects of envenomation.

Epidemiological (de Silva 1976a, 1980, 1981, 1986b, 1987b; de Silva & Ranasinghe 1983; de Silva, Jayatilaka & Ranasinghe 1983; de Silva & Hewage 1987, Sawai et al 1983; Swaroop & Grab 1954) and clinical studies (Jeyarajah 1984; Jahubar, Subramaniam & James 1984; Karunaratne 1970; Karunaratne & Anandadas 1973; Sreeharan & Ganeshamoorthy 1984; Visuvaratnam, Vinayagamoorthy & Balakrishnan 1970; Yoganathan 1973) show that snake bite is an important medical problem and an occupational hazard in Sri Lanka. At present the mortality rate (per 100,000 population) from snake bite is one of the highest in the world.

Closer examination of the results of epidemiological, clinical, ecological, topographical and sociological studies on snake bite in Sri Lanka, revealed that the following facts influence the high morbidity and mortality in the island.

Incidence by species

As regards to the incidence of bites according to species, de Silva & Ranasinghe (1983) gave an approximate index arrived from collation of published literature and those which the authors have collected from hospitals and traditional snake bite physicians. According to this, the highest incidence (27%) of bites is caused by *Hypnale* species (Table 2).

TABLE 2
Species of snakes responsible for bites.

	Bungarus	Naja	V.russelli	Hypnale species	Others	NR
No. of bites	494	686	1001	1553	1661	331
Percentage	8.6	12.0	17.5	27.1	29.0	5.8

NR - Not recorded.
Source - De Silva and Ranasinghe, 1983.

Snakes responsible for fatalities

Species of snakes that caused death are given in Table 3. According to this data *Vipera russelli* is responsible for nearly 40% of deaths. Recent clinical studies (Jeyarajah 1984, Perumainar 1978, Sreeharan & Ganeshamoorthy 1984) support these findings.

TABLE 3
Distribution of snakes responsible for deaths

	Bungarus	Naja	V.russelli	Hypnale	NR	Total
No. of bites	87	178	207	14	33	519
Percentage	17	34	40	3	6	100

NR - Not recorded.
Source - De Silva, 1976a.

Mortality

Mortality data due to snake bite is maintained by the Registrar General and is available for the past century. However, from January 1950 to December 1979, snake bite fatalities were classified in accordance with the international list of disease and cause of death, and were registered under 'Accidents caused by bites and stings of venomous animals and insects'. Deaths due to stings by wasps and hornets are also included under this category. The latter however are only a few. Nevertheless, the data maintained by the Registrar General provides a clear pattern of the death rate.

Sex of victims

Table 4 shows some mortality data of snake bite available with the Registrar General (Registrar General, personal communication, October, 1987). According to this data and epidemiological studies (de Silva 1976a, 1980, 1981, de Silva & Ranasinghe 1983; de Silva & Hewage 1987) it is evident that males are more exposed to snake bite than females, the ratio being 2:1.

TABLE 4
Deaths due to snake bite* by sex

Year	Males	Females	Total
1975	469	205	674
1976	464	223	687
1977	482	229	771
1978	601	261	862
1979	573	248	821

* Including stings of insects.
Source - Registrar General, personal communication Oct. 1987.

Age of victims

Epidemiological and clinical studies indicate that nearly 50% of people between the age 15 — 40 years are bitten more often by snakes. In a recent study (de Silva & Hewage 1987) 60% (n = 227) of bites involved those between 20 — 39 years of age, with a mean age of 27.24. In Sri Lanka, snake bite is not uncommon among children below 15 years of age and in fact, 26% of deaths due to snake bite were in this age group. Further, our studies indicate that infants one month to one year too fall victim to snake bites (de Silva 1976a, de Silva, Jayatilaka & Ranasinghe 1983).

Circumstances of bite

The circumstances under which people were bitten by snakes in most (42 — 85%) instances were, while engaged in agriculture fields like weeding, harvesting, guarding fields etc.. Further in Sri Lanka, the majority of people live in rural areas (79% during the 1981 Census). Thus snake bite in the tropics is a rural and an occupational hazard (Reid 1968).

Anatomical site of bite

Many studies (de Silva 1976a, 1980, 1981; Sawai et al 1983; Visuvaratnam et al 1970) show that the most (73 — 74%) vulnerable body site, is below the knee (toes, foot, ankle and leg). This was mainly due to accidental treading on snakes, which may be well camouflaged in the undergrowth or not seen in the dark. The other common bodily site are the fingers and hand. This usually happens during harvesting, weeding, clearing and while cutting grass. Bites on head, trunk and genitals are not uncommon. This was specially evident in krait bites.

Time of bite

Though the majority of snakes are nocturnal in habits, about 40% of bites by nocturnal snakes (mainly vipers) occurred during the day (between 6 am and 6 pm). This is mainly due to occupational accidents and not to the active movements of these snakes. However, a characteristic biting pattern was observed with *Bungarus caeruleus* and *B. ceylonicus*. Studies (de Silva 1981,

1986a and 1987b; Green 1908; Fernando & Dias 1982; Ponnambalam 1939), dealing exclusively with *Bungarus* bites or which include *Bungarus* bites showed that all the bites took place during the night (between 6 pm and 6 am) and mainly on people asleep in houses. Further it was evident from the above data that the victims of *Bungarus* species run a greater risk of death than from any other snakes in Sri Lanka (de Silva 1981).

Seasonal variation of bites

No distinct seasonal pattern was observed for Sri Lanka (de Silva 1976a, 1981) except for *Bungarus* bites. Nevertheless, a slight increase was observed during harvesting seasons (de Silva 1981, Kirupanathan 1970). This was also observed during ecological studies of snakes. However, in case of *B. caeruleus* bites, a distinct seasonal pattern was observed (de Silva 1981, 1986a, 1987b) (Table 5). This corresponded with its biological habits. The other factors which influence the incidence of snake bite in Sri Lanka are its climatic zones, topography and demographic trends. It was evident in ecological and snake bite studies carried out by de Silva (1976a, 1980, 1981, 1986a), that there were less venomous snakes in the third peneplain and more bites in the first peneplain.

TABLE 5

Biting pattern of *Bungarus caeruleus*

Reproductive cycle	Month	No of bites	Percentage
Normal activity	January-August	19	22.1
Mating period	September-November	36	41.9
Gestation and incubation	December-March	15	17.4
Hatching	April-May	16	18.6

Source – De Silva, 1986.

Type of treatment and fatality rate

It was observed that snake bite victims with systemic signs (like acute renal failure, respiratory distress, and haemorrhagic manifestations) die without proper medical attention at their homes, thus showing that proper treatment will reduce the fatality rate.

Snake Bite Treatment In Sri Lanka

A number of medical systems exist in Sri Lanka and each has its own management of snake bite poisoning. The different systems are: Indigenous (Ayurvedic), Allopathy (Western), Sidda, Unai, Homeopathy, Ahikuntaka (Sri Lanka Gypsies) and Veddah (Aborogines of Sri Lanka). Of these, the Indigenous (Ayurvedic) system and Allopathic (Western) system are sought by people presently in case of snake bite. Hence in this presentation only the Indigenous system and allopathy (western) system are discussed.

Indigenous (Ayurvedic) system

The Indigenous system is the oldest (more than 2,500 years old) and well established part of the Sri Lanka culture (de Silva & Uragoda 1983; de Silva 1987). One of the earliest legends of traditional treatment of snake bite in the island is when the famous warrior King Dutugemunu (161-137 BC) was bitten by a cobra on three different occasions. He has been treated by a snake bite physician known as Kapurunada (Liyanarachchi 1972) but on the third instance it was fatal (Wimalabuddhi 1966).

Literature

The early literature on Indigenous treatment are in Sanskrit, Pali, Sinhala and Tamil written on Palm leaves or ola. *Sarartha Sangrahaya* is the earliest existing work to originate in Sri Lanka, and was written by the physician king Buddadasa (340-368 AD). It contains a chapter on the treatment of snake bite envenoming. From the 4th century to 19th century, many works on different aspects of medicine, were written. In these, some contain a chapter on snake bite treatment whilst a few deal exclusively with snake bite treatment.

The first printed book in Sinhala dealing exclusively with snake bite treatment was published in 1876. Between 1876 and 1985 nearly 100 Sinhala books and papers on snake bite treatment were published.

The indigenous system is practiced mainly by a group of about 7,000 of which nearly 2,000 are registered with the government as snake bite physicians. A few graduates of the College of Ayurveda too practice this art.

Hospitals

Some of the Government Ayurveda Hospitals have special wards for the treatment of snake bite patients. There are some 'Snake bite Hospitals' run by Indigenous snake bite physicians. Some of these receive financial assistance from the government.

Treatment

The traditional system records 24 techniques of treating a snake bite envenomed person. The physician uses one or many according to the degree of envenomation.

Present status

At present the Indigenous snake bite physicians are well organised and established. In spite of the readily available modern western medical facilities, traditional indigenous practices continue to be the widely sought form of treatment. This is clearly evident from the following studies. Of 393 snake bites recorded from one particular (Anuradhapura) district for the year 1979, 385 (98%) sought Indigenous treatment (de Silva 1981). A study of 110 fatal cases from the same district for the years 1980, 1981 and 1982 showed that all have first sought indigenous treatment. However, 27 (25%) of them have gone to the government hospital at a critical stage (Sawai et al 1983). In a study of 22

Russell's viper bites, it was shown that all had first sought indigenous treatment (Jeyarajah 1984). From hospital admissions, for the years 1980, 1981 and 1982, the total number of deaths due to snake bite reported from most allopathic hospitals were 36, 53 and 85 respectively. But the reports of the Registrar General for the same years indicate 821, 798 and 574 deaths due to snake bite suggesting that the majority died out of hospitals.

At present there are a few indigenous snake bite physicians who administer polyvalent antivenom serum and hydrocortisone successfully. They promptly refer their patients to hospitals if there are signs of impending complications (renal failure and respiratory paralysis). Hence it is felt that a selected number of indigenous physicians from rural areas who are more scientifically oriented, should be given training on modern allopathic techniques of management of snake bite patients. Presently there is an alarming shortage of allopathic physicians in the remote rural areas, where the incidence of snake bite is highest.

It is highly felt that a detailed study is necessary to establish the efficiency of indigenous drugs, their therapeutic values and the venom neutralising capabilities of the native medicaments.

Allopathic or Western system

Although the allopathic system came to Sri Lanka around the 16th century, it appears that there are no records of treating a snake bite victim allopathically until the early 19th century. Even some of the important contributions on Sri Lanka made by Baldaeus (1672), Knox (1681), Rebeiro (1685) mentioned only traditional treatment of snake bites.

However, in early 19th century, Davy (1821) mentioned the use of oil, arsenic and eau de luse. According to him, "oil seems to have been useful, both applied externally, and taken internally, for many instances of the bite of the viper, and arsenic seems to have done good, in some instances of the bite of the hooded snake", and of eau de luse, Davy (1821) states that it does not deserve the 'high character that was first given to it'. Eau de luse mentioned by Davy are not traditional herbal medicines used by the native physicians hence it may be assumed that these could be some of the early allopathic drugs used in the management of snake bite treatment in Sri Lanka. Further, by Davy's statement 'high' character that was first given to eau de luse', it is clear that this had been a popular allopathic drug used in case of snake bite envenomation from possibly late 18th century. In fact Bennett (1843) refers to one John Tranchell, a Swede who lived in South Sri Lanka (Weligama), treating snake bite patients with eau de luse.

Lyophilized polyvalent antisnake-venom serum effective against the venoms of Indian, *Naja naja*, *Bungarus caeruleus*, *Vipera russelli* and *Echis carinatus*, has been imported to Sri Lanka from Haffkine Institute, Bombay, since 1952 (Superintendent, Medical Stores, Colombo 1972, personal communication). This does not mean that snake bite was not treated in hospitals earlier. On the contrary, patients had been managed in allopathic hospitals even a century ago (Administrative report 1880). In the year 1879 one snake bite patient had been treated and in 1880, three cases. At present nearly 5,000 patients are managed in Allopathic hospitals in Sri Lanka. Recently (1982), the Sri Lanka Medical Association formed a snake bite expert committee. This committee published their first report (Ceylon Medical Journal 28(3), 1983). This important contribution for the country contains papers dealing with medically important snakes, first aid, epidemiology of snake bite and management. It is also proposed to manufacture antivenom serum in Sri Lanka using venoms of Sri Lankan snakes.

Acknowledgements

I wish to thank Dr Sarath Edirisinghe for reading and commenting on the manuscript, Mr Michihisa Toriba of Japan Snake Institute for the photograph of *Echis carinatus* and for providing some relevant literature, Dr Sarath Kotagama for the photograph of *Balanophis ceylonensis*, Messrs Samson Premasiri and Cyril Wijesundara for providing me with some rare specimens for photographing; Dr P. Gopalakrishnakone for inviting me to write on snakes of Sri Lanka for this book and Prof. Malcolm A. Fernando for this continued encouragement. Finally I wish to thank Miss Priyani Peiris for her patience and excellent typing.

References

Abercromby, A.F. (1910). The snakes of Ceylon. Murrary and Co. London, 89 p.

Abercromby, A.F. (1911). The effects of the bite of 'Ancistrodon hypnale, *Spolia Zeylanica*, 7(28); 205

Abercromby, A.F. (1913). Distribution of snakes of Ceylon, *Spolia Zeylanica*. 8(32); 304-305.

Administrative Report (1880) Report of the Acting Principal Civil Medical Officer and Inspector General of Hospitals. Medical Part IV, p. 208.

Amaratunga, B. (1972). Middle cerebral occlusion following Russell's viper bite, *Journal of Tropical Medicine and Hygiene*, 75(5); 95-97.

Baldaeus, Philip (1672). A true and exact description of the most celebrated East-India coast of Malabar and Cormandel, as also of the Isle of Ceylon, Vol 3, Amsterdam, p. 827-829.

Bennet, J.W. (1843). Ceylon and its capabilities, W.H. Allen and Co., London, p. 113-120.

Biddell, W.H. (1951). The Quest, *Loris*, 6(1); 311-312.

Bobeau, G. (1912). The venom of snakes, *Spolia Zeylanica*, 8(30); 116-121.

Bobeau, G. (1913). On the minute structure of the poison-gland of the cobra (Naja tripudians), *Spolia Zeylanica*, 9(33); 16-20.

Burger, W.L. (1974) A case of mild envenomation by the mangrove snake, Boiga dendrophila, *Snake*, 6(2); 99-100.

Census and Statistics, Dept. (1986) Statistical Pocket Book of the Democratic Socialist Republic of Sri Lanka, Colombo.

Constable, J.D. (1949). Reptiles from the Indian Peninsula in the Museum of comparative Zoology, *Bulletin of the Museum of Comparative Zoology*, 103(2); 59-160.

Crusz, H. (1984). Parasites of endemic and relict vertebrates: A biogeographical review, IN *Ecology and Biogeography in Sri Lanka*, Ed. C.H. Fernando, Junk Publishers, The Hague, p. 321-351.

Davy, J. (1821). An account of the interior of Ceylon and of its inhabitants with Travels in the island, Longman, Hurst, Rees, Orma and Brown, London.

Davy, J. (1839). On the poison of three of the poisonous snakes of Ceylon, IN: Researches, Physiological and Anatomical, Vol. 1, Smith, Elder and Co. London, p. 113-134.

Da Silva M.V. and M.A. Buononato (1983/84). Relato clinico de envenonamento Humano por PhiLodrayas olfersii, *Memorias do Instituto Butantan*, 47/48; 121-125.

Deraniyagala, P.E.P. (1945). Some New Races of the Python, Chrysopela, Binocellate cobra and Tith Polonga inhabiting Ceylon and India, *Spolia Zeylanica*, 24(2); 103-112.

Deraniyagala, P.E.P. (1951). Some New Races of the snakes Eryx, Calliophis and Echis, *Spolia Zeylanica*, 26(2); 147-150.

Deraniyagala, P.E.P. (1954). Two new snakes from Ceylon, *Proceedings Ceylon Association for Advancement of Science*, 10th Annual Sessions Part I, Sectional Programmes and Abstracts, Sec D, Colombo, p.24.

Deraniyagala, P.E.P. (1955). A coloured Atlas of some vertebrates from Ceylon, Vol 3, Serpentoid Reptilia, Ceylon National Museums, Colombo, 107 p.

Deraniyagala, P.E.P. (1960). The effects of the venom of *Echis carinata sinhaleya* the saw scaled viper of Ceylon, *Spolia Zeylanica*, 29(1); 33-34.

Deraniyagala, P.E.P. (1975). A new fossorial snake of the Genus Rhinophis Hemprich, *Spolia Zeylanica*, 33(1), 535-536.

De Silva, Anslem (1973). The cobra concept in Sinhala art and sculpture, *Tourists Ceylon*, 1(1), 32-38.

De Silva, Anslem (1976). Venomous snakes of Sri Lanka, *Snake*, 8; 31-42.

De Silva, Anslem (1976a). The pattern of snake bite in Sri Lanka, *Snake*, 8; 43-51.

De Silva, Anslem (1979). The Ceylon Krait. Record of a large specimen, *Loris*, 15(2); 97-98.

De Silva, Anslem (1980). Snake bites and antivenom treatment in Sri Lanka. Proc. International Seminar on Epidemiology and treatment of snake bite, Japan, p. 134-137.

De Silva, Anslem (1980a). An annotated bibliography of snakes of Sri Lanka, *Snake*, 12; 61-108.

De Silva, Anslem (1981). Snake bite in Anuradhapura District, *Snake*, 13; 117-130.

De Silva, Anslem (1982). Rare snakes of Sri Lanka, *Loris*, 16(1); 19-22.

De Silva, Anslem (1982a). Some cólour variations of the Green pit viper (*Trimeresurus trigonocephalus*), Loris, 16(2); 61-63.

De Silva, Anslem and Aloysius, D. (1983). Moderately and mildly venomous snakes of Sri Lanka, *Ceylon Medical Journal*, 28(3); 118-127.

De Silva, Anslem and Ranasinghe, L. (1983). Epidemiology of snake bite in Sri Lanka: A Review, *Ceylon Medical Journal*, 28(3); 144-154.

De Silva, Anslem, Kumari Jayatillake and Lakshman Ranasinghe (1983). Epidemiology of snake bite in Sri Lankan children, *Ceylon Medical Journal*, 28(3); 155-162.

De Silva, Anslem and C.G. Uragoda (1983). Traditional methods of snake bite treatment in Sri Lanka, *Ceylon Medical Journal*, 28(3); 170-174.

De Silva, Anslem (1983). Reproductive habits of *Trimeresurus trigonocephalus* (Sonnini et Latreille), *Snake* 15; 16-21.

De Silva, Anslem (1983a). *Trimeresurus trigonocephalus* bites, *Snakes*, 15; 91-94.

De Silva, Anslem and M. Toriba (1984). Reproductive habits of *Hypnale hypnale* (Merrem) Sri Lanka, *Snake*, 16; 135-138.

De Silva, Anslem (1984). Snakes of Sri Lanka: Endangered? *Loris,* 16(5); 221-222.

De Silva, Anslem (1986). Snakes of Sri Lanka: A Review (Part I), *Loris,* 17(3); 126-129.

De Silva, Anslem (1986a). Reproductive behaviour and biting patterns of Krait *(Bungarus caeruleus), Proceedings of the Kandy Society of Medicine,* 9; 14-16.

De Silva, Anslem (1986b). Snakes and snake bite in Sri Lanka: Recent Findings, Primary Health Care — Information, Education and Communication, Health Education Bureau, 5 p.

De Silva, Anslem (1987). Indigenous snake bite physicians and their management of snake bite in Sri Lanka, *Ayurveda Sameekshawa,* 1(3); 102-106.

De Silva, Anslem (1987a). Ecological notes on *Bungarus ceylonicus* Gunther, 1864, *Snake,* 19; 59-66.

De Silva, Anslem (1987b). Some epidemiological and clinical aspects of *Bungarus caeruleus* bite, *Proceedings of the Kandy Society of Medicine,* 10; 113-115.

De Silva, Anslem and Hewage, P. (1987). Snake bite in Mahaweli System H area: Galnewa, *Proceedings of the Kandy Society of Medicine,* 10; 115-116.

De Silva, Anslem and Lionel Pereira (1987). A large *Bungarus ceylonicus* Gunther, *Snake,* 19, 143.

De Silva, Anslem (1989) Hypnale nepa bite: First Record. *Proceedings of the Kandy Society of Medicine,* 11; 8-10

De Silva, PHDH (1969). Taxonomic studies on Ceylon snakes of the Family colubridae, *Spolia Zeylanica,* 31(2); 431-546.

De Silva, PHDH (1980). Snake Fauna of Sri Lanka with special reference to skull, dentition and venom in snakes, National Museums of Sri Lanka, Colombo, 472 p.

Eisenberg, J.F. and G.M. McKay (1970). An annotated checklist of the recent mammals of Ceylon with keys to the species, *Ceylon Journal of Science* (Biological Science), 8; 69-99.

Ferguson, William (1877). The order of snakes: Ophidia IN Reptile Fauna of Ceylon, Govt Printer, Colombo, 17-26.

Fernando, B (1977). Kraits and wolfsnakes the karawalas(s), *LORIS ,* 14(3); 157-159.

Fernando, E.C. (1962). The occurrence of *Echis carinata,* the saw-scaled viper in the Southern Province, *Loris,* 9(3); 215-216.

Fernando, P. and Dias, S. (1982). Indian Krait bite poisoning, *Ceylon Medical Journal,* 27; 39.

Fletcher, T.B. (1908). Notes on snakes from Diyatalawa, *Spolia Zeylanica,* 5(18); 98-101.

Gans, Carl and Fetcho J.R. (1982). The Sri Lanka genus *Aspidura* (Serpentes, Reptilia Colubridae), *Annals of Carnegie Museum,* 51(14); 217-316.

Gaussen, H., P. Legris, M. Viart and L. Labroue (1964). Vegetation map of Ceylon, International map of the vegetation. Ceylon Survey Department.

Gloyd, H.K. (1977). Descriptions of new taxa of crotalid snakes from China and Ceylon (Sri Lanka). *Proceedings Biological Society of Washington,* 90(4); 1002-1015.

Gnanawimala, Rev. Kirielle (1943) Prayoga — Ratnavali, Mahabodhi Press, Colombo.

Goonaratne, B.M.W. (1968). The poisonous land snakes of Ceylon, *Ceylon Medical Journal,* 13(1); 19-25.

Gopalakrishnakone, P. and Jayatilaka A.D.P. (1974). Light and Electron microscopic observations on the glands of some snakes, *Proceedings, Ceylon Association for Advancement of Science,* Section A, Colombo, 24-25.

Gopalakrishnakone, P and Jayatilaka, ADP (1975). Electron Microscopic studies on renal lesions caused by *Trimeresurus trigonocephalus* (Green Pit Viper) venom. *Proceedings, Sri Lanka Association for advancement of science,* Colombo, 13.

Gopalakrishnakone, P and Jayatilake, A.D.P. (1975a). Electrone Microscopic study of the skeletal muscle associated with the venom gland of *Naja naja* (cobra) *Proceedings, Sri Lanka Association for advancement of science,* Colombo, 13-14.

Gopalakrishnakone, P. (1981). Snake venom and local necrosis, *Proceedings of the Kandy Society of Medicines,* 4;210.

Gopalakrishnakone, P., Reid H.A. and Theakston R.D.G. (1981). Histopathological study of the disseminated intravascular coagulation (D.I.C.) caused by the saw-scaled or carpet viper *(Echis carinatus)* in experimental animals, *Proceedings 37th Annual Sessions, Sri Lanka Association for Advancement of Science,* Section A. p. 10.

Green, E.E. (1908). Note on the death of a Cooly from snake bite, *Spolia Zeylanica,* 5(18); 103.

Green, E.E. (1910). A case of snake bite, *Spolia Zeylanica,* 7(25); 54.

Gunther, G.A.C.L. (1858) Catalogue of Colubrine snakes in the collections of the British Museum, British Museum, London, XVI + 281.

Gunther, G.A.C.L. (1864) Reptiles of British India, Ray Society, London, XXVII + 444.

Gunther, G.A.C.L. (1869) Report on two collections of Indian Reptiles, *Proceedings Zoological Society London,* 500-507.

Gyi, Ko Ko (1970). A revision of colubrid snakes of the subfamily Homalopsinae, *University of Kansas 'museum of Natural History,* 20(2); 47-223.

Haly, Amyrald (1886). First report on the collection of snakes in the Colombo Museum, National Museum, Colombo 18 p.

Hayashi, Y. and H. Tanaka (1982). A battery-operated stunning rod for immobilizing the venomous snake, Habu, *Trimeresurus flavoviridis, Japan Journal of Experimental Medicine,* 52(1); 49-50.

Henry, G.M. (1925). Notes of *Ancistrodon hypnale,* the hump-nosed viper, *Spolia Zeylanica,* 13(2); 257-258.

Jahubar, M., Subramaniam S. and James R.F. (1984). An analysis of snake bite in Base Hospital Mannar, Abstracts, *Jaffna Medical Assocaiation,* 2nd Annual Sessions, p. 9.

Jayatilake, A.D.P., Gopalakrishnakone, P. and Alcorn D. (1981). Electron microscopic study of the pathological lesions produced by viper venom in experimental animals, *Proceedings, Sri Lanka Association for Advancement of Science,* Part I, 11.

Jeyarajah, R. and Gopalakrishnakone, P. (1981). A study of 13 snake bite patients in Peradeniya, *Proceedings, Kandy Society of Medicine,* 4; 8.

Jeyarajah, R. (1984). Russell's viper bite in Sri Lanka, a study of 22 cases, *American Journal of Tropical Medicine and Hygiene,* 33(3); 506-510.

Karunaratne, K.E. de S. (1970). Snake bite poisoning experiences in General Hospital Jaffna, *Jaffna Medical Journal,* 10(2); 119-124.

Karunaratne, K.E. de S. and Anandadas J.A. (1973). The use of antivenom in snake bite poisoning, *Ceylon Medical Journal,* 18(1); 37-43.

Khan, M.S. and Tasnim, R. (1986) Balling and Caudal luring in young Bungarus caeruleus, *Snake,* 18(1); 42-46.

Kirupannthan, S. (1970). Snake bites in Kilinochchi Hospital, 1969-1970, *Jaffna Medical Journal,* 10(2); 115-118.

Knox, Robert (1681). An historical relation of the island of Ceylon, in the East Indies, Richard Chiswell, London, p 29-30.

Kono, H. and Sawai, Y. (1975) Systemic poisoning from the bite of Rhabdophis tigrinus, *Snake,* 7(1), 38-39.

Kumaranayake, C.S. (1971). Pathological findings in viper bites, *Ceylon Medical Journal,* 16(1); 47-50.

Linnaeus, C. (1758) System Naturae, i, 10th Ed. Stockholm.

Liyanarachchi, S. (1972). *Visa veda muthuhara*, Author, Diamond Printer, Colombo, 502 p. (Text in Sinhala).

Mahendra, B.C. (1984). Handbook of the snakes in India, Ceylon, Burma, Bangladesh and Pakistan, *The Annals of Zoology*, 22, 412 p.

Malnate, E.V. (1960) Systemic division and evolution of the colubrid snake genus Natrix, with comments on the sub family Natricinae, *Proceedings Academy of Natural Sciences Philadelphia*, 112 (3), 41-71.

Malnate, E.V. and Minton, S.A. (1965) A redescription of the Natricine snake Xenochrophis cerasogaster, with comments on its taxonomic status; *Proceedings, Academy of Natural Sciences Philadelphia*, 117(2); 19-43.

Mamonov, G. (1977). Case report of envenomation by the mountain racer *Coluber ravergieri* in USSR, *Snake*, 9; 27-28.

Mangili, Guglielmo (1959). I Veleni ofidici is a coagulazione del sangue, *Archivio Zoological Italiano*, 44; 165-214.

Maretic, Z and Russell F.E. (1979). An unusual nonvenomous snake bite, *Toxicon*, 17(4); 425-427.

Mather, H.M., S. Mayne and T.M. McMonagle (1978). Severe envenomation from 'harmless' pet snake, *British Medical Journal*, 1; 1324-1325.

Mertens, R. (1968). Die arten und unterarten der schmuckbaumschkangen (Chrysopelea), *Senckenb Biology*, 49; 191-217.

Minton, Sherman A (1978). Beware Nonpoisonous snakes, *Natural History*, 87(9); 56-60.

Moore, J.C. (1960). Squirrel geography of the Indian subregion, *Syst. Zool.* 9; 1-17.

Moorman, F.R. and Panabokke, C.R. (1961) Soils of Ceylon, *Tropical Agriculturalist.* 117, 161-172.

Munasinghe, D.R. and Kulasinghe, P. (1965). Snake bite, a case report, *Ceylon Medical Journal*, 10 (2 and 3); 140-143.

Nicholls, Lucius (1929). The identification of the land snakes of Ceylon, *Ceylon Journal of Science*, (D), 2(3); 91-157.

Nimalasuriya, A. (1971) Anti-cholinesterases in the control of the neurological manifestations of RV bite, *Journal of Colombo General Hospital*, 2(4); 186-188.

Obst, F.J. (1983). Zur Kenntnis der schlangengathung vipera, *Zoologische Abhandlungen*, 38(13); 229-234.

Ogawa, H. and Y. Sawai (1986). Fatal bite of the Yamakagashi *(Rhabdophis tigrinus)*, *Snake*, 18; 53-54.

Pearless, S.H. (1909). Snakes at Badulla, *Spolia Zeylanica*, 6(21); 54-55.

Peiris, Gerald (1976). The physicial environment, IN: *Sri Lanka a Survey*, Ed. K.M. de Silva, Horst and Co. London, p. 3-30.

Pereira, D.H. (1875). A chapter on the natural history of Ceylon, Third paper: Venomous snakes, *Ceylon Friend*, 2nd series, 6(72); 265-270.

Perumainar, M. (1973). The effects of Russell's viper venom on the rat kidney, *Proceedings, Ceylon Association for Advancement of Science*, Section A, Colombo 40.

Perumainar, M. (1975). Renal damage following hump-nosed viper bite, *Proceedings, Sri Lanka Association for Advancement of Science*, 31st Annual Sessions, Part I, Programme and Abstracts, p. 14.

Perumainar, M. (1975a) Pathogensis of micro clots formation following viper bites, *Proceedings Sri Lanka Association for Advancement of Science*, 31st Annual Sessions, Part 1, Sectional Programmes and Abstracts, p. 14.

Perumainar, M. (1978). Acute renal failure following Russells viper bite, *Proceedings Kandy Society of Medicine*, 1; 22.

Ponnambalam, C. (1939). Notes on fatal case of Krait poisoning, *Ceylon Journal of Science*, Section D, 5(2); 37-38.

Ponnambalam, C. (1960). Ceylon snakes, *Loris*, 8(6); 378-381.

Reid, H.A. (1968). Snake bite in the tropics, *British Medical Journal*, 3, 359-362.

Ribeiro, J. (1685). History of Ceilao (Translated). P.E. Pieris.

Russell, Patrick (1796) An account of Indian Serpents collected on the coast Coromandal; London 90p.

Sawai, Y., M. Toriba, H. Itokawa, Anslem de Silva, G.L.S. Perera and M.B. Kottegoda (1983) Death from snake bite in Anuradhapura district, *Ceylon Medical Journal*, 28(3); 163-169.

Senanayake, F. Ranil; M, Soule and J.W. Senner (1977). Habitat values and endemicity in the vanishing rain forests of Sri Lanka, *Nature*, 265; 351-354.

Smith, M.A. (1938). The Nucho-Dorsal glands of snakes, *Proceedings of the Zoological Society London*, 108(3); 575-583.

Smith M.A. (1943). The Fauna of British, India, Ceylon and Burma, including the whole of the Indo-Chinese sub-region, Reptilia and Amphibia, Vol. 3 Serpentes, Taylor and Francis, London, 568 p.

Somanader, S.V.O. (1957). Hump-nosed viper (Kunakatuwa), *Loris*, 7(5); 422-423.

Spaar, A.E. (1910). The bite of the Russell's viper, *Spolia Zeylanica*, 6(24); 188-190.

Sreeharan, N. and Ganeshamoorthy, J. (1984). Management of envenomised snake bites low dose antivenom, *Abstracts XI International Congress of Tropical Medicine and Malaria*, Calgary, Canada, p. 146.

Stejneger, L. (1893). The poisonous snakes of North America (as quoted by Taub, 1967).

Stemmler, Gyger O. (1965). Zur Biologie der rassen von *Echis carinatus* (Schneider) 1801, *Salamandra*, 1; 29-46.

Swaroop, S and Grab B. (1954) Snake bite Mortality in the World, *Bulletin of the World Health Organization*, 10, 35-76.

Taub, Aaron M. (1966). Ophidian cephalic glands, *Journal of Morphology*, 118(4); 529-542.

Taub, Aaron M. (1967). Comparative histological studies on Duvernoy's gland of colubrid snakes, *Bulletin of the American Museum of Natural History*, 138(1); 1-50.

Taylor, E.H. (1947). Comments on Ceylonese snakes of the genus Typhlops with descriptions of New Species, *University Kansas Science Bulletin*, 31(13); 283-298.

Taylor, E.H. (1950). A brief review of ceylonese snakes, *University Kansas Science Bulletin*, 33(14); 519-603.

Thanabalasundrum, R.S. and Vidyasagara, N.W. (1969). Snake bite and its treatment, *Ceylon Medical Journal*, 14(4); 188-191.

Varagunam, T. and Panabokke, R.G. (1970). Bilateral cortical necrosis of the kidneys following snake bite, *Postgraduate Medical Journal*, 46(537); 449-451.

Visuvaratnam, M., Vinayagamoorthy, C. and Balakrishnan, S. (1970). Venomous snake bites in North Ceylon — A study of 15 cases, *Journal of Tropical Medicine and Hygiene, 73(9);* 9-14.

Vitanage, P.W. (1972). Post-precambrian uplifts and neotectonic movements in Ceylon, *24th International Geological Congress*, Sec. 3, 642-654.

Wall, F. (1905). Notes on snakes collected at Hakgala, Ceylon, *Spolia Zeylanica*, 3(10); 144-147.

Wall, Frank (1921). Ophidia Taprobanica or the snakes of Ceylon, Govt. Printer, Colombo, 581 p.

Wall, Frank (1923). Notes on snakes collected on Annasigalla Estate from August, 1920 to December, 1921, *Spolia Zeylanica*, 12(46); 252-270.

Wall, Frank (1924). Notes on Ceylon snakes collected by Mr W.W.A. Phillips, *Spolia Zeylanica*, 13(1); 71-88.

Warrell, D.A. (1983). Venoms and toxins of animals and plants, IN: *Oxford Textbook of Medicine*, Eds. Weatherall, D.J., Ledingham, J.G.G. and Warrell, D.A., Oxford Medical Publications, Oxford.

Warrell, D.A. (1986). Tropical snake bite: clinical studies in South-East Asia, IN: *Natural Toxins, animal plant and microbial*, Ed. J.B. Harris, Clarendon Press, Oxford, 25-45.

Whitaker, Romulus (1978). Common Indian snakes, a field guide, Macmillan Co. of India Ltd., New Delhi, 154 p.

Wijesinghe, T.M.K. (1981) Agro-ecological map of Sri Lanka, Land and Water use Division, Department of Agriculture, Peradeniya, ITC, Enschede, Netherlands.

Willey, Arthur (1903). Some rare snakes of Ceylon, *Spolia Zeylanica*, 1(3); 81-89.

Wimalabuddhi, Rev. Balagalle (1966). Sinhala Thupavansa, Rathna Publishers, Colombo, p. 161 (Text in Sinhala).

Yoganathan, S. (1973) Clinical manifestations and treatment of snake bite in Vavuniya, *Ceylon Medical Journal*, 18(2); 86-92.

Venomous Snakes And Snake Bite In Thailand

Chulalongkorn Hospital and Thai Red Cross
Bangkok, Thailand

Contributors:

Piboon Jintakune, : Scientist, Science Division, Thai Red Cross
Sakchai Limthongkul : Associate Professor of Medicine,
Department of Medicine, Chulalongkorn Hospital
Suebsan Mahasandana : Assistant Professor of Medicine,
Department of Medicine, Chulalongkorn Hospital
Kesorn Meemano, : Physician, Department of Medicine,
Chulalongkorn Hospital
Charn Pochanugool, : Associate Professor of Medicine,
Department of Medicine, Chulalongkorn Hospital
Visith Sitprija, : Professor of Medicine, Department of Medicine,
Chulalongkorn Hospital

SECTION A

Venomous Snakes of Thailand

[Piboon Jintakune, Charn Pochanugool, Sakchai Limthongkul, Suebsan Mahasandana, Kesorn Meemano and Visith Sitprija]

Thailand has more than 160 species of snakes belonging to 9 families. Of these, only 46 species or 2 families are deadly venomous. Twenty-four are land snakes, and the rest, sea snakes.

It has been estimated that in Thailand, more than 10,000 people are bitten by snakes in each year and 600 of these die. Ten species of these snakes represent the greatest threat (see classification).

The Siamese cobra (*Naja kaouthia*) is the most well known venomous snake of Thailand (Fig. 1). The bite of this species is very dangerous with a mortality rate which appears to be higher than that of other venomous snakes. This snake is widely distributed throughout the country. The cobra is well known for its characteristic hood. It serves as a threat display when the cobra is frightened or annoyed. The hood markings are monocellate.

The spitting cobra(*Naja sputatrix*) has developed the ability to spit venom over a distance of several feet. Its hood may be unmarked or have a binocellate marking. The ability to spit is due to the fact that the opening of the fangs' groves are towards the front, while the fangs' opening of the non-spitting Siamese cobra is near the tip. Spitting cobras usually spit the venom towards the head or face of an enemy. If the venom enters the eyes, there is an immediate burning pain with inflammation and permanent blindness may result.

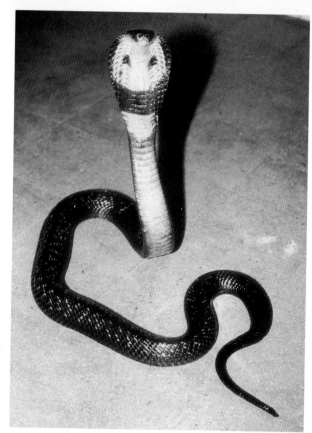

Figure 1
Cobra *(Naja kaouthia)*

Figure 2
King cobra
(Ophiophagus hannah)

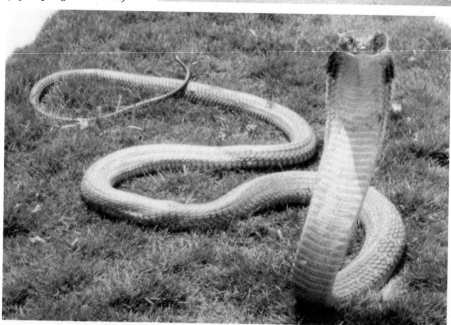

The king cobra *(Ophiophagus hannah)* is the longest venomous snake of Thailand and perhaps in the world (Fig. 2). The largest king cobra ever caught in Thailand was trapped in Nakhon Sri Thammarat province in the South. It measured 5.59 metres long. Most king cobras, however, grow to a length of 3 to 4 metres. The king cobra is found in all parts of Thailand but mainly in the South. The generic name *Ophiophagus* indicates that it feeds mainly on other snakes. It hunts both day and night. It hisses to warn its victim and can strike a person even when its hood is expanded, a technique the other cobras do not possess. The bite of a large king cobra is likely to be rapidly fatal, as fast as 3 minutes in one report. In fact, there are very few instances of natural king cobra bites recorded in Thailand, primarily because the king cobra lives deep in jungles and hilly areas where only very few people venture.

The banded krait *(Bungarus fasciatus)* is the least aggressive of Thailand's venomous snakes (Fig. 3). It is shy and inoffensive, rarely bites a man unless severely provoked. The normal behaviour for a banded krait when caught is to coil up and hide its head. Most banded krait bites recorded are the result of people stepping on them or handling them. The venom is a potent neurotoxin. Most kraits are nocturnal and their principal food are smaller snakes. The banded krait is found in rice fields and lowlands, in all parts of Thailand, but commonly in the central region.

The Malayan krait *(Bungarus candidus)* is smaller than the banded krait but it is more aggressive (Fig. 4). Like its cousin, it is a nocturnal animal. It lives in lowlands and moist areas. It is found in every part of the country but commonly in the South and Southeast of Thailand.

The Russell's viper *(Vipera russelli siamensis)* is quite aggressive when disturbed, it makes a fearsome hissing warning sound which may be followed by a lightning strike (Fig. 5). It feeds at night on rodents, birds and frogs. It lives in jungle and lowland areas of the central region of Thailand. This species is very dangerous.

The green pit vipers *(Trimeresurus* sp.) also take an important position among Thai venomous snakes. The name pit viper comes from a special structure which appears as a deep groove between the nostril and eye on each side of the head and which is called the pit organ. It functions as a thermoreceptor very sensitive to changes of temperature. The pit vipers use the pit organ for searching for warm blooded prey such as small rodents or birds. Most green pit vipers *(Trimeresurus)* are bush and land dwellers and nocturnal in habit. Eleven species of *Trimeresurus* have been recorded in this country (Taylor, 1965). The most dominant of them are the white-lipped green pit viper *(T. albolabris)* (Fig. 6) and the Pope's green pit viper *(T. popeorum)* (Fig. 7). Both of them are distributed throughout the country. They do not appear to be especially dangerous and very few fatalities have been reported from their bite.

The Malayan pit viper *(Agkistrodon rhodostoma* or *Calloselasma rhodostoma)* is widely distributed throughout the country but mainly in the South (Fig. 8). Normally, it is not aggressive and usually lies motionless under fallen leaves or in grasses. If disturbed, it could make a very quick strike. It

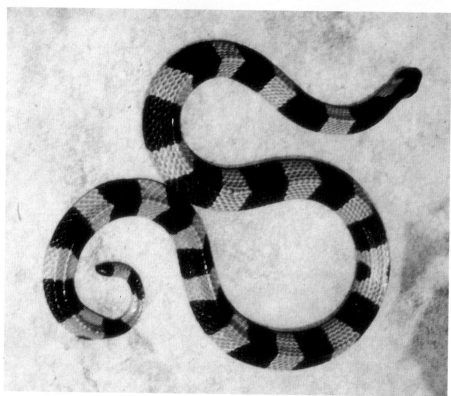

Figure 3
Banded krait *(Bungarus fasciatus)*

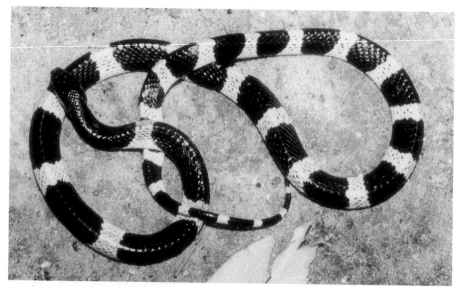

Figure 4
Malayan krait *(Bungarus candidus)*

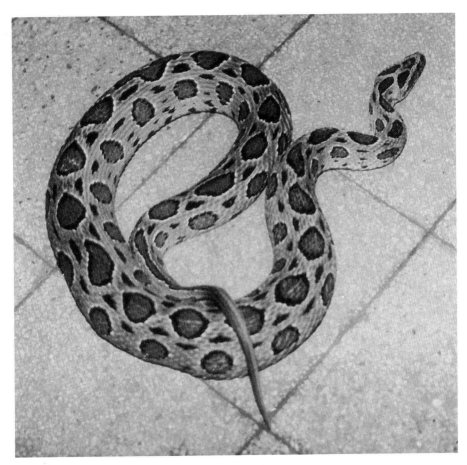

Figure 5
Russell's viper *(Vipera russelli siamensis)*

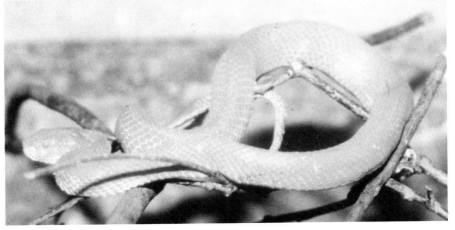

Figure 6
White-lipped green pit viper *(Trimeresurus albolabris)*

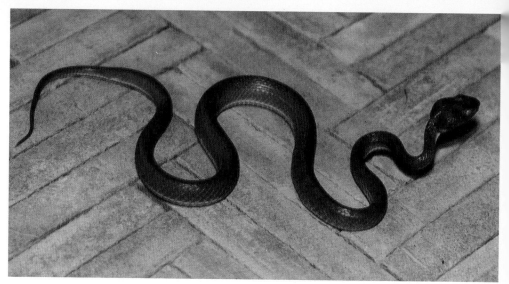

Figure 7
Pope's green pit viper *(Trimeresurus popeorum)*

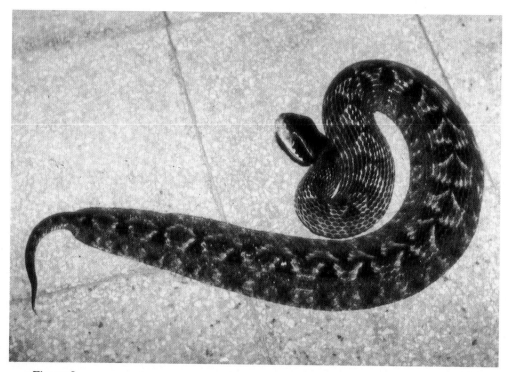

Figure 8
Malayan pit viper *(Agkistrodon rhodostoma* or *Calloselasma rhodostoma)*

accounts for a significant number of snake bites in Thailand. Fortunately, the mortality rate is quite low.

The sea snakes spend most of their lives in coral reefs, in water near muddy flats or in the deep sea. They have loose skin and a flat or paddle-shaped tail for swimming. They feed on eels and small fish. Twenty-two of Thailand's 23 varieties of sea snakes, are venomous. The commonest among all Thai venomous sea snakes is the Hardwick's sea snake *(Lapemis hardwicki)*. Other common species which are usually found in Thailand's waters are the blue-banded sea snake *(Hydrophis cyanocinctus)*, the beaked sea snake *(Enhydrina schistosa)*, the small headed sea snake *(Microcephalophis gracilis)* and the black and yellow sea snake *(Pelamis platurus)* (Fig. 9).

Classification of the venomous snakes of Thailand

The classification is based on the work of Taylor (1965) and Phelps (1981).

Class	— Reptilia
Order	— Squamata
Sub-order	— Serpentes

1.	F. — Viperidae	2.	F. — Elapidae	3.	F. — Colubridae
	Sf. — Viperinae		Sf. — Elapinae		Sf. — Colubrinae
	Sf. — Crotalinae		Sf. — Hydrophinae		Sf. — Homalopsinae
			Sf. — Laticaudinae		

In Thailand, only the first and second families are medically important venomous snakes. The third family, Colubridae, are the rear-fanged snakes which can be considered harmless in Thailand.

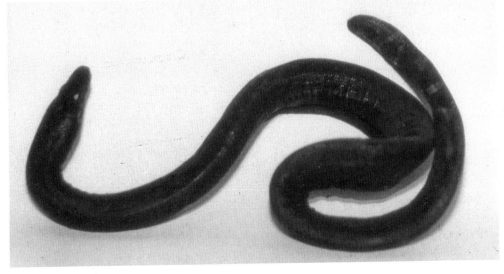

Figure 9
Sea Snake *(Pelamis platurus)*

Elapidae

The snakes in this family have a pair of permanently erect and enlarged fangs in the front of the upper jaw. The fangs have a deep enclosed vertical groove through which the venom is injected when the snake bites. Sub-families of the Elapidae are:

1. Elapinae — Cobras and Kraits
2. Hydrophinae — Sea snakes
3. Laticaudinae — Sea snakes

Viperidae

Snakes in the family have very large fangs at the front of their upper jaws. The fangs are movable and have a hollow canal running through them which act like a hypodermic needle. Sub-families of the Viperidae are:

1. Viperinae — Vipers
2. Crotalinae — Pit vipers

Habits of some important venomous snakes (Reitinger and Lee, 1978):

Siamese cobra and spitting cobra —	They are normally terrestrial but may climb. Found from sea level up to 800 m, but mainly in lowland areas.
King cobra —	Open hilly areas and jungles. Mainly terrestrial but climbs fairly well.
Banded krait —	Open areas and fields. Often found near water. Does not climb.
Malayan krait —	Hilly areas. Often found near water. Does not climb.
Russell's viper —	Plains and hills. Terrestrial and seldom climbs.
Malayan pit viper —	Hilly areas, rubber fields. Terrestrial and does not climb.
White-lipped green pit viper —	Found from sea level up to over 1,000 m. Seems to prefer hilly areas near streams, but may venture into urban areas for food. Rather terrestrial but climbs very well.
Pope's green pit viper —	Same as white-lipped green pit viper.
Sea snakes —	Marine dwellers.

Snake Bite In Thailand: A General View

[Charn Pochanugool, Kesorn Meemano, Sakchai Limthongkul, Suebsan Mahasandana, Piboon Jintakune and Visith Sitprija]

Snake bite is one of the national health problems of Thailand, an agricultural country in Southeast Asia. The low central plains along the Chao Phya river, the mountainous forests, semi-arid plateau and the tropical monsoon forests are suitable habitats for venomous snakes. There are 7 kinds of venomous snakes that pose the medical problems: cobras *(Naja kaouthia, Naja sputatrix)*, king cobras *(Ophiophagus hannah)*,Russell's vipers *(Vipera russelli siamensis)*, Malayan pit vipers *(Calloselasma rhodostoma)*, green pit vipers *(Trimeresurus* species*)*, kraits *(Bungarus fasciatus* and *Bungarus candidus)*, and sea snakes (Hydrophinae).

There are no accurate statistics of snake bite in Thailand. However, it is estimated to be about 10,000 cases with 600 deaths each year. In Chulalongkorn Hospital, a general hospital where most of the cases of snake bite are seen, there are 2,000 patients with snake bite each year, accounting for 3.2% of total patients in the emergency room. Sixty percent of the cases are envenomated by venomous snakes. Green pit viper bites are most common, followed in order by cobra bites, Russell's viper bites, Malayan pit viper bites and krait bites. Sea snake bite poisoning is least common. Most of the victims are bitten at night. In some species such as Malayan krait, the bite usually occurs while the victim is asleep. However, it is interesting that in cobra bite the patients are bitten mostly during the day. Fishermen are bitten from time to time by *Lapemis hardwicki* which has a less potent venom. Envenomation from this kind of sea snake is therefore seldom observed. Sea snake poisoning is mainly caused by the bite of *Enhydrina schistosa* (Reid, 1975). Snake bite occurs throughout the year, although it is somewhat more common between May and December with more rain and cool weather.

The lower limbs are usually affected since the victims are bitten during walking or working. In green pit viper bite, the hand is often the site of bite. In suburbs of Bangkok, most patients can reach the hospital within one to two hours following the bite. This can be a problem in the rural areas with poor transportation.

Clinical symptoms

The symptoms of snake bite usually result from a combination of fear, anxiety and envenomation. The symptoms produced by fear and anxiety are those of sympathetic stimulation. First aid treatment from the local primary care such as tourniquet application or traditional medicine may cause local reactions and infection at the site of bite. Besides the general symptoms such as pain, nausea, vomiting, palpitation and fainting, the symptoms and signs resulted from envenomation fall into 2 categories.

Neuromuscular symptoms

Neuromuscular symptoms usually are caused by the bite of Elapinae (cobras and kraits) and Hydrophinae (sea snakes). The common symptoms consist of ptosis of the eyelids, blurred vision, paresthesia, headache, increased salivation, trismus and paralysis of the muscle of deglutition, tongue and vocal cord. Respiratory muscle paralysis is life threatening. Local tissue necrosis at the site of bite is common in cobra bite. In sea snake bite, muscular tenderness can occur a few hours following the bite. Myoglobinuria is observed and renal failure may develop.

Haematological symptoms

Epistaxis, haematemesis, haematuria, ecchymosis of the skin, haemorrhage in the mucous membrane and brain may be observed in viper bites. Local symptoms with swelling, haemorrhage and even gangrene are more severe in green pit viper bite and Malayan pit viper bite than in Russell's viper bite. Intravascular haemolysis and haemoglobinuria may be observed. Signs of increased vascular permeability such as oedema and severe proteinuria, as observed in Russell's viper bite in Burma (Myint-Lwin et al, 1985), has not been the experience in Thailand. Neuromuscular symptoms with ptosis of the eyelids, described in Russell's viper bite in Ceylon (Jeyarajah, 1984), has not been observed. Russell's viper bite is often complicated by acute renal failure.

The venom of Colubridae also produces haematological symptoms. Although *Rhabdophis subminiata* is common, the bite has not been reported.

Management of snake bite

Attention is given to the kind of snake brought to the doctor by the patient, the site of the bite and the symptoms. Since symptoms and signs depend on the amount of venom injected, snake bite does not necessarily produce the symptoms.

The poisonous snake is characterised by the presence of 2 fangs on the front of the upper jaw. The fangs of Elapidae are permanently erected, while the Viperidae have a pair of larger movable fangs. The presence of the 2 fang marks at the site of bite signifies the bite by venomous snake. However, there is reservation to this since in our experience only 67% of cobra bites had 2 definite fang marks. In 33% the fang mark was either not definite or there was only one fang mark.

Local treatment consists of proper cleaning of the site of bite. Tourniquet application should be used only for the early phase of neurotoxic snake bite, and should be released for 15 seconds every 30 minutes. Antivenom administration is the treatment of choice when there is systemic symptoms. Supportive treatment for pain and respiratory care are necessary. In neurotoxic snake bite, respiratory support with assisted ventilation can be life saving especially when the antivenom is not available (Pochanugool et al, to be published). Haemodialysis has been shown to improve the muscular symptoms in sea snake bite (Sitprija et al, 1971), and exchange blood transfusion has been effective in Russell's viper bite (Peiris et al, 1969). Further clinical study is warranted in these areas.

Neurotoxic Snake Bite

[Charn Pochanugool, Sakchai Limthongkul, Suebsan Mahasandana, Kesorn Meemano, Piboon Jintakune and Visith Sitprija]

There are 4 kinds of snakes with neurotoxic venom in Thailand, belonging to the family Elapidae. They are *Naja naja* (cobra), *Ophiophagus hannah* (King Cobra), *Bungarus fasciatus* (banded krait) and *Bungarus candidus* (Malayan krait). Cobra bites are most common in this group, but bites by kraits and king cobras are occasionally observed. Males are more at risk than females.

Local signs and symptoms

The presence of 2 fang marks at the site of bite is characteristic of venomous snake bite. However, not all victims with serious effect have 2 definite fang marks. In our experience only 67% of cases of cobra bite have 2 definite fang marks, while 19% have one fang mark and 14% have no definite fang mark. There are mild pain and swelling at the site of bite. The tissue around the fang marks shows discoloration and becomes necrotic between one hour and 32 hours with the mean of 13 hours. The diameter of the necrotic area ranges from 0.5 to 15cm. The necrosis involves only skin and subcutaneous tissue. No muscle is effected. The early necrosis indicates that enzymatic processes are involved (Iddon et al, 1987). However, in some cases with delayed development of tissue necrosis, bacteria might play a role. Local necrosis is an important feature in cobra bite, occurring in 46% of cases and requiring one to two months to heal. Cases with indefinite fang marks show less necrosis than those with definite fang marks despite the same systemic symptoms. The distance between the 2 fang marks also shows positive correlation with tissue necrosis. This local tissue necrosis at the site of bite is occasionally observed in krait bite.

Systemic symptoms

Systemic symptoms include headache, nausea, vomiting and abdominal pain in some cases. The earliest and definite sign indicating neurotoxic snake bite is ptosis with palpebral fissure less than 0.5 cm. The other symptoms and signs are slurred speech, salivation, dysphagia, ocular muscle paralysis, respiratory paralysis and paralysis of extremities. Since respiratory muscle paralysis occurs at the higher percentage and earlier than paralysis of the extremities, muscles of respiration thus seem to be more sensitive to neurotoxic venoms than the muscles of extremities.

There is no complete paralysis when the distance between fang marks is less than 1 cm. The incidence of muscle paralysis is up to 50% when the distance is more than 1 cm. However, the development of tissue necrosis in the cases with assisted ventilation is earlier when compared with those which did not need assisted ventilation.

Management

1. Prevention: Theoretically, ground snake bite can be prevented by wearing gloves and boots while working in the rice field or in the jungle and by not placing the hand into any place where one cannot see. Those who work with snakes must be very careful. We see from time to time snake bite in workers who handle snakes in the snake farm.

2. First aid: Tourniquet application may be used in neurotoxic snake bite. The use of bandage over and above the bite site with splint and immobilization of the affected part are recommended (Sutherland et al, 1979). Herbal medicine is to be avoided. The patients must be carried to a nearby hospital, as soon as possible. Cutting or sucking the wound is absolutely prohibited.

3. Management in the hospital: The following principles are used in treating neurotoxic snake bite.

a) Observe closely the patient bitten by a neurotoxic snake.

b) Treat as soon as possible when there are definite signs and symptoms of neurotoxic nature.

In practice, when the patient arrives in the hospital and there are no symptoms and signs of neurotoxic envenomation (ie. no ptosis, no slurred speech, no difficulty in opening the mouth) the tourniquet is to be removed, the bite area is cleaned with normal saline or distilled water and antiseptic. The patient is then observed closely. If the patient develops signs and symptoms of neurotoxic envenomation or when the patients come to the hospital with signs and symptoms of neurotoxic envenomation, the antivenom should be given immediately after the intravenous line has been established (Mitrakul et al, 1984). With the tourniquet already applied the antivenom must be given before removing the tourniquet or cleaning the wound. At the same time the apparatus for intubation and assisted ventilation must be ready to be used in case the symptoms and signs progress to respiratory failure.

The indications for intubation and assisted ventilation are (Limthongkul et al, in press):

a) Dysphagia or aspiration which indicates that the muscles of deglutition are fatigued. If measured, the vital capacity is less than 1.5 litres and the peak flow is less than 200 lites/minute.

b) Paradoxical abdominal movement or respiratory alternans which indicates grade II respiratory muscle-diaphragm fatigue.

Therefore while observing the patients, measurement of peak flow should be done every 10 — 15 minutes. Intubation and assisted ventilation are performed promptly if there is any indication as stated above. While the patient is intubated and ventilation is assisted, other symptomatic and supportive measures should be given. Adequate fluid and calories are given by intravenous infusion to keep fluid, electrolytes and acid base in balance and to provide adequate calories.

In the year 1982, when there was shortage of neurotoxic antivenom in Chulalongkorn Hospital, we could save 5 neurotoxic snake bite victims by assisted ventilation and supportive care (Pochanugool et al, to be published). From 1982 to 1984, we treated 51 cases of cobra bite without antivenom and managed them symptomatically with only respiratory supportive care. All recovered completely except one who had respiratory arrest and died on arrival at the hospital. The findings are of great interest. A comparative study between those patients receiving antivenom and those without antivenom therapy is being conducted.

Administration of antivenoms

Antivenoms from Queen Saovapha Memorial Institute are used. The initial dose is 40 — 100 ml intravenously, followed by 20 — 30 ml every 10 — 15 minutes according to signs and symptoms of the patients. In practice the requirement of the antivenom range from 100 — 400 ml per case with an average of 200 ml. The dosage is the same either for the bite of cobra, king cobra or krait. Corticosteroid has no clinical effects on the outcome (Trishnanonda, 1979).

Before antivenom administration a skin test with subcutaneous injection of 0.2 ml of antivenom should be performed. If the diameter of the wheel is more than 1 cm, methyl prednisolone (100 mg) is intravenously given with the antivenom hourly for 3 doses. Adrenalin must be at hand for treating the possible anaphylactic reaction.

Anticholinesterase

Prostigmine and edrophonium chloride have been used with both favorable and unfavorable results (Banerjee et al, 1972; Campbell 1964; Warrell et al, 1983). Yet, anticholinesterase may serve as an adjuvant treatment along with antivenoms. In this respect further critical clinical study is needed.

Local lesion

In 46% of cobra bite cases, tissue necrosis develops. Tissue necrosis occurs early and requires debridement (Fig. 10). Skin graft helps in shortening the duration of hospitalization. Of the cobra bite patients with tissue necrosis, 88% require skin graft. Appropriate antibiotics should be given.

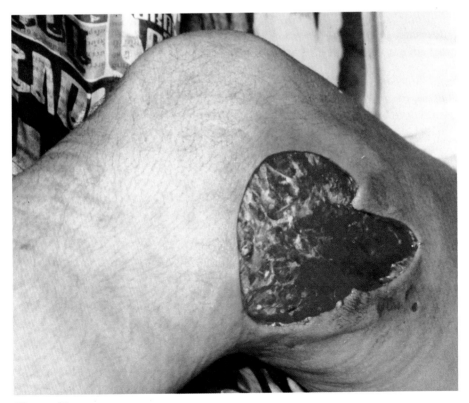

Figure 10
Local tissue necrosis in cobra bite after debridement

Viper Bite

[Suebsan Mahasandana, Charn Pochanugool, Sakchai Limthongkul, Kesorn Meemano, Piboon Jintakune and Visith Sitprija]

Viper bites are most common among poisonous snake bites in Thailand with a broad spectrum of clinical manifestations.

Generally there are many effects of viper venom on organs with the main actions being vasculotoxicity (Bonta et al, 1979; Rothchild et al, 1979) and haemostatic defects (Nahas et al, 1964). The coagulant effect of Russell's viper venom is by the thromboplastin-like action (Mitrakul, 1979) through the activation of factor X and V which subsequently provoke disseminated intravascular coagulation (DIC) (Mahasandana et al, 1980; Than et al, 1987). For the crotalids the major coagulant fraction has a thrombin like action (Mitrakul, 1973, 1979; Talalak, 1977; Gaffney et al, 1979) causing hypofibrino-genemia (Chan, 1979; Mahasandana et al, 1980; Mitrakul, 1982) and thrombocytopenia in serious cases (Mahasandana et al, 1980; Mitrakul, 1982).

Clinical manifestations of viper bite

Clinical manifestations are the results of local and systemic effects of the venoms. General complaints following the bites include pain, nausea, vomiting, diarrhoea, palpitation and fainting. Local pain occurs in all cases. The rare symptoms such as myalgia and transient disorientation are occasionally found in Russell's viper bite. The signs besides transient hypotension (in some cases) are oedema, ecchymosis, blisters and necrosis of the affected limbs (Maha-sandana et al, 1980; Mitrakul, 1982; Myint-Lwin et al, 1985; Ho et al, 1986). Other uncommon signs are lymphadenitis, lymphangitis and cellulitis. Non-clotting blood is the cardinal sign of systemic envenomation following viper bites. There is spontaneous systemic haemorrhage of various organs leading to gingival bleeding, haematemesis. hematuria and subconjunctival haemorrhage (Mahasandana et al, 1980; Ho et al, 1986). Clinical manifestations following viper bites, therefore, vary greatly from mild degree of oedema to serious systemic haemorrhage depending upon the amount of venom injected. Patients admitted soon after the bites are usually found with local effects and in severe cases systemic haemorrhage occurs. Those who are not treated immediately may develop complications. The immediate complications are angioedema (Mahasandana et al, 1980) shock, confusion and compartmental syndrome (Warrell et al, 1986). The delayed complications include necrosis, thrombo-phlebitis, lymphangitis, cellulitis, glomerulopathy and acute renal failure. Bleeding into central nervous system is a major cause of death. Russell's viper bite has a higher mortality rate than the crotalid envenomations.

In the clinical approach of viper bite victims, considerations must be given to specific snake species, degrees of severity, complications and fang mark size. The definite diagnosis requires the detection of venom antigen in the serum or urine (Theakston et al, 1977; Coulter et al, 1980; Dhaliwal et al, 1983; Ho et al, 1986; Silamut et al, 1987). Because there are wide ranges in degrees of envenomation following viper's bite, close observation for the signs of specific envenomation is mandatory when the venom antigen cannot be detected on admission. In rural areas where the antigen detection is not possible, the geographical area where the patients are bitten, typical symptoms and signs and laboratory indicators of coagulopathies are the important clues in making a diagnosis of the snake species.

Russell's viper bite
(Vipera russelli siamensis)

The victims of this snake are mostly farmers in the paddy fields of the central part of Thailand. The clinical presentations other than the previous mentioned are transient hypotension and tightness in the chest. Usually Russell's viper bite patients have a lesser degree of local swelling than the crotalid victims (Mahasandana et al, 1980). Blisters and necrosis are also less common than the crotalid's victims. Other signs such as conjunctival oedema, shock from pituitary haemorrhage and chronic hypo-pituitarism reported in Burma (Myint-Lwin et al, 1985; Tun-Pe et al, 1987) have not been observed in Thailand. Gingival bleeding and haematemesis are the two common systemic haemorrhages. The laboratory findings in severe cases are compatible with disseminated intravascular coagulation (DIC), characterized by unclotted blood, prolonged PTT, PT, TT, depletion of factors X, V, II and fibrinogen, thrombocytopenia and secondary increased fibrinolysis (Mahasandana et al, 1980; Than-Than et al, 1987). In some cases besides the unclotted blood from DIC, there are massive intravascular haemolysis (ie. haemoglobinemia and haemoglobinuria) and microangiopathic-haemolytic anaemia. There is a high percentage of acute renal failure in severe cases (Mahasandana et al, 1980; Myint-Lwin et al, 1985), the causes of which are multiple (Sitprija and Boonpucknavig 1977; Aung-Khin, 1978; Date et al, 1981, 1982). Conventional treatment of acute renal failure should be prescribed. Some patients may need peritoneal dialysis or haemodialysis. The mortality rate is minimal, the causes of death are central nervous system bleeding (Mahasandana et al, 1980; Myint-Lwin et al, 1985) and acute pulmonary oedema in some cases (Jeyarajah, 1984). If the unclotted blood and renal complication are corrected appropriately patients usually have complete recovery, and rarely chronic disability.

Malayan pit viper bite
(Calloselasma rhodostoma or Agkistrodon rhodostoma)

The prominent physical signs following this snake bite are multiple blisters (Fig. 11) and a severe degree of local necrosis of the affected limb (Fig. 12) (Reid et al, 1963; Chan, 1979; Ho et al, 1986). Multiple haemorrhagic blisters develop very rapidly. Gingival bleeding is most common. The most serious emergency complication is compartmental syndrome (Warrell et al, 1986) which requires urgent fasciotomy. This complication occurs as early as 12 — 24 hours after the bite necessitating the urgency of correction of uncoagulable blood by specific antivenin administration. The other serious local complication is tissue necrosis that may even require amputation of the affected limb (Ho et al, 1986; Warrell et al, 1986). Renal complication has not been observed, except

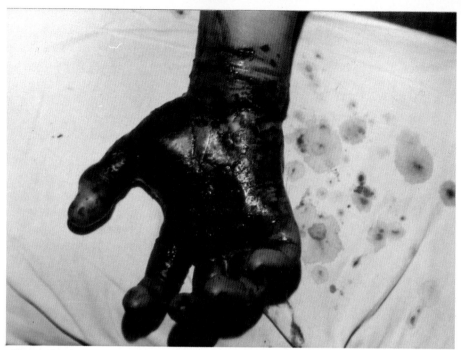

Figure 11
Tissue necrosis of hand in Malayan pit viper bite

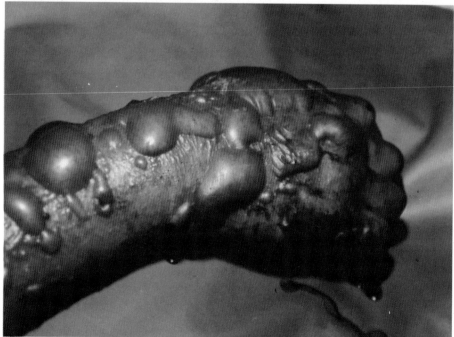

Figure 12
Multiple blisters in Malayan pit viper bite.

for haematuria. However, chronic disability from local necrosis and unrecognized compartmental syndrome can be considerable. All the victims should be closely observed for a certain period of time ie. 48 hours, because some patients may develop non-clotting blood while under observation. The essential haematological laboratory data in severe cases besides anaemia are hypofibrinogenemia or afibrinogenemia, thrombocytopenia and increased plasma fibrin degradation products (Warrell et al, 1986). After correction of non-clotting blood by antivenin administration some patients may develop recurrence of venom antigenemia which is due to slow absorption of the venom (Ho et al, 1986). Recurrence tends to occur in the patient with the high level of circulating venom on admission (Ho et al, 1986). Infection of the necrotic wound is not uncommon. Mortality is low and central nervous system bleeding is the usual cause of death. In dealing with Malayan pit viper bite, attention should be aimed at preventing the quick progression of local necrosis that may cause chronic disability to the victim.

Green pit viper bite
(Trimeresurus species)

There are two common species of Green pit vipers in Thailand: *T. albolabris* and *T. popeorum*. Since bushes and creepers are the common habitats of these gardeners and children are frequently the victims. The most striking local effect is oedema which varies from mild to severe affecting the whole limb (Mitrakul et al, 1973; Mahasandana et al, 1980; Mitrakul, 1982). Oedema may persist as long as 4 weeks in some cases. Gingival bleeding is common. Clinical patterns can be divided into mild, moderate and severe cases. In mild cases there is only oedema. There are oedema (Fig. 13) and ecchymosis (Fig. 14) in moderate cases. For severe cases there is spontaneous systemic haemorrhage in addition to oedema and ecchymosis. There is good correlation between ecchymosis of the affected limb and clinical severity (Mahasandana et al, 1987). The other clinical effects such as blister (Fig. 15) and necrosis do not correlate with degree of severity (Mahasandana et al, 1987). Necrosis occurs more common on the digits than on other bitten sites (Fig. 16) (Mahasandana et al, 1980). Renal complication is rare. The patients may have the chronic disability from gangrene at the bitten site especially in the digits. Central nervous system bleeding may be the cause of death but is uncommon (Mahasandana et al, 1980). The degree of hypofibrinogenemia varies from mild to afibrinogenemia depending on the severity of envenomation. Thrombocytopenia correlates well with higher degrees of severity (Mahasandana et al, 1980; Mitrakul, 1982; Mahasandana et al, 1987). Increased plasma fibrin degradation product is the usual laboratory finding.

Management of viper bite.

The aims for the treatment of viper bites are prevention of venom reaching the systemic circulation, neutralization of circulating venom, correction of venom induced abnormalities and general supportive cares.

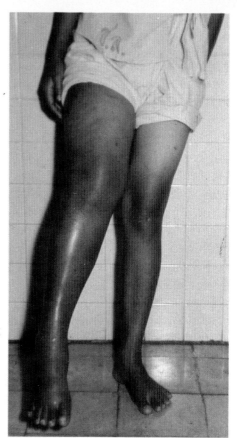

Figure 13
Oedema of the right leg following the bite of a green pit viper.

Figure 14
Ecchymosis of the skin in green pit viper bite

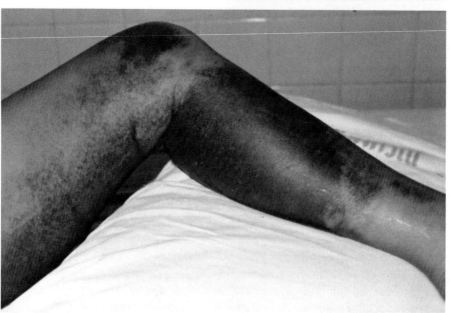

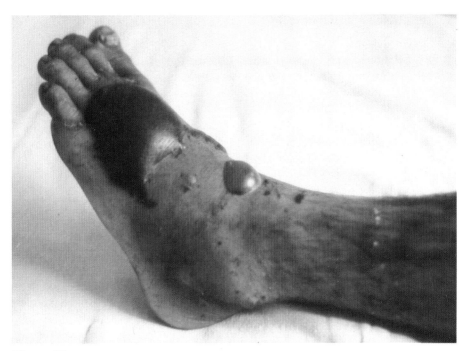

Figure 15.
Haemorrhagic blisters of the foot in green pit viper bite.

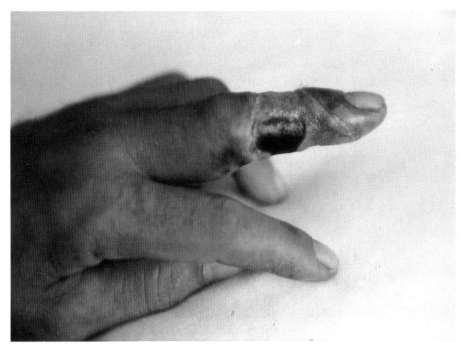

Figure 16.
Tissue necrosis of the finger in green pit viper bite

The outline is as follows:

1. First aid
   1.1 Pressure and immobilization (Sutherland et al, 1979)
   1.2 Admission to hospital as soon as possible.
   1.3 Avoidance of trauma at the bitten area such as wound incision or suction of the wound.
2. Hospital management
   2.1 Patient evaluation
       2.1.1 specific species identification
       2.1.2 degree of severity
       2.1.3 emergency complications
   2.2 Medical treatment of snake bite
       A.   General care
            1. Reassurance
            2. Snake bite chart: consists of vital signs, date/time of snake bite, fang mark size, symptoms, local effects (oedema, ecchymosis, blister, necrosis), signs of systemic haemorrhage
            3. Obtain blood or urine specimen of snake venom antigen detection (if available)
            4. If (3) is not available perform the indicator of coagulopathies as follows:
               4.1 Venom clotting time (Lee & White): if special laboratory is available, perform PTT, PT, TT, FDP or specific factor assay if indicated.
               4.2 Platelet count or estimation
               4.3 Blood smear examination
            5. Wound cleaning
            6. Avoidance of further bleeding ie. I.M. injection, apply local pressure long enough after venepuncture
            7. BUN, creatinine, electrolytes
            8. Record fluid intake/output
            9. Medication: analgesic (avoidance of aspirin), tranquilizer
            10. Fluid replacement: 5% D/N/2 2,500-3,000 ml. per day (normal renal function) if there is evidence of acute renal failure the fluid administration should be restricted.

       B.   Specific treatment
            1. Criteria for specific antivenom administration : The non-clotted blood or venous clotting time lasts longer than 30 minutes
            2. Monovalent antivenom 4 — 6 vials in 5% D/N/2 250 ml. I.V. infusion over 30 minutes and repeated every 6 hours if indicated clinically.
            3. Skin test for hypersensitivity should be performed before antivenom administration.
            4. Heparin infusion may be considered in Russell's viper bite.

5. Blood components therapy (PRC, FFP, platelet concentrates) for supportive care if indicated clinically.
C. Treatment of the following complications
   1. Immediate complications : angioedema, hypotension, shock, compartmental syndrome, acute renal failure.
   2. Delayed complications : debridement of the blisters, wound care, antibiotic if indicated and tetanus prophylaxis.

References

Aung-Khin, M. (1978). Histological and ultrastructural changes of the kidney in renal failure after viper envenomation. Toxicon 16:71.

Banerjee, B.N., Sahni, A.L., Chacko, K.A. Neostigmine in the treatment of Elapidae bites. J. Assoc Physicians India 20:503.

Bonta, I.L., Vargaftig, B.B., Bohm, G.M. Snake venoms as an experimental tool to induce and study model of microvessel damage. In : Chen-Yuan Lee (ed.) Handbook of Experimental Pharmacology. Vol 52. Snake venom. Berlin : Springer-Verlag, 1979. 664-674.

Campbell, C.H. (1964). Venomous snake bite in Papua and its treatment with tracheostomy, artifical respiration and antivenin. Trans. R. Soc. Med. Hyg. 58:263.

Chan, K.E. (1979). Bleeding after Malayan pit viper bites. Proceeding of congenital and acquired bleeding disorders in tropical areas. Southeast Asian Trop. Med. Publ. Hlth. 10:276.

Coulter A.R., Harris, R.D., Sutherland, S.K. (1980). Enzyme immunoassay for the rapid clinical identification of snake venom. Med. J. Aust. 1:433.

Date, A., Shastry, J.C.M. (1981). Renal ultrastructure in cortical necrosis following Russell's viper envenomation. J. Trop. Med. Hyg. 84:3.

Date, A., Shastry, J.C.M. (1982). Renal ultrastructure in acute tubular necrosis following Russell's viper envenomation. Pathology 137:225.

Dhaliwal, J.S., Lim, T.W., Sukumaran, K.D. (1983). A double antibody sandwich MICRO-ELISA Kit for the rapid diagnosis of snake bite. Southeast. Asian J. Trop Med. Publ. Hlth. 14:367.

Gaffney, P.J., Marsh, N.A., Talalak, P. (1979). Snake venoms and haemostasis : Some suggested mechanisms of action. (Proceedings of congenital and acquired bleeding disorders in tropical areas). Southeast Asian J. Trop. Med. Publ. Hlth. 10:258.

Ho, M., Warrell, D.A., Looareesuwan S., Phillips, R.E., Chantavanich, P., Krabwang, J., Supanaranond, W., Viravan, C., Hutton, R., Vejcho, S. (1986). Clinical significance of venom antigen levels in patients envenomated by Malayan pit viper (*Calloselasma rhodostoma*).Am. J. Trop. Med. Hyg. 35:579.

Ho, M., Warrell, M.J., Warrell, D.A. Bidwell, D., Voller, A. (1986). A critical reappraisal of the use of enzyme-linked immunosorbent assay in the study of snake bite. Toxicon 24:211.

Iddon, D., Theakston, R.D.G., Ownby, C.L. (1987). A study of pathogenesis of local skin necrosis induced by *Naja nigricollis* (spitting cobra) venoms using simple histological staining technique. Toxicon 25:665.

Jeyarajah, R. (1984). Russell's viper bite in Sri-Lanka. Am., J. Trop. Med. Hyg. 33:506.

Limthongkul, S., Pochanugool, C., Benyajati, C., Meemano, K. Respiratory muscle fatigue in cobra bite treated patients. J. Med. Assoc. Thai. In press.

Mahasandana, S., Rungruhsirivorn, V., Chantarankul, V. (1980). Clinical manifestations of bleeding following Russell's viper and Green pit viper bites in adults. Southeast Asian Trop. Med. Publ. Hlth. 11:285.

Mahasandana, S., Ratananda, S., Akkawat, B. (1987). Ecchymosis as a clinical predictor in Green pit viper bites. Presented at 1st Asian-Pacific Congress on Animal, Plant and Microbial Toxins, Singapore. June 24-27, 1987.

Mitrakul, C. (1973). Effect of Green pit viper *(Trimeresurus erythrurus* and *Trimeresurus popeorum)* venoms on blood coagulation, platelets and fibrinolytic enzyme system. Studies in vivo and in vitro. Am. J. Clin. Pathol 60:654.

Mitrakul, C., Impan, C. (1973). The haemorrhagic phenomena associated with Green pit viper *(Trimeresurus erythrurus* and *Trimeresurus popeorum)* bites in children. A report of studies to elucidate their pathogenesis. Clin. Paediat. 12:215.

Mitrakul, C. (1979). Effect of five snake venoms on coagulation, fibrinolysis and platelet aggregation. (Proceedings of congenital and acquired bleeding disorders in tropical area). Southeast Asian J. Trop. Med. Pub. Hlth., 10:266.

Mitrakul, C. (1982). Clinical features of viper bites in 72 Thai children. Southeast Asian J. Trop. Med. Pub. Hlth., 13:628.

Mitrakul, C., Dhamkrongart, A., Futrakul, P. et al (1984). Clinical feature of neurotoxic snake bite and response to antivenin in 47 children. Am. J. Trop. Med. Hyg. 33:1259.

Myint-Lwin, Warrell, D.A., Phillips, R.E., Tin-Nu-Swe, Tun-Pe, Maung-Maung Lay (1985). Bites by Russell's viper *(Vipera russelli siamensis)* in Burma : Haemostatic, vascular, and renal disturbances and response to treatment. Lancet 2 (8467):1259.

Nahas, L., Macfarlane, R.G., Denson, N.W.E. (1964). A study of coagulant action of eight snake venoms. Thromb. Diath. Haem. 12:355.

Peiris, O.A., Wimalaratne, K.D.P., Nimalasuriya, A. (1969). Exchange transfusion in the treatment of Russell's viper bite. Postgrad. Med. J. 45:627.

Phelps, T. (1981). Poisonous snakes. Blandford Press Ltd, London.

Reid, H.A., (1975). Epidemiology of sea snakes bites. J. Trop. Med. Hyg. 78:106.

Reid, H.A., Thean, P.C., Chan, K.E. Baharom, A.R. (1963). Clinical effects of bites by Malayan pit viper *(Agkistrodon rhodostoma)*. Lancet 1:6 17.

Reitinger, F.F., Lee J.K.S. (1978). Common Snakes in South East Asia and Hong Kong. South China Printing Co Ltd, Hong Kong.

Rothchild, A.M., Rothchild, Z. Liberation of pharmacologically active substances by snake venoms. In : C.Y. Lee (ed). Handbook of Experimental Pharmacology. Vol. 52. Snake Venom, Berlin : Springer-Verlag, 1979. 592-620.

Silamut, K., Ho, M., Looareesuwan, S., Viravan, C., Wuthiehanun, V., Warrell, D.A. (1987). Detection of venom by enzyme-link immunosorbent assay (ELISA) in patients bitten by snake in Thailand. Br. Med. J. 29-402.

Sitprija, V., Boonpucknavig, R. (1977). The kidney in tropical snake bite. Clinical Nephrol. 8:377.

Sitprija, V., Sribhibhadh, R., Benyajati, C., (1971). Haemodialysis in poisoning by sea snake venom. Br. Med. J. 3:218.

Sutherland, S.K., Coulter, A.R., Harris, R.D. (1979). Rationalization of first-aid for elapid snake bite. Lancet 1:183.

Talalak, P. (1977). Action of *Trimeresurus erythrurus* and *Trimeresurus popeorum* venom on blood coagulation. J. Med. Assoc. Thai. 60:9.

Taylor, E.H. (1965). The Serpents of Thailand and Adjacent Waters. The University of Kansas Science Bulletin, Vol. 45, No. 9.

Than-Than, Khin Ei Han, Hutton, R.A., Myint-Lwin, Tin-Nu-Swe, Phillips, R.E., Warrell, D.A. (1987). Evolution of coagulation abnormalities following Russell's viper bite in Burma. Br. J. Haematol. 65:193.

Theakston, R.D.G., Lloyd-Jones, M.J., Reid, M.A. (1977). MICRO-ELISA for detection and assaying snake venom and venom-antigody. Lancet 2:639.

Trishnanonda, M. (1979). Incidence, clinical manifestation and general management of snake bite. Southeast Asian J. Trop. Med. Publ. Hlth. 10:148.

Tun-Pe, Phillips, R.E. Warrell, D.A., Moore, A.A. Tin-Nu-Swe, Myint-Lwin (1987). Acute and chronic pituitary failure resembling Sheehan's syndrome following bites by Russell's viper in Burma. Lancet 2 (8562):763.

Warrell, D.A., Looareesuwan, S., Theakston, R.D.G., Phillips, R.E., Chantavanich, P., Virvan, C., Supanaranond, W., Krabwang, J., Ho, M., Hutton, R.A., Vejcho, S. (1986). Randomized comparative trial of three monospecific antivenom for bites by the Malayan pit viper *(Calloselasma rhodostoma)* in southern Thailand: Clinical and laboratory correlation. Am. J. Trop. Med. Hyg. 35:1235.

Warrell, D.A., Looareesuwan, S., White, N.J., Theakston, R.D.G., Warrell, M.J., Kosakarn, W., Reid, H.A. (1983). Severe neurotoxic envenoming by the Malayan krait *Bungarus candidus* (Linnaeus):response to antivenom and anticholinesterase. Br. Med. J. 286:678.

SECTION B

Renal Involvement of Snake Bite

[Visith Sitprija, Charn Pochanugool and Suebsan Mahasandana]

Being a highly vascularized organ, the kidney is commonly involved in snake bite. A broad spectrum of renal involvement has been described (1-3). In this section clinical renal problems, renal pathological changes and pathogenesis will be covered.

Clinical Renal Manifestations

The clinical spectrum varies from mild urinary sediment changes to renal failure.

Proteinuria

Proteinuria with mild urinary sediment changes is observed in 4% of snake-bite patients (4). In most cases proteinuria is less than 1 g/24h, and disappears very quickly. Although nephrotic syndrome has been described in the literature, the cause-effect relationship has not been substantiated (5). In our extensive experience with snake bite we have not encountered any patient with nephrotic syndrome. However, in Burma the bite by Russell's viper can produce heavy proteinuria due to increased glomerular permeability (6). Again, this is a transient phenomenon and disappears upon recovery of clinical symptoms. Hemoglobinuria may be observed in Russell's viper bite, and myoglobinuria usually occurs in sea snake bite.

Hematuria

Microscopic hematuria has been observed in a variety of bites and may accompany mild proteinuria. Gross hematuria is common in viper bite. Bleeding, due to coagulation abnormality and vasculotoxicity of the viper venom, is usually of short duration and never alarming. Renal infarction may account for gross hematuria with back pain. Nephritic syndrome is observed occasionally in green pit viper bite (7). This is characterised by edema, hematuria and hypertension. Mild renal failure may occur in this clinical setting.

Renal failure

Renal failure is common in various snake bites including sea snake, Russell's viper, puff adder, saw scale viper, *Bothrops jararaca*, crotalid snake, *Cryptophis nigrescens*, tiger snake, boomslang, dugite, gwardar and Agkistrodon snake (8). In Thailand, the bites of Russell's viper, sea snake and green viper are responsible for renal failure and the incidence is high in Russell's viper bite.

Disseminated intravascular coagulation is common. Intravascular hemolysis and hemoglobinuria are occasionally seen. Renal failure usually occurs soon after the bite. The occurrence of renal failure in Russell's viper bite is about 70% of the cases. Nonoliguric renal failure is not uncommon. In occasional cases myoglobinuria may occur. The duration of renal failure varies from one week to several weeks. Severe oliguria and anuria should be suspected in those patients with cortical, necrosis, acute interstitial nephritis (9) or extracapillary proliferative glomerulonephritis (10).

In sea snake bite renal failure is associated with rhabdomyolysis, muscular paresis and myoglobinuria. Hyperkalemia can be alarming and requires prompt treatment. Hyperuricemia, hyperphosphatemia and hypocalcemia are associated laboratory findings. Hemodialysis has been shown to improve muscular symptoms (11).

Rarely, renal failure may be seen in green pit viper bite. This is glomerular rather than tubular in origin. Diffuse proliferative glomerulonephritis has been observed (7, 12).

Renal Pathological Changes

There is a broad spectrum of pathological changes.

Glomerular lesions

Mild mesangial proliferative glomerulonephritis is common in snake bite. When renal histological study is performed later in the course of the disease there may be immune complex deposition with IgM and C3. Mesangiolysis has been observed following the envenomation of Habu snake (13), Russell's viper (12) and Agkistrodon snake (14). Focal mesangial proliferative glomerulonephritis has been described. (13). Diffuse proliferative glomerulonephritis may be seen occasionally in green pit viper bite (12), and extracapillary proliferative glomerulonephritis has been reported in Russell's viper bite. (10).

Vascular lesions

Arteritis of interlobular artery can be seen in Russell's viper envenomation (1). There is deposition of C3 in the arterial wall where the lesion is located. Thrombophlebitis of interlobular vein is noted in both Russell's viper bite and green pit viper bite.

Tubulointerstitial lesions

Tubular necrosis with various degrees of interstitial changes is a common pathological counterpart of acute renal failure. This has been noted in Russell's viper bite and sea snake bite. Heme casts are seen when there is associated intravascular hemolysis. Myoglobin pigment is observed when there is rhabdomyolysis especially is sea snake bite. Tubular degeneration and necrosis are diffuse, but are more prominent in the distal and collecting tubules.

Several diffuse interstitial changes with mononuclear cell infiltration is occasionally observed in Russell's viper bite (9).

Cortical necrosis and renal infarct

Rarely is cortical necrosis seen in our experience with Russell's viper bite.

This is in contrast to the experience in India where cortical necrosis is found more often (2). This could be related to the delayed treatment in India. Renal infarct is also seldom.

Pathogenesis of Renal Lesions

Three main factors are responsible for the pathogenesis of renal changes: nonspecific inflammatory effects, immunologic mechanism and direct nephrotoxicity (15).

1. Nonspecific inflammatory effects

Several factors in the process of inflammation are nonspecific, being shared by various diseases, but can compromise microcirculation leading to renal ischemia and impairment of renal function. At the clinical level these risk factors include hypovolemia, intravascular hemolysis, intravascular coagulation, myoglobinuria, blood hyperviscosity and cardiac dysfunction.

Various chemical mediators such as prostaglandins, kinins, histamine, serotonin, leukotrienes, catecholamines, renin, angiotensin, thromboxane A2 and cytokines are released in inflammation. Some are vasodilators and some are vasoconstrictors. Yet, the net result is vasoconstriction and renal ischemia. Complement activation and oxygen radical release further contribute to the renal injury.

2. Immunologic mechanism

Immune complex type of glomerulonephritis has been observed in the patients who receive antivenom prior to renal biopsy. This is not surprising. However, immune complex glomerulonephritis has also been demonstrated in those patients who do not receive any antivenom when the renal biopsy is performed later in the course of the disease (7). This is interesting, and is interpreted to indicate that the venom antigen is implanted to the glomeruli and the antibody later acquired binds with the antigen already deposited. The findings are suggestive of in situ immune complex glomerulonephritis. Yet, glomerulonephritis of this type is usually mild and presents no significant clinical manifestations except for mild proteinuria.

3. Direct nephrotoxicity

Viper venoms are vasculotoxic causing vasculitis and glomerulonephritis. The demonstration mesangiolysis, diffuse proliferative and extracapillary proliferative glomerulonephritis without deposition of immune complex indicates glomerulotoxicity of the venom.

Tubulotoxicity of Russell's viper venom is reflected by the decreased potential difference across the proximal tubular membrane of *Triturus* kidney in isolated renal perfusion when the kidney is perfused with the venom (16). The increase in urine flow, urine sodium excretion and urine N — acetyl β glucosaminidase without any alteration of renal blood flow and glomerular filtration rate is indicative of tubular injury (17).

Renal involvement in snake bite thus varies widely. All renal structures can be involved, giving various clinical renal manifestations. The causes are multiple. Renal failure is the result of several factors operating in concert.

References

1. Sitprija V, Boonpucknavig V: The kidney in tropical snakebite Clin Nephrology 8:377, 1977.
2. Chugh KS, Pal Y, Chakravarty RN, Datta BN, Mehta R, Sakhuja V, Mandal AK, Sommers SC: Acute renal failure following poisonous snake bite. Amer J Kidney Dis 4:30, 1984
3. Aung-Khin M: Histological and Ultrastructural changes of the kidney in renal failure after viper envenomation. Toxicon 16:71, 1978
4. Sitprija V: Renal disease in snakebite. In "Natural Toxins", Eaker D, Wadström T (eds), Pergamon Press, Oxford and New York, 1980, p.43
5. Steinbeck AW: Nephrotic syndrome developing after snakebite. Med J Aust 1:543, 1960.
6. Lwin M, Warrell DA, Phillips RE, Swe TN, Pe T, Lay MM: Bites by Russell's viper (Vipera russelli siamensis) in Burma: haemostatic, vascular and renal disturbances and response to treatment. Lancet 2:1259, 1985
7. Sitprija V, Boonpucknavig V: Glomerular changes in tropical viper bite in man. Toxicon 21 (Suppl) : 401, 1983
8. Sitprija V: The kidney in acute tropical disease. In "Tropical Nephrology", Kibukamusoke JW (ed), Citforge Pty, Canberra, Australia, 1984, p. 148.
9. Sitprija V, Suvanpha R, Pochanugool C, Chusil S, Tungsanga K: Acute interstitial nephritis in snake bite. Am J Trop Med Hyg 31:408, 1982
10. Sitprija V, Boonpucknavig V: Extracapillary proliferative glomerulonephritis in Russell's viper bite. Br Med J 2:1417, 1980
11. Sitprija V, Sribhibhadh R, Benyajati C: Haemodialysis in poisoning by sea snake venom. Br Med J 3:218, 1971
12. Sitprija V, Boonpucknavig V: Tropical diseases and glomerulonephritis. Proceedings of The 3rd Asian-Pacific Congress of Nephrology, Singapore 1986, p.262
13. Cattel V, Bradfield JWB: Focal mesangial prolifeative glomerulonephritis in the rat caused by Habu snake venom. Am J Pathol 87:511, 1977
14. Sakurai N, Sugimoto K, Sugihara H, Shirasawa H, Muro H, Kaneko M, Nikai T, Shibata K: Glomerular injury in mice induced by Agkistrodon venom. Am J Pathol 122: 240, 1986
15. Sitprija V, Thamaree S, Chaiyabutr N: Renal Pathogenesis of snake bite. Proceedings of The First Asia-Pacific Congress on Animal, Plant and Microbial Toxins, Singapore, 1987, p. 108
16. Chaiyabutr N, Sitprija V, Sugino N, Hoshi T: Russell's viper venom-induced depolarization in the proximal tubule of Triturus kidney. ICMR Annals 5:181, 1985
17. Thamaree S, Chaiyabutr N, Leepipatpaiboon S, Buranasiri K, Tosukowong p, Sirivongs P, Sitprija V: Effects of indomethacin on renal hemodynamics, urinary enzymes and thromboxane B_2 following envenomation of Russell's viper in dogs. Chula Med J 31:387, 1987

The Highly and Potentially Dangerous Elapids of Papua New Guinea

The identification, ecology and distribution of venomous species, and the clinical diagnosis and treatment of snakebite

by Mark T. O'Shea

BSc., FRGS

46 Buckingham Road, Penn, Wolverhampton, WV4 5TJ, England

Introduction

The Second Largest Island in the World

Papua New Guinea constitutes the eastern half of the World's second largest island and it has, in the past, been governed by German, British, Japanese and Australian administrations. The western half of the island, known today as West Papua or Irian Jaya, was formerly a Dutch colony but now constitutes the largest territory in the Republic of Indonesia. Papua New Guinea received its full Independence in 1975 and ow comprises nineteen provinces, incorporating several large archipelagoes to the north and east of the mainland, and the National Capital District surrounding the capital, Port Moresby.

The popular view of mainland Papua New Guinea is of a region of impenetrable, and relatively unexplored, montane rainforests clinging precariously to steep, unscalable ridges and peaks with rushing, torrential whitewater rivers gouging their way through the rock and vegetation as they race towards the coasts. Since much of central Papua New Guinea is comprised of a soaring montane backbone, which rises to over 4000m (13,130ft), this description is accurate when applied to the Highland Provinces but large areas of both northern and southern Papua are covered by lowland rainforests, monsoon forests, and vast arid *Eucalyptus* savanna woodlands which bear more resemblance to the drier areas of neighbouring Australia. There are also extensive freshwater swamps and coastal and estuarine mangrove entanglements. Enormous areas of Papua New Guinea are extremely low-lying and flat, especially the huge expanses of Western Province between the Fly River and the Irian Jaya border which barely rise more than 200m above sea-level. Because this region is subject to extensive seasonal flooding it was necessary to site the administrative centre on the offshore island of Daru. Further east in Central and Milne Bay Provinces the mountains rise almost straight from the sea. There are two major river systems; the Fly-Strickland in the southwest and the Sepik in the northwest.

There are several large archipelagoes to the north and east of the Papua New Guinea mainland the most noteworthy being the large island Provinces of East and West New Britain and New Ireland, the Admiralty Island Group in Manus Province to the north and the Trobriand, D'Entrecasteaux and Louisiade Archipelagoes of Milne Bay Province to the southeast. North Solomons Island Province, containing Bougainville Island, to the far east borders the archipelagoes of the independent Solomon Islands.

The population, comprising mainly Papuans and Melanesians, is believed to number some three million, mostly centred in the Highlands Provinces and the major lowland towns of Port Moresby, Lae, Madang and Rabaul. The country boasts over 700 languages but the main tongues are English, Pidgin, Hiri and Police Motu. Outside the major centres most of the population subsist by slash and burn garden horticulture and hunting and are, therefore, often isolated by many miles from larger villages or main communication routes. Most of the population move about on foot or in small canoes although larger private and Government boats travel along the coasts, between the islands and for considerable distances up the more navigable rivers. An increasing number of settlements are becoming linked by roads, especially around Port Moresby, Madang, Lae, Wewak, Mt Hagen and Popondotta. However, most of these road systems are not interlinked and the major connections between isolated communities remains the extensive air network. Unfortunately internal air travel in Papua is fairly expensive.

The climate is equatorial monsoon with distinct wet and dry seasons but the variation in relief brings about localised differences in climate with the central mountainous backbone receiving 225-575cm of rainfall annually compared to the southern coast which lies in a rainshadow zone and receives only 100cm annually and the majority of low-lying Western Province which receives 150cm of rain per year, hence the considerable variations in vegetational cover. Lowland temperatures vary from 70°F to 90°F (21°C — 32.2°C) and relative humidity varies from 70-90%.

A Unique Fauna.

The fauna of New Guinea is ostensibly Australasian sharing many species, genera and families with that huge continent, but numerous taxa of Indonesian or Pacific origin are also represented here together with a unique collection of endemic species and genera. There are no monkeys, no native jungle cats and no hornbills. Instead, fantastic birds of paradise, tree kangaroos, flightless cassowaries and spiny egg-laying echidnas are found. Even amongst the herpetofauna several taxa are conspicuous by their absence, namely the venomous solenoglyphous family Viperidae, and the non-venomous/mildly venomous family Colubridae, which are so diverse elsewhere in the tropics, are poorly represented. Other groups have diversified and speciated greatly, in particular the skink lizards, family Scincidae, the pythons, subfamily Pythoninae, and the venomous proteroglyphous family Elapidae. This study concerns this latter family as, although it is well known that Australia is the only country in the world with more species of venomous than non-venomous snakes, it is often not realised that New Guinea shares several of Australia's most venomous species and also boasts a few highly venomous endemic species.

Snakebite As A Hazard In Papua New Guinea.

In the majority of the World's tropical regions all elapids are considered a potential threat to human life, whether they are cobras, mambas, kraits or coral snakes, but in Australia and New Guinea the situation is quite different. When it is realised that the Australasian elapids have diversified and speciated widely, to occupy the vacant niches which are otherwise inhabited by the numerous harmless colubrid species throughout the rest of the world, it can be seen that many of the small, secretive, burrowing species of the genera *Toxicocalamus* and *Unechis*, with their inoffensive manners, small mouths and weak venom, are no more dangerous to man than the tiny non-venomous or only mildly venomous colubrid species which they mirror ecologically such as the Indo-Chinese *Calamaria* or Neotropical *Tantilla*.

Twenty-six species of terrestrial elapids have been recorded from New Guinea and the archipelagoes to the east, including the Solomon Islands. This constitutes 35% of the total known ophiofauna, excluding seasnakes. Only nine species in six genera are considered to be highly dangerous to man — 12% of the recorded Papuan snake fauna. All of these species are confined to the mainland provinces and they will be dealt with individually in the following sections. However, caution is still advised regarding some of the moderately sized insular elapids, with unknown and, therefore, potentially harmful venom. It should be noted that Kinghorn and Kellaway (1943) reported the death adder *(Acanthophis)* from New Britain but the author is unable to locate any further records and de Haas (1950) omits this locality whilst including Indonesian Torres Strait islands. Papuan insular species to be treated with respect include Muller's snake, *Aspidomorphus muelleri* (max. length 640mm), found throughout much of the mainland and the New Britain and New Ireland Provinces, Hediger's snake, *Parapistocalamus hedigeri* (300mm), *Salomonelaps par* (750mm), and the Banded small-eyed snake, *Loveridgelaps elapoides* (800mm), from Bougainville, North Solomons Provinces, and the Solomon Islands. Manus Province has no terrestrial elapids.

Many of the dangerous elapids are confined to the lowland savanna/ woodland regions of southern Papua, with the notable exception of the ubiquitous Death adders, *Acanthophis spp.*, and the elusive rainforest New Guinea small-eyed snake, *Micropechis ikaheka*. Death adders are responsible for many serious snakebites in the Ramu River Valley, Madang Province and the small-eyed snake is the cause of the alarming incidence of snakebite accidents on the north coast of Madang Province and on neighbouring Karkar Island. However, many venomous snakebites occur in low-lying southern localities and most of the documented and medically treated bites take place in or around Port Moresby which possesses both a large resident and itinerant human population and a wide variety of suitable habitats for the four species of dangerous elapids known to occur in coastal Central Province. Whilst certain areas of Western Province may accommodate more species of highly venomous snakes the population is more scattered and bites are less likely to come to the attention of the authorities. Before a specific antivenom was produced for the death adder Tidswell (1906) estimated that the Australian mortality rate from this single species was as high as 50%. Even so, notified deaths due to snakebite in Papua during Campbell's time never exceeded eight per year or 1.7/100 000 population.

During a two month visit to Western Province in 1986 the author received reports of ten 'serious' bush snakebites; two of these were confirmed as venomous snakebites. One terminated fatally, possibly due to a combination of venom and the over-exuberant use of knives by villagers to bleed the venom from the patient. This 'first aid' treatment was prevented on the second occasion by an expedition nurse who intervened on the victim's behalf.

Campbell reported that the Papuan blacksnake, *Pseudechis papuanus*, was the main cause of serious snakebites in southern Papua. This somewhat biased assertion was based on identification of the snake by the victim rather than by a qualified person. The Papuan blacksnake seems to instill an almost mythological dread into the people of the Trans-Fly to the point where almost any dark unicolour snake is called a 'Pap black' by Western Province villagers. The author collected a number of battered Papuan blacksnake cadavers which were really harmless colubrid species; *Amphiesma mairii* or *Dendrelaphis punctulatus*. Some Papuans do not differentiate between the blacksnake and the taipan *(Oxyuranus scutellatus)*, although Togo villagers believe they are female and male, respectively of the same species (Parker, 1982). It is, therefore, extremely probable that many envenomations by taipans or whipsnakes *(Demansia spp.)*, together with symptomless bites from aggressive non-venomous species, such as the diurnal treesnake *Dendrelaphis punctulatus*, will be blamed on the Papuan blacksnake by rural snakebite victims.

It might be true that the Papuan blacksnake was once more common than it is today and, therefore, more deserved of its reputation. However, it now seems likely that the situation has changed and this species is extremely rare, if not extinct, in certain parts of its range. In two months in Western Province the author examined 116 snakes but only saw one *Pseudechis papuanus*. The reason for the probable decline of the blacksnake population is most likely to be the introduction of the cane or marine toad, *Bufo marinus* from South America, into areas of Papua New Guinea and Australia as a biological crop pest control in the 1930's and 1940's. The threats posed by this toad on resident frog-eating snakes, such as the Papuan blacksnake and most other Australo-Papuan elapids, with the notable exception of the taipan, are threefold. First, none of the frogs normally preyed upon by these snakes contain any toxins which could harm the snake but bufonid toads, (naturally absent from Australasia), posses a powerful bufotoxin which is at its most potent in *B. marinus*. There are snakes in the Americas which can cope with these toxins but Papuan elapids die rapidly from their effects. Because these toads have no natural enemies they are able to breed in large numbers and invade new habitats without any control. The second and third effects of the marine toad on the snake fauna of Papua concern the eating habitats of the toads themselves. They eat not only the frogs that the snakes would have otherwise preyed upon, but they also devour the young snakes. Together with habitat destruction, reclamation of land and cutting of woodland which all affect the status of the snakes and their amphibian prey, blacksnake populations are almost certain to decline. The taipan, *Oxyuranus scutellatus*, however, being a strict mammal-eater is not only relatively unaffected by the increasing populations of *B. marinus*, but destruction of woodland for building is likely to attract both the taipan's rodent prey and, therefore, the snake itself. This situation is mirrored in Queensland where taipan numbers have risen, or at least remained stable, whilst anurophagous species have declined (Covacevich & Archer, 1975; Shine & Covacevich, 1983). Taipans appear to be more common than blacksnakes around Port Moresby and on Daru Island, Western Province, where *B. marinus* is well established. However, the status of the toad and the blacksnake in mainland Western Province would make an interesting study.

The small-eyed snake should also be treated with extreme caution. Its habitats and the effects of its venom are little understood. It is probably a much more dangerous species than is currently believed, especially in Madang Province and on nearby Karkar Island where the snake is known as the 'white snake', and only its secretive nocturnal nature prevents more human bites. Seven probable fatalities due to this species have been reported (Blasco and Hornabrook, 1972).

The highly venomous seasnakes are extremely common in the surrounding Pacific Ocean. Approximately twenty species have been reported from Papuan coastal waters. Most are inoffensive, totally marine and rarely encountered, except by fishermen hauling in nets. However, some species of seasnakes, particularily the highly venomous common beaked seasnake *Enhydrina schistosa*, have been recorded as travelling for many miles up the larger tidal rivers. *E.schistosa* has been responsible for several serious bites in the Ramu River, Madang Province (Hudson & Fromm, 1986) and the author collected a specimen believed to be *E.schistosa* sixty kilometres inland on the Oriomo River, Western Province. In addition, whilst most seasnakes are helpless when removed from their aquatic environment, the sea kraits, *Laticauda colubrina* and *L.laticaudata*, actually venture onto land to lay their eggs. These black and gunmetal banded snakes may be encountered on coral or rocky beaches or in mangrove swamps and, although they are generally placid and rarely bite, the toxicity of their venom means that they must be considered potentially dangerous. For the purposes of the study discussion of seasnakes will be confined to the population of *E.schistosa* in the Ramu River System.

Parker (1982), also records the presence of an undescribed species' of aquatic snake from southern Trans-Fly, Western Province which is said to be 'normal' with smooth brown or yellow-brown scales, enlarged ventrals and a short cylindrical tail but which possesses venom which is believed to cause death within minutes. This snake is considered to be extremely rare and

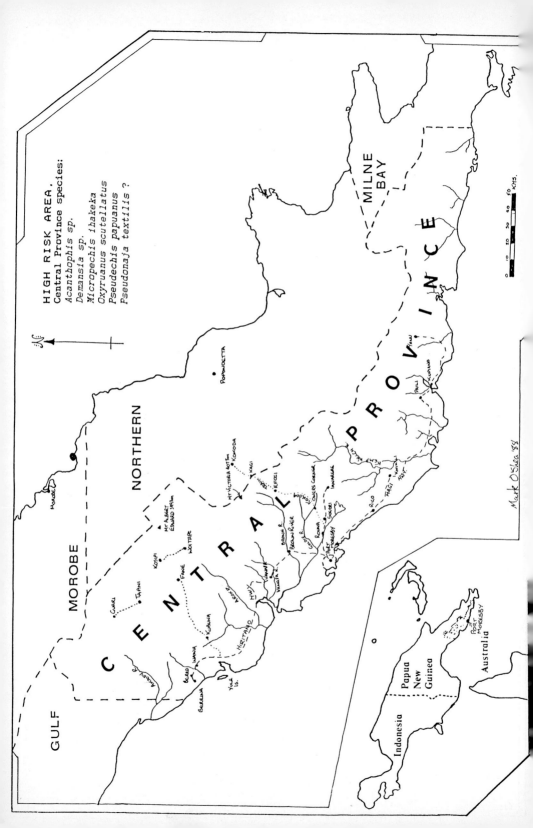

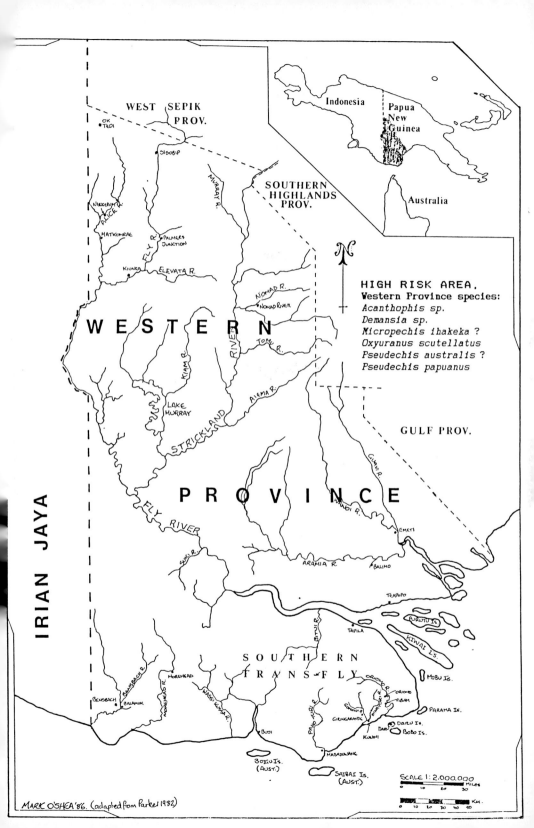

thought only to inhabit the muddy bottoms of small freshwater streams and sago swamps, occasionally emerging onto dry land to bask. With a maximum length of two metres, this snake is thought to have been responsible for the extremely rapid deaths of three young girls who were bathing in the Ouwe Creek near Wipim. Neither Parker, nor this author, has been able to locate a specimen of this snake despite visits to Wipim and interviews with villagers. However, the Ouwe Creek does feed into the Oriomo River, in which this author located a *Hydrophis*, so the possibility of some form of land-locked seasnake being the cause of the deaths cannot be dismissed.

It should, of course, be noted that not all riverine or estuarine snakes are dangerous seasnakes. Two species of harmless file snakes, *Acrochordus* (family Acrochordidae), and five mildly venomous members of the subfamily Homalopsinae (family Colubridae), (Parker 1982; O'Shea 1986), also inhabit these environments.

History Of Snakebite In Papua New Guinea.

The Statistics of Snakebite.

Much of the important early work on snakebite in southern 'Papua' concerns cases of elapine snakebite treated at Port Moresby General Hospital and studied by Campbell (1966; 1967; 1969), during the six years period, October 1959 to November 1965, when he was a general physician. Campbell submitted his exhaustive study on the subject as a thesis towards his degree as a Doctor of Medicine at the University of Sydney in 1969 and also published several important papers based on his findings in *The Medical Journal of Australia, Toxicon* and other journals. Other relevant papers in this area include Price and Campbell's (1979) study of snakebite admissions to PMGH between 1967 and 1971 and Brian and Vince's (1987) work on snakebites amongst children, aged 2 to 16, admitted to PMGH between 1981 and 1984. In contrast few papers have appeared regarding snake envenomation in northern 'New Guinea' other than Blasco and Hornabrook (1972) and Hudson and Pomat's (1988) survey of snakebite in Madang Province and admissions to Madang General Hospital between 1977 and 1986. These studies of the clinical signs and symptoms of Papua New Guinean snakebite have been drawn on extensively here as this author is a tropical herpetologist with a primary interest in the ecology, taxonomy, distribution and venoms of snakes from a zoological, rather than a medical, standpoint.

Prior to the Second World War few hospitals existed in Papua and snakebite admissions were quite infrequent. The largest single yearly quota for snakebite admissions was six amongst a total of ninety-one admissions to Port Moresby Hospital during 1906-07. Fatalities also rarely featured in the statistics, although undoubtedly they occurred in rural areas. Campbell reports that the *Annual Report of the Territory of Papua*, (which does not include New Guinea north of the mountainous backbone), records three deaths each in the years 1915-16, 1926-27 and 1934-35 and also occasional reports from *The Papuan Villager* during the late 1920's and early 1930's. The statistics obtained following World War Two are equally misleading as the *Annual Reports of*

Papua records numerous snakebites from non-venomous species or bites which did not result in envenomation, together with the serious cases, under the same heading: "Poisoning by Snake Bite", or later as "Effects of Poison" which include other causes of clinical poisoning.

Campbell spent a great deal of time sifting through the available data and statistics and he was finally able to present a series of data for snakebite admission and deaths in Papuan hospitals. This data is summarised here but it must be remembered first, that many snakebite victims never seek medical attention and are, therefore, not included in these statistics, and second, that the New Guinea districts, where at least three dangerous species occur, are not represented in Campbell's data.

Campbell estimated that during the late 1950's and 1960's snakebite, or suspected snakebite, was thought to be responsible for 155 admissions (6.3 per 1000 admissions), annually to Papuan hospitals (Table 1), excluding the hospitals in the Southern Highlands. Snakebites, therefore, accounted for five to ten percent of admissions in outstation hospitals and up to thirty-five percent of admissions to Port Moresby Hospital. Campbell also concluded that the fatality rate amongst admissions to PMGH was 7% and Brian and Vince (1987) reported a similar death rate (7.7%) amongst all children but a much higher rate of mortality (21%) for children under five.

Of 482 suspected snakebite admission to Port Moresby General Hospital over a six years period, Campbell determined that only 123 of these admissions showed definite signs of envenomation. The other cases ranged from possible snakebites with no envenomation to accidents with inanimate objects. Hudson and Pomat considered 175 admissions to Madang General Hospital which were believed to be as a result of possible or definite snakebites but case notes were only available for 129 of these patients and in only 64 of those were symptoms of envenoming recorded. It is, therefore, dangerous to rely too much on the available medical records and statistics although they may be useful as a rough guide. In addition, many indigenous Papuans, in common with many rural peoples throughout the world, place considerable faith in traditional medicines, in preference to 'modern' medical techniques and prefer to remain in their own villages rather than to travel considerable distances to unfamiliar hospitals. Since data is only available for hospital snakebite admissions and deaths the true status of snakebite in rural Papua New Guinea is not known.

In an attempt to understand the statistics of snakebite and be able to predict high risk groups, activities and times of day, Campbell restricted his interest to the 123 patients with unequivocal bites by venomous snakes but Hudson and Pomat considered their entire group of 129 possible and definite snakebites for which case notes were available. Within Campbell's test group 111 patients developed systemic symptoms whilst of 64 of Hudson and Pomat's group showed positive signs of envenoming . Campbell's twelve who showed no signs of envenomation were bitten by snakes which were subsequently killed and identified as venomous. Brian and Vince's study of snakebite amongst children records 63 admissions but case notes were missing for nine patients. Of the remaining 54 patients all but two showed definite signs of envenoming.

TABLE 1
Snakebite Admissions for Papua 1961-67

District 1961-67	Snakebite admissions[1] Total no. admissions	No. per 1000 admissions
Western	85/10066	8.4
Gulf	132/11085	11.9
Central[2]	673/78514	8.6
Central excl, NCD	182/12774	
Port Moresby NCD	491/65740	
Milne Bay	3/25227	0.1
Northern	40/23709	1.7
Total[3]	933/148601	6.3

1. Complete data for several years from certain hospitals was unavailable.
2. Five to ten seriously envenomated patients transferred annually from outstation hospitals to Port Moresby Hospital are recorded twice.
3. Southern Highlands District was omitted. No highly venomous snakes are known to occur in Southern Highlands,

adapted from Campbell 1969

TABLE 2
Notified Deaths due to Snakebite in Papua 1959–67

Year	Deaths
1959-60	8
1960-61	1
1961-62	4
1962-63	2
1963-64	7
1964-65	5
1965-66	3
1966-67	5
1959-67	35

adapted from Campbell 1969.

Two of the nine omitted children subsequently died from snakebite envenoming.

Campbell's study group mostly originated from Central Province with only one patient each from Western, Gulf and Milne Bay Provinces. Most of the 120 Central Province bites occurred along the coastal lowlands of the province with the majority, seventy persons, being bitten within twenty miles of Port Moresby. Only six bites took place at an appreciable distance inland, four between the Brown River and Mt Victoria and two near Tapini in the north of the province. When the writer interviewed locals in Tapini only the death adder was reported to be found in the surrounding mountains and valley. Hudson and Pomat's study concerns patients from throughout the province since MGH is the major referral hospital for Madang town and 27 rural heath centres.

Campbell discovered that the sex ratio of the Port Moresby study group snakebite victims was four males to one female with males between five and forty-five and females between five and thirty-five receiving bites. Two additional males aged three and fifty-five, outside the main age groups, were also bitten. The highest risk group were males aged twenty to twenty five, as this group tended to travel more extensively hunting or looking for work. Brian and Vince's juvenile study group in the same area demonstrated a closer male: female ratio (almost 3:2) since the daily routine of children probably varies little between the sexes. The highest risk group was the under fives. Hudson and Pomat's Madang sexual ratio for all age groups is also much closer than Campbell's Port Moresby ratio (less than 2:1).

As would be expected from a study of the natural history of southern Papuan elapids, most of Campbell's venomous snakebites admitted to PMGH were inflicted during the hours of daylight with 108 bites taking place between 05.30 and 18.30 and only eight bites occurring between 18.30 and 22.00; only one bite occurred in the early morning. With the exception of the secretive death adder and small-eyed snake, the large, dangerous Papuan elapids are mainly diurnal or crepuscular (active at dusk). They only become nocturnal in the hottest weather so encounters are unlikely, especially when it is realised that the fear of sorcery and the dark keeps a large proportion of the population at home during the night. However, the time of envenoming was one of the major discrepancies to occur between the work of Campbell at PNGH and Hudson and Pomat at MGH. Only the death adder and the small-eyed snake occur in Madang Province and since both are nocturnal or crepuscular species a higher number of nocturnal bites would be expected (42 bites, 33%). Diurnal bites were still more frequent with 80 bites (62%) occurring during the day. In seven cases the time of the snakebite was not recorded. Diurnal bites from apparently nocturnal species can be explained by: a) considerably increased human movements during the hours of daylight, b) cryptically patterned death adders sleeping on forest trails used by barefoot travellers, and c) bites to the hands or arms resulting from snakes uncovered during forest or garden brushwood or log clearance.

In common with other countries where most of the indigenous population moves around unshod, most bites (Campbell 112; Hudson & Pomat 105), occurred on the lower limb with most of those (Campbell 82; Hudson & Pomat 92), on the foot, compared to bites to the upper limb and hand (Campbell 11; Hudson & Pomat 10). Campbell also analysed the circumstances of the bite. Sixty-six bites took place whilst the victim was walking and 28 whilst working, usually in the gardens which are often located some distance from the living quarters, or hunting. Neither series of circumstances is surprising as many paths in lowland Papua New Guinea are fringed, and in places, overhung by dense razor-grass which provides an ideal habitat for the large diurnal elapids such as the taipan or Papuan blacksnake. Gardens too, are often overgrown and debris left lying on the ground for any period of time is likely to become occupied by sheltering snakes. The author received numerous reports of large, fast moving diurnal snakes in these garden habitats. Few bites occur actually within the village confines and the author noted that the Kiwai people of southern Western Province deliberately keep the grass around the houses very short to discourage snakes. Interestingly, few bites amongst the indigeous peoples, only four in Campbell's study, originate from deliberate attempts to pick up snakes, yet this is a the major cause of snakebite in adolescent males in Europe, U.S.A., South Africa and Australia.

Campbell also considered whether snakebite was more likely in any particular month of the year. From his six year study he concluded that victims were admitted to hospital throughout the year but in any particular year a month may go past without a single admission for snakebite. Hudson and Pomat, however, reported almost three times as many snakebite admissions during the wet season (92 October-May) than during the dry season (37 June-September) It is, therefore, difficult to predict months of greatest risk although snakes are generally believed to be more common during the wet season. This last fact is born out from the author's experiences of catching snakes throughout the Tropics.

The Melanesian Attitude to Snakes and Snakebite.

Snakes, particularly venomous species, feature strongly in the imaginations and stories of the indigenous people of Papua New Guinea. The author encountered several interesting beliefs concerning harmless species such as the wart snake *(Acrochordus arafurae)*, carpet python *(Morelia spilota)*, and brown cat snake *(Boiga irregularis)*, but the snake which has the strongest hold over the villagers of southern Western Province is undoubtedly the 'Pap blak'. This snake is feared to the point of hysteria if it, or another black coloured snake, is discovered near a village. Snakes are seen as totems, religious deities, protectors of property, signs or omens of impending disaster, reincarnations of dead relatives, avengers of broken taboos and the instruments of sorcery. Some peoples attribute certain snakes, encountered under particular circumstances, with magical powers whilst other people see the snakes merely as the tools of the magic men; the Mega Mega Auri (the man who sends snakes), or Ove-devenar (the black snake man of the Trans-Fly). The author met one such magic man who claimed to be able to call out snakes at will. Other sorcerers are said to turn themselves into snakes to injure the intended victim.

Snakesbites are viewed initially, like any other illness or disease, as a retribution upon that person for the breaking of a strict taboo or ancient law by either himself or a close relative. Attempts are made by the native practitioner, or Hedura Tauna, to treat the bite with local herbs and incantations whilst family members are questioned to determine the nature of the broken taboo. Should the patient's condition deteriorate, sorcery is believed to be the cause and an attempt to discover the name of the magic man concerned will be made.

If the sorcerer is located he will be offered gifts and requested to reverse the sickness. Various herbal medications and occult practices will be used but if signs such as build up of mucus in the back of the mouth, repeated bite marks or bleeding from mouth or wounds occur, the magic man will consider the case hopeless. The first of these is a symptom of the onset of advanced paralysis, the second a frequent characteristic of taipan bite and the third is a common sign of Papuan blacksnake bite so there would be little chance of survival for the victim at this stage. If death occurs it is always considered to be due to sorcery.

This almost fatalistic approach to snakebite with its reliance on herbs, incantation and the power of the magic men, coupled with the enormous distances involved in reaching hospital and the poor routes of communication in the interior, could indicate that many more snakebite deaths occur than the medical doctors examine or Government officials are able to record.

Campbell suggested that as the intervention of the native practitioner, or the sorcerer, could delay modern 'medical' treatment of a patient suffering from severe elapine envenomation, some form of compromise whereby the native practioner and the medical doctor collaborate over the case would be adviseable.

Dangerous New Guinea Elapids.

Species of the following terrestrial elapid genera have been recorded on the New Guinea mainland: *Acanthophis, Aspidomorphus, Demansia, Glyphodon, Micropechis, Oxyuranus, Pseudechis, Pseudonaja, Toxicocalamus* and *Unechis*. To assist readers referring to out-dated papers on the subject of the elapids of New Guinea it should be explained that the genus *Pseudapisto-calamus* is now considered to be a synonymy of *Apistocalamus* which, together with *Ultrocalamus*, is regarded as a subgenus of *Toxicocalamus* (McDowell, 1969). Likewise the New Guinean members of *Denisonia* and *Suta* are currently synonymised with *Unechis*. In addition the genera *Loveridgelaps, Parapistocalamus* and *Salomonelaps* are known from Bougainville Island and the Solomon Islands to the far east (McDowell, 1970; McCoy, 1980). However, most of the species within these minor genera are small, secretive and inoffensive with tiny mouths incapable of administering a dangerous bite, and they pose no serious threat to man. Care should still be taken, however, with little known species as there always remains the possibility that a bite from a larger specimen could have alarming, if not life threatening effects (ie, a bite from Muller's snake, *Aspidomorphus muelleri*, has been recorded as causing vomitting and sweating (Campbell, 1969). Although totally aquatic and not strictly elapids, seasnakes of the monotypic genera *Enhydrina* have been recorded in freshwater Papuan river systems. As only the underlined genera are considered likely to constitute a threat to human life in Papua New Guinea only species contained within those genera will be considered here. Since *E.schistosa* occurs in large numbers in the Ramu River system where it's bite poses a serious potential threat this species has been included whilst exclusively marine species or occasional river invaders have been omitted.

Highly Dangerous New Guinea Elapids:

> *Acanthophis antarcticus* and *A.praelongus* (Death Adders);
> *Oxyuranus scutellatus canni* (Papuan Taipan);
> *Pseudechis australis* (Mulga or King Brownsnake);
> *Pseudechis papuanus* (Papuan Blacksnake);
> *Pseudonaja textilis* (Eastern Brownsnake).

Potentially Dangerous New Guinea Elapids:

> *Demansia atra* and *D.papuensis* (Papuan Black Whipsnakes)
> *Micropechis ikaheka ikaheka* (Small-eyed or Ikaheka Snake).
> *Enhydrina schistosa* (Common Seasnake)

The taxonomy of the six terrestrial genera is far from simple as the number of recognised New Guinea species and subspecies within these genera varies from six to ten depending on the authority. These problems are summarised below and it is left to the reader to decide on the validity of each issue.

Taxonomic Problems of Dangerous New Guinea Elapids
Acanthophis

The death adders are easily distinguished from all other snakes within their geographical range, except perhaps from the ground boa *(Candoia aspera)*, which also occurs in New Guinea and has a relatively short stout body. However, within the genus *Acanthophis* there are certainly taxonomic problems and many name combinations and couplings have been used in the past; *A.antarcticus antarcticus* and *A.antarcticus pyrrhus* for Australia (Worrel 1963), *A.antarcticus* and *A.pyrrhus* (Cogger 1975; Mirtschin & Davis 1982), *A.laevis* from Western Province, Papua New Guinea (Macleay 1877), *A.antarcticus rugosus* from Merauke, Irian Jaya, and *A.antarcticus antarcticus*, (including Macleay's *A.laevis)*, from Australia and Papua New Guinea (Loveridge 1948; de Haas, 1950). Storr (1981), records three species for Australia: *A.antarcticus*, *A.pyrrhus* and *A.praelongus*, with the note that the third of these species also occurs in southern New Guinea. It seems likely that more than one species does occur in New Guinea and this author captured death adders in Western and Central Provinces which certainly appeared to possess different scalation, head shape and degrees of supraocular adornment. It seems quite likely that both *Acanthophis antarcticus* and *A.praelongus* may inhabit New Guinea and only further field work, examination of New Guinea specimens, chromosomal and electrophoretic studies will solve the problem (see key for morphological differences between the two species).

Demansia

Formerly all Papuan whipsnakes were recognised as representing either a subspecies of *Demansia psammophis* (Loveridge 1945; Slater 1956), or the subspecies *Demansia olivacea papuensis* (Worrell 1963; Klemmer 1963; Slater 1968). This second subspecies was eventually elevated to species level but is still considered closely related to both Australian species, *D.psammophis* and *D.olivacea*. The situation is further complicated as Cogger (1975), records the Australian species, *Demansia atra*, as occurring in southern Papua. Authors are divided as to whether Papua is inhabited by one or other of the species, *D.atra* or *D.papuensis* (Cogger 1975; Scott, Parker & Menzies 1977; Whitaker & Whitaker 1982), or possibly both species (Storr 1978; Parker 1982; Golay 1985). Storr (1978), differentiates between Australian specimens of these two species on ventral pigmentation, head coloration, size and combined ventral and subcaudal scale counts but Parker (1972; 1982), reports that McDowell considered these characters of dubious value when they were used to define Papuan species. This author collected several specimens in Western Province which would appear to be *D.atra* based on Storr's characteristics.

Micropechis

Klemmer (1963), considered the New Guinea populations of *Micropechis ikaheka* to be *Micropechis i.ikaheka* whilst he confined the subspecies *M.i.fasciatus* to Aru Island to the southwest of Irian Jaya. This is the generally accepted view for this species but Slater (1956; 1968), differentiated between northern and southern races on the mainland allocating the subspecies accordingly; northern race, *M.i.ikaheka*, and southern race, *M.i.fasciatus*. For the purposes of this study only *Micropechis i.ikaheka* is recognised for New Guinea, following Klemmer.

Oxyuranus

The Australian taipan, *Oxyuranus scutellatus*, is known to occur in Queenland and Northern Territory and the New Guinea population was considered to represent simply extralimital distribution of an Australian snake species. However, Slater (1954; 1956), described the New Guinea taipan as a separate subspecies, *Oxyuranus s. canni*, based on its more pronounced scale keels, the ventral red-orange stripe and possibly also the greater size that Papuan specimens are said to attain.

Pseudechis

No taxonomic problems exist regarding the endemic Papuan blacksnake, *Pseudechis papuanus*, but the presence or absence of a second species, the Australian *Pseudechis australis*, in southern Irian Jaya, and possibly also southwestern Papua, is viewed with some doubt by some authors. Worrell (1963), is dubious of the presence of *P.australis* in New Guinea due to its close apparent relationship with *P.papuanus* with which it would need to exist sympatrically. However, recent studies suggest that *P.papuanus* is more

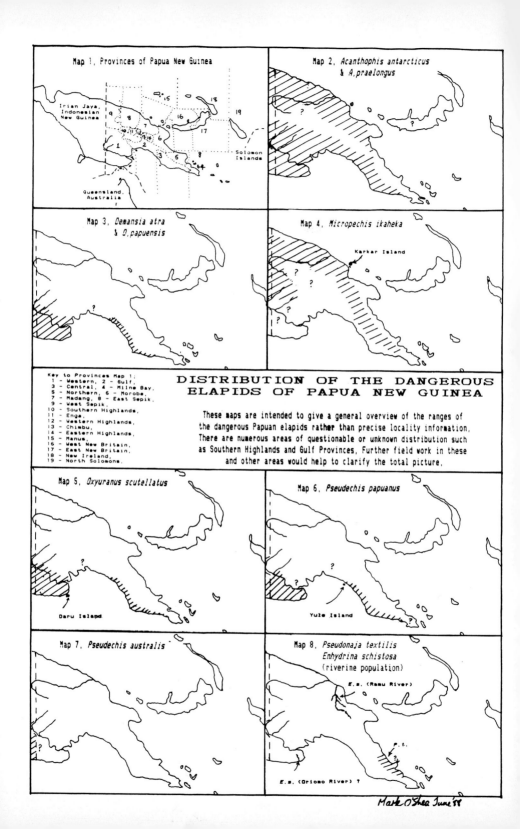

Map 1, Provinces of Papua New Guinea

Irian Jaya, Indonesian New Guinea

Queensland, Australia

Solomon Islands

Map 2, *Acanthophis antarcticus* & *A.praelongus*

Map 3, *Demansia atra* & *D.papuensis*

Map 4, *Micropechis ikaheka*

Karkar Island

Key to Provinces Map 1;
1 - Western, 2 - Gulf,
3 - Central, 4 - Milne Bay,
5 - Northern, 6 - Morobe,
7 - Madang, 8 - East Sepik,
9 - West Sepik,
10 - Southern Highlands,
11 - Enga,
12 - Western Highlands,
13 - Chimbu,
14 - Eastern Highlands,
15 - Manus,
16 - West New Britain,
17 - East New Britain,
18 - New Ireland,
19 - North Solomons.

DISTRIBUTION OF THE DANGEROUS ELAPIDS OF PAPUA NEW GUINEA

These maps are intended to give a general overview of the ranges of the dangerous Papuan elapids rather than precise locality information. There are numerous areas of questionable or unknown distribution such as Southern Highlands and Gulf Provinces. Further field work in these and other areas would help to clarify the total picture.

Map 5, *Oxyuranus scutellatus*

Daru Island

Map 6, *Pseudechis papuanus*

Yule Island

Map 7, *Pseudechis australis*

Map 8, *Pseudonaja textilis*
Enhydrina schistosa
(riverine population)

E.s. (Ramu River)

P.t.

E.s. (Oriomo River) ?

Mark O'Shea June '88

closely related to the Australian species, *P.colletti* (Mengden, Shine & Moritz, 1986). Other authors also agree that *P.australis* probably does occur in the Irian Jaya/Papua frontier region (Slater, 1968; Parker, 1982; Mengden *et al* 1986; Shine, 1987).

Pseudonaja

Pseudonaja textilis is an Australian species which has subsequently been recorded from a number of northeastern coastal and inland localities in Milne Bay and Northern Provinces (McDowell, 1967 records specimens collected by the Archbold Expeditions of 1953, and both Worrell and Cogger have examined and confirmed identification of *P.textilis* material originating from Papua New Guinea). It is, however, strangely absent from apparently suitable sites in Central and Western Provinces which lie between its disjunct Papuan collection sites and its more familiar continental Australian distribution. It has been suggested by Slater (1968), that these Papuan records originate from specimens or eggs accidentally introduced by Australian military forces during the 1940's. However, the Papuan specimens often appear to be darker (even black) than the usual Australian species and they have a slightly higher maxillary tooth count (12 rather than 9-11, McDowell, 1967).

Individual Species Accounts
Highly Dangerous Species:

NEW GUINEA DEATH ADDERS *Acanthophis antarcticus* Shaw and *Acanthophis praelongus* Ramsey

Average/Maximum length:
300-500mm/1000mm (1-1½ft/3ft)

Description
a) physique:
An elapid which has evolved to fill the niche in Australasia which is occupied elsewhere by the viperids. Characterised by a short, stumpy viper-like body; rough, strongly or weakly keeled, or smooth scales; short tail with comb-like terminal spinal process; broad viper-like head; occasionally raised horn-like supraocular scales and either keeled rugose or smooth scales; relatively long and mobile fangs and vertically elliptical pupil.

b) colouration:
Highly variable dorsally; red, brown or greyish, either uniform or with alternating broad or narrow, pale and dark transverse bands, spotted with black; ventrally either immaculate or spotted with black, tail black white or yellow tipped; head as body, brown or red with darker transverse streaks above with white labials, spotted with black, and white chin, also spotted with black. (Fig. 1)

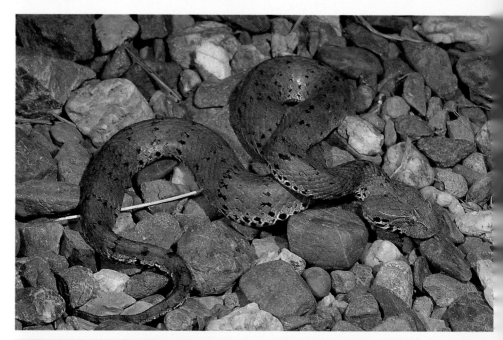

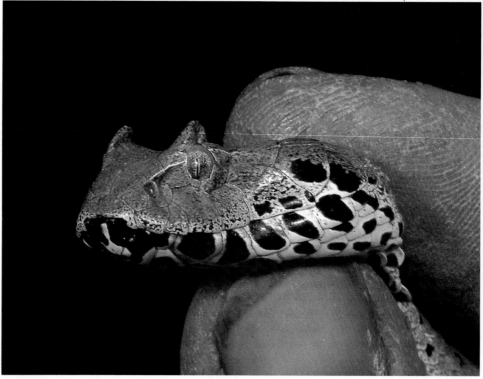

Figure 1
Acanthophis praelongus

c) scalation:

21, or rarely 23, rows, (*A. antarcticus*), or 23 rows, (*A. praelongus*), at midbody; 110-124, (*A. antarcticus*), or 122-134, (*A. praelongus*); subcaudals 36-50, (*A. antarcticus*), or 47-57, (A. *praelongus*), anteriorly single, posteriorly paired; anal plate single; loreal scale absent; subocular scales present.

Habitat:

Widespread in monsoon and rainforest habitats, both lowland and fairly highland, and occasionally in savanna woodland and upland grassland valleys.

Habits:

Commonly encountered on paths and trails asleep during the day when it poses a considerable threat as it will respond by biting if trodden on. Following the initial bite the death adder will often hang on, not attempting to flee in the manner of the other elapids, so it is frequently killed by its victim. Usually bites, below the ankle. Considered most common at the end of the wet season. Ovoviviparous.

Dial period of activity:

Nocturnal, sluggish during the day.

Prey preferences:

Terrestrial skinks, birds or small mammals and possibly frogs, using wiggling tail tip to attract prey.

Distribution within PNG:

Wide-spread throughout mainland Papua New Guinea excepting Northern, Milne Bay, Enga and Southern Highlands Provinces and extreme altitudes above 1800m in other highland provinces. Small montane race known from Henganofi, Eastern Highlands, and large one metre specimens known from the Sepik and Markham River regions. Kinghorn and Kellaway (1943) report specimens from New Britain but record is doubtful.

Extralimital distribution:

Indonesia from Irian Jaya to Ceram, Tanimbar and the Aru Islands in the Moluccas (de Rooji, 1917; de Haas, 1950). Doubtful records from Borneo. Both 'species' occur in Australia together with a third species, *Acanthophis pyrrhus* (Storr, 1981).

Fang length:

5-8.3mm (Fairley, 1929)

Average/Maximum venom yield:

42-84.7mg/235.6mg[A] (Fairley & Splatt, 1929)

[A] = data obtained from Australian specimens

Lethal subcutaneous dose:

0.015mg (100gm Guinea pig Campbell, 1969); 0.025-0.15mg/kg (man, Kellaway, 1929)

Toxicity LD$_{50}$:

0.338mg/kg^A (mouse, Broad, Sutherland & Coulter, 1979)

Toxicity LD$_{100}$:

0.5-0.7mg/kg (mouse s.c., Trethewie, 1971)

Active effects of venom:

Strongly to moderately neurotoxic; weakly haemolytic, possibly anticoagulant (Kellaway, 1929) and cytotoxic. Coagulant factor incomplete prothrombin activator only functioning in presence of factor V (Mebs, 1978). Wounds do not bleed and no clinical haemotoxic effects on blood. Not haemorrhagic. Neurotoxic action, postsynaptic causing peripheral curare-like neuromuscular block (Kellaway, Cherry & Williams, 1932), is reversible. Neurotoxin isolated from *A. antarcticus* (acanthophin A, Sheumack *et al*, 1979; Sutherland, 1980).

Antiserum/initial dose:

CSL Monovalent Death Adder/6000 units (CSL Med.H/b 1979; 1985; Mirtschin & Davis, 1982).

PAPUAN TAIPAN *Oxyuranus scutellatus canni* (Slater)

Average/Maximum length:

1830-2440mm/3355mm (6-8ft/11ft)

Description
a) physique:

A large slender species with elongated 'coffin-shaped' head, distinct from narrow neck; tail long and whip-like; eye moderate-sized with round pupil; supraocular scale over eye sharply shelved giving snake scowling expression.

b) colouration:

Dorsum of body olive, dark brown or dark grey, usually with an orange or pinkish stripe evident in interstitial skin of vertebral scale rows; venter cream to off-white, either immaculate or speckled with orange; head coloured as dorsum or paler, especially in juveniles, snout and labials usually lighter; iris of eye brown. (Fig. 2)

c) scalation:

21, or 23, rows at midbody, anteriorly keeled; ventrals 220-250; subcaudals 45-80, all paired; anal plate single; loreal and subocular scales absent.

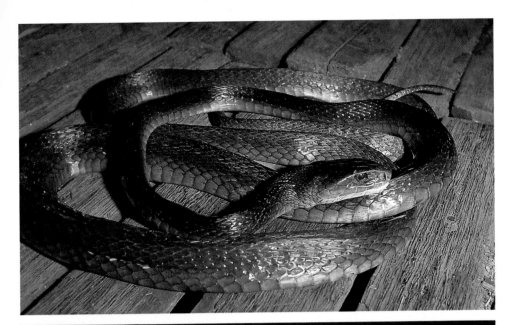

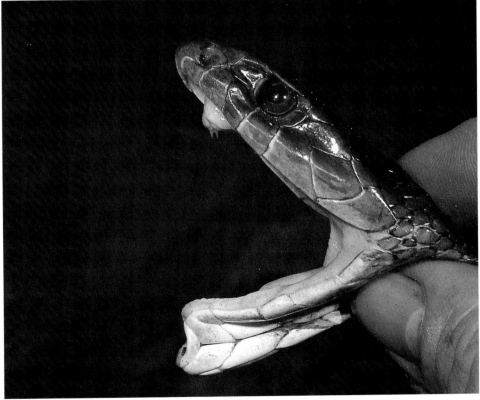

Figure 2
Oxyuranus scutellatus canni

Habitat:

Lowland savanna and savanna woodland.

Habits:

Nervous and retiring but will strike with speed and aggression if startled, threatened or molested, arching the body back, flattening the head and striking forward and upwards, often biting more than once in quick succession. Moves rapidly over the ground, often with head and forepart of body raised. Possesses very acute sense which usually prevent human encounters, but when aroused known for characteristic rapid and multiple "strike and release" bites which may lead to enormous quantities of venom being injected. Commonest during wet season. Oviparous.

Dial period of activity:

Diurnal and crepuscular, but nocturnal in warm weather.

Prey preferences:

Mammals, rats, bandicoots, and possibly ground nesting birds.

Distribution within PNG:

Confined to lowland southern coastal localities in Western, Central, (Kukipi to east of Marshall Lagoon and inland to 1,100ft on Sogeri Plateau), and Milne Bay Provinces. May also occur in Gulf Province although not yet recorded there. Known from mainland Milne Bay Province as far east of Samarai but not recorded from islands of D'Estrecasteaux and Louisiade Archipelagoes. Particularily common on Oriomo Plateau in southern Trans-Fly region, on Daru Island and in the vicinities of Morehead, Lake Murray and Balimo, Western Province and around Port Moresby, NCD, in Central Province.

Extralimital distribution:

Endemic New Guinea subspecies confined to Papua, (although may subsequently be recorded in southeastern Irian Jaya), but close relative, *Oxyuranus scutellatus scutellatus*, occurs in Queensland and Northern Territory, Australia.

Fang length:

13mm[A] (Kellaway, 1932).

Average/Maximum venom yield:

100-200mg/400mg[A] (Campbell, 1967); 500mg (Trethewie, 1971).

Lethal subcautaneous dose:

0.0025mg[A] (100gm Guinea pig, Morgan 1956); 0.0034mg[A] (25gm mouse); 0.1mg/kg (man,Kellaway, 1929; Morgan, 1956).

Toxicity LD$_{50}$:

0.002mg/kg (Guinea pig, Campbell, 1969); 0.02mg/kg (Guinea pig s.c., Trethewie, 1971a); 0.064mg/kg (mouse, Broad *et al*, 1979); 0.12mg/kg (mouse s.c., Trethewie, 1971a).

Active effects of venom:

Strongly neurotoxic and coagulant; weakly haemolytic, also possibly cytotoxic, myotoxic and cardiotoxic causing heart failure (Habermehl, 1981). Coagulant factor complete prothrombin activator converting prothrombin to thrombin in presence or absence of factor V (Denson, 1969; Mebs, 1978). Neurotoxin isolated from taipan (taipoxin, Fohlman *et al*, 1976) is second most potent terrestrial snake neurotoxin known, causing presynaptic blockade (Sutherland, 1980) and myolysis (Harris *et al*, 1977).

Antiserum/initial dose:

CSL Monovalent Taipan/12 000 units (CSL Med. H/b., 1979; 1985; Mirtschin & Davis, 1982).

Mulga or King Brownsnake *Pseudechis australis (Gray)*

Average/Maximum length:

2440mm/2745mm (8ft/9ft)

Description
a) physique:

A heavy bodied species with a broad head which is slightly distinct from the neck, especially in large specimens which may have bulbous cheeks; eye small with round pupil.

b) colouration:

Yellow, red or tan brown dorsally both head and body; venter yellowish cream.

c) scalation:

17 rows at midbody, smooth; ventrals 185-225; subcaudals 50-75, all single except extreme posterior few which are paired; anal plate normally divided; loreal and subocular scales absent.

Habitat:

Savanna and savanna woodlands but also in tropical forests and deserts in Australia.

Habits:

A slow moving species but capable of injecting huge quantities of venom which, although not as toxic as that of the eastern *P.papuanus*, constitutes a considerable danger. Reputed to be unpredictable and inclined to hold on when it bites this species will flatten its head and strike with rapidity and aggression. Ovoviviparous but may be oviparous in some areas.

Dial period of activity:

Diurnal or crepuscular becoming nocturnal in hot weather and not active during the heat of the day.

Prey preferences:

Small mammals, frogs and reptiles, including other snakes.

Distribution within PNG:

Probably present in Western Province west of the Fly River, especially in the Morehead region near the frontier with Irian Jaya.

Extralimital distribution:

Throughout most of Australia, except extreme southwest, southeast and Tasmania, in a wide variety of habitats. Also from southeastern Irian Jaya in the vicinities of Etna Bay and Merauke (Loveridge, 1948) near frontier with Papua New Guinea.

Fang length:

?

Average/Maximum venom yield:

180mg/600mg (Worrell, 1963).

Lethal subcutaneous dose:

0.16mg[A] (100 gm Guinea pig, Campbell, 1969).

Toxicity LD$_{50}$:

1.91mg/kg[A] (mouse, Broad et al, 1979).

Active effects of venom:

Strongly haemolytic and cytotoxic; weakly neurotoxic and myotoxic affecting heart muscle (Campbell, 1969). Potent myotoxin isolated (mulgo-toxin, Leonardi et al, 1979). Reported to be anticoagulant (Kellaway, 1938; Kellaway & Williams, 1929; Cogger, 1971) or contain anticoagulant properties (Marshall & Herrmann, 1983). Possibly haemorrhagic (Campbell, 1967). Causes continual wound bleeding (Sutherland, 1983).

Antiserum/initial dose:

CSL Monovalent Blacksnake/18 000 units (CSL Med. H/b., 1979; 1985; Mirtschin & Davis, 1982).

PAPUAN BLACKSNAKE *Pseudechis papuanus* Peters & Doria

Average/Maximum length:

2135mm/2440mm (7ft/8ft)

Description

a) physique:

A strong, stout bodied species with a broad, flat head, distinct from neck; tail fairly long; eye small with round pupil; supraocular not distinctly shelved.

b) colouration:

Dorsum of body uniformly glossy jet black, rarely brown; venter blue-grey or gunmetal-grey; head as dorsum above but may be lighter on labials; neck yellow to off-white with black specklings. (Fig. 3)

c) scalation:

19, or rarely 21, rows at midbody, all smooth; ventrals 221-230; subcaudals 49-63 with first 25-45 single and remainder paired; anal plate divided; loreal and subocular scales absent.

Habitat:

Lowland savanna and savanna woodland but showing a greater preference for damper, swampy ground and also extending further into forests than the taipan.

Habits:

Nervous and inclined to flee at man's approach but when cornered the blacksnake will attack with power and tenacity apparently unrivalled by any other Australo-Papuan species. More commonly encountered in late dry season. Oviparous.

Dial period of activity:

Diurnal and crepuscular but avoiding hottest part of day.

Prey preferences:

Small mammals and possibly also frogs and ground nesting birds.

Distribution within PNG:

Probably confined to southern coastal lowlands. The species is recorded from the Irian Jaya frontier region and from Morehead, Lake Murray and the Oriomo Plateau, west of the Fly River in Western Province, and from lowland localities around Port Moresby, Marshall Lagoon and Amazon Bay in Central Province. It also occurs along the southern Milne Bay Province but has not been recorded from Northern Province although it may occur in Gulf Provinces. Recorded from Yule Island but not Daru Island. Formerly thought to be much

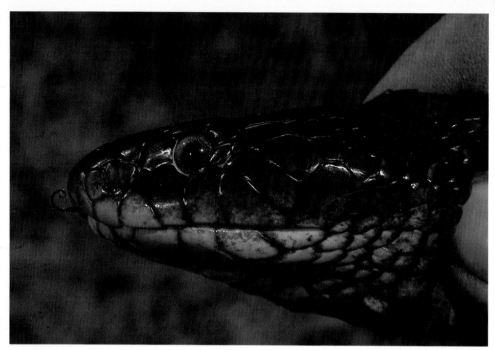

Figure 3
Pseudechis papuanus

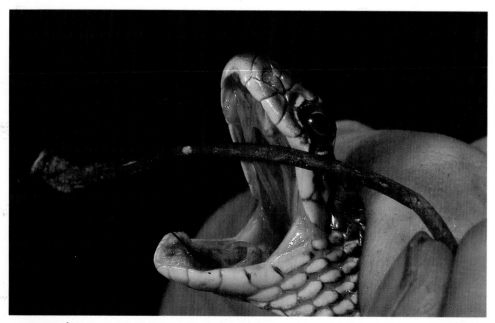

Figure 4
Demansia atra

more common than it is today, possibly due to the introduction of the highly toxic-skinned cane toad, *Bufo marinus (see Snakebite as a Hazard in Papua New Guinea).*

Extralimital distribution:

New Guinea endemic also occurring in Irian Jaya along southern coast to Prince Frederik Hendrik Island.

Fang length:

6.1mm

Average/Maximum venom yield:

200mg/494mg (Campbell, 1967).

Lethal subcutaneous dose:

0.02mg (100gm Guinea pig, Campbell, 1967).

Toxicity LD$_{50}$:

?

Active effects of venom:

Very strongly haemolytic and neurotoxic; possibly haemorrhagic (Campbell, 1967). Probably not procoagulant (Marshall & Herrmann, 1983) but not necessarily anticoagulant, opinions vary greatly.

Antiserum/initial dose:

CSL Monovalent Papuan Blacksnake/18 000 units (Mirtschin & Davis, 1982), Polyvalent Papuan/40 000 units (CSL, 1985).

EASTERN BROWNSNAKE *Pseudonaja textilis* **(Dumeril & Bibron)**

Average/Maximum length:

1830mm/2135mm (6ft/7ft)

Description
a) physique:

A slender snake with its head barely distinct from the neck; tail moderate length; eye medium-sized with round pupil.

b) colouration:

Dorsally the body is yellow brown, dark brown or black, often with darker crossbands which are particularly evident in juveniles; venter off-white to creamy-yellow, speckled with pink, brown or grey; head coloured as body with lighter throat.

c) scalation:

17 rows at midbody, all smooth; ventrals 185-235; subcaudals 45-75, usually all paired but occasionally with anterior few single; anal plate divided; loreal and subocular scales absent.

Habitat:

Upland grasslands and sandy or rocky heathlands but also in swamplands and cultivated areas.

Habits:

Very fast moving and inclined to flee from human approach but prepared to defend itself vigorously if molested with a raised coiled neck and mouth open wide in readiness for the strike. May strike several times in quick succession from the S-stance. Common in very warm weather. Oviparous.

Dial period of activity:

Usually diurnal.

Prey preferences:

Small lizards and frogs but also small mammals.

Distribution within PNG:

Northeastern Papua New Guinea from Dogura, Cape Vogel and Mori Biri Bay, Milne Bay Province, to Embogo and Popondetta, Northern Province, possibly a human introduction from Australia.

Extralimital distribution:

Eastern Queenland, New South Wales, Victoria and southern South Australia. Also isolated localities in Northern Territory.

Fang length:

2.8mm (Campbell, 1969).

Average/Maximum venom yield:

2-5mg/40-67.2mg[A] (Sutherland, 1983).

Lethal subcutaneous dose:

0.0025mg[A] (100gm Guinea pig, Campbell, 1969).

Toxicity LD$_{50}$:

0.041mg/kg[A] (mouse, Broad et al, 1979).

Toxicity LD$_{100}$:

0.25mg/kg (mouse, Trethewie, 1971a).

Active effects of venom:

Strongly coagulant and neurotoxic; weakly haemolytic and cytotoxic; also myotoxic. Coagulant strongly diffusible causing thrombosis and haemorrhage from mucus membranes (Kellaway, 1938). Coagulant factor of venom complete prothrombin activator causing conversion of prothrombin to thrombin in presence or absence of factor V (Denson, 1969; Mebs, 1978). Strongest known terrestrial snake neurotoxin isolated (textilon, Coulter *et al*, 1979).

Antiserum/initial dose:

CSL Monovalent Brownsnake/1000 units (CSL Med.H/b., 1979; Mirtschin & Davis, 1982); Monovalent Taipan.

Potentially Dangerous Species:
PAPUAN BLACK WHIPSNAKES *Demansia atra* (Macleay) and *Demansia p. papuensis* (Macleay)

Average/Maximum length:

658mm/1148mm (2ft/3ft8in.) *(D.atra)* 630mm/1515mm (2ft/5ft) *(D.papuensis)*

Description
a) physique:

Slender, rapidly moving snakes with narrow head distinct from neck; tail long and whip-like; eye large with round pupil.

b) colouration:

Dorsally olive brown or dark brown to black lightening towards tail which may be red-brown; interstitial skin yellow to white; venter blue-grey, darkening posteriorly; head dorsally spotted with dark pigment but labials lighter, white or yellowish, spotted with brown; chin white; eye with brown iris surrounded by circumorbital ring of yellow on preocular and postocular scales. (Fig. 4)

c) scalation:

15 rows at midbody, all smooth; ventrals 160-225; subcaudals 69-105, paired; anal plate divided; loreal and subocular scales absent.

Habitat:

Savanna and savanna woodland but also in cultivated gardens.

Habits:

Probably the fastest snake in New Guinea moving across the ground so rapidly that the eye has difficulty following it. Not an aggressive species but specimens which are molested will bite rapidly. Most common in the drier season.

Dial period of activity:

Diurnal and often seen abroad during the hottest part of the day when other species are not in evidence. Not seen at night. Oviparous.

Prey preferences:

Lizards are possibly frogs and small mammals.

Distribution within PNG:

Differentiating between the New Guinea species of *Demansia* presents considerable difficulties for the taxonomist but representatives of the genus occur throughout the southern savanna lowlands from the extensive grasslands to the west of the Fly River to Balimo in Western Province and also in coastal lowland localities of Central Province. Whether *Demansia* is represented in Gulf Province has yet to be determined.

Extralimital distribution:

D.atra occurs in Western Australia, Northern Territory and Queensland, and a subspecies of *D.papuensis*, *D.papuensis melaena*, has been recently described for Western Australia and Northern Territory. *Demansia spp.* also inhabit the southern savanna of Irian Jaya.

Fang length:

?

Average/Maximum venom yield:

?

Lethal subcutaneous dose:

?

Toxicity LD$_{50}$:

14.2mg/kg[A] (saline, mouse, Broad *et al*, 1979)

Active effects of venom:

Neurotoxic and possibly haemorrhagic and coagulant (Campbell, 1969).

Antiserum/initial dose:

CSL Monovalent Tiger Snake/3000 units (Mirtschin & Davis, 1982); Monovalent Brownsnake; Polyvalent Papuan.

NEW GUINEA SMALL-EYED OR IKAHEKA SNAKE *Micropechis i. ikaheka* (Lesson)

Average/Maximum length:

1500mm/2000mm (4½ ft/6ft)

Description

a) physique:

Fairly stocky bodied species with relatively short tail; head narrow but distinct from neck; eye small with round pupil.

b) colouration:

Dorsally, body may be yellowish anteriorly with increasingly darker scales edged with cream posteriorly, (northern race), especially recognisable as yellow or white snake in Madang or Karkar Island, or with increasingly more apparent dark crossbands towards the hind part of the body and onto the tail and scattered dark spots.on neck, (southern race); tail black with yellow ventral blotches, (northern race), or banded black and brown with cream blotches on belly (southern race); ventrals creamish yellow edged with black, (northern race), or brown, (southern race); head dorsally black or grey with lighter brown or yellow labials, throat and chin.

c) scalation:

15 rows at midbody, all smooth; ventrals 178-223; subcaudals 37-55, all paired; anal divided; loreal and subocular scales absent.

Habitat:

Confined to monsoon and rainforest areas and swamps, but not apparently dry savanna woodlands, from sea level to 15 000m. This species has also been recorded from plantations and commonly encountered under old coconut husks.

Habits:

Generally a secretive semi-fossorial, (burrowing), species inhabiting leaf litter or loose soil and usually only encounted when it ventures onto the surface in a clearing or when uncovered under a decaying log. Reacts with aggression if handled or molested. Most commonly encountered in the drier months. Oviparous.

Dial period of activity:

Both diurnal and nocturnal but usually venturing abroad after dark.

Prey preferences:

Little known but earthworms have been recorded and small burrowing frogs and lizards are also possibilities

Distribution within PNG:

Widespread throughout mainland Papua New Guinea's forests but not recorded from Gulf, Southern Highlands, Western Highlands and Enga Provinces. A problem in northern coastal Madang Province and nearby Karkar Island.

Extralimital distribution:

Throughout Irian Jaya including some of its neighbouring islands to the north and west. A second subspecies, *Micropechis i fasciatus*, is recorded from Aru Island to the southeast of Irian Jaya.

Fang length:

?

Average/Maximum venom yield:

?

Lethal subcutaneous dose:

0.5-1.0mg (25gm mouse, Campbell, 1969).

Toxicity LD$_{50}$:

?

Active effects of venom:

Highly myotoxic causing myalgia, muscle tenderness, severe neuromuscular paralysis and myoglobinuria (Sutherland, 1983; Hudson & Pomat, 1988). rhabdomyolysis (Blasco & Hornabrook, 1972; Hudson & Pomat, 1988); oliguria, renal failure and cerebral hypoxia (Sutherland, 1983), minor symptoms of nausea, severe headache and prolonged weakness. Capable of causing unconsciousness and ceasation of respiration in just over two hours and death in 6½ hours although the original onset of symptoms may be greatly delayed (Blasco & Hornabrook, 1972).

Antiserum/initial dose:

CSL Movovalent Tiger Snake in large doses (Tscharke *in* Blasco & Hornabrook, 1972).

COMMON OR BEAKED SEASNAKE *Enhydrina schistosa* (Daudin)

Average/Maximum length:

950-1150mm/1400mm (3-4ft/4ft 8in.)

Description
a) physique:

Body elongate and narrow anteriorly; head small, barely distinct from neck; tail laterally compressed and paddle-like.

b) colouration:

Dorsally blue-grey to grey with dark grey or dark annuli laterally, broadest dorsolaterally, often masked by dark dorsal pigment in adult specimens; venter white.

c) scalation:

49-66 scale at midbody, imbricate or subimbricate, weakly keeled; ventrals 239-322; preanals feebly enlarged; characterised by elongate mental shield.

Habitat:

Coastal marine but also estuarine and frequently encountered in freshwater systems. Not found in deep water far from land.

Habits:

A graceful, rapid swimmer but helpless on land. Noted for its aggression (Habermehl, 1981). Viviparous.

Dial period of activity:

Diurnal or nocturnal.

Prey preferences:

Fish.

Distribution within PNG:

Probably throughout Papuan coastal waters and in certain freshwater river system. Recorded for coastal Gulf Province by Whitaker and Whitaker (1982) and the Ramu River System, Madang Province, by Hudson and Fromm (1986). A seasnake collected in the Oriomo River, Western Province, by the author was believed to be a *Hydrophis* but unfortunately the specimen was lost.

Extralimital distribution:

Northwest to the Persian Gulf and the coast of East Africa, India, Malaysia and Indonesia and south to northern Australia (Smith, 1926). In freshwater captured in Tonle Sap Lake, Kampuchea (Bourret, 1934). Absent from Solomon Islands, Philippines, southern China and Japan (Barme, 1968).

Fang length:

3mm (Minton & Minton 1971).

Average/Maximum venom yield:

8.5/79mg (Habermehl, 1981); 15mg (Worrell, 1963)

Lethal subcutaneous dose:

0.05mg/kg (man, Trethewie, 1971a); 1.5mg (man, US Navy, 1962).

Toxicity LD$_{50}$:

0.0021-0.0025mg (2.1-2.5μg) (20gm mouse dry wt.i.p., Carey & Wright, 1960); 0.057mg (57μg) (rabbit); 0.061mg (61μg) (Guinea pig); 0.02mg (20μg) (frog) Barme, 1968.

Toxicity LD$_{100}$:

0.0025mg (2.5μg) (20gm mouse i.v., Barme, 1963); 0.026mg/kg (26ug) (Barme, 1958).

Active effects of venom:

Strongly myotoxic and rhabdomyolytic (Hudson & Fromm, 1986; Hudson & Pomat, 1988) causing general muscular weakness, proteinuria, myoglobinuria, neuromuscular respiratory paralysis, cyanosis, terminal hypertension and renal failure (Trethewie, 1971). Also contains a postsynaptic neurotoxin (Walker & Yeoh, 1974; Mebs. 1978). No localised pain in area of bite.

Antiserum/initial dose:

CSL Seasnake ?

TABLE 3

Venom Yield and Potency for Papuan Elapids

Species	Venom yield mg average/maximum	LD$_{50}$ mg/kg mouse	LSD[1] mg/100gm guinea pig	LSD[1] mg/25mg mouse	LSD[1] mg/kg man
Acanthophis antarcticus (& *A,praelongus?*)	42-85/235	0.338	0.015		0.025-0.15
Demansia atra & D. papuensis	?	14,2[(saline)2]			
Micropechis ikaheka	?			0,5-1,0	
Oxyuranus scutellatus	100-200/400	0.064	0.0025	0.0034	0.1
Pseudechis australis	180/600	1.91	0.16		
Pseudechis papuanus	200/494		0.02		
Pseudonaja textilis	2-5/67	0.041	0.0025		
Enhydrina schistosa	8.5/79	0.0025			0.05

1. LSD = certain lethal subcutaneous dose
2. saline value not comparable with other values in table

Clinical Features Of Papuan Elapid Snakebite.
Examination of the Wound.

In cases of true viper or pit viper bites the large fangs, which may measure up to 30mm, frequently leave obvious puncture wounds surrounded by extensive areas of swelling, oedema, discolouration and tenderness. However, the fangs of elapids are much smaller, rarely exceeding 10mm, and many of the accompanying symptoms may be absent. The small puncture wounds made by small fangs may easily close up and, unless accompanied by serum weeping or bleeding, they may become impossible to locate, especially on the bare feet of native people with their tough skins and numerous abrasions, cuts and other day-to-day injuries. If bite injuries are identified they may consist of lacerations or puncture wounds. Lacerations may be the result of a bite from a non-venomous species such as a python, a large specimen of which can cause a fearsome injury. Puncture wounds may be single, double, treble or multiple. Treble puncture wounds are common in single bite situations as many venomous snakes have a reserve fang ready to replace an old fang which will soon be shed. The bite will, therefore, consist of two close punctures, side-by-side or one behind the other, together with a third puncture wound a short distance away. Multiple bites from taipans or Papuan blacksnakes will be indicated by one, two or more pairs of equidistant puncture wounds. First aid lacerations will often obscure all puncture wounds. Small ecchymoses around apparent puncture injuries, slight oedema and localised swelling do not necessarily indicate a venomous snakebite as non-venomous bites may produce these signs and oedema may occur as a result of torniquet application. In approximately 50% of elapid bite cases there is often no envenoming (Russell, 1980). However, continued wound bleeding indicates injection of a coagulant snake venom.

The Early Symptoms.

The early symptoms of elapid snakebite in Papua New Guinea fall into three categories as defined by Campbell (1969);

Non-specific symptoms: vomiting, headache, pain in the lymph nodes, abdominal pain, loss of consciousness, general weakness, visual difficulties, sweating, pallor and diarrhoea.

Clinical bleeding symptoms: bleeding from the gums or gingival sulci, vomiting of blood, spitting or coughing of blood stained sputum, wound bleeding and passage of bloody urine.

Muscular paralysis symptoms: difficulty in moving or operating jaw, tongue, eyes, eyelids, limbs or in swallowing.

Non-specific symptoms.

Campbell reported that the commonest early symptom of Australasian elapid envenoming is vomiting, or the desire to vomit, adding that it occurred in exactly half of his study group of 68 patients with positive envenoming (31 patients vomited and three demonstrated their desire to vomit) between half an hour and twelve hours after the bite. In 27 patients this was the first symptom which indicted a venomous snakebite and it could, therefore, be a useful indicator that envenoming has taken place. However vomiting could be caused by other factors such as fear or shock which may easily arise in patients who have been bitten by either venomous or non-venomous species. In addition, vomiting would be expected if the patient had previously been treated using traditional emetic herbal methods. Only if there is no history of this remedy can vomiting be considered important as an early sign of systemic envenoming.

The presence of blood in the vomit may also indicate that a venomous bite has occurred but this appears to be rare; it was recorded in only two of

Campbell's patients. Bites from the following Papuan species have been observed to cause vomiting in patients; death adder, taipan, Papuan blacksnake, small-eyed snake, eastern brownsnake and Muller's snake. This latter species of the genus *Aspidomorphus* is not included in this study as it is not considered a life-threatening species but bites have occurred and victims have experienced unpleasant symptoms.

Campbell records that headaches were common features of envenoming but that they varied greatly in severity and duration and also that their onset can occur anytime during the first four hours after elapine snakebite. He reports that headache is rare in Melanesian society and, therefore, such a symptom is of more importance in Papua New Guinea than it would be in the West. Envenomation from taipan, Papuan blacksnake, death adder, eastern brownsnake and small-eyed snake have all been recorded as causing headaches in Papua New Guinea.

Campbell goes to great lengths to emphasise the extreme importance of these first two symptoms in the diagnosis of envenoming by dangerous elapids in Papua New Guinea, or Australia, especially as these features may soon disappear or diminish. The danger is that if these symptoms are not recognised as signs of envenoming the patient may go on to develop more severe paralytic symptoms.

Localised pain in the lymph nodes is a common feature of snakebite, particularly the bites of viperid snakes, and it has also been recorded following bites from death adder, taipan and Papuan blacksnakes. In common with vomiting and the onset of headache it may be the first obvious symptom; it usually persists for longer than the other two symptoms, for up to two and a half days even after the administration of antivenom, with varying severity.

Abdominal pain was reported by Campbell. He commented that it could be either localised or generalised, mild or severe and extremely variable in its duration, often remaining after antivenom treatment. Pain in abdominal lymph nodes was also noticed in patients. This symptom was common and severe in envenoming resulting from the Papuan blacksnake but was also recorded from the taipan and eastern brownsnake.

Either rapid and sudden unconsciousness or a gradual loss of consciousness, preceded by visual difficulties, may occur following envenoming by the taipan, death adder, Papuan blacksnake and eastern brownsnake from a few minutes to one hour after the bite. Periods of unconsciousness have lasted for periods of less than one hour to up to twelve hours some patients have failed to recover consciousness and have subsequently died. The presence of a clammy, cold or sweaty skin and a weak pulse led Campbell to postulate that the venom may have had an effect on the circulatory system which resulted in unconsciousness but he also reports that in some cases the loss of consciousness may be caused by the action of the venom on the brain. Loss of consciousness frequently precedes the dangerous paralytic stage of envenoming which usually becomes apparent when the patient regains consciousness and is unable to move. Blasco and Hornabrook (1972) reported a case of small-eyed snake bite in which the patient became unconscious and suffered respiratory arrest within five minutes of admission to hospital, just over two hours after the envenoming. Other early symptoms included vomiting, cyanosis of lips and gums, heaviness of limbs and shortness of breath. This patient failed to respond to death adder antivenom or resuscitation and subsequently died.

Drowsiness, often cited as a characteristic of Australian elapid poisoning, is an unreliable sign of envenoming since it may be caused by other factors including the consumption of alcohol or genuine tiredness. However, apparent drowsiness, suggested by general weakness or fatigue and ptosis, may be caused by the paralytic effects of the venom on the muscles. Patients who appeared to be 'drowsy', and who went to sleep, frequently awoke later in a totally paralysed state. Campbell is equally sceptical of the value of irritability as a symptom as it may be as much the product of fear as of the effects of envenoming. Convulsions have also occurred following venomous snakebites in Papua New Guinea but these may be the result of hypotension rather than a direct cause of the venom.

The venom of the small-eyed snake is recorded by Slater as causing diarrhoea, but although this has occurred as a result of other snakebites in Australia, Campbell did not witness it and it does not appear to be a common symptom of Papuan snakebite.

Clinical bleeding symptoms.

Bleeding from the gums and gingival sulci is an important symptom of systemic envenoming and blood stained sputum or vomit has been recorded following envenoming by taipan or eastern brownsnake. These symptoms are not observed following death adder envenoming. Both taipan and brownsnake have strongly coagulant venoms. Campbell reported similar symptoms following bites from "Papuan blacksnakes" but it is now thought that the taipan was probably the species responsible. Marshall and Herrmann (1983) deny procoagulant activity in the venoms of both Papuan blacksnake (*P.papuanus*) and mulga brownsnake (*P.australis*). Campbell reports that the venom of the mulga or king brownsnake is powerfully anticoagulant but authorities are divided as to whether any of the genus *Pseudechis* possess anticoagulant qualities in their venoms. However, Marshall and Herrmann (1983) reported that three species of interest here; *Pseudechis australis, P.papuanus* and *Acanthophis antarcticus*, did demonstrate the possession of a powerful unknown anticoagulant factor which was neither antithrombin nor fibrinogenolytic. Some snake venoms *in vitro* may be demonstrated to possess both coagulant and anticoagulant properties depending on the concentration of venom tested (Mebs, 1978) and incoagulable blood *in vivo* does not necessarily indicate an anticoagulant venom since coagulant factors will also cause bleeding via a defibrination syndrome. However, the anticoagulant properties of many Australasian venoms are probably of little clinical significance. Regardless of whether the venom is coagulant or anticoagulant positive envenoming can be diagnosed if continued bleeding or serum weeping from the fang puncture wounds or 'first aid' lacerations is observed.

Dark urine may also be observed but it should be tested to determine whether the cause in haemoglobinuria or myoglobinuria. Although rectal bleeding and melaena have been reported following Australian elapine snakebites, neither has been reported from Papua New Guinea.

Muscular paralysis symptoms.

Early symptoms of muscle paralysis due to envenoming may manifest as difficulties in moving the eyelids, eyes, jaw, tongue or in swallowing and as a general weakness of the limbs, but it is not indicative of a bite from any particular species of Papuan elapid since the entire group is characterised by the possession of neurotoxins in the venom.

On occasions none of the above symptoms is seen and the first sign of envenoming may be severe peripheral curare-like neuromuscular paralysis of the respiratory and chest muscles. This usually indicates that either a death adder or a small-eyed snake was responsible but occasionally a taipan bite may proceed to neuromuscular paralysis without early symptoms becoming apparent.

In conclusion it is recommended that the first two symptoms, vomiting and headache, should not be ignored or disregarded as they are frequently the earliest features of a potentially serious, life-threatening snakebite. If they are overlooked the patient may subsequently suffer loss of consciousness and paralysis. Continual observation of the patient is essential as many of these symptoms, including the two most important, are only temporary, often of short duration and may be misinterpreted.

The Clinical Signs.
Enlargement and/or tenderness of lymph nodes.

One or both of these signs can occur within the first few hours after a bite and may endure for up to two days even after administration of antivenom. Although reported as a common feature of 'Papuan blacksnake' bites, tenderness of lymph nodes is not confined to envenoming by that species and may follow bites from taipan or death adder. Lymph node tenderness is due to the action of the lymphatic system in the absorption of venoms with high molecular weight such as those of the vipers and pit-vipers of America, Asia and Africa and many Australian elapids. Campbell (1969), provides details of a lymph node biopsy carried out at the Kanematsu Memorial Institute of Pathology in Sydney Hospital following envenoming from an elapid which was probably a small-eyed snake. He quotes Professor ten Seldam of the Department of Pathology at the University of Western Australia who reports that the severe dilation of the peripheral sinusoids with oedema in the lymph node surroundings and areas of haemorrhage and necrosis within the lymph node, without severe inflammation, indicated that a very toxic substance had entered the lymph node and caused a similar reaction to that seen in lymph node biopsies from two fatal Indonesian snakebites.

Abdominal pain and muscle guarding.

Both tenderness and muscle guarding may be mild or severe, general or localised following the bite of the Papuan blacksnake, and possibly also the taipan, and the tenderness in the region of the inguinal ligament was also recorded by Campbell following a death adder bite. The tenderness may be due to the effect of the venom on the abdominal lymphatic system. Without a history of snakebite the patient may be diagnosed as suffering from acute appendicitis.

Muscular paralysis and the neurotoxic effects.

Paralysis of the voluntary muscles is a common sign of elapid envenoming, often commencing either soon after the bite has occurred, or later, after admission to hospital, and continuing for up to thirty hours with increasing severity until it becomes potentially life-threatening. Slight ptosis and other difficulties in ocular muscle movement are usually the first signs of elapid-invoked paralysis followed by visual difficulties and muscular paralysis of the jaw, tongue, palate and pharynx. Complete ptosis, if it occurs, may not take place until much later. Pupil reactions to light can still, however, be observed at all times, even in cases of total eye paralysis.

The early signs of myasthenia gravis may occur. This neuromuscular disorder, which is characterised by the weakness and fatigability of ocular, bulbar and proximal limb muscles, is caused by a decrease in available acetylcholine receptors at the neuromuscular junctions. In severe instances it may result in the impairment of respiratory activity (Drachman, 1987).

If the patient is in a recumbent position jaw muscle paralysis may cause the lower jaw to drop back slightly and it may become impossible for the patient to extend his tongue. Speech deteriorates until it becomes impossible and drooling of saliva indicates that swallowing is also difficult. In a recumbent patient there is a danger of inhalation of saliva.

The next muscles to show signs of paralysis are usually the facial muscle, controlling expression, but complete paralysis of the facial muscles may take many hours to occur. A general weakness of the limbs is an early sign of general muscle paralysis. In the early stages the standard reflex actions can still be registered but later these too will become subdued. Whilst a severely paralysed patient may not be able to sit up, roll over or turn his head, and may even appear moribund, with almost totally closed eyes and expressionless face, he may still have control over movements of his fingers and toes and be able to slightly twist the pelvis. Cutaneous sensation seems to remain intact except for a small area surrounding the actual bite area.

Paralysis of the chest muscles and the muscles of the diaphragm is obviously a serious sign and respiration may cease even before limb paralysis is complete.

Respiratory obstruction may result from oral or chest secretions draining into the lungs from where the patient is unable to cough them up or spit them out. Also obstruction of the airway by the paralysed tongue can be dangerous and it may be necessary to insert an artifical airway. These problems, coupled with decreased respiratory activity caused by the effect of the venom on the respiratory chest muscles and the diaphragm, eventually result in cyanosis, anoxia, unconsiousness and death due to asphyxia. In most instances of severe paralysis it is necessary to initiate endotracheal intubation or to perform a tracheotomy and remove sputum from the airway. Campbell estimated that most patients would not survive for more than one or two hours beyond the point where a tracheotomy was indicated. Tracheotomies were performed from three to 96 hours after envenoming and the time at which they became necessary could be used as an indicator of the degree of severity of the bite and the probable dosage of venom injected. Campbell reported that although antivenom administered during the early stages of envenoming was frequently successful in reversing or diminishing the degree of muscle paralysis, in the later stages only patients with bites resulting from death adders showed a significant response to antivenom and it would appear that in the cases of Papuan blacksnake or taipan bites, where antivenom is often not capable of reversing paralysis, intubation, tracheotomy and life-support by other means are essential in order to preserve life.

Even so, elapid snake venoms, which contain powerful neurotoxins, are capable of causing extremely powerful, and sometimes irreversible, peripheral neuromuscular blockages. Sutherland (1983) suggests that venoms containing postsynaptic neurotoxins such as the deaths adders *(Acanthophis sp.)* probably causes a more rapid onset of paralysis than the venoms with presynaptic components such as the Australian tiger snake *(Notechis scutatus)*. However, postsynaptic neurotoxins are more easily reversed with antivenom than that caused by presynaptic venoms.

Haemotoxic effects.

In the section on *clinical bleeding symptoms* it was noted that both anticoagulant and coagulant properties may be present in the same venom and both may cause the blood to become incoagulable. However, the effects of the anticoagulant factors do not seem to have any serious bearing on the clinical effects and treatment of the envenoming and the dangerous haemotoxic effects of Australo-Papuan elapine snakebite result more from the procoagulant factors of the venom.

Strongly procoagulant venoms such as those of the taipan and the eastern brownsnake are very diffusible and cause a conversion of prothrombin to thrombin resulting in afibrinogenaemia (Sutherland, 1983). Both of these species possess venoms which are complete prothrombin activators capable of converting prothrombin to thrombin in either plasma deficient in factor V or in normal plasma (Denson; 1969, Mebs, 1978) but the venoms of the death adder and the Australian tiger snake *(Notechis scutatus)* are incomplete prothrombin activators which cause coagulation only in the presence of factor V (Mebs, 1978). A thrombosis may cause death through extensive haemorrhaging from the mucus membranes (Kellaway, 1938) but the presence of incoagulable blood does not necessarily result in haemorrhagic symptoms. Many coagulant venoms will not cause haemorrhage unless a secondary factor is involved such as a medical history of stomach ulcers or damage to the actual blood vessels through the actions of another venom factor, a haemorrhagin. Haemorrhagins are not generally considered common factors in Australasian snake venoms. Even so, due to the incoagulability of the blood there will be continued bleeding from the fang puncture marks and also from any 'first aid' incisions or tracheotomy wounds.

The defibrination of the blood by a procoagulant venom can also cause symptoms such as bleeding from the gums and coughing and spitting of blood stained sputum which have already been recorded as important early symptoms of venomous snakebite.

Campbell carried out numerous haematological tests, including the now out-dated rabbit anti-fibrin test, (RAF), on patients admitted to Port Moresby Hospital with snakebite envenoming. He found many of the usual blood tests were of limited value in determining the type of snake responsible and the degree of envenoming. However, the simple bedside whole blood clotting test is a quick and useful technique for determining whether the patient has received a bite from a species possessing a coagulant venom.

Campbell also conducted fibrinogen titres to determine the amount of fibrinogen present in the patient's plasma. He reports that whereas the normal titre for a Caucasoid is 1 in 64, the normal titre for a Melanesian is 1 in 32, the addition of EACA raises the Melanesian titre to that of a Caucasoid but the presence of a coagulant venom such as that of the taipan will reduce the titre to 1 in 16 or even zero.

Prolonged whole blood coagulation and a low fibrinogen titre would suggest that the snake concerned was one of those species with a strongly coagulant venom. Antiserum is usually effective in reversing these effects.

Haemolysis of the blood corpuscles is a further consequence of certain Papuan elapine bites. The venom of the blacksnake, and possibly also the mulga brownsnake, is reported to be strongly haemolytic and it is capable of causing high levels of haemoglobinuria. The taipan is thought to be weakly haemolytic but there has been at least one case of a taipan bite in Papua New Guinea resulting in haemoglobinuria. Death adder and eastern brownsnake venoms are also weakly haemolytic. Antiserum also has a powerful effect in reversing these haemolytic symptoms.

Proteinuria and Haemoglobinuria.

Proteinuria may be a consequence of Papuan elapine envenoming but urine samples tested soon after poisoning rarely register any significant level of proteinuria. Similarly, after administration of antivenom the level of any apparent proteinuria may drop off dramatically.

In addition, blacksnake and taipan venoms may have a severely damaging effect on the kidneys if antivenom is delayed or not given. In cases of the late administration of antivenom it is frequently necessary to maintain dialysis due to the renal damage caused by the venom prior to its administration. If antivenom therapy has been greatly delayed the renal damage may be severe and irreversible.

Haemoglobinuria may be evident quite early in the history of envenoming usually before severe paralysis has occurred, and it is normally associated with a high level of proteinuria. Haemoglobinuria is a sure sign that a severe envenoming has taken place and is usually a strong indication of either a Papuan blacksnake or taipan bite. There is also a record of haemoglobinuria from a possible Australian mulga brownsnake bite, (Campbell, 1969), a species which may yet be recorded in Western Province and which is closely related to the Papuan blacksnake, both members of the genus *Pseudechis* (Mengden, Shine & Moritz, 1986). The relationship between haemoglobinuria and anuria causing renal failure is not clear.

The absence of proteinuria or haemoglobinuria does not preclude the possibility that a venomous snakebite has occurred. For example, death adder bites rarely cause proteinuria and never haemoglobinuria. These signs may also be missed if the patient is not seen until some time after antivenom has been administered.

Myotoxic effects.

The venom of the little known small-eyed snake is believed to be highly myotoxic causing myalgia, muscle tenderness and severe neuromuscular paralysis. Since small-eyed snake venom does not demonstrate coagulopathy the presence of 'dark' urine will indicate myoglobinuria rather than haemoglobinuria (Sutherland, 1983). Hudson and Pomat (1988) report 16 cases of envenoming from Madang Province, 11 of which demonstrated 'dark' urine. Six of these patients subsequently suffered renal failure probably caused by the delay between the venomous bite and the administration of antivenom. These 16 cases exhibited signs of myotoxicity or rhabdomyolysis (striated muscle destruction) and since 15 of these bites were from terrestrial snakes and the venom of the only other dangerous elapid in the region, the death adder, is non-myotoxic in its effects it must be considered that these symptoms occurred as a result of small-eyed snake envenoming. In three of the cases the description of a 'long white snake' suggests that the small-eyed snake was responsible. If untreated the consequence of myoglobinuria may be oliguria within 24 hours leading to renal failure and death several days later (Sutherland, 1983). This species has been responsible for several serious human accidents and at least one documented and several other suspected deaths (Blasco & Hornabrook, 1972 and Hudson & Pomat, 1988). Myoglobinuria frequently also causes cerebral hypoxia in severely envenomed patients (Sutherland, 1983).

The venom of the common seasnake *(Enhydrina schistosa)*, also causes myotoxic or rhabdomyolytic signs and symptoms, in common with many other hydrophiids, which may be accompanied by neuromuscular paralysis (Hudson & Fromm, 1986). Muscle tenderness is a very prominent clinical feature of envenoming by *E.schistosa* (Sutherland, 1983) together with myoglobinuria (Reid, 1961). The hyaline lysis and necrosis of the skeletal muscle is a common pathological feature of *E.schistosa* envenoming (Marsden & Reid, 1961). Other signs and symptoms of sea snake envenoming include paresis; aching and muscular stiffness and weakness; ptosis; thirst; cold and sweating; vomiting and nasal regurgition; failing vision and eventual respiratory paralysis and cyanosis. Severe necrosis of the kidneys and eventual renal failure may occur in patients who are still alive after 48 hours (Mebs, 1978) most deaths occurring during the first 24 hours (Barme, 1968).

The venom of the mulga or king brownsnake, together with many other Australasian elapine snakes, is also reported to contain a powerful myotoxin (Sutherland, 1983) having a severely damaging effect on the skeletal muscle.

Cardiovascular effects.

The only Papuan-Australian snake venom thought to be severely cardiotoxic is that of the mulga or king brownsnake which is only weakly neurotoxic. Whether the venom of the Papuan blacksnake has any cardiotoxic qualities is unknown although Campbell reports normal ECGs from six cases of blacksnake bite.

The cardiotoxic effects of snake venoms are thought to be partially due to the presence of a phospatidase and proteolytic enzymes or a neurotoxin but the situation is not clear with regard to Australian snake carditoxins which also release adenosine, a powerful cardiac depressant, into the heart (Trethewie, 1971 p.89).

Hypotension may occur rapidly in Papuan-Australian elapine bites either with or without the patient losing consciousness or developing convulsions. This is termed primary hypotension and it is signified by pallor, a bloodless face with blueing lips and extremities, cold clammy skin, a slow, weak pulse and almost undetectable respiration. Although the patient may appear quite moribund recovery can be extremely rapid and total.

It is believed that this sudden drop in blood pressure is caused by the autopharmacological effects of the venom on the release of substances from the tissues and cells into the blood. Various venoms cause the release of histamine, "slow-reacting substance", adenyl compounds and anaphylatoxins which have differing effects on the homeostasis of the victim. The venoms of many viperids (Mebs, 1970) and Australian elapids (Warrell, *pers.comm.*) release bradykinin into the plasma, from the protein precursor bradykininogen, through the action of specific venom enzymes called kininogenases (Rocha e Silva, 1970). The effects of the release of bradykinin into the plasma are smooth muscle stimulation, vasodilatation, increased capillary permeability and pain (Rocha e Silva, 1970). If large quantities of these substances are introduced into the circulation the result will be a rapid drop in blood pressure and 'shock'. Bradykinin has a very short half-life and the effects of the primary hypotension wear off rapidly (Mebs, 1978). Other "slow-reacting substances" may also be responsible for causing autopharmacological changes and effects in Australo-Papuan snakebite victims but in many cases their mechanisms are not fully understood.

Although the hypotension caused by Australasian elapine venoms resembles an anaphylatic reaction, Campbell points out that the sudden and complete recoveries from primary hypotension are not typical of anaphylaxis.

Pretreatment with an anti-histamine does not apparently prevent primary hypotension.

If sufficient damage has been done to the circulatory system by either the haemorrhagic qualities or some other factor of the venom a secondary form of hypotension may occur due to fluid loss into the tissues. This is a common feature of viper and pit-viper venoms but the only snakes of interest to this survey which may contain sufficient quantities of haemorrhagin in their venom are members of the genus *Pseudechis* (Campbell, 1969 p.167)

Campbell reported that anoxia was also a major cause of secondary hypotension in severely paralysed patients suffering from "Papuan blacksnake" (possibly taipan) envenoming and correct and intensive nursing procedures could prevent such an occurence. Even changing the patient's posture in the bed so that a tracheotomy can be performed has resulted in secondary hypotension with fatal results. Pulmonary oedema due to over-transfusion of blood and normal saline has also been responsible for causing death through secondary hypotension in blacksnake bite regardless of the effects of the venom itself.

Treatment Of Papuan Snakebite.

This section is only intended as a brief resume of advice proffered by Campbell and Sutherland regarding the treatment of elapid snakebite in Papua New Guinea since the current theories and techniques for the treatment of venomous snakebite will be covered in more detail by another author (see Warrell, this volume). Sutherland (1983), describes in detail the treatment of envenoming in Australo—Papuan elapine snakebite victims.

First Aid.

Reassurance of the patient is extremely important, especially in the case of children, and aspirin or alcohol given in extreme moderation may be helpful as a calming influence according to Reid (1980). Possibly a placebo medication could also be considered. Above all the patient should be discouraged from exerting himself. The bitten limb should be elevated, if possible, and the victim should be taken to seek medical help as soon as possible. If should be remembered that Australia and Papua New Guinea contain some of the World's most venomous snakes and that the neurotoxins of some species do not respond well to antivenom once a significant amount of time has elapsed. The identity of the snake is extremely important but frequently overlooked at this stage. If the snake has been killed it should be taken with the patient to hospital. However, further injury should not be risked in a fruitless search for the reptile by either the patient or his companions as some species are capable of delivering several fatal bites. A severely injured and apparently 'dead' snake should not be handled as it may 'come back to life' momentarily and administer a serious bite. Even a decapitated head can deliver a bite should a jaw muscle be stimulated. The body of the reptile should be lifted with a stick into a secure box or glass jar, not a bag which may be sat upon, for the journey to hospital where it should be identified by a competent person. In the absence of the snake's body the patient should be interviewed regarding the snake's approximate length, colouration, body shape, mode of attack and the habitat, locality and time of day when the bite occurred. This information should be noted down accurately as it will be required to assist with probable identification of the species responsible. It should be remembered that in certain regions of Papua New Guinea, every snake is a 'Papuan blacksnake' so the positive identification of this species as the snake responsible, by the victim is of limited value.

Over-exuberant bush techniques such as incision and bleeding of the fang puncture wounds should be strongly discouraged as these practises may lead to excessive blood loss (especially in cases where the venom is strongly procoagulant and has caused widespread defibrination); damage to nerves and tendons (Reid, 1980); delayed healing and the possibility of infection and the obscuring of recognisable fang wounds. In addition, wound cutting and the sight of blood in children is likely to lead to intense fright, panic and increased heart beat and circulation which will further increase the possibilities of a tragic outcome. It is unlikely that suction will remove a significant quantity of the venom, especially if injected into tissue, and bleeding will probably open up more blood vessels for venom absorption. Tourniquets are also unpopular due to their frequent misuse. A more acceptable alternative might be a crepe-type pressure bandage designed to slow down circulation in the bitten limb but not restrict it entirely. However, if a large quantity has been injected a tourniquet may be necessary (Reid, 1980) but it is important to relieve the pressure at regular short intervals. To prevent movement in the bitten limb it should be splinted with a suitable piece of wood.

The patient should be observed for the early symptoms of serious envenomation as detailed in the clinical section; vomiting, headache, ptosis etc. The airway must be kept clear of mucus and respiration must be maintained, if necessary by tracheotomy and artifical respiration in very serious cases and the patient dispatched to hospital by the most rapid means possible.

Excessive quantities of alcohol, emetic herbal remedies and potentially hazardous tribal magical techniques should be avoided if possible but care must be taken to avoid distrust and infringment of tribal taboos. It may be necessary to work in collaboration with the village tribal magic man rather than risk alienation, resentment and the possible withdrawal of assistance or transportation.

A pamphlet on First Aid for Snakebite in Australia (Sutherland, 1988) is available from the Commonwealth Serum Laboratories, Victoria which is also applicable for Papua New Guinea.

Hospitalisation.

Campbell advises that all suspected venomous snakebite victims should be admitted to hospital and put under regular hourly observations for pulse rate, respiration rate and blood pressure and the presence of the early symptoms of snakebite envenoming. If symptoms are present already or subsequently appear, the patient should be checked for difficulty in swallowing or breathing. All urine should be tested for protein and blood and the colour noted.

The aims of the physician should be to:

a. neutralise the effects of the venom using antivenom,

b. relieve respiratory obstruction and maintain an airway, by endotracheal intubation or tracheotomy if necessary,

c. deal with respiratory insufficiency, by artifical respiration if necessary.

If the signs and symptoms of envenoming occur the patient should be treated with antivenom following the recommendations of the manufacturers. Antivenom for use in Papua New Guinea is produced by the Commonwealth Serum Laboratories in Victoria, Australia. Depending on the identity of the snake the practitioner can administer Monospecific Death Adder, Taipan, Blacksnake or Brownsnake antivenoms. In cases where the snake was not positively identified, a Polyspecific Papuan antivenom is available. Tiger snake antivenom is also, reportedly, effective in the treatment of certain Papuan snakebites. CSL also developed a Venom Detection Kit (chap.5, Sutherland, 1983) which was intended to make it possible to identify the snake species responsible for an envenoming in a very short time and allow the use of the correct monospecific antivenom. The kits comprised a series of colour coded capillary tubes attached to a fine syringe. Each section was coated with a specific antivenom and the venom's identity was indicated by a colour change in the section coated with antivenom specific to that species, or group of related species. However, they have not proved to be very successful due to the occurrence of paraspecific reactions and false positive results (Warrell, *pers.comm.*) and whether such a finely-tuned technique, if fully reliable, would be of much value in a small Papuan clinic must also be queried.

The elapsed time between the snakebite and the administration of antivenom is extremely important in the treatment of Papuan elapid bites. It is reported that cobra bites respond well to antivenom even if administered extremely late in the treatment, when the patient is moribund and lifeless (Ahuja & Singh, 1954) and it seems likely that the effects of death adder venom may respond similarly (Campbell, 1967). However, taipan and blacksnake venoms are very different and late administration of the either polyspecific or monospecific antivenom frequently has little effect on the neurotoxic component of the venom although it may reverse the effects of the haemolytic and procoagulant venom factors. The recommended antivenom dose is intended to neutralise the average venom yield of the species concerned. In cases of taipan or blacksnake envenomation, where multiple bites are not uncommon, Campbell (1967), suggests that up to ten times the recommended dose may be required to even stand a chance of reversing paralysis, especially if antivenom is not administered until a considerable time after the occurrence of the bite.

The Tensilon (edrophonium) test for myasthenia gravis, caused by a decrease in acetylcholine receptors at the neuromucuslar junctions, is useful in determining whether skeletal muscle weakness and general fatigue are due to snakebite envenoming with a neurotoxic venom. A bolus of 10mg of edrophonium, an anticholinesterase, is injected intravenously following a test dose of 1-2mg (Clarke, 1987). A rapid improvement lasting 2-3 minutes indicates a positive result but the test should also be performed using a control substance such as normal saline to eliminate error. Care should also be taken when conducting the Tensilon test as it may cause bronchial obstruction and syncope (Clarke, 1987). Facilities for resuscitation should therefore be available. Considerable success has been reported for this technique in determing neurotoxic snake bite envenoming by Australian elapids (Warrell, *pers.comm.*) ie. in foals bitten by Eastern brownsnakes, *Pseudonaja textilis*, and in humans receiving bites from Philippine cobras, *Naja naja philippinensis*, (Watt *et al*, 1986).

Blood gases can be estimated regularly in large hospitals to test for respiratory insufficiency caused by ongoing neuromuscular paralysis but in smaller field clinics adequate results can be obtained using peak flow metres to measure vital capacity and expiration.

To reduce the chance of anaphylaxis caused by the intravenous introduction of antivenom it should be administered either by slow direct pulse injection (Malasit *et al*, 1986), or by slow infusion over thirty minutes, together with a glucose or saline solution of equal volume, via an infusion giving set. In case of anaphylaxis, or some other allergic reaction, it is advisable for the practitioner to have adrenaline, (0.5ml of 1:1000 adrenaline), and the necessary equipment for emergency resuscitation standing by.

Allergic reactions may vary from severe and sudden anaphylaxis to abdominal pain, lasting and widespread urticaria or shivering and a rise in body temperature. In the long term serum sickness may occur up to nine days after antivenom treatment and administration of steroids may be necessary.

Following the administration of antivenom the patient should continue to be observed as antivenom may not immediately arrest the onset of life-threatening paralysis, particularly in the case of taipan or blacksnake bites. If partial paralysis of the chest, palate or pharynx occurs the patient should be nursed on one side and observed closely in case endotracheal intubation or a tracheotomy is required. A build up of oral secretions in the pharynx will indicate that immediate action is necessary. Campbell estimated that if reliance was placed solely on administration of antivenom at least 25% of patients, who could be saved if adequate and unimpeded respiration was maintained, would die. Following the operation, close and constant nursing and monitoring for blockage of the airway will also be necessary. In serious cases of paralysis artifical respiration may become essential and the need for continual and skilled nursing and medical supervision cannot be over emphasised. Eventually, under these conditions, even severe paralysis should diminish although this may take up to seven days of intensive care.

Appendix One:

Key to Papuan Snake Families.

Five of the World's ten families of snakes are respresented in the herpetofauna of New Guinea. The taxonomic position and relationships of highly venomous sea snakes and the dangerous land snakes of Australasia have long been a cause of controversy. Smith, Smith and Sawin, (1977) confined the usage of the family name Elapidae to the terrestrial proteroglyphous snakes of Africa, Asia and America and the amphibious sea kraits of the genus *Laticauda* together termed "Palatine Erectors". The true sea snakes and all terrestrial Australasian proteroglyphs received a separate family, the Hydrophiidae, the "Palatine Draggers". Although this classification has found many followers (Golay, 1985) it is perhaps misleading in that it suggests a strong relationship between Smith *et al's* terrestrial Elapids and *Laticauda* which has not been proven (McCarthy, 1985).

1a. Tail enlarged and laterally compressed, paddle-shaped or body banded blue and black.

Marine Elapidae (Laticaudinae, sea kraits, and Hydrophiinae, sea snakes)

1b. Tail not compressed into paddle-shape, usually cylindrical.   2

2a. Ventral scales not enlarged, similar in size to dorsal scales.   3

2b. Ventral scales broader than long, at least three times width of dorsal scales.   4

3a. Less than forty scales at midbody, all smooth; eyes vestigal and often barely visible.

Typhlopidae (blind snakes)

3b. In excess of eighty scales at midbody, rough and tubucular; skin very loose; eyes well developed.

Acrochordidae (wart or file snakes)

4a. In excess of thirty midbody scale rows; heat sensitive labial pits usually present.

Boidae (Pythoninae — pythons)

4b. Less than thirty scale rows at midbody.   5

5a. One or more loreal scales present between nasal and preocular, if loreal scale absent, then 23 or more scales at midbody and divided anal plate.

Colubridae (Colubrinae, Natricinae and Homalopsinae — typical snakes)

5b. Loreal scale absent, anal entire if 23 scale rows at midbody.

Terrestrial Elapidae (Elapinae)

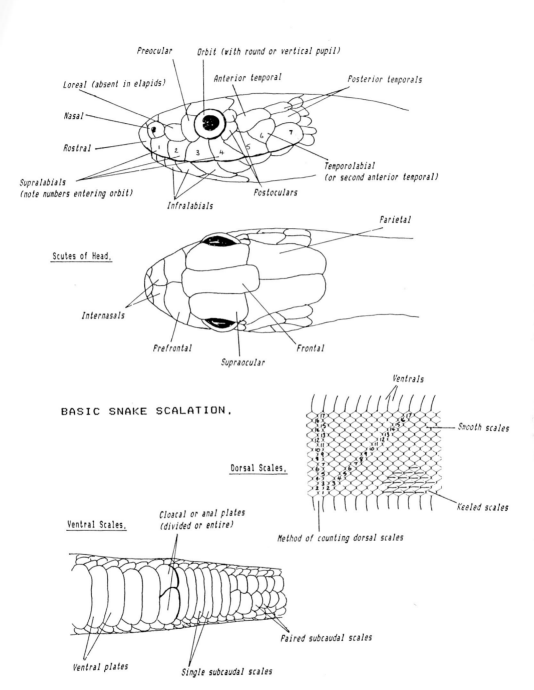

Preocular

Orbit (with round or vertical pupil)

Loreal (absent in elapids)

Anterior temporal

Posterior temporals

Nasal

Rostral

Temporolabial
(or second anterior temporal)

Supralabials
(note numbers entering orbit)

Postoculars

Infralabials

Farietal

Scutes of Head.

Internasals

Prefrontal

Supraocular

Frontal

Ventrals

BASIC SNAKE SCALATION.

Smooth scales

Dorsal Scales.

Keeled scales

Method of counting dorsal scales

Cloacal or anal plates
(divided or entire)

Ventral Scales.

Paired subcaudal scales

Ventral plates

Single subcaudal scales

633

Appendix Two:

Key to the Dangerous Papuan Elapids

1a.   Body short, stout viper-like with short tail; total length less than one metre; head angular and viper-like and very distinct from neck; two or three subocular scales present separating supralabials from orbit; comb-like spine on tip of tail; scales of body and head smooth or rugose; scale rows at midbody 21 or 23; anal plate entire; subcaudals anteriorly single, posteriorly paired; supralabials number six or seven with temporolabial contacting or failing to contact lip; eight infralabials; pupil of eye vertically elliptical.   2

1b.   Body not stout or viper-like; head not angular, not viper-like, distinct or indistinct from neck; no suboculars separating supralabials from orbit; no comb-like tip to tail; scales of head smooth and of body smooth or, occasionally, partially keeled; scale rows at midbody 13 to 23; anal plate entire or divided; subcaudals usually paired, occasionally partially or totally single; supralabials number four, five, six or seven (if seven with sixth supralabial as temporolabial failing to contact lip); six or seven infralabials; pupil of eye round or vertically elliptical.   3

2a.   Scutes of head smooth or weakly rugose; anterior dorsals weakly keeled or smooth, supralabials boldly patterned with black, or dark brown, and white; free edge of supraocular not usually raised; dorsal scale rows usually not fewer on neck than at midbody.

                                         Acanthophis antarcticus

2b.   Scutes of head moderately rugose; anterior dorsals usually strongly keeled; supralabials not boldly patterned; free edge of supraocular often raised; dorsal scale rows fewer on neck than midbody.

                                         Acanthophis praelongus

3a.   Total length less than one metre; always six infralabials; usually 15 scale rows at midbody, occasionally 13 or 17, (17 rows on Fergusson and Woodlark Islands, Milne Bay Prov., only); subcaudals all or mostly paired, (if all single first subcaudal always divided into pair, Rossel Island, Milne Bay Prov., only); anal plate usually divided but if entire, then supralabials either number four or five with second and third entering orbit; otherwise supralabials usually number six with third and fourth entering orbit; temporolabial scale absent.

                            Genus *Toxicocalamus* (9 species)

3b.   Total length varies from less than one metre to over three metres; always seven infralabials; 15 or more scale rows at midbody; subcaudals all single, all paired or combined single and paired; anal plate divided or entire; supralabials usually number six or seven, usually with third and fourth entering orbit; temporolabial scale present or absent.   4

4a.   Total length less than two metres; scale rows at midbody number 15.   5

4b.   Total length from less than one metre to over three metres; scale rows at midbody number 17 or more.   9

5a.   Small snakes, total length less than 0.5 metre; anal plate entire; subcaudals single; pupil of eye round.   Genus *Unechis* (1-2 species)

| 5b. | Small to medium snakes, total length up to two metres; anal plate divided; subcaudals all paired; pupil of eye round or vertically elliptical. | 6 |

5b. Small to medium snakes, total length up to two metres; anal plate divided; subcaudals all paired; pupil of eye round or vertically elliptical. 6

6a. Eye very small with round pupils; total length up to 2 metres; dorsum of body banded or progressively darker towards posterior; midbody scale rows not reducing in number towards cloaca. ***Micropechis ikaheka***

6b. Eye medium to large with elliptical or round pupil; total length up to 1½ metres; dorsum either immaculate, mottled, flecked or striped; midbody scale rows reducing or not reducing in number towards cloaca. 7

7a. Midbody scale rows not reducing in number towards cloaca, 15-15; subcaudals number forty or less; body and tail not elongate; canthus rostralis absent; eye medium with vertically elliptical pupil, either obvious or barely discernible; total length less than 0.7 metres.
Genus *Aspidomorphus* (3 species)

7b. Midbody scale rows reducing in number towards cloaca, 15-13; subcaudals number sixty or more; body and tail elongate; canthus rostralis present; eye large with round pupil, total length up to 1½ metres. 8

8a. Ventrals and subcaudals number 257-270; head unspotted.
Demansia atra

8b. Ventrals and subcaudals number 281-322; head pale brown with darker brown spots. ***Demansia papuensis***

9a. Scale rows at midbody number 17. 10

9b. Scale rows at midbody number more than 17. 12

10a. Small to medium sized snake, total length less than one metre; broad contact of prefrontal with second supralabial prevents contact of nasal with preocular; temporolabial present; subcaudals all paired; dorsum grey to gunmetal, occasionally with lighter band across nape of neck.
Genus *Glyphodon* (1 species)

10b. Medium to large snakes, total length up to 2¾ metres; contact between prefrontal and supralabials confined to point contact, not preventing point contact between nasal and preocular; temporolabial present or absent, subcaudals usually combined single and paired; dorsum usually dark or light brown without visible nape markings. 11

11a. Subcaudals either totally paired or mostly paired with few anterior single subcaudals; temporolabial absent moderately slender body; eye medium sized. ***Pseudonaja textilis***

11b. Subcaudals mostly single with paired subcaudals posteriorly; temporolabial present; heavy stout body; eye small. ***Pseudechis australis***

12a. Scale rows at midbody usually 19 rarely 21, all smooth and glossy; dorsal colouration deep black; supraocular not protruding over eye; anal plate divided; subcaudals mostly single with paired subcaudals posteriorly; heavy stout body; eye small. ***Pseudechis papuanus***

12b. Scale rows usually 21, occasionally 23, keeled anteriorly, not glossy; dorsal colouration usually brown with lighter head and red vertebral stripe; supraocular protruding as distinct shelf over eye; anal plate entire; subcaudals all paired; moderately slender body; eye large.
Oxyuranus scutellatus

Acknowledgements

The author is extremely grateful to Profesor David A. Warrell (Nuffield Dept. of Clinical Medicine, John Radcliffe Hospital, Oxford); Dr R. David G. Theakston (WHO Collaborative Centre for the Control of Antivenoms, Liverpool School of Tropical Medicine) and Dr Victor W. Johnson (Consultant Physician, New Cross Hospital, Wolverhampton) for agreeing to critically review the manuscript and offer invaluable advise on its content and style. Grateful thanks for assistance in the field go the Venturers and Staff of the Papua New Guinea phase of Operation Raleigh and to Karol M. Kisokau (Secretary to the Conservator of Fauna, PNG Dept. of Environment and Conservation) for permission to carry out the field work. Also thanks to Jim Menzies (National Museum of PNG); Dr John Pernetta and Peter Lambley (University of PNG); Dr Straun K. Sutherland (Commonwealth Serum Laboratory, Victoria); Eibleis Fanning and Nick Payne of Operation Raleigh Research in London; Fred Parker of Townsville, Queensland; Campbell Smith (Burns Philp Shipping) and to Philip Willmott-Sharpe (Royal PNG Constabulary) and Douglas Airways for arranging the flight up to Tapini. Valuable assistance and local advice was also received from Bishop David Hand; Aliya Gageya at Wipim; Headley Douglas at Tapini and Ken and Kerry in Woitape amongst many other persons, both Papuan nationals and expatriots. Finally thanks should go to the villagers of Oriomo; Wipim; Kunini; Giringarande; Tapini and many other localities who stayed their hands from their machetes enabling the author to obtain another live specimen.

Bibliography

Ahuja M.L., and Singh G. (1954) Snake Bite in India. *Ind. J. Med. Res.* 42:661.

Archer R. 1977 Snakebite: Nursing care study. *Nursing Times* p. 206–209.

Barme M. (1958) *Bull. Soc. Pathol. Exotique 51:258.*

──────(1968) Venomous Sea Snakes (Hydrophiidae). chap.11 in *Venomous Animals and Their Venoms Vol.1* (Bucherl, Buckley and Deulofeu eds.) Academic Press: p.285-308.

Blasco P., and Hornabrook R.W. (1972) A neglected but potentially dangerous New Guinea snake — the small-eyed snake *(Micropechis ikaheka). Papua New Guinea Med. J. 15*:155-165.

Bourett R. (1934) Les Serpents marins de l'Indochine francaise. Note No.25. *Inst. Oceanographique Vietnam.*

Brian M.J. and Vince J.D. (1987) Treatment and outcome of venomous snake bite in children at Port Moresby General Hospital, Papua New Guinea. *Trans. Roy. Soc. Trop. Med. Hyg. 81*:850-852.

Broad A.J., Sutherland S.K., and Coulter A.R. (1979) The lethality in mice of dangerous Australian and other snake venoms. *Toxicon 17*:661-664.

Campbell C.H. (1964) Venomous snake bite in Papua and its treatment with tracheotomy, artifical respiration and antivenene. *Trans. Roy. Soc. Trop. Med. Hyg. 58*:263.

──────(1966) The Death Adder *Acanthophis antarcticus:* The effect of the bite and its treatment. *Med. J. Aust. 1966 (2)*: 922-925.

──────(1967) The Taipan *(Oxyuranus scutellatus)* and the effect of its bite. *Med. J. Aust. 1967 1*:735-738.

──────(1967) Antivenene in the treatment of Australian and Papuan snake bite. *Med. J. Aust 1967 2*:106.

──────(1967) The Papuan Black Snake *(Pseudechis papuanus)* and the effect of its bite. *Papua and New Guinea Med. J. 10 4*:117-121.

──────(1969) Clinical Aspects of Snake Bite in the Pacific Area. *Toxicon 7*:25-28.

──────(1969) *A Clinical Study of Venomous Snake Bite in Papua. PhD. Thesis, Dept. Med. Uni. Sydney.*

──────, and Young L.N. (1961) The symptomatology, clinical course and successful treatment of Papuan elapine snake envenomation. *Med. J. Aust. 1961 1*:479.

Caras R.A. (1964) *Dangerous to Man.* Barrie & Jenkins.

Carey J.E. and Wright E.A. (1960) The toxicity and immunological properties of some sea-snake venoms with particular reference to that of *Enhydrina schistosa. Trans. Roy. Soc. Trop. Med. Hyg.* 54:50-67.

──────(1961) The site of action of the venom of the sea snake *Enhydrina schistosa. Trans. Roy. Soc. Trop. Med. Hyg.* 55:153-160.

Clarke C.R.A. (1987) Neurology and Muscle Disease. in *Clinical Medicine* (Kumar and Clark eds.) p.864-865. Bailliere Tindall.

Cogger H.G. (1971) The Venomous Snakes of Australia and Melanesia. chap.23 in *Venomous Animals and Their Venoms Vo.2* (Bucherl and Buckley eds). Academic Press. p.35-77.

──────(1975) *Reptiles and Amphibians of Australia.* Reed.

Commonwealth Serum Laboratory Medical Handbook (1979)

Commonwealth Serum Laboratory pamphlet (1985) *Treatment of Snake Bite in Australia and Papua New Guinea using Antivenom.*

Coulter A.R., Broad A.J. and Sutherland S.K. (1979) in *Neurotoxins, Fundamental and Clinical Advances* (Chubb and Geffen eds.) Adelaide Uni. Union Press.

Covacevich J. and Archer M. (1975) The distribution of the cane toad, *Bufo marinus*, in Australia and its effects on indigenous vertebrates. *Mem. Queensland Mus.* *17*:305-310.

de Haas C.P.J. (1950) Checklist of the Snakes of the Indo-Australian Archipelago. *Treubia 20 (3)*:511-625.

de Rooji N. (1971) *The Reptiles of the Indo-Australian Archipelago, II. Ophidia.* Brill, Leiden.

Denson K.W.E. (1969) Coagulant and anticoagulant action of snake venoms. *Toxicon* *7*:5-11.

Druchman D.B. 1987 Myasthenia Gravis in *Encyclopedia of Neuroscience Vol.2* p. 726-727. (Adelman G. ed.)

Fairley N.H. (1929) The dentition and biting mechanism of Australian snakes. *Med. J. Aust. 1929 1*:313.

_____ and Splatt B. (1929) Venom yields in Australian poisonous snakes. *Med. J. Aust. 1929 1*:336.

Fohlman J., Eaker D, Karlsson E. and Thesleff S. (1976) *Eur. J. Biochem. 68*:457.

Golay P. (1985) *Checklist and keys to the Terrestrial Proteroglyphs of the World.* Elapsoidea Spec. Pub. Geneva.

Gow G.F. (1976) *Snakes of Australia.* Angus & Robertson.

Habermehl G.G. (1981) *Venomous Animals and Their Toxins.* Springer-Verlag, Berlin.

Harding K.A. and Welch K.R.G. (1980) *Venomous Snakes of the World. A Checklist.* Pergamon Press.

Harris J.B., Johnson M.A. and Macdonell C. (1977) *Br. J. Pharmac. 61*:133.

Hudson B.J. (in press) The small-eyed snake *(Micropechis ikaheka)*: a review of current knowledge. *Papua New Guinea Med. J.*

_____ and Fromm T. (1986) Bites due to sea snakes in the Ramu River system. *Twenty-second Ann. Symp. Papua New Guinea Med. Soc.*

and Pomat K. (1988) Ten years of snake bite in Madang Province, Papua New Guinea. *Trans. Roy. Soc. Trop. Med. Hyg. 82*:506-508.

Kellaway C.H. (1929) The venom of *Notechis scutatus. Med. J. Aust. 1929 1*:348.

_____ (1929) Observations on the certainly lethal dose of venom of the Death Adder *(Acanthophis antarcticus)* for the common laboratory animals. *Med. J. Aust 1929 1*:764.

_____ (1932) Venomous Land Snakes in Australia. *Bull. Antivenin Inst. Amer. 5*:53.

_____ (1938) *Med. J. Aust. 1938 2*:585-589.

_____ Cherry R.O. and Williams F.E. (1932) The peripheral action of Australian snake venoms: 2. The curari-like action in mammals. *Aust. J. Exp. Biol. Med. Sci. 10*:181.

_____ and Williams F.E. (1929) The venoms of *Oxyuranus Maclennani* and of *Pseudechis Scutellatus. Aust. J. Exp. Biol. Med. Sci. 6*:155.

Kinghorn J.R. and Kellaway C.H. (1943) *The Dangerous Snakes of the South West Pacific Area.* Army Handbook.

Klemmer K. (1963) Liste der rezenten Gifschlangen. in *Die Gifschlangern der Erde, Marburg.*

Leonardi T.M., Howden M.E.H. and Spence I. (1979) *Toxicon 17*:549.

Lindgren E. (1975) *Wildlife in Papua New Guinea.* Frederick Muller.

Loveridge A. (1945) *Reptiles of the Pacific World.* Macmillan.

_____ (1948) New Guinean Reptiles and Amphibians in the Museum of Comparative Zoology and United States National Museum. *Bull. Mus. Comp.Zool. 101 2*:307-430.

Macleay W. (1877) The ophidians of the Chevert Expedition. *Proc, Linn, Soc N.S.W. 1(2)*:33-41.

Malasit et al (1986) *Br. Med. J.* 292:17-20.

Marsden A.T.H. and Reid H.A. (1961) Pathology of sea-snake poisoning. *Br. Med. J. iv:* 1290-1293.

Marshall L.R. and Herrmann R.P. (1983) Coagulant and Anticoagulant Actions of Australian Snake Venoms. *Thromb. Haemostas (Stuttgart) 50(3):*707-711.

McCarthy C. J. (1985) Monophyly of elapid snakes (Serpentes: Elapidae). An assessment of the evidence. *Zool. J. Linn. Soc. 83:*79-93.

McCoy M. (1980)*Reptiles of the Solomon Islands. Wau. Ecology Inst. Handbook No. 7.*

McDowell S.B. (1967) *Aspidomorphus,* a genus of New Guinea snakes of the family Elapidae, with notes on related genera, *J. Zool. Soc. Lond. 151:*497-543.

_____ (1969) *Toxicocalamus,* a New Guinea genus of snakes of the family Elapidae, *J. Zool. Soc. Lond. 159:*443-511.

_____ (1970) On the status and relationships of the Solomon Island elapid snakes. *J. Zool. Soc. Lond. 161:*145-190.

McPhee D. (1979) *The Observer's Book of Snakes and Lizards of Australia.* Methuen.

Mebs. D. (1970) A comparative study of enzymes activity in snake venoms. *Int. J. Biochem. 1:*335-342.

_____ (1978) Pharmacology of Reptilian Venoms, chap.4 in *Biology of The Reptilia Vol 8B Physiology* (Gans and Gans eds.) p.437-560.

Mengden G.A., Shine R. and Moritz C. (1986) Phylogenetic relationships within the Australian venomous snakes of the genus *Pseudechis. Herpetologica 42:(2):*215-229.

Mikua C.K. (1974) *Animals of Waigani. No.1 Snakes.* UPNG Biol. Dept.

Minton S.A. Jr. and Minton M.R. (1971) *Venomous Reptiles.* George Allen and Unwin.

Mirtschin P. and Davis R. (1982) *Dangerous Snakes of Australia*, Rigby.

Morgan F.G. (1956) The Australian Taipan *Oxyuranus scutellatus scutellatus* (Peters) in *Venoms*, (Buckley and Porges eds.) N.Amer. Assoc. Adva. Sci. Wash. :359.

O'Shea M.T. (1986) Snakes of the Homalopsinae from the Southern Trans-Fly, Papua New Guinea. *Herptile 11(4):*155-162.

Parker F. (1972) Snakes of the Elapid genus *Suta* in New Guinea. *Papua New Guinea Sci, Soc.Proc. 23:*13-17.

_____ (1982) *The Snakes of Western Province. Wildlife in Papua New Guinea No.82/1* Dept. Lands and Environment, Konedobu.

Price M. and Campbell C.M. (1979) Snake bite admissions Port Moresby General Hospital (1967-1971, *Papua New Guinea Med. J. 19:*155

Reid H.A. (1961) Myoglobinuria and sea-snake bite poisoning. *Br. Med. J. iv.:*1284:1289.

_____ (1970) The Principles of Snakebite Treatment. *Clin, Tox, 3(3):*473-482.

_____ (1980) *Incision and Suction as First-Aid Treatment in Snake Bite*, pamphlet WHO Coll. Centre for Control Antivenoms, Liverpool Sch. Trop. Med.

_____ (1983) *Clinical Effects of Snake Bite and Medical Treatment of Snake Bite in the Tropics*, pamphlet Liverpool Sch. Trop. Med.

_____ and Theakston R.D.G. (1983) The management of snake bite *Bull. WHO. 61(6):*885-895.

Rocha e Silva M. (1970) *Kinin Hormones, with Special Reference to Bradykinins and Related Kinins*, C.C.Thomas, Springfield, I11.

Russell F.E. (1980) *Snake Venom Poisoning.* Lippincott, Philadelphia p.285-287.

Scott F., Parker F. and Menzies J.I. (1977) *A checklist of the Amphibians and Reptiles of Papua New Guinea.* Wildlife in Papua New Guinea No. 77/3 Dept. of Lands and Environment, Konedobu.

Sheumack D.D., Howden M.E.H. and Spence I. (1979) *Toxicon 17:*609

Shine R. (1987) The Evolution of Viviparity: Ecological Correlates of Reproductive Mode within a genus of Australian Snakes *(Pseudechis:* Elapidae) *Copeia 1987 (3):* 551-563.

Shine R. & Covacevich J. (1983) Ecology of Highly Venomous Snakes: the Australian Genus *Oxyuranus* (Elapidae). *J. Herpetology 17(1):*60-69.

Slater K.R. (1954) A brief account of the snakes of the Port Moresby area. *Papua New Guinea Sci. Soc. Ann. Rep. & Proc.* 6:51

_____ (1956) On the New Guinea Taipan. *Mem. Nat. Mus. Vict. 20:*201-205.

_____ (1968) *A Guide to the Dangerous Snakes of Papua.* V.P.Bloink, Port Moresby.

Smith H.M., Smith R.B. and Sawin H.L. (1977) A summary of snake classification (Reptilia: Serpentes). *J. Herpetology 11(2):*115-121.

Smith M.A. (1926) *A Monograph of the Sea Snakes. Br. Mus. Monographs.* P.36-40.

Storr G.M. (1978) Whip snakes *(Demansia,* Elapidae) of Western Australia. *Rec. West. Aust Mus. 6(3):*287-301.

_____ (1981) The Genus *Acanthophis* (Serpentes: Elapidae) in Western Australia. *Rec. West. Aust. Mus. 9(2):*203-210.

Sutherland S.K. 1976 Treatment of Snakebite in Australia and Papua New Guinea. *Aust. Family Physician 5:* 272-288.

Sutherland S.K. (1980) The biochemistry and actions of some Australian venoms with some notes on first aid. *Chemistry in Australia 47(9):*351-356.

_____ (1981) When do you remove first aid measures from an envenomed limb. *Med. J. Aust. 1981:*542-544.

_____ (?) Snake Bite in Remote Areas. *Med. J. Aust.* p.620.

_____ (1983) *Australian Animal Toxins. The Creatures, Their Toxins and Care of the Poisoned Patient.* Oxford Uni. Press, Melbourne.

_____ (1988) *Biochemistry and Pharmacology Notes. The main actions of some important Australian venoms and toxins.* Comm. Serum Labs. Victoria.

_____ (1988) *First Aid for Snakebite in Australia.* Comm. Serum Labs. pamphlet. Victoria.

Tidswell F. (1906) *Researches on Australian Venoms, Snake-Bite, Snake-Venom and Antivenene: The Poison of the Platypus; the Poison of the Red-Spotted Spider.* N.S.W. Dept. Public Health, Sydney: 27.

Trethewie E.R. (1971) The Pharmacology and Toxicology of the Venoms of the Snakes of Australia and Oceania. chap.24 in *Venomous Animals and Their Venoms Vol.2* (Bucherl and Buckley eds.) Academic Press. p.79-101.

_____ (1971) The Pathology, Symptomatology, and Treatment of Snake Bite in Australia. chap.25 in *Venomous Animals and Their Venoms Vol.2* (Bucherl and Buckley eds.) Academic Press. p.103-113.

US Navy (1962) *Poisonous Snakes of the World.* A manual for use by U.S. amphibious forces.

Walker M.J.A. and Yeoh P.N. (1974) The *in vitro* neuromuscular blocking properties of sea snake *(Enhydrina schistosa)* venom. *Eur. J. Pharmac. 28:*199-208.

Watt G. et al 1986 Positive response to edrophonium in patients with neurotoxic envenoming by cobras *(Naja naja philippinensis).* A placebo-controlled study. *NEJM 315:*1444-8.

Whitaker R. and Whitaker Z. (1982) *Reptiles of Papua New Guinea.* Wildlife in Papua New Guinea No.82/2. Dept. of Lands and Environment, Konedobu.

Worrell E. (1963) *Reptiles of Australia.* Angus & Robertson.

Treatment of Snake Bite in the Asia-Pacific Region: A Personal View

David A. Warrell

Professor of Tropical Medicine & Infectious Diseases,
University of Oxford

Introduction

The preceding chapters in this compendium testify to the medical importance of snake bite in many parts of the Asia-Pacific region. Particularly striking are the data from Sri Lanka, India, Burma and Papua New Guinea. In Sri Lanka, the incidence of snake bite has increased to more than 400 per 100,000 population per year with an incidence of snake bite mortality of more than six per 100,000 per year (Phillips et al 1988). In Burma, Russell's viper bite still claims around 1,000 lives each year and has been the fifth commonest among all causes of death in the country (Myint-Lwin et al 1985). In India more than 20,000 deaths per year were reported at the end of the nineteenth century and recent figures suggest similar totals with consistently more than 1,000 deaths per year in Maharashtra State alone (Deoras 1981 pp. 1–3). The impact of snake bite on primitive indigenous communities was revealed to Gajdusek during his surveys for kuru in the Fore Highlands of Papua new Guinea: in villages in the kuru region where kuru was rare, snake bite was the commonest cause of death (Gajdusek 1977).

Despite the evident importance of snake bite, there is very little sound clinical evidence on which to base recommendations for treatment. As a result a variety of conflicting views have emerged. This chapter does not attempt to review the therapeutic controversies but to present a personal view based on published data and personal experience in the region.

First aid treatment

All patients bitten by snakes require urgent assessment by trained medical staff. First aid is the emergency treatment given immediately by the victim or by others at the scene of the bite. The aims of first aid are

1. to deliver patients as quickly as possible to a place where they can be seen by medical staff.
2. To delay the evolution of life-threatening envenoming at least until they reach a place where they can receive medical care.
3. To alleviate severe early symptoms of envenoming.

First aid treatment must not be confused with medical treatment for, in the vast majority of cases, those present when and where the patient is bitten will not be medically trained. Most snake bites occur in the rural tropics as unexpected and unpredictable accidents, although there are times of year and occupations associated with a greatly increased risk of snake bite. For example, in Burma, most snake bites are inflicted on rice harvesters during the period October to December. Zoos, snake farms and well organised expeditions can provide themselves with first aid equipment such as splints, crepe bandages, tourniquets, analgesics and other simple drugs, but most snake bite victims will have to extemporize, using materials which come to hand at the scene of the accident (Figure 1). High risk groups such as farmers, plantation workers, fishermen and their families should be taught about the prevention and first aid treatment of snake bites.

General recommendations for the first aid

1. *Reassure the patient:* many people bitten by snakes are terrified, fearing sudden death. They may behave irrationally, for example cutting off the bitten digit. A few become frankly hysterical. The basis of reassurance is the effectiveness of modern treatment for snake bite, the relatively slow progression to severe envenoming, which usually allows time to reach hospital, and the fact that venomous snakes often bite humans without injecting venom.
2. *Do not tamper with the bite wound* in any way except to wipe it once with a damp cloth to remove surface venom.
3. *Immobilise the bitten limb* as far as is practicable using a makeshift splint or sling. If available, crepe bandaging of the splinted limb (Sutherland 1980) is the most effective method.
4. *Transport the patient*, as quickly as possible, to the nearest place where they can be seen by a medically-trained person (health station, dispensary, clinic or hospital). Avoid exercising the bitten limb which will promote the spread of venom. If no motor vehicle or boat is available, the patient can be carried on a stretcher or hurdle, on the pillion or crossbar of a bicycle or on someone's back.
5. *Take along the dead snake* for identification but make sure that it really is dead (some species can feign death), do not touch it with bare hands and do not risk further bites by pursuing the culprit into the undergrowth. Severed snake heads, both fresh and preserved, have inflicted severe and even fatal bites (Kitchens et al 1987; Griffin & Donovan 1986).
6. *Do not apply tourniquets*, ligatures or constricting bands except when the snake is identified as a dangerous species capable of neurotoxic envenoming such as

   Elapids (cobras and kraits)
   Australasian "elapids" (genera Acanthophis, Micropechis, Oxyuranus, Pseudechis and Pseudonaja)
   Sea snakes

7. *Avoid potentially harmful traditional first aid measures* such as cauterisation, incision, excision or amputation of the bite site, suction by mouth, vacuum pump or syringe, combined incision and suction by "Venom-

ex" apparatus, injection or instillation of compounds such as potassium permanganate, phenol (carbolic soap) and trypsin, application of electric shocks or ice (cryotherapy), use of tradition herbal, folk and ayurvedic remedies such as ingestion of emetic plant products and parts of the snake, multiple incisions and tattooing, insufflation of oily substances into the trachea and application of irritants to the conjunctivae.

Dangers of tourniquets, compression bandages and other occlusive methods

Reported complications include the following:

1. Ischaemia and gangrene (Figure 2).
2. Damage to superficial peripheral nerves, especially the lateral popliteal (common peroneal) nerve at the neck of the fibula (Figure 3).
3. Increased fibrinolytic activity in the occluded limb (Klenerman et al 1977).
4. Congestion, swelling and increased bleeding from the occluded limb (Bhat 1974).
5. Shock on releasing a tight tourniquet (Pugh and Theakston 1987; Tun-Pe et al 1987).
6. Intensification of local effects of venom in the occluded limb (Frost 1981).

Because of these dangers, occlusive methods should only be used after bites by neurotoxic elapids and sea snakes (see above). In these cases, a compressive method may hinder the spread of venom and delay the development of respiratory paralysis until the patient reaches medical care. If a splint and crepe bandage are available, the least painful way to apply compression and the most effective method of ensuring immobilisation of the bitten limb is to use the method described by Sutherland (1980). It is said that a firmly applied crepe bandage, exerting a compression of approximately 55 mmHg, can be left in place for several hours, but Sutherland (1983a) cautions against prolonged use especially after the patient has arrived in hospital. Exaggerated local effects of envenoming, such as muscle spasms and necrosis, have been described in crepe bandaged limbs (Frost 1981; Sutherland 1983a). In the absence of a crepe bandage, a tight constricting band can be applied around the upper arm or thigh. Tourniquets applied tightly enough to obliterate the arterial pulse are painful and must be released for at least one minute after an hour. If reapplied they should be finally removed after two hours, preferably after an intravenous infusion has been established in hospital or dispensary, with antivenom available and other drugs and resuscitation equipment in readiness for immediate use.

Dangers of other traditional first aid methods

Cauterisation, excision or amputation of the bite site are damaging and unwarranted in view of the uncertainty of envenoming after snake bite and the risk of secondary infection and persistent bleeding. Likewise, methods which combine incision and suction are of uncertain benefit and carry the risks of damaging nerves, blood vessels and tendons, introducing infections including tetanus and leading to uncontrolled bleeding in patients with incoagulable

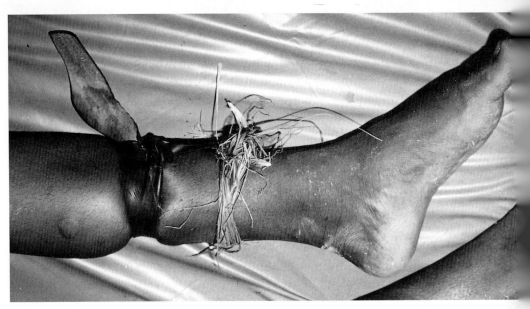

Figure 1
Typical tourniquet made out of car tyre inner tube applied by a farmer in Burma.

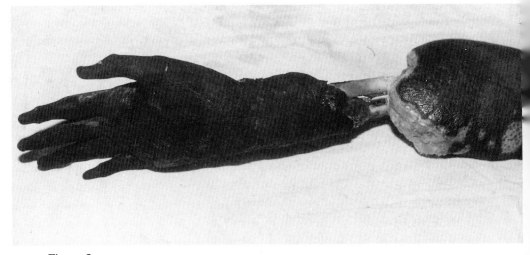

Figure 2
Gangrene following the use of a tight tourniquet. The patient applied a tight tourniquet above the elbow for more than three hours after being bitten by a Malayan pit viper (*Calloselasma rhodostoma*). He sought herbal treatment and came to hospital three weeks later.

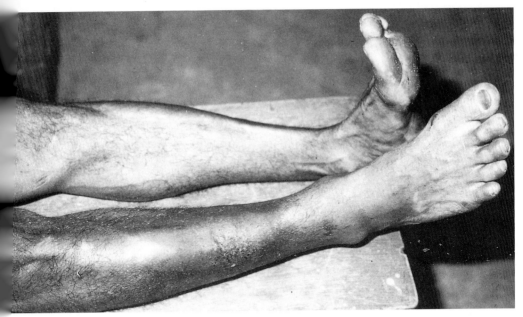

Figure 3
Right lateral popliteal nerve palsy after use of a tight below knee tourniquet following Russell's viper bite in Burma. The patient is attempting to dorsiflex both feet.

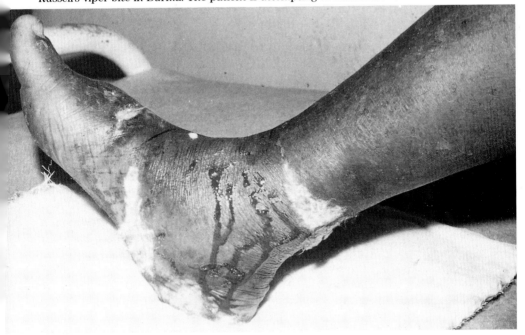

Figure 4
Persistent bleeding from multiple razor incisions in a patient with incoagulable blood after bite by *Echis carinatus*. The patient was severely anaemic as a result of this blood loss.

blood (Figure 4). Powerful suction, chemicals such as potassium permanganate and phenol, and cryotherapy can cause tissue necrosis in addition to that resulting from the venom itself. There is no reliable experimental support for the use of electric shocks. Irresponsible recommendations of this method, based on uncontrolled clinical observations, have exposed patients to the dangers of electrocution.

Treatment of early manifestations of envenoming (before the patient reaches hospital)

Fear, may produce trembling, tachycardia and tachypnoea resulting in respiratory alkalosis with acroparaesthesia, carpopedal spasm, dizziness and even syncope. Frightened patients occasionally become extremely agitated and even hysterical, simulating coma. Treatment is by reassurance and sedation with chlorpromazine or some other tranquilizing drug.

Pain in the bitten limb may be severe. Oral paracetamol is preferable to aspirin, which commonly causes gastric erosions even in healthy people, and could lead to persistent gastric bleeding in patients with incoagulable blood.

Vomiting is a common early symptom of severe systemic envenoming by elapids, Australasian snakes, sea snakes and vipers. It is sometimes the result of ingested emetic herbal remedies. Aspiration of vomitus is particularly likely if a patient is becoming drowsy or comatose. Patients should be laid on their side in a head down position. Persistent vomiting can be treated with chlorpromazine given in a dose of 25–50 mg for adults, 1 mg/kg for children, by mouth, injection or suppository (see below for caution about injections).

Anaphylaxis. Within a few minutes of bites by some species of *Vipera* and Australasian "elapids", patients may develop manifestations of systemic anaphylaxis such as hypotension, shock, angio-oedema of the mouth, gums, lips and face, breathlessness, bronchospasm, abdominal colic, vomiting and diarrhoea with other signs of autonomic nervous system stimulation such as sweating and gooseflesh. These features are attributable to autopharmaco-logical effects of venom, releasing endogenous mediators or activating precursors such as bradykinin. On rare occasions, people who have been bitten or exposed in other ways to a specific snake venom, may become sensitized and develop true immediate-type I hypersensitivity after a bite or contact of mucosae, such as the lips and mouth with venom when applying suction to a wound. The essential treatment of systemic anaphylaxis is adrenaline (see below under treatment of antivenom reactions). Hypotensive patients should be tipped head downwards and those with severe bronchospasm, dyspnoea or cyanosis should be given oxygen by any available means.

Vasovagal syncope. In the same way that some healthy and robust individuals develop vaso-vagal syncope in response to simple venepuncture, some patients bitten by snakes develop immediate transient profound bradycardia and hypotension. In severe cases they may lose consciousness, begin to twitch or even have generalised convulsions and become cyanosed. The best treatment is head down tilt.

Bulbar and respiratory paralysis. Early signs of neurotoxicity may develop within 20 to 30 minutes of a snake bite, but significant bulbar and respiratory paralysis are unusual sooner than one to two hours after the bite. The earliest manifestations of neurotoxicity are difficulty in focussing and a feeling that the eyelids are heavy. Eyebrows may be raised by frontalis contraction before there is demonstrable ptosis. Later signs include external ophthalmoplegia, inability to open the mouth, protrude the tongue, speak and swallow. Paralysis of the jaw and tongue may result in upper airway obstruction and aspiration. Later, respiratory muscle paralysis may lead to respiratory failure. Early treatment consists of laying patients on their sides and keeping the airway clear by elevating the jaw and inserting an oral airway if this is available. Patients who are cyanosed or who have respiratory distress should be given oxygen and if clearing the airway does not produce immediate relief, artificial ventilation must be given. In the absence of any special equipment, mouth-to-mouth or mouth-to-nose ventilation can be life-saving. Manual ventilation by ambu bag and anaesthetic mask is rarely effective. If the patient is unconscious and no femoral or carotid pulse can be felt, external cardiac massage and mouth-to-mouth ventilation should be started without delay.

Medical treatment in health stations, dispensaries, hospitals etc.

Ideally, all patients bitten by snakes should be assessed by medically-trained staff. Uncertainties such as the species responsible, the amount of venom injected and the likely time course for development of signs, demand that patients should be kept under observation for at least 24 hours. The only exception should be in the case of those bitten by unequivocally non-venomous species (for example legless lizards, Boidae, Typhlopidae and some colubrids). Snake bite is a medical emergency and the normal sequence of history-taking, examination and treatment may have to be compressed so that the three are carried out simultaneously. The doctor or other medically qualified person must decide quickly whether the patient has been bitten by a snake, whether there are signs of envenoming and whether antivenom and ancillary treatment is needed. There are three important preliminary questions:

1. In which part of your body were you bitten?
2. How long ago were you bitten?
3. Have you brought the snake and, if not, can anyone describe it or say what kind of snake bite it was? If the dead snake was left behind, someone should be sent to collect it immediately. If no one saw the snake, the circumstances may provide a clue. For example, the snake most likely to be responsible for biting people while they are asleep in their huts in southern Asia is a *Bungarus* species (krait); cobras are usually responsible for biting freshwater fisherman and other species cause particular occupational hazards (for example *Calloselasma rhodostoma* for plantation workers in South East Asia, *Vipera russelli* for rice farmers).

History

Patients should be asked to describe the evolution of symptoms, for example, local pain, the spread of swelling and tenderness up the bitten limb, pain in regional lymph nodes, systemic bleeding, paralytic symptoms etc. Patients should be asked specifically about important symptoms of systemic envenoming: vomiting, fainting, muscular pain and weakness, abdominal pain and bleeding. Effects of pre-hospital treatment can confuse the interpretation of symptoms and signs. Thus, ingested remedies may cause vomiting, irritants rubbed in the eye can cause intense conjunctivitis, even blindness, and oily material blown through a tube into the trachea can cause ruptured eardrums, laryngospasm and pneumonitis.

Examination

The absence of discernible fang marks does not exclude snake bite, but the discovery of two discrete puncture marks does suggest a bite by a venomous snake. Unfortunately, the pattern of fang punctures is rarely helpful as there may be marks by accessory fangs, other teeth and sometimes multiple bites. The distance between the fang marks is proportional to the size of the snake. Local swelling and tenderness and lymph node involvement are usually the earliest sign of envenoming, but factitious swelling may be caused by a tourniquet. However, although most cases of significant envenoming by Viperidae and Asian cobras are associated with the development of local swelling within two hours of the bite, it is salutary that 9% and 18% of case of systemic envenoming by *Vipera russelli* in Burma and Sri Lanka respectively, showed absolutely no local swelling (Myint-Lwin et al 1985; Phillips et al 1988). A number of species with neurotoxic venoms, such as sea snakes, kraits and some Australasian elapids such as *Acanthophis* produce virtually no local effects. Rapidly spreading swelling and early local blistering suggests severe envenoming. The gingival sulci should be examined meticulously as these are usually the first site of spontaneous sustemic bleeding. Bleeding from recent wounds, venepuncture sites and skin lesions suggests that the blood is incoagulable. Shock is indicated by collapse, impaired consciousness, sweaty, cold, cyanosed extremities and a low blood pressure. The foot of the bed should be raised and an intravenous infusion of a plasma expander started immediately (see below). Patients should be examined repeatedly for ptosis, an early sign of neurotoxicity. If there is any suggestion of respiratory muscle weakness, attempts should be made to monitor this objectively (for example, by measuring peak expiratory flow, vital capacity or expiratory pressure using the mercury manometer of a sphygmomanometer). Coma is usually secondary to respiratory failure or shock. Muscle tenderness, resistance to passive muscle stretching and trismus suggest rhabdomyolysis caused by venoms of sea snakes, some Australasian elapids, and Sri Lankan/south Indian *Vipera russelli*. Patients may become oliguric within a few hours of being bitten by *Vipera russelli* and much later in the course of severe envenoming by other species. Haemorrhagic venoms (Viperidae, some Australasian elapids) can cause microscopical or frank haematuria. Massive intravascular haemolysis results in black urine (Sri Lankan and Indian *Vipera russelli)*, while, in the absence of haemoglobinuria, urine containing a high concentration of myoglobin has a very dark mahogany colour and may settle as a dark brown curd (Sutherland 1983b p. 203).

A simple test for gross consumption coagulopathy is to take a few mls of blood into a clean, dry, glass test tube and leave it undisturbed for 20 minutes at ambient temperature. If the blood runs out when the tube is tipped at the end of that time severe hypofibrinogenaemia can be inferred.

The above clinical assessment will indicate whether antivenom is needed immediately or whether the patient should be kept under observation. The following signs should be checked at least every hour:

1. Level of consciousness.
2. Presence or absence of ptosis.
3. Pulse rate and rhythm.
4. Blood pressure.
5. Respiratory rate.
6. Extent of local swelling.
7. New symptoms or signs.

Antivenom treatment

The single most important decision in any patient bitten by a snake is whether or not to give antivenom, the only specific antidote to venom. Antivenom is the hyperimmune serum of animals, usually horses, immunized with snake venom. Most commercial antivenoms consist largely of $F(ab)_2$ fragments of immunoglobulin obtained by pepsin digestion and ammonium sulphate precipitation. Antivenom should never be used routinely and indiscriminately for the following reasons:

1. All commercial antivenoms carry a risk of potentially serious serum reactions.
2. Antivenom is not always necessary: many patients are bitten by non-venomous snakes and a large proportion of those bitten by venomous snakes are not envenomed.
3. Antivenoms have a range of specific and paraspecific neutralizing activity and are useless for venoms outside that range. Specific antivenoms are not available for treatment of envenoming by some important species (for example *Bungarus candidus* in South East Asia).
4. Antivenom is expensive, always in short supply and has a limited shelf life. Supplies must not be squandered.

Indications for antivenom

A Systemic envenoming

1. Haemostatic disturbances: spontaneous systemic bleeding (e.g. gums, epistaxis), coagulopathy (e.g. incoagulable blood, prolonged clotting time, elevated FDP or thrombocytopenia).
2. Cardiovascular abnormalities: shock, hypotension, abnormal electrocardiogram, arrhythmia, cardiac failure, pulmonary oedema.

3. Neurotoxicity.
4. Generalised rhabdomyolysis.
5. Impaired consciousness of any cause.
6. In patients with definite signs of local envenoming, the following indicate significant systemic envenoming: neutrophil leucocytosis, elevated serum enzymes such as creatine phosphokinase and aminotransferases, haemoconcentration, uraemia, hypercreatininaemia, oliguria, hypoxaemia, acidosis and vomiting.

B Severe local envenoming

Local swelling involving more than half the bitten limb, or associated with extensive blistering or bruising, especially in patients bitten by species whose venoms are known to cause local necrosis (e.g. many Viperidae, Asian cobras). Bites on digits (which carry a high risk of necrosis).

Contraindications to antivenom

There is no absolute contraindication to antivenom in patients with life-threatening systemic envenoming. However, patients with an atopic history (asthma, hay fever, vernal conjunctivitis, eczema, food and drug allergies) and those who have had reactions to equine antiserum on previous occasions have an increased risk of severe reactions. In these cases, pretreatment with subcutaneous adrenaline and intravenous antihistamine and corticosteroid may prevent or diminish the reaction. Rapid desensitization is not recommended.

Hypersensitivity testing

Intradermal, subcutaneous or intraconjunctival tests with diluted antivenom have no predictive value for early (anaphylactic) or late (serum sickness type) antivenom reactions and should no longer be used (Malasit et al 1986).

Timing of antivenom treatment

Antivenom should be given as soon as signs of systemic or severe local envenoming are evident (see above). The average times between bite and death are eight hours (range 12 minutes to 120 hours) for Asian cobras, 18 (3-63) hours for *Bungarus caeruleus*, three days (15 minutes to 264 hours) for *Vipera russelli* and five days (25 hours to 41 days) for *Echis carinatus*. In the majority of cases of snake bite, antivenom can be given well within these bite-death intervals. It is almost never too late to try antivenom treatment; it has proved effective up to two days after sea snake bites and 10 days or more after *Echis carinatus* bites. When patients arrive in hospital with a tourniquet or other constricting band in place, antivenom treatment, if it is thought necessary, should be started before these are loosened. Otherwise there is a risk of severe envenoming when the pent up blood from the occluded limb is released into the circulation.

Antivenom specificity

When the biting species is known, optimal treatment consists of mono-specific antivenom. However, in areas where the venoms of a number of different species produce similar clinical manifestations, polyspecific anti-venoms are necessary for use in the majority of patients who do not bring the dead snake for identification. Some antivenoms display a wide range of para-specific activity. Commonwealth Serum Laboratories "tiger-sea snake" anti-venom raised against venoms of Australian tiger snake (*Notechis scutatus*) and beaked sea snake (*Enhydrina schistosa*) neutralizes the venoms of three terrestrial Australasian snakes and at least 12 different species of sea snakes. Antivenom solutions which have become opaque should not be used as protein precipitation is associated with loss of activity and an increased risk of reactions.

Administration

Antivenom is most effective when given intravenously. Freeze-dried (lyophilized) antivenom is dissolved in water. Antivenom can be given by intravenous injection at a rate of about 5 ml/minute or, diluted in isotonic fluid and infused over 30-60 minutes. The incidence and severity of antivenom reactions is the same with these two methods (Malasit et al 1986). The advantage of intravenous infusion is ease of control, but intravenous push injection requires less expensive equipment, is quicker to set up and ensures that someone remains at the patient's side during the crucial first 10-15 minutes after the start of treatment when early reactions are most likely to occur.

When intravenous administration is impossible, antivenom can be given by deep intramuscular injection at multiple sites in the anterior and lateral aspects of the thighs, followed by massage to promote absorption. Absorption from intragluteal injection is unreliable. However, there is a limit to the volume of antivenom that can be given by this route and there is a risk of haematoma formation in patients with incoagulable blood. A general rule in the treatment of snake bite is to avoid injections other than by the intravenous route. Intramuscular and subcutaneous injections carry the risk of local bleeding in patients with impaired haemostasis. Venepuncture sites must be dressed with a pressure bandage to prevent oozing of blood. Injection of antivenom into the fang marks seems rational but is difficult, painful and hazardous, especially in the case of bites on digits or into other tight fascial compartments, and has not proved effective in animal studies.

Dosage

Guidelines for initial dosage based on clinical studies are available for some important antivenoms in the region (Table 1). However, in most cases, manufacturer's recommendations are based on mouse assays which may not correlate with clinical findings. The initial dose of antivenom, however large, may not completely neutralize the depot of venom at the site of injection. Patients should be observed for several days even if they show a good clinical response to the initial dose of antivenom. Continuing absorption of venom may

Table 1
Guide to initial dosage of some important antivenoms for bites in the Asia-Pacific region

Species		Approximate Manufacturer, antivenom	initial dose
Latin name	English name		
Acanthophis antarcticus	Death adder	CSL,[a] monospecific	3000-6000 units
Bungarus caeruleus	Indian krait	Haffkine polyspecific	100 ml
Calloselasma (Agkistrodon) rhodostoma	Malayan pit viper	Thai Red Cross (Saovabha), Bangkok, monospecific	100 ml
		Thai Government Pharmaceutical Organization, monospecific	50 ml
		Twyford Pharmaceutical	10 ml
Echis carinatus	Saw-scaled or carpet viper	SAIMR,[b] *Echis*, monospecific	20 ml
		Behringwerke, *Bitis-Echis-Naja*, polyspecific	100 ml
Hydrophiidae	Sea snakes	CSL, *Enhydrina schistosa*	1000 units
Naja kaouthia	Monocellate Thai cobra	*Thai Red Cross, monospecific*	100 ml
Naja naja	Indian cobra	*Haffkine, Kasauli, polyspecific*	100 ml
Pseudonaja textilis	Eastern brown snake	CSL, *monospecific*	3000-6000 units
Trimeresurus albolabris	Green pit viper	*Thai Red Cross, monospecific*	100 ml
Vipera palaestinae	Palestine viper	*Rogoff Medical Research Institute, Tel Aviv, Palestine viper monospecific*	50-80 ml
Vipera russelli	Russell's viper	*Burma Pharmaceutical Industry, monospecific*	40 ml
		Haffkine polyspecific	100 ml

a   Commonwealth Serum Laboratories, Australia;
b   South African Institute for Medical Research.

652

cause recurrent neurotoxicity or coagulopathy after the serum antivenom concentration has declined (Ho et al 1986).

There is no evidence that snakes vary the dose of venom injected with the age or size of their victim and so the dose of antivenom should be the same for patients of all ages and sizes, i.e. *CHILDREN MUST BE GIVEN THE SAME DOSE OF ANTIVENOM AS ADULTS.*

Response to antivenom

Neurotoxic signs often respond slowly or unconvincingly. There are reports of dramatic improvement within 30 minutes of antivenom treatment in the case of envenoming by *Acanthophis* (Campbell 1966) and *Naja kaouthia* (Trishnananda et al 1978). Cardiovascular effects such as hypotension and sinus bradycardia may respond within 10-20 minutes. Spontaneous systemic bleeding usually stops within 15 to 30 minutes and blood coagulability is restored within one to six hours of an adequate neutralizing dose of antivenom. The simple clotting test (see above) repeated at six hour intervals is a convenient method of monitoring the dose of antivenom when a defibrinating venom has been injected. The initial dose of antivenom should be repeated if severe cardiovascular or neurotoxic symptoms persist for more than 30 minutes and incoagulable blood persists for more than six hours after the first dose. Bites by exceptionally large and venomous species may require enormous doses of antivenom, for example, 1,150 ml of specific antivenom was given to a patient bitten by *Ophiophagus hannah*, the world's largest poisonous snake (Ganthavorn 1971).

Antivenom reactions

There are three types of reactions: early (anaphylactic), pyrogenic and late (serum sickness type).

1. *Early reactions* usually occur between 10 and 60 minutes after starting intravenous administration of antivenom. Symptoms include cough, tachycardia, itching (especially of the scalp), urticaria, fever, palpitations, nausea, vomiting and headache. The incidence and severity of these reactions "are directly proportional to the speed and quantity with which the healing antiserum reaches its 'target'" (Lancet 1980). Although there are undoubted differences in the incidence of reactions to antivenoms refined by various methods and given by different routes, much of the wide range of reported incidences must be attributable to variations in the quality of clinical observation during the three hours after treatment. Mild reactions may be missed completely and deaths misattributed to snake bite rather than antivenom-induced anaphylaxis. More than 5% of patients with early reactions develop manifestations of severe systemic anaphlaxis such as hypotension, bronchospasm and angiooedema, but there are few reports of deaths reliably attributed to these reactions.

   Mechanism of early reactions. Early reactions have been termed immediate hypersensitivity reactions on the assumption that they represented type I,

IgE-mediated hypersensitivity to equine serum. However, these reactions are not predicted by hypersensitivity tests (Malasit et al 1986) and usually occur in patients who have not been sensitized to equine protein in the past. The anticomplementary activity of commercial antivenoms *in vitro* (Sutherland 1977), like the anticomplementary activity of homologous human immuno-globulin *in vivo*, is attributable to IgG aggregates and immune complex formation. In recent years, anaphylactic reactions to human immunoglobulin have been virtually eliminated by modifying the refinement process. Pepsin digestion has been replaced by passage through ion exchange columns and the final product is free of IgG aggregates.

Treatment. The essential treatment of anaphylaxis is adrenaline (epinephrine) 0.1% (1 in 1000) in a dose of 0.5 to 1.0 ml for adults, 0.01mg/kg for children. Adrenaline should be given by subcutaneous injection at the first sign of a reaction. In severe cases the same dose can be given by intra-muscular injection or, during cardiac resuscitation, by slow intravenous or even intracardiac injection. This should be followed by an intravenous injection of antihistamine, such as chlorpheniramine maleate (10 mg for adults, 0.2 mg/kg of children) to combat the effects of massive histamine release during the reaction.

2. *Pyrogenic reactions.* Symptoms are those of an endotoxin reaction developing one to two hours after treatment. There is an initial chill with cutaneous vasoconstriction, gooseflesh and shivering. Temperature rises sharply during the rigors and there is intense vasodilatation, widening of the pulse pressure and eventually a fall in mean arterial pressure. Temperature falls with profuse sweating and there may be associated gastrointestinal symptoms such as vomiting and diarrhoea. In children, febrile convulsions may occur at the peak of fever.

Treatment. The patients should lie flat to prevent postural hypotension. Temperature can be reduced by fanning, tepid sponging, hypothermia blankets or antipyretic drugs such as paracetamol (15 mg/kg) given by mouth, suppository or via nasogastric tube.

3. *Late reactions (serum sickness type).* The incidence and speed of development of these reactions increases with the dose of antivenom. About seven days after treatment (range 5-24 days), there is itching, urticaria, 'flu-like symptoms with fever, arthralgia which may include the temporman-dibular joint, lymphadenopathy, periarticular swellings, albuminuria and neurological symptoms including neuralgic amyotrophy, mononeuritis multiplex usually of the radial nerve, Guillain-Barre syndrome, polyneuropathy and rarely encephalopathy.

Mechanism is an inflammatory response to immune complex deposition.

Treatment. Antihistamines alone may contain the milder attacks: chlorpheniramine 2 mg four times a day for adults, 0.2 mg/kg per day in divided doses for children or terfenadine 60 mg twice a day for adults or terfenadine suspension 5 ml (30 mg) twice a day for children. Severe cases, including those with neurological symptoms, should be given prednisolone (5 mg four times a day for five days in adults, 0.7 mg/kg per day in divided doses for five days in children).

Efficacy of antivenom

The concept of immunization with venom was introduced by Sewall more than a hundred years ago (Sewall 1887) and antivenoms have been used to treat envenomed humans since the end of the nineteeth century (Calmette 1896; Vital Brazil 1987). Antivenoms have reduced snake bite mortality. For example, from 8% to 2.4% in bites by *Bothrops* in Costa Rica, from 74% to 12% after bites by *Crotalus durissus terrificus* in Brazil (WHO 1981); from approximately 20% to less than 3% in *Echis ocellatus* bites in Nigeria (Warrell 1979) and in Australia from 50% for *Acanthophis*, 45.5% for *Notechis scutatus* and 18.7% for *Pseudonaja textilis* to very low levels (Sutherland 1983 p. 186). Most clinicians have no doubt about the life-saving efficacy of antivenoms. This impression has been given abundant support by recent studies which have documented the rapid elimination of venom antigenaemia after antivenom treatment (Khin-Ohn-Lwin et al 1984; Ho et al 1986; Phillips et al 1988). Claims that envenomed patients can be managed adequately without antivenom are totally unconvincing. At Chulalongkorn Hospital in Bangkok, Benyajati and his colleagues kept alive patients with severe neurotoxic envenoming by *Naja kaouthia* by mechanical ventilation (Benyajati et al 1961; Limthongkul et al 1987). They believed that antivenom was harmful and that venom could be eliminated by forced diuresis. This approach has received no experimental confirmation and 46% of the patients denied antivenom developed local necrosis, 87.5% requiring skin grafting (Pochanugool et al 1987). However, generations of students taught at this famous medial school have been inculcated with the idea that antivenom is unnecessary and are now implementing this policy in various parts of the country.

Ancillary treatment

As emphasised above, antivenom is by far the most important element in the medical treatment of snake bite. The following discussion of ancillary treatments assumes that specific antivenom has been given promptly and in adequate quantities.

Treatment of local envenoming

Most of the local effects of snake bite are attributable to cytolytic and other activities of the venom itself, but the fangs of wild and captive snake can introduce bacterial infection into the wound, although some venoms are antibacterial (Stocker and Traynor 1986).

The risk of secondary infection is greatly increased if the wound is incised with an unsterile instrument or if the tissue becomes necrotic. Pathogens responsible for secondary infection of snake bite wounds include organisms peculiar to the snake's oral cavity (Jorge et al 1988), and usual wound pathogens such as *Staphylococcus aureus* and *Clostridium tetani* (Warrell et al

1986). These infections should be prevented with penicillin or erythromycin and a booster dose of tetanus toxoid should be given. If the wound has been tampered with or there is evidence of local necrosis, an aminoglycoside such as gentamicin should be added. The wound should be cleaned with antiseptic. Bullae can be aspirated to dryness with a fine sterile needle, rather than allow them to rupture and leak incontinently into the bedclothes. Snake bitten limbs should be nursed in the most comfortable position derived by trial and error. The most comfortable position for the envenomed arm may be suspended in a sling, while, for the lower limb, it may be with the knee flexed and supported on pillows. The wound should be examined frequently for evidence of necrosis. This occurs most commonly after bites on the digits. Early signs of necrosis include blistering, blackening or blanching of the skin, loss of sensation and a characteristic smell of putrefaction. There is a high risk of secondary infection and so the necrotic tissue should not be allowed to slough spontaneously but should be debrided by a surgeon under general or local anaesthesia as soon as possible (Figure 6). Skin appearances may be deceptive, for necrosis can extend along fascial planes and into deeper structures beneath apparently normal skin. Large areas may be denuded of skin; recovery can be accelerated by applying split skin grafts immediately after debridement, provided that the

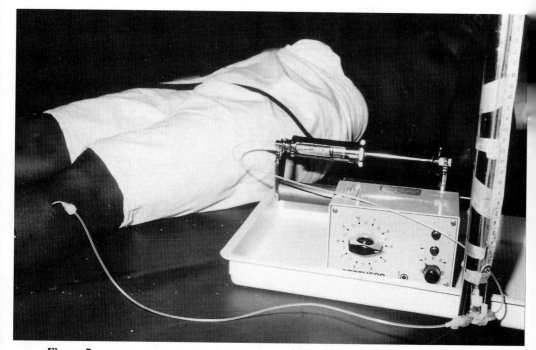

Figure 5

Measurement of intracompartmental pressure in a patient with suspected anterior tibial compartment syndrome after a bite by a Malayan pit viper (*Calloselasma rhodostoma*). A teflon cannula is inserted into the compartment and connected to a saline manometer and slow infusion pump. The "opening pressure" at which saline begins to flow into the compartment indicates intracompartmental pressure.

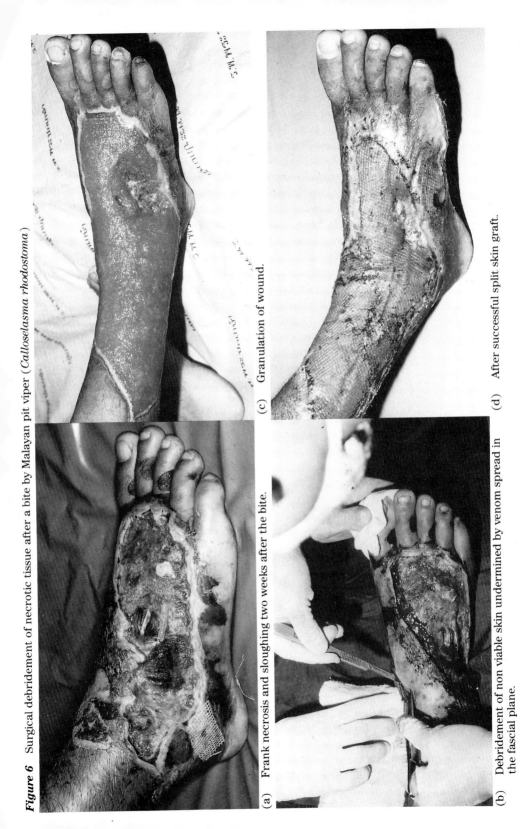

Figure 6 Surgical debridement of necrotic tissue after a bite by Malayan pit viper (*Calloselasma rhodostoma*)

(a) Frank necrosis and sloughing two weeks after the bite.

(b) Debridement of non viable skin undermined by venom spread in the fascial plane.

(c) Granulation of wound.

(d) After successful split skin graft.

wound is not infected (Figure 7). Debrided tissue, serosanguineous discharge and pus should be cultured and the patient treated with appropriate antimicrobials.

The development of very severe pain, especially in the lower leg, may indicate intracompartmental syndrome or thrombosis of a major artery.

Intracompartmental syndromes result from swelling of muscles within tight fascial compartments, such as the anterior tibial compartment, such that tissue pressure exceeds venous pressure and ischaemic damage is added to the effects of the venom. Signs, other than excessive pain, include weakness of the muscles contained by the compartment, pain when they are passively stretched, hyperaesthesia of areas of skin supplied by nerves running through the compartment and obvious tension of the compartment (Matsen 1980). Palpable distal arterial pulses do not exclude intracompartmental ischaemia. Pressure inside the fascial compartment could be measured by introducing a fine cannula connected to a pressure transducer and infusion pump (Figure 5). Intracompartmental pressures above 45 mmHg (60 cm of water) are associated with a high risk of ischaemic necrosis and, if encountered in accident surgery, would be regarded as an indication for fasciotomy. However, in animal experiments, fasciotomy did not prove effective in saving envenomed muscles (Garfin et al 1984). Fasciotomy must not be performed before blood coagulability has been restored by antivenom. Return to normal haemostasis can be speeded up by transfusion of fresh whole blood or clotting factors. Provided that adequate antivenom treatment is given as soon as possible after the bite, fasciotomy will rarely if ever be needed. A possible exception is bites to the digits, especially involving the finger pulps which are frequently complicated by necrosis. Expert surgical advice should be sought, especially if the thumb or index finger is involved.

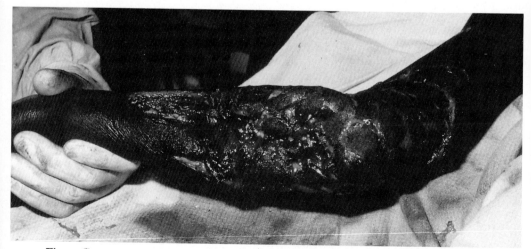

Figure 7
Immediate application of "postage stamp" split skin grafts from the thigh to a large area debrided after bite by African spitting cobra (*Naja nigricollis*).

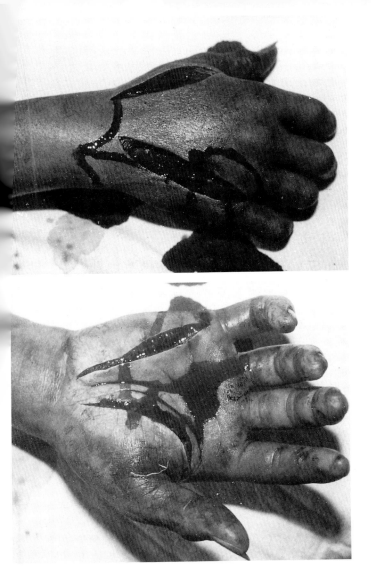

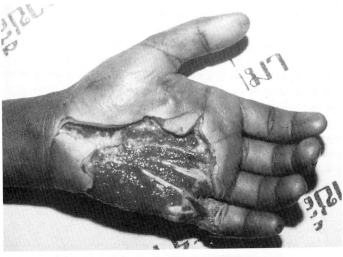

Figure 8
(a) and (b) Unnecessary
fasciotomy of dorsum and
palm of hand in a patient
with mild local envenoming
and defibrination following
bite by green pit viper
(*Trimeresurus albolabris*) in
Thailand.
(c)   Resulting skin loss.
*(By courtesy of
Dr. Sornchai Looareesuwan)*

Intracompartmental syndromes appear particularly common following bites by *Calloselasma rhodostoma* in Thailand and *Trimeresurus okinavensis* in Okinawa. In some countries, fasciotomy is carried out frequently and unnecessarily in patients with simple local swelling without evidence of increased intracompartmental pressure (Figure 8). Complications of fasciotomy include delayed healing, protracted convalescence and permanent disfigurement and impaired function, damage to nerves, tendons and other important tissues, and, if the procedure is carried out while blood is still incoagulable, persistent massive blood loss (Figure 9).

Arterial thrombosis is a rare complication which is difficult to diagnose. Many intensely swollen snake bitten limbs are cold and cyanosed with arterial pulses impossible to palpate through the oedema. Excessive pain of rapid onset, with sharply demarcated cold area and arterial pulses that are undetectable by doppler ultrasound probe (Figure 10), suggests a diagnosis of arterial thrombosis. This can be investigated by arteriography once haemostasis has been restored. There may be a possibility of thrombectomy or reconstructive arterial surgery.

Haemostatic abnormalities

Once specific antivenom has been given to neutralize venom procoagulants, fibrinolytic factors, antiplatelet factors and haemorrhagins, restoration of haemostasis may be accelerated by giving fresh whole blood, fresh frozen plasma, cryoprecipitates (containing fibrinogen, Factor VIII, fibronectin and some Factors V and XIII) or platelet concentrates. The role of heparin has been discussed since the 1940s but it has never proved convincingly beneficial in clinical use and in individual cases has exaggerated the haemostatic problem with disastrous results. Addition of heparin did not accelerate recovery from coagulopathy in patients envenomed by *Echis ocellatus* Nigeria (Warrell et al 1976). The antifibrinolytic agent, epsilon aminocaproic acid, has been used without demonstrable benefit in patients envenomed by *Calloselasma rhodostoma* (Reid 1965).

Neurotoxic envenoming

Bulbar and respiratory paralysis can lead to aspiration, airway obstruction and respiratory failure. The airway must be kept clear by positioning the patient head down lying on their side with the jaw elevated to prevent the tongue blocking the upper airway and an oral airway in place. If respiratory distress develops tracheostomy should be performed and a cuffed tube inserted or a cuffed endotracheal tube should be introduced (Figure 11), although the latter may be more distressing for the majority of patients who remain fully conscious. Patients have recovered completely after 30 days of manual ventilation by ambu or anaesthetic bag (Lin-Zhen-Yao and Ou-Ming 1976) and after 10 weeks of mechanical ventilation (Patten et al 1985). Fayrer first suggested the use of artifical respiration in snake bite in 1872 (Ewart et al 1874), but there are still new reports in the literature of patients dying of untreated respiratory failure. Some specific antivenoms may act too slowly to

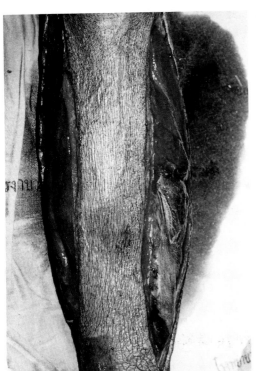

Figure 9
Fasciotomy of leg in a defibrinated patient bitten by a Malayan pit viper (*Calloselasma rhodostoma*). Surgery was performed before adequate antivenom treatment had been given to restore blood coagulability. Bleeding persistent for 10 days and required transfusion of 20 units of blood.

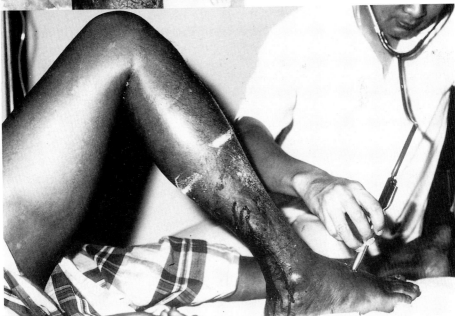

Figure 10
Doppler ultrasound probe in use to detect impalpable dorsalis pedis pulse in a patient with a tensely swollen limb after a bite on the calf by Malayan pit viper (*Calloselasma rhodostoma*).

prevent death from respiratory failure even when given in very large doses. However, patients treated with artificial ventilation alone may develop severe local envenoming and other life-threatening manifestations of envenoming such as cardiovascular collapse.

In eight out of 46 fatal cases of snake bite in Thailand, artifical ventilation was not attempted despite the development of respiratory failure (Looareesuwan et al 1988). However, patients who are intubated and mechanically ventilated require careful nursing. In the same series of 46 fatal cases, five died as a result of blockage of the airway and adequate mechanical ventilation was not achieved in a further 10 cases.

Use of anticholinesterases

Paralytic effects of neurotoxic South American venoms were not reversed by prostigmine (Barrio and Brazil 1951) but Banerjee et al (1972) demonstrated a dramatic and sustained response in patients with neurotoxic envenoming from Indian *Naja naja*. This was confirmed in a double-blind trial in patients envenomed by *N. n. philippinensis* (Watt et al 1987). Variable responses have been reported in victims of *Bungarus candidus* (Warrell et al 1982) (Figure 12) and *B. caeruleus* (Sethi & Rastogi 1981). There was no response in patients envenomed by sea snakes (Reid 1979), but foals envenomed by *Pseudonaja textilis* were improved by neostigmine (Pascoe 1975). In general, clinical response seems more likely if post synaptic (alpha) neurotoxins predominate in the venom, but the effect is so rapid and potentially so valuable that *all patients with neurotoxic symptoms should be given the benefit of a "Tensilon" (edrophonium) test as in the case of patients with suspected myasthenia gravis.* Atropine sulphate (0.6 mg for adults, 50 μg/kg for children) is given first by intravenous injection to block unpleasant muscarinic effects of acetylcholine such as increased secretions and abdominal colic. Edrophonium chloride (10 mg in adults, 0.25 mg/kg in children) is then given by intravenous injection, 2 mg at first, followed after 45 seconds by the remaining 8 mg if there is no effect. Ideally, the response should be measured objectively: duration of lid retraction on upward gaze, maximum interdental distance on mouth opening, forced expiratory pressure or vital capacity. Patients who respond convincingly can be maintained on neostigmine methylsulphate (50-100 μg/kg) and atropine sulphate (15 μg/kg) by sub-cutaneous injection every four hours or by continuous intravenous infusion. Patients who can swallow tablets may be maintained on neostigmine (initial adult dose 15 mg four times a day) or pyridostigmine (initial dose 60 mg four times a day) with atropine (0.6 mg twice a day) or propantheline hydrochloride (15 mg twice a day). Overdosage of anticholinesterase drugs may lead to cholinergic crises presenting with increasing muscle weakness which may cause respiratory failure. In some cases of neurotoxic envenoming, especially by Asian cobras, anticholinesterases may provide a fast-acting and valuable adjunct to specific antivenom, sparing the patient the need for assisted ventilation.

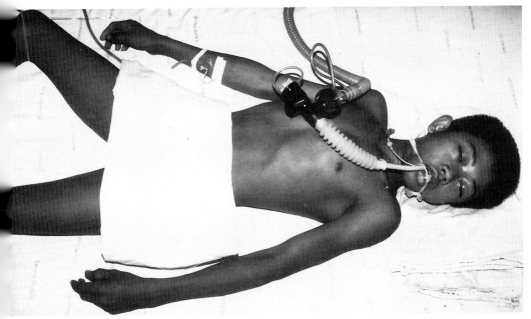

Figure 11
Endotracheal intubation and mechanical ventilation of a patient with total flaccid paralysis after envenoming by a Malayan krait (*Bungarus candidus*).
(By courtesy of Dr. Sornchai Looareesuwan)

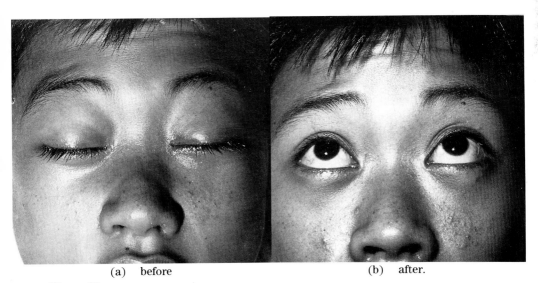

(a)   before   (b)   after.

Figure 12
Response to edrophonium in the patient (Figure 11) envenomed by *B. candidus*

Generalised rhabdomyolysis or myonecrosis

Some venoms containing phospholipases A2 with presynaptic (beta) neurotoxic activity can cause generalised breakdown of skeletal muscle resulting in myoglobinaemia, myoglobinuria, hyperkalaemia, hyperphosphataemia, and hypocalcaemia. Concentrations of serum enzymes such as creatine, phosphokinase and aspartate aminotransferase may be greatly elevated. Physical signs suggesting rhabdomyolysis include generalised muscle tenderness, pain on passive stretching of muscles, generalised weakness and trismus associated with the passage of dark reddish brownish or black urine. To prevent myoglobinuric nephropathy, alkaline diuresis is recommended (Ng and Suki 1980 p. 251). For adults, 25 g of mannitol and 100 milliequivalents of sodium bicarbonate are added to one litre of 5% dextrose which is infused over four hours while central venous pressure and urine output are monitored. This can be followed by an intravenous injection of frusemide 240 mg over 15 minutes if there is no diuresis. Potential dangers of mannitol are hyponatraemia, fluid overload and hyperkalaemia, while bicarbonate may exacerbate hypocalcaemia.

Hypotension and shock

Specific antivenom can reverse direct myocardial effects of some snake venoms (for example causing sinus bradycardia and electrocardiographical abnormalities) and venom induced vasodilatation, but in patients who have leaked large amounts of blood and plasma into the bitten limb and elsewhere a plasma expander, such as fresh whole blood or fresh frozen plasma, will be needed to correct hypovolaemia. The foot of the bed should be raised in an attempt to improve cardiac filling while an intravenous infusion and pressure monitoring is established. The safest way to restore circulating volume without incurring fluid overload is to monitor central venous pressure through a long catheter inserted percutaneously at the antecubital fossa and advanced until its tip is in the superior vena cava (Figure 13), or to monitor pulmonary arterial wedge pressure (indirect left atrial pressure) with a Swan-Ganz catheter. Systemic blood pressure should be measured frequently using a sphygmomanometer.

Other causes of hypotension should be considered such as haemorrhagic shock following a massive concealed bleed into the gastrointestinal tract, a cardiac arrhythmia and anaphylaxis caused by an antivenom reaction or an autopharmacological effect of the venom. If there is any possibility of an antivenom reaction, adrenaline should be given forthwith (see above).

Patients who remain hypotensive and shocked (poor peripheral circulation, impaired consciousness, reduced urine output) despite the use of antivenom and restoration of a central venous pressure of between 0 and +3 cm or a mean pulmonary capillary wedge pressure of up to 10 mmHg by infusing plasma expanders should be given dopamine by continuous infusion through the central venous catheter in an initial dose of 2 μg/kg/minute.

Shock of various causes can occur in severe envenoming by many species of snakes, but is seen most commonly in this region in patients bitten by Viperidae,

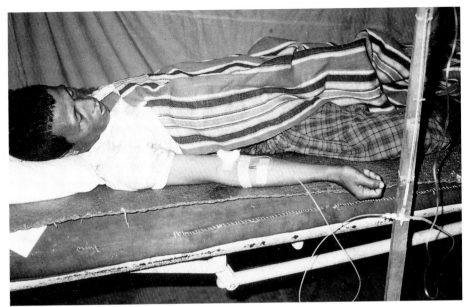

Figure 13
Central venous pressure monitoring in a rural hospital in Burma using a saline manometer and 70 cm catheter (Vygon) inserted at the antecubital fossa using the Seldinger method.

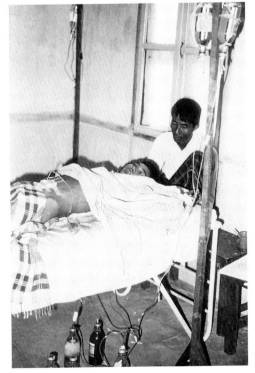

Figure 14
Peritoneal dialysis in a victim of Russell's viper being carried out in a rural hospital in Burma.

especially *Vipera russelli*, and as an early autopharmacological phenomenon in patients bitten by snakes of the genus Vipera and some Australasian "elapids".

Renal failure

Causes of acute renal failure following snake bite include haemonhage into the kidney; ischaemia resulting from hypotension, disseminated intravascular coagulation and renal vasoconstriction; the controversial pigment nephropathies resulting from intravascular haemolysis (haemoglobinuria) and rhabdomyolysis (myoglobinuria); direct nephrotoxicity and immune complex glomerulonephritis caused by antivenom reactions. Renal failure can occur as a rare complication in any case of severe envenoming but is the major cause of death in patients bitten by *Vipera russelli*. Urine output and fluid balance (or at least daily weight) should be recorded in all patients with severe envenoming. If the urine output falls below 400 ml/24 hours, central venous pressure should be monitored and a urethral catheter inserted. Cautious rehydration with isotonic fluid (to increase the central venous pressure to +3 cmH$_2$0) can be followed by the use of high doses of frusemide (up to 100 mg intravenously) and finally low doses of dopamine (2.5 μg/kg/minute) by continuous infusion into a central vein. If these measures fail to increase urine output, patients should be managed conservatively until dialysis is indicated. In Rangoon, where *Vipera russelli* bite is the commonest medical cause of acute renal failure, mortality has been reduced to 27% by peritoneal dialysis (Figure 14). Most patients respond to 72 hours of continuous dialysis (Figure 15). Blood coagulability should be restored with adequate doses of antivenom and, if necessary, by replacement of clothing factors before peritioneal dialysis is started.

Snake venom ophthalmia

Populations of "Spitting" cobras (for example *N. n. sputatrix, N. n. philippinensis, N. n. sumatrana, N. n. samarensis*) occur in Thailand, Malaysia, Indonesia and the Philippines. Venom spat into the eye can cause intense conjunctivitis and there is a risk of secondary infection of corneal erosions. First aid treatment is the same as for any other chemical conjunctivitis. Venom should be washed from the eye or mucous membranes as soon as possible using large volumes of water or any other available bland fluid. Unless a corneal abrasion can be excluded by slit lamp examination or fluorescein staining, the patient should be treated as if they had a corneal injury. A topical antimicrobial agent (tetracycline or chloramphenicol) should be applied or instilled frequently and the eye should be closed with a dressing pad.

Other drugs in the treatment of snake bite

Despite their widespread use, there is no convincing evidence for the use of corticosteroids and antihistamine other than in the treatment of antivenom reactions. There is a challenging array of traditional herbal remedies but none has yet been proved to be beneficial in patients.

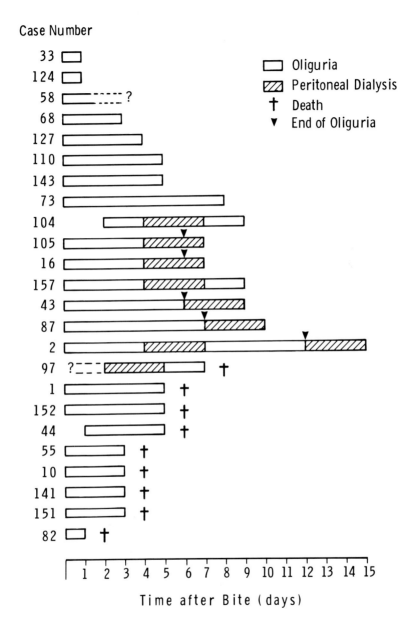

Figure 15

Results of peritoneal dialysis in eight out of 24 victims of Russell's viper bite with oliguric acute renal failure. Note early onset of oliguria after the bite. Cases arranged in increasing order of severity from top to bottom.

References

Banerjee RN, Sahni AL, Chacko KA (1972). Neostigmine in the treatment of Elapidae bites. J Ass Physns India *20* (7) 503-9.

Barrio A, Brazil OV (1951). Acta Physiol Latinoam *1* 291.

Benyajati C, Keoplung M, Sribhibhadh R (1961). Experimental and clinical studies on glucocorticoids in cobra envenomation. J Trop Med Hyg *64* 46-49.

Bhat RN (1974). Viperine snake bite posioning in Jammu. J Indian Med Ass *63* (12)383-392.

Calmette A (1896). The treatment of animals poisoned with snake venom by the injection of antivenomous serum. Lancet *ii* 449-450.

Campbell CH (1966). The death adder (*Acanthophis antarcticus*): the effects of the bite and its treatment. Med J Aust *2* (20) 922-925.

Deoras PJ (1981). Snakes of India. National Book Trust, New Delhi, India. 4th edition.

Ewart J, Richard V, Mackenzie SC (1874). Report on the effects of artificial respiration, intravenous injection of ammonia and administration of various drugs etc. in Indian and Australian snake-poisoning; and the physiological, chemical and microscopical nature of snake poisons. Calcutta, Bengal Secretariat Press.

Frost J (1981). Tiger snake envenomation and muscle spasm. Med J Austr *2* (11) 579.

Gajdusek DC (1977). *In*: Symposium on Health and Diseases in Tribal Societies. London, Ciba Foundation Symposium. New Series, No. 49, New York, Elsevier.

Ganthavorn S (1971). A case of king cobra bite. Toxicon *9* (3) 293-4.

Garfin SR, Castilonia RR, Mubarak SJ, Hargens AR, Russell FE, Akeson WH (1984). Rattlesnake bites and surgical decompression: results using a laboratory model. Toxicon *22* 177-182.

Griffen D, Donovan JW (1986). Significant envenomation from a preserved rattlesnake head (in a patient with a history of immediate hypersensitivity to antivenin). Anns Emerg Med *15* 955-8.

Ho M, Warrell DA, Looareesuwan S, Phillips RE, Chanthavanich P, Karbwang J, Supanaranond W, Hutton RA, Vejcho S (1986). Clinical significance of venom antigen levels in patients envenomed by the Malayan pit viper (*Calloselasma rhodostoma*). Am J Trop Med Hyg *35* (3) 579-587.

Ho M. Warrell MJ. Warrell DA, Bidwell, D, Voller A (1986). A critical reappraisal of the use of ELISA in the study of snake bite. Toxicon *24* (3) 211-221.

Jorge MT, Ribeiro LA, Mendonca JS, Silva MLR, Kusano EJU, Cordeiro CLS (1988). Bacterial flora from *Bothrops jararaca* mouth and from abscesses depending on snake bites. XII International Congress of Tropical Medicine and Malaria, Amsterdam.

Khin-Ohn-Lwin, Aye-Aye-Myint, Tun-Pe, Theinghe-Nwe, Min-Naing (1984). Russell's viper venom levels in serum of snake bite victims in Burma. Trans R Soc Trop Med Hyg *78* 165-8.

Kitchens CS, Hunter S, Van Mierop LHS (1987). Severe myonecrosis in a fatal case of envenomation by the canebrake rattlesnake (*Crotalus horridus atricaudatus*). Toxicon *25* (4) 455-458.

Klenerman L, Mackie I, Chakrabarti R, Brozovic M, Stirling Y (1977). Changes in haemostatic system after application of a tourniquet. Lancet *i* 970-972.

Lancet (1980). Antivenom therapy and reactions. Lancet *i* 1009-1010.

Limthongkul S, Pochanugool C, Meemano K (1987). Respiratory failure and its non-antivenin treatment in 37 adult neurotoxic snake-bite patients. *In:* Progress in Venom and Toxin Research, Faculty of Medicine, National University of Singapore pp. 52-59.

Lin-Zhen-Yao, Ou-Ming (1976). The cure of a patient with respiratory paralysis for thirty days after *Bungarus multicinctus* bite. New Traditional Chinese Med 4 24-8.

Looareesuwan S. Viravan C, Warrell DA (1988). Factors contributing to fatal snake bite in the rural tropics: analysis of 46 cases in Thailand. Trans R Soc Trop Med Hyg 82 930-34.

Malasit P, Warrell DA, Chanthavanich P, Viravan C, Mongkolsapaya J, Singhthong B, Supich C (1986). Prediction, prevention, and mechanism of early (anaphylactic) antivenom reactions in victims of snake bites. Brit Med J 292 17-20.

Matsen FA (1980). Compartmental Syndromes. Grune & Straton: P. 162.

Myint-Lwin, Warrell DA. Phillips RE, Tin-Nu-Swe, Tun-Pe, Maung-Maung-Lay (1985). Bites by Russell's viper (*Vipera russelli siamensis*) in Burma: Haemostatic, vascular and renal disturbances and response to treatment. Lancet *ii* 1259-1264.

Ng RCK, Suki WN (1980). Treatment of acute renal failure. *In*: Acute Renal Failure (eds.) Brenner BM, Stein JH, Churchill Livingstone, New York: pp. 229-273.

Pascoe RR (1975). Brown snake bite in horses in south-eastern Queensland. J S Afr Vet Assoc 46 (1) 129-31.

Patten BR, Pearn JH, De Buse P, Burke J, Covacevich J (1985). Prolonged intensive therapy after snake bite: a probable case of envenomation by the rough-scaled snake. Med J Austr 142 467-9.

Phillips RE, Theakston RDG, Warrell DA, Galigedara Y, Abeysekera DTDJ, Dissanayaka P, Hutton RA, Aloysius DJ (1988). Paralysis, rhabdomyolysis and haemolysis caused by bites of Russell's viper (*Vipera russelli pulchella*) in Sri Lanka: failure of Indian (Haffkine) antivenom. Quart J Med 68. 691–716.

Pochanugool C, Limthongkul S, Meemano K (1987). Clinical features of 37 non-antivenin treated neurotoxic snake bite patients. *In*: Progress in Venom and Toxin Research (eds.) Gopalakrishnakone P, Tan CK. Faculty of Medicine, National University of Singapore.

Pugh RHN, Theakston RDG. (1987). Fatality following use of a tourniquet after viper bite envenoming. Anns Trop Med Parasitol 81 (1) 77-8.

Reid HA (1965). E-aminocaproic acid and fibrinolysis in viper bite defibrination. Lancet *ii* 5-7.

Reid HA (1979). Symptomatology, pathology and treatment of the bites of seasnakes. *In*: Snake Venoms. Handbook of Experimental Pharmacology 52 922-955 (ed.) Lee C-Y. Springer-Verlag, Berlin.

'Sethi PK, Rastogi JK (1981). Neurological aspects of ophitoxemia (Indian krait) - a clinico-electromyographic study. Indian J Med Res 73 269-276.

Sewall H (1887). Experiments on the preventive inoculation of rattlesnake venom. J Physiol VIII 203-210.

Stocker JF, Traynor JR (1986). The action of various venoms on *Escherichia coli*. J Appl Bacteriol 61 383-88.

Sutherland SK (1977). Serum reactions: an analysis of commercial antivenoms and the possible role of anticomplementary activity in denovo reactions to antivenoms and antitoxins. Med J Austr Apr 23 613-5.

Sutherland SK (1980). First aid for snakebite in Australia with notes on first aid for bites and strings by other animals. CSL booklet, Australia.

Sutherland SK (1983a). Prolonged use of pressure immobilisation after after snake bite, Med J Austr Jan 22, p 58.

Sutherland SK (1983b). Australian animal toxins. The creatures, their toxins and care of the poisoned patient. Oxford University Press, Melbourne.

Trishnananda M. Yongchaiyudha S, Chayodom V (1978). Clinical observations on glucocorticoids in cobra envenomation. SE Asian Trop Med Pub Hlth 9 (1) 71-3.

Tun-Pe, Tin-Nu-Swe, Myint-Lwin, Warrell DA, Than-Win (1987). The efficacy of tourniquets as a first aid measure for Russell's viper bites in Burma. Trans R Soc Trop Med Hyg *81* 403-405.

Vital Brazil O (1987). History of the primordia of snake-bite accident serotherapy. Mem Inst Butantan *49* (1) 7-20.

Warrell DA (1979). Clinical snake bite problems in the Nigerian savanna region. Technische Hochschule Darmst Schriftenreihe Wissenschaft und Technik *14* 31-60.

Warrell DA, Looareesuwan S, Theakston RDG, Phillips RE, Chanthavanich P, Viravan C, Supanaranond W, Karbwang J, Ho M, Hutton RA, Vejcho S (1986). Randomized comparative trial of three monospecific antivenoms for bites by the Malayan pit viper (*Calloselasma rhodostoma*) in southern Thailand: clinical and laboratory correlations. Am J Trop Med Hyg *35* (6) 1235-1247.

Warrell DA, Looareesuwan S, White NJ Theakston RDG, Warrell MJ, Kosakarn W, Reid HA (1983). Severe neurotoxic envenoming by the Malayan krait *Bungarus candidus* (Linnaeus): response to antivenom and anticholinesterase. BMJ *286* 678-680.

Warrell DA, Pope HM, Prentice CRM (1976). Disseminated intravascular coagulation caused by the carpet viper (*Echis carinatus*): trial of heparin. Br J Haematol *33* 335-342.

Watt G. Theakston RDG, Hayes CG, Yambao ML, Sangalang R, Ranoa CP, Alquizalas E, Warrell DA (1986). Positive response to edrophonium in patients with neurotoxic envenoming by cobras (*Naja naja philippinensis*). A placebo-controlled study. N Engl J Med *315* 1444-8.

WHO (1981). Progress in the characterization of venoms and standardization of antivenoms. WHO Offset Publication No. 58, Geneva.

SCIENTIFIC INDEX